Nutrition, Immunity, and Infection in Infants and Children

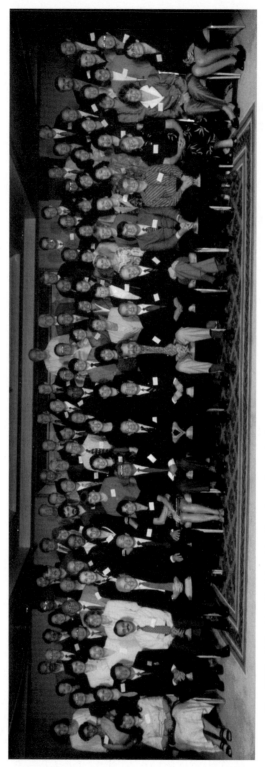

The 45th Nestlé Nutrition Workshop, Nutrition, Immunity, and Infection in Infants and Children, was held in Bangkok, Thailand, 29 March–1 April 1999.

Nestlé Nutrition Workshop Series
Pediatric Program Volume 45

Nutrition, Immunity, and Infection in Infants and Children

Editors

Robert M. Suskind   *Dean, Professor of Pediatrics, The Chicago Medical School, Finch University of Health Sciences, North Chicago, Illinois 60064, U.S.A*

Kraisid Tontisirin   *Director, Institute of Nutrition, Mahidol University, Salaya, Phutthamonthon, Nakhom Pathom 73170, Thailand*

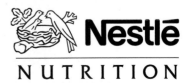

LIPPINCOTT WILLIAMS & WILKINS

Acquisitions Editor: Beth Barry
Developmental Editor: Zebulon Spector
Production Editor: Melanie Bennitt
Manufacturing Manager: Benjamin Rivera
Compositor: Maryland Composition
Printer: Maple Press

Nestec Ltd., 55 Avenue Nestlé
CH-1800 Vevey, Switzerland
Lippincott Williams & Wilkins,
530 Walnut Street
Philadelphia, PA 19106 USA
LWW.com

Printed in the USA

Library of Congress Cataloging-in-Publication Data

Nutrition immunity, and infection in infants and children/editors, Robert M. Suskind, Kraisid Tontisirin.
    p.; cm — (Nestlé Nutrition workshop series; v. 45. Pediatric Program)
  Based on the 45th Nestlé Nutrition Workshop.
  Includes bibliographical references and index.
  ISBN 0-7817-3079-1
    1. Nutritional disorders in infants—Congresses. 2. Nutritional disorders in children—Congresses. 3. Infants—Diseases—Immunological aspects—Congresses. 4. Children—Diseases—Immunological aspects—Congresses. 5. Developmental immunology—Congresses. 6. Infection in children—Congresses. 7. Immunological diseases in children—Congresses. I. Suskind, Robert M., 1937- II. Kraisid Tontisirin. III. Nestlé Nutrition S.A. IV. Nestlé Nutrition Workshop (45th : 1999 : Bangkok, Thailand) V. Nestlé Nutrition workshop series; .45. VI. Nestlé Nutrition workshop series Pediatric Program.
  [DNLM: 1. Infant Nutrition Disorders—immunology—Congresses. 2. Child Nutrition Disorders—immunology—Congresses. 3. Communicable Diseases—Child—Congresses. 4. Communicable Diseases—Infant—Congresses. WS 120 N97657 2000]
  RJ390 .N88 2000
  618.92'3079—dc21

                                           00-058297

10 9 8 7 6 5 4 3 2 1

Preface

This 45th Nestlé Nutrition Workshop served as an invigorating forum for scientists engaged in the fundamental and applied aspects of research in the area of nutrition, immunity, and infection in infants and children. By enhancing knowledge of the prevention and treatment of childhood malnutrition and infectious disease, one recognizes the positive impact that nutrition can have on initiatives which catalyze on disease processes. Practical clinical research initiatives, which catalyze action in the field of nutrition and health, should be undertaken with clear goals in mind. In addition, basic research, which provides fundamental and newer insights into the malnutrition/disease process, should be actively pursued. A working plan armed with practical action for achieving substantial change in the field is necessary as our infants and children enter the new millennium.

At the outset, the workshop reviewed the global burden of malnutrition and infectious diseases in children as evidenced from the not only alarming associated morbidity and mortality, but also from the ever-present threats to children's well being. Low birth weight (LBW) and nutritional deficiencies, in particular, have adverse effects on child survival and development, and serve as an important risk factor for a number of adult diseases. Childhood malnutrition leads to growth deficiency in adult life, resulting in reduced work output and a decrease in the individual's, and therefore society's, development and productivity. The pathophysiology of malnutrition in the young child leads to changes in the malnourished child, many of which are reversible, except for those related to mental development. It is well established that there are strong influences of early malnutrition on subsequent mental development.

Malnutrition also affects susceptibility to infection, with documented evidence that cellular immunity, humoral immunity, and the complement system are markedly impaired in malnourished children. These changes, fortunately, are reversed with improved nutrient intake. The pathologic effect of infection on the development of an appropriate immune response, including the acute phase response, is well established. The clinical balance between microbes and the host defence system in malnourished children needs to be more clearly defined. Ultimately, nutrition modulated events in host-pathogen interactions are vital to understanding where exactly nutrition fits in. In particular, the role of micronutrients is important not only in the therapy but in the prevention and control of malnutrition.

The methodologies for evaluating the impact of nutrition on function includes identifying phenotype abnormalities, molecular defects, gene defects, and errors in gene transcription that occur in the malnourished host. There is clearly a need to use immunological tools available in the differential diagnosis of primary and secondary immune abnormalities. Under the subject of molecular and immunologic evaluation of nutritionally at-risk hosts, the mutual influences of nutrition on the immune response and the effect of immunity on infection merit attention. A practical testing structure that includes a three-tiered system needs to be developed to obtain immunological information in different nutritional states. Relationships between body weight and immunity, the impact of the immune response on nutrient requirements and more specifically, the dietary management of immune incompetence are further areas of study.

The presentations then focused on various aspects of nutrition and immunity. Recent literature is emerging on "immune enhancing" formulas for feeding, a field which needs further research. The definition of adverse nutritional outcome, the immune assessment of botanicals and the development of diets to improve immune systems are subjects for further exploration. Expansion, quantification, and application of standardized immunologic tests become imperative, especially for human populations to understand the "host response" in realistic field situations. Development of specific bio-markers is required to enable translation of immunologic indices into specific benefits and outcomes. This has valuable implications in refining methodologies for assessing the immune system in states of malnutrition as well as disease. A public health approach must be adopted to address the multifactorial factors affecting the nutritional status of the host.

With respect to nutritional concerns such as low birth weight and its consequences on susceptibility to infection and immunity, the future research agenda calls for specific measures of immune function in this population of children at risk. Methodologies need further improvement, disaggregation of stunting and wasting and the development of practical and sustainable nutrition intervention for LBW infants are urgent priorities. The interrelationships of LBW and the immune deficiency response, and specifically, the impact of trace element merits further exploration of supplementation. The effects of varying types and levels of dietary lipids, specifically oils, were presented as areas for future research and practice. The alteration of host defence by specific fatty acids such as fish oil need to be resolved in humans in view of the marked nutritional benefits demonstrated in animal models. The manifestation of essential fatty acid deficiency is well known to impair the development of the immune system. Additional areas of exploration include the impact of a reduction of fat in human diets to enhance lymphocyte proliferation. Immune competence must be appreciated and understood in the context of endocrine reorganization of metabolism in PEM. Exercise, stress, and nutrition in the context of the immune response needs to be more clearly defined.

Micronutrient malnutrition in its broadest sense alters the immune system; the most affected responses include cell–mediated immunity, phagocyte function, the complement system, mucosal immunity, and the humoral immune response. The complexity and interdependence of the immune response and the sensitive and functional effects of nutrient intake and nutritional status on the immune response and susceptibility to infection was reviewed. Deficiencies of vitamins E and A have been shown to impair both the humoral and the cell-mediated responses in animal models, while in humans, indirect evidence indicates an increased susceptibility to infection. Serum vitamin E levels in children with AIDS reportedly are lower than those of HIV controls. Lower serum tocopherol levels have also been reported to be associated with persistent human papillomavirus infection and pulmonary tuberculosis. Beneficial effects of vitamin A supplementation in reducing morbidity and mortality from measles in children with low vitamin A status exist. However, the benefits in infants as well as in the timing of the administration of the vitamin and the co-administration with childhood vaccines remain controversial. It has recently been shown to adversely affect antibody production and limit the protection afforded by vaccination. Vitamin A supplementation is beneficial in reducing the severity of diarrheal diseases, while the evidence for its impact on malarial infection is equivocal and needs further investigation. An update was also presented relating immunocompetent cells and cytokines, which are involved in the evolution and alterations of nutritional status to eating disorders and infectious diseases.

A new understanding has emerged into the mechanisms involved in the development of allergic sensitization. IgE antibodies are the host components responsible for triggering the allergic reaction. Allergic reactions can occur at any age, though regulation of the immune response is modified with maturation of the immune system through gradual changes of fetal and newborn responses. Infections, vaccines, and exposure to allergens influence the development of allergies. There is a need to develop suitable allergy prevention programs. In addition, there is a need to understand more closely who is at risk for developing allergies, what is the allergic risk, and what is the relationship between the history of allergy and skin test results. Demonstration among large-scale populations is required. Prevention of allergy and infectious disease in general populations is crucial over the long term.

The presentation of nutrition and infection reiterated that while much of the impact of infectious disease is reflected in the prevalence of malnutrition, the effects on nutritional status of chronic sub-clinical or "inapparent" infections have recently been appreciated. The metabolic effects of infection, which are mediated through cytokine activation and the ensuing amplification of host defense mechanisms, favor partitioning and redistribution of dietary and endogenous nutrients away from the maintenance of host nutritional status, body composition and growth toward support of the immune system and the acute phase response.

Infection confounds clinical assessment of nutritional status, blurs the distinction between dietary and infectious etiologies of impaired nutritional status, and thus complicates intervention. There is a need to learn more about the extent to which low-grade subclinical infections cause a re-orientation of amino acid metabolism, to the extent that growth and/or micronutrient status, are altered. While the relationship between infection, undernutrition, and growth retardation in infants and young children is well-established, there is a need to know whether growth retardation relates solely to anorexia and reduced food intake or whether there is an independent effect of infection/inflammation on growth and development. Mechanisms by which pro-inflammatory cytokines generate during infection and the mechanism by which inflammation impairs growth and development were summarized.

Gastrointestinal illnesses have a higher probability of occurring in children with pre-existing nutritional deficits. Episodes in malnourished children are more likely to be of longer duration, greater severity and to lead to increased mortality in malnourished children. Results of community-based supplementation trials using zinc, vitamin A, or iron were described. Populations at high risk of zinc deficiency are likely to have a reduced incidence of diarrheal disease upon receiving supplemental zinc. Vitamin A may also confer similar benefits with regard to diarrhea, especially in populations with vitamin A deficiency. The possibility of iron supplementation increasing the risk of diarrhea, however, is uncertain.

Interactions of acute respiratory infections, measles, and nutritional status failed to show consistent beneficial impacts of vitamin A supplementation on the incidence, prevalence, or mortality from acute lower respiratory infections in children between the ages of 6 months and 5 years. While low plasma zinc appears to be associated with lower respiratory tract infections, zinc supplementation does not reduce childhood mortality. Malnutrition was clearly shown to affect HIV transmission and progression. Energy balance, food intake, nutrient malabsorption, cytokines, hormonal changes, and metabolic alterations all play a role in the etiology of malnutrition during HIV infection. Parasitic infections have also been shown to severely affect host nutrition as a result of the blood loss associated with malaria or hook worm infections and the enteropathy associated with gastrointestinal infections and its effects upon digestion and absorption.

All presentations were followed by fruitful discussions, which supported the viewpoint of the experts. This volume, which documents most of the issues and discussions of the workshop, is intended to provide valuable reference material for practitioners and researchers in the field of clinical nutrition. We hope that this will pave the way for newer and exciting research for translation at the field level so that childhood nutrition and health can be improved in countries throughout the world.

My co-chairman, Dr. Robert Suskind, and I thank all the participants for their enlightening contributions to this meeting. We are grateful to Prof. Ferdinand Haschke and Dr. Anne-Lise Carrié-Faessler, Nestec Ltd., Vevey, Switzerland, Mr. Giorgio Albertini, Nestlé Italiana S.p.A., Milano, Italy, and Mr. Thomas Coley, Nestlé (Thailand) Ltd., for their strong support of our endeavors towards making this workshop a meaningful one.

Prof. Kraisid Tontisirin, Thailand
Prof. Robert M. Suskind, USA

Foreword

Primary protein-energy malnutrition is still common in developing countries, and physicians and healthworkers throughout the world are becoming increasingly aware of malnutrition secondary to diseases such as AIDS. More than 50% of the world's children who suffer from malnutrition live in Southeast Asia. It was, therefore, important to organize the 45th Nestlé Nutrition Workshop in Thailand, where clinical research in this field was coordinated by the World Health Organization (WHO) collaborating center at Mahidol University, Bangkok.

Substantial recent advances have increased our ability to understand and evaluate the immune system of children in health and disease. Clinical immunology has increased the ability to recognize immunological abnormalities and now permits better diagnosis and treatment of many immunological abnormalities due to infections with HIV or malnutrition.

.The participants of the meeting proposed to establish international project platforms for further coordination of research in the field of nutrition and immunology. Among the priority projects were the development of a standardized questionnaire to evaluate diseases in relation to nutrition and immunology, as well as the standardization of field studies and animal work.

I thank the two Chairmen, Prof. Kraisid Tontisirin and Prof. Robert Suskind, for putting the program together and inviting experts to present their opinions on selected topics in the field of nutrition and immunity. The invited scientists from 32 countries substantially contributed to the discussions that are published in the book. Mr. Tom Coley's team from Nestlé Thailand provided all logistical support and all participants enjoyed a taste of Thai hospitality. Dr. Carrié-Faessler from the Nutrition Division in Vevey, Switzerland was responsible for the scientific coordination. Her excellent cooperation with the Chairmen was fundamental to the success of this Workshop.

PROFESSOR FERDINAND HASCHKE, M.D.
Vice-President
Nestec Ltd.
Vevey, Switzerland

Contents

Global Burden of Malnutrition and Infection in Childhood 1
K. Tontisirin and L. Bhattacharjee

The Malnourished Child: An Overview 23
R. M. Suskind, L. Lewinter-Suskind, K. K. Murthy, D. Suskind,
   D. Suskind, and D. Liu

Nutrition, Immunity, and Infectious Diseases in Infants and Children:
   An Overview 45
G. T. Keusch

A Review of the Immune System: Methodology for Evaluating the
   Impact of Nutrition on Its Function 55
R. U. Sorensen, B. Butler, and L. E. Leiva

The Molecular and Immunologic Evaluation of Nutritionally At-Risk
   Hosts 69
J. Powell, S. H. Yoshida, J. Van de Water, and M. E. Gershwin

The Effect of Protein-Energy Malnutrition on Immune Competence 89
B. Woodward

Low Birthweight Infants, Infection, and Immunity 121
A. Ashworth

The Effect of Dietary Fatty Acids on the Immune Response and
   Susceptibility to Infection 137
P. C. Calder

Stress, Nutrition, and the Immune Response 173
J. S. Kennedy

Iron-Zinc, Immune Responses, and Infection 201
R. K. Chandra

The Effect of Vitamin Deficiencies (E and A) and Supplementation
   on Infection and Immune Response 213
S. N. Meydani, W. W. Fawzi, and S. N. Han

Eating Disorders (Obesity, Anorexia Nervosa, Bulimia Nervosa),
   Immunity, and Infection 243
A. Marcos, A. Montero, S. López-Varela, and G. Morandé

Allergy and Infection 263
R. U. Sorensen and M. C. Porch

The Metabolic Effects of Infection on Nutritional Status 281
C. R. Fjeld

Anorexia and Cytokines in the Acute Phase Response to Infection . 303
M. J. G. Farthing and A. B. Ballinger

Relations Between Gastrointestinal Infections and Childhood
    Malnutrition 319
K. H. Brown

The Interaction of Acute Respiratory Infections, Measles, and
    Nutritional Status 337
H. M. Coovadia and A. Coutsoudis

Nutrition and Infection: Human Immunodeficiency Virus Infection,
    Tuberculosis, and Melioidosis 359
G. E. Griffin and D. Macallan

Malnutrition and HIV Infection 371
W. W. Fawzi and E. Villamor

The Interactions of Nutritional Status and Parasitic Diseases 407
D. Wakelin

Concluding Discussion: The Future Perspectives and the Next
    10 Years 425
R. M. Suskind and K. Tontisirin

Subject Index 433

Contributing Authors

Speakers

Ann Ashworth
Reader in Community Nutrition
Public Health Nutrition Unit
London School of Hygiene
and Tropical Medicine
Keppel Street
London WC1E 7HT
United Kingdom

Kenneth H. Brown
Professor, Department of Nutrition
Director, Program in International
Nutrition
University of California at Davis
One Shields Avenue
Davis, California 95616
USA

Philip C. Calder
Reader in Human Nutrition
Institute of Human Nutrition
University of Southampton
Bassett Crescent East
Southampton, SO16 7PX
United Kingdom

Ranjit K. Chandra
Prof. Janeway Child Health Center
Memorial University of Newfoundland
St. John's Newfoundland,
A1A 1R8
Canada

Hoosen M. Coovadia
Department of Paediatrics and Child
Health.
Faculty of Medicine
University of Natal
Private Bag #7
Congella 5013
South Africa

Michael J. G. Farthing
Digestive Diseases Centre
St. Bartholomew's & the Royal London
School of Medicine & Dentistry
Turner Street
London E1 3AD
United Kingdom

Wafaie W. Fawzi
Assistant Professor
Department of Nutrition and Epidemiology
Harvard School of Public Health
665 Huntington Avenue, SPH 2
Boston, Massachusetts 02115
USA

Carla R. Fjeld
Fjeld and Associates
8213 Lilly Stone Drive
Bethesda, Maryland 20817
USA

M. Eric Gershwin
Professor
Department of Internal Medicine
University of California at Davis
TB 192
Davis, California 95616
USA

George E. Griffin
Department of Infectious Diseases
St. George's Hospital Medical School
London SW17 ORE
United Kingdom

Jeff Kennedy
Department of Cancer Immunology &
AIDS
Dana Farber Cancer Institute, Dana 516
44 Binney Street
Boston, Massachusetts 02115
USA

Ascensión Marcos
Instituto de Nutrición y Bromatología
Facultad de Farmacia
Ciudad Universitaria
Madrid 28040
Spain

Simin N. Meydani
Professor, School of Nutrition Science and
* Policy*
Sackler Graduate School of Biomedical
* Sciences*
Tufts University
711 Washington Street
Boston, Massachusetts 02111
USA

Ricardo U. Sorensen
Professor and Chairman
Department of Pediatrics
Louisiana State University Health
* Sciences Center*
1542 Tulane Avenue
New Orleans, Louisiana 70112
USA

Robert M. Suskind
Dean
Professor of Pediatrics
The Chicago Medical School
Finch University of Health Sciences
3333 Green Bay Road
North Chicago, Illinois 60064
USA

Kraisid Tontisirin
Director
Institute of Nutrition,
Mahidol University
Salaya, Phulihamonihon
Nakhom, Pathom 73170
Thailand

Derek Wakelin
Professor
School of Life and Environmental Sciences
University of Nottingham
University Park
Nottingham NG7 2RD
United Kingdom

William D. Woodward
Professor
Department of Human Biology and
* Nutritional Sciences*
University of Guelph
Guelph, Ontario
N1G 2W1
Canada

Session Chairmen

A. Valyasevi/*Thailand*
P. Tantibhedhayangkul/*Thailand*
P. Jirapinyo/*Thailand*
S. Lolekha/*Thailand*
U. Thisyakorn/*Thailand*

Invited Attendees

Don Robertson/*Australia*
Fadheela Al-Mahroos/*Bahrain*
Chowdhury Badruddin Mahmood/*Bangladesh*
Evandro Alves Prado/*Brazil*
Nelson Augusto Rosario Filho/*Brazil*
Koum Kanal/*Cambodia*
Joanne Embree/*Canada*
Elizabeth Rousseau/*Canada*
Fang Feng/*China*
Li Tingyu/*China*
Yang Yi/China
Yang Xiaoguang/*China*
Abdalla Ahmed/*Egypt*
Abu-Zekry Mona/*Egypt*
Anne Ormisson/*Estonia*
Vas Novelli/*Great Britain*
Julikw Thomas/*Great Britain*
Kwan Yat Wah/*Hong Kong*
Tse Kong/*Hong Kong*
Tse Lai Yin/*Hong Kong*
Agnes Kalmar/*Hungary*
Eva Micskey/*Hungary*
Gabriele Ambrosioni/*Italy*
Antonio Marini/*Italy*
Antonio Russo/*Italy*
Giuseppe Zoppi/*Italy*
Malak Hussein Kalawi/*Kuwait*
Dace Gardovska/*Latvia*
Joseph Haddad/*Lebanon*
Vytautas Baciulis/*Lithuania*
Romeo Rodriguez/*Mexico*
Abderrahim Baroudi/*Morocco*
Touhami Ouazzani/*Morocco*
Chit Ko Tin/*Myanmar*

Khin Mya Aye/*Myanmar*
Phyu Phyu Aung/*Myanmar*
Than Tun Myint/*Myanmar*
Tin Tin Nwe/*Myanmar*
Sally Gatchalian/*Philippines*
Hermana Gregoria/*Philippines*
Jacek Mrukowicz/*Poland*
Piotr Socha/*Poland*
Henrique Carmona da Mota/*Portugal*
Joao Gomes-Pedro/*Portugal*
Larissa Scheplyagina/*Russia*
Saad Abdullah Al Saeidi/*Saudi Arabia*
Vanessa Tan Chung Cheng/*Singapore*
Anna Coutsoudis/*South Africa*
Faiza Benkebil/*Switzerland*
Martine Cuny/*Switzerland*
Philippe Eigenmann/*Switzerland*
Chen Wendy Wei-Win/*Taiwan*
Tzu Chia-Hsiang/*Taiwan*
Chomchak Chuntrasakul/*Thailand*
Chaleerat Derekwatanachai/*Thailand*

Chantana Jutiteparak/*Thailand*
Sungkom Jongpipatvanich/*Thailand*
Ladda Mo-Suwan/*Thailand*
Daranee Mukhajonpun/*Thailand*
Jarungchit Ngamphaiboon/*Thailand*
Chanchai Panthongviriyakul/*Thailand*
Chulaporn Roongpisuthipong/*Thailand*
Sonchai Siriwanabus/*Thailand*
Umaporn Sutudworavuth/*Thailand*
Prasong Teinboon/*Thailand*
Siriwat Tiptaradol/*Thailand*
Vichai Tunpichit/*Thailand*
Chongjit Ungkathavanich/*Thailand*
Pakit Vichyanond/*Thailand*
Nualanong Visitsuntorn/*Thailand*
William Cochran/*USA*
Bill Klish/*USA*
Nguyen Cong Khanh/*Vietnam*
Nguyen Van Dung/*Vietnam*
Tran Tan Tram/*Vietnam*
Tran Thi Phuong Mai/*Vietnam*

Nestlé Representatives

Giorgio Albertini   Nestlé Italiana S.p.A., Milano, Italy
Anne-Lise Carrié-Faessler   Nestec Ltd, Vevey, Switzerland
Lajos Hanzel   Nestlé Hungaria Kft., Budapest, Hungary
Ferdinand Haschke   Nestec Ltd, Vevey, Switzerland
Linda Hsieh   Nestlé USA, Inc., Glendale, CA, USA
Milagros Virginia Lim   Nestlé Philippines, Inc., Manila, Philippines
Liu Ke Lan   Nestlé (China) Ltd., Beijing, China
Olga Netrebenko   Nestlé Food LLC, Moscow, Russia
Ulrich Preysch   Nestlé Suisse SA, Vevey, Switzerland
Lesley Scharf   Nestlé Canada Inc., Vevey, Switzerland
Marie-Christine Secretin   Nestec Ltd, Vevey, Switzerland

Nestlé Nutrition Workshop Series
Pediatric Program

Volume 45: Nutrition, Immunity and Infection in Infants and Children
Robert M. Suskind and Kraisid Tontisirin, Editors; 464 pp., 2001.

Volume 44: Risk Assessment in the Food Chain of Children
Peter J. Aggett and Harry A. Kuiper, Editors; 304 pp., 2000.

Volume 43: Nutrition of the Very Low Birthweight Infant
Ekhard E. Ziegler, Alan Lucas, and Guido E. Moro, Editors; 288 pp., 1999.

Volume 42: Probiotics, Other Nutritional Factors, and Intestinal Microflora
Lars Å. Hanson and Robert H. Yolken, Editors; 320 pp., 1999.

Volume 41: Nutrition and Bone Development
Jean-Philippe Bonjour and Reginald C. Tsang, Editors; 304 pp., 1999.

Volume 40: Clinical Trials in Infant Nutrition
Jay A. Perman and Jean Rey, Editors; 304 pp., 1998.

Volume 39: Placental Function and Fetal Nutrition
Frederick C. Battaglia, Editor; 288 pp., 1997.

Volume 38: Diarrheal Disease
Michael Gracey and John A. Walker-Smith, Editors; 368 pp., 1997.

Volume 37: Feeding from Toddlers to Adolescence
Angel Ballabriga, Editor; 320 pp., 1996.

Volume 36: Long-Term Consequences of Early Feeding
John Boulton, Zvi Laron, and Jean Rey, Editors; 256 pp., 1996.

Volume 35: Diabetes
Richard M. Cowett, Editor; 320 pp., 1995.

Volume 34: Intestinal Immunology and Food Allergy
Alain L. de Weck and Hugh A. Sampson, Editors; 320 pp., 1995.

Volume 33: Protein Metabolism During Infancy
Niels C.R. Räihä, Editor; 264 pp., 1994.

Volume 32: Nutrition of the Low Birthweight Infant
Bernard L. Salle and Paul R. Swyer, Editors; 240 pp., 1993.

Volume 31: Birth Risks
J. David Baum, Editor; 256 pp., 1993.

Volume 30: Nutritional Anemias
Samuel J. Fomon and Stanley Zlotkin, Editors; 232 pp., 1992.

Volume 29: Nutrition of the Elderly
Hamish N. Munro and Günter Schlierf, Editors; 248 pp., 1992.

Volume 28: Polyunsaturated Fatty Acids in Human Nutrition
Umberto Bracco and Richard J. Deckelbaum, Editors; 256 pp., 1992.

Volume 27: For a Better Nutrition in the 21st Century
Peter Leathwood, Marc Horisberger, and W. Philip T. James, Editors; 272 pp., 1992.

Volume 26: Perinatology
Erich Saling, Editor; 208 pp., 1992.

Volume 25: Sugars in Nutrition
Michael Gracey, Norman Kretchmer, and Ettore Rossi, Editors; 304 pp.,
1991.

Volume 24: Inborn Errors of Metabolism
Jürgen Schaub, François Van Hoof, and Henri L. Vis, Editors; 320 pp.,
1991.

Volume 23: Trace Elements in Nutrition of Children—II
Ranjit Kumar Chandra, Editor; 248 pp., 1991.

Volume 22: History of Pediatrics 1850–1950
Buford L. Nichols, Jr., Angel Ballabriga, and Norman Kretchmer, Editors;
320 pp., 1991.

Volume 21: Rickets
Francis H. Glorieux, Editor; 304 pp., 1991.

Nutrition, Immunity, and Infection in Infants and Children, edited by Robert M. Suskind and Kraisid Tontisirin. Nestlé Nutrition Workshop Series, Pediatric Program, Vol. 45. Nestec Ltd., Vevey/Lippincott Williams & Wilkins, Philadelphia ©2001.

Global Burden of Malnutrition and Infection in Childhood

Kraisid Tontisirin and Lalita Bhattacharjee

Institute of Nutrition, Mahidol University (INMU), Thailand

Malnutrition and infection play a major role in causing the preventable deaths and disabilities that occur in much of the developing world, especially among young children. Malnourished children suffer loss of precious mental capacity, fall ill more often, and grow up with lasting mental or physical disabilities. Most nations at the 1990 World Summit for Children pledged, among various goals for children's improvement, to reduce mortality in infants and children aged younger than 5 years by one third of the 1990 levels or to 50–70/1,000 live births, and to reduce severe and moderate malnutrition among children aged less than 5 years (under-5) by half. Despite concerted efforts catalyzed by both international and national initiatives at various levels toward nutritional improvement, the global impact on nearly all forms of malnutrition is falling far short of that required to meet the health goals for children by the year 2000.

Viewed globally, however, the improvements in infant and child health in the past 50 years have been spectacular, and overall reductions in under 5 and infant mortality are accelerating in much of the world. Nevertheless, regional and even national data on malnutrition and infection in children often hide variations between and within countries (1).

In this chapter, we will consider the situation relating to malnutrition and infection, their consequences and burden, from a global and regional perspective. Such an assessment would provide a clear understanding of the impact of malnutrition and infection, which is essential in the management of nutrition-related health research and action programs designed to prevent and control childhood malnutrition.

MALNUTRITION–INFECTION SYNERGISM

Inadequate dietary intake, both in quantitative and qualitative terms, and disease are immediate causes of malnutrition and deaths of young children. They reinforce each other synergistically. Malnutrition causes debility and children in particular are susceptible to developing infections that can become extensive and serious. Also, certain infections and parasitic diseases have a profound influence on nutritional status, mediated by changes in dietary intake, absorption, nutritional requirements (especially for energy and protein), and loss of endogenous nutrients. Malnutrition takes several forms, which often appear in combination and make a mutual contribution to the overall picture, including protein-energy malnutrition and deficiencies of micronutrients such as vitamin A, iron, iodine, and other related trace minerals. Infants and young children have immature immune systems, and they may be vulnerable to the immunodepressive effects of marginal or moderate hypovitaminosis. For instance, although vitamin A status influences the response to infection, infections can also induce a state of vitamin A deficiency, a fact that has been well documented during measles infection in developing countries. More recently, low plasma retinol concentrations have also been reported in a substantial proportion of children with measles in the United States (2). Iron deficiency also depresses immunity. Zinc deficiency has a general effect on infectious disease, again at least partly through the immune system. Whereas much of the attention paid to iodine deficiency has been related to its effects on brain development, it appears also to have an effect on immunity.

Protein-energy malnutrition is known to have a depressant effect on the immune system. Deficiencies of vitamin A, riboflavin, iron, and zinc, which are often associated with protein-energy malnutrition, have a profound influence both on the host's response to infection and on rates of microbial proliferation. Even mild forms of malnutrition have been shown to have an adverse effect on immunocompetence and, hence, on morbidity and mortality. The mechanisms leading to growth failure and clinical malnutrition operate through anorexia, changes in metabolism, malabsorption, and behavioral changes affecting feeding practices, leading eventually to malnutrition in the face of limited nutritional reserves (3,4).

CAUSES OF MALNUTRITION

An understanding of the complex causes of malnutrition helps one appreciate the magnitude of the problem. Malnutrition is not a simple problem with a single, simple solution. A multitude of interrelated determinants is implicated in its cause, which necessitate a series of multifaceted and multisectoral approaches in addressing malnutrition. Among the factors that precipitate conditions leading to childhood malnutrition, infection, and death are poverty, ignorance, and disease; inadequate food; an unhealthy environment; social stress; and discrimination, most of which persist throughout much of the developing world.

Interest in the relations between nutrition and infection, and in the environment in which they occur, was stimulated by Scrimshaw *et al.* (5) (Fig. 1). A conceptual framework of the causes of malnutrition, developed in 1990 as part of the United Nations Children's Fund (UNICEF) nutrition strategy, finds application in this context (6). In this framework, the causes of malnutrition are multisectoral, embracing food,

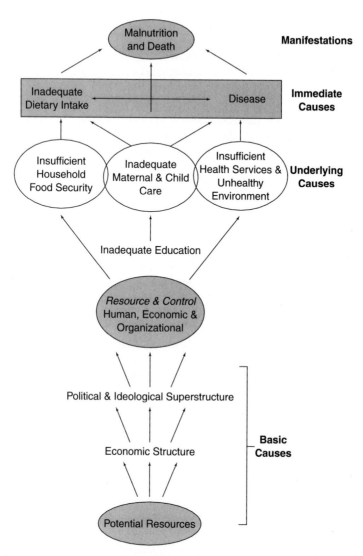

FIG. 1. Conceptual framework of the causes of malnutrition. From United Nations Children's Fund (6).

health, and caring practices. They are also classified as immediate causes (individual level), underlying causes (household or family level), and basic causes (societal level), whereby factors at one level influence those at the other levels. Among the underlying causes of inadequate dietary intake and infectious disease, inadequate access to food at the family level, insufficient health services, an unhealthy environment, and lack of proper care for children and women are most evident. At the basic level, malnutrition is a consequence of disease and inadequate dietary intake, but many other factors—social, political, economic and cultural—are involved apart from the physiologic causes.

This framework has been used at national, district, and local levels to help plan effective actions to improve nutrition in children. Thus, while viewing the global burden of malnutrition and infection, the interplay between the two most significant immediate causes of malnutrition—inadequate dietary intake and illness, which create a vicious circle—must be carefully considered. A malnourished child whose resistance to illness is compromised, falls ill and malnutrition worsens. Children who enter this malnutrition–infection cycle, as commonly occurs in developing countries, quickly enter a potentially fatal cycle as one condition feeds off the other.

GLOBAL MAGNITUDE OF CHILD MALNUTRITION

Low Birthweight

Nearly one third of all babies born in the world are of low birthweight. Globally, the World Health Organization (WHO) estimates that 25 million low birthweight infants (weight at birth < 2,500 g) are born each year, constituting 17% of all live births, nearly 95% of them in the developing world. The incidence of low birthweight varies between regions of the world, with levels of 32% in South Asia (but 9% in eastern Asia), 11% to 16% in Africa, and 10% to 12% in Latin America and the Caribbean. Born underweight and fed with suboptimal breast-feeding practices, low birthweight infants are at increased risk of protein-energy malnutrition and illness. Low birthweight is an important indicator of fetal–intrauterine nutrition and can lead to stunting in the young child. Low birthweight is a major problem in Asian countries, associated with both neonatal and postneonatal mortality. Analyses in selected Asian countries reveal very high rates of low birthweight in Bangladesh and India (50% and 30%, respectively) (1,7).

Protein-Energy Malnutrition

It is estimated that 168 million children under 5 years of age, or 27% of the world's children in this age group, are currently malnourished, as measured by weight-for-age (−2 SD National Center for Health Statistics (NCHS) median). Currently, more than 76% of these live in Asia (mainly southern Asia), 21% in Africa, and 3% in Latin America. As many as 206 million children are stunted—shorter than they should be for their age—and shorter than could be accounted for by any genetic variation in developing countries (1).

The prevalence of childhood malnutrition in various regions is shown in Table 1 (8–10). South Asia suffers by far the worst incidence of child undernutrition among all the regions in the developing world, including Sub-Saharan Africa. Some 17% of under-5 children were found to be wasted during the period 1985–1995, as compared with an average of only 9% in developing countries as a whole and 7% in Sub-Saharan Africa. Similarly, as many as 60% of children in south Asia were stunted, compared with 41% in the developing world and 39% in Sub-Saharan Africa.

TABLE 1. *Regional variation in childhood malnutrition*

	Low weight for height (% wasted)	Low height for age (% stunted)	Low weight for age (% underweight)	Low birthweight babies (% LBW)
South Asia	17.1	59.5	58.3	33
Bangladesh	15.5	64.6	65.8	50
Bhutan	4.1	56.1	37.9	—
India	19.2	62.1	63.9	33
Maldives	6.3	—	—	20
Nepal	14.0	69.0	70.0	26
Pakistan	9.2	50.0	40.4	25
Sri Lanka	12.9	27.5	38.1	25
East and South-East Asia	5.2	33.3	23.6	11
Sub–Saharan Africa	7.0	38.8	30.2	16
Middle East/North Africa	8.8	32.4	25.3	10
Latin America/Caribbean	2.6	22.7	12.0	11
Developing countries	9.1	40.7	33.9	19

LBW, low birth weight
From UNDP (8), UNICEF (9), FAO (10).

The prevalence of underweight is seen in Table 2. More than half the world's underweight children are found in south Asia: 85 million of a global total estimated at about 160 million (11). Underweight, even in mild form, increases the risk of death, inhibits cognitive development in children, and leads to reduced fitness and productivity among adults. It perpetuates the problem from one generation to the next, through malnourished women having low birthweight babies.

Figure 2 shows prevalence trends of underweight among children between 1985 and 1995 and the projection up to 2010 (11). Figure 3 indicates the percentage of malnourished children from 1993 projected up to 2020 (12). In South Asia (of which India accounts for more than 70% of the population), the prevalence is approximately 50%. This is 50% higher than in the next region, South-East Asia, where approximately one third (32% in 1995) of the children are underweight. It appears that the global rate of progress is inadequate for achieving the 1990 World Summit Year 2000 goal of reducing levels of moderate and severe malnutrition. The rate of reduction in malnutrition worldwide during successive intervals since 1980 shows a relative decrease but falls far short of what is required. The persistently slow reduction in the

TABLE 2. *Underweight children (0–60 months) by region, 1985–1995*

Region	Percent underweight (millions)				Numbers underweight (millions)				Trends (pp/yr)	
	1985	1990	1993	1995	1985	1990	1993	1995	1985–90	1990–95
South Asia	55.3	50.1	49.6	48.8	87.2	84.5	86.5	85.2	−1.04	−0.26
South-East Asia	39.8	34.2	33.1	32.4	22.3	19.8	19.5	19.1	−1.12	−0.36
China	22.7	17.8	16.6	15.0	23.0	21.1	18.4	16.6	−0.98	−0.56
Total	34.3	30.7	30.4	29.3	163.8	160.5	161.9	158.0	−0.72	−0.28
Total 0–4 population					476.6	523.3	533.5	537.4		

From United Nations (11).

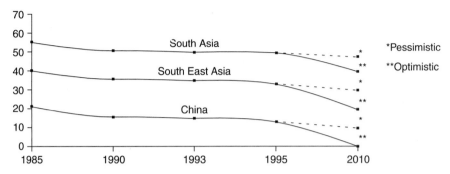

FIG. 2. Trends in prevalence of underweight children, 1985–1995, and projection of underweight children, 2010.

magnitude of global malnutrition is alarming, owing to its powerful impact on infant and young child mortality.

Micronutrient Deficiencies

Deficiencies in the intake or absorption of vitamin A, iron, and iodine have serious consequences for health and mental and physical function. The estimated prevalences and numbers affected by these three deficiencies are given by region in Table 3 (13–15). At the other end of the malnutrition spectrum are found the nutritional problems arising from childhood obesity, which will also be discussed below.

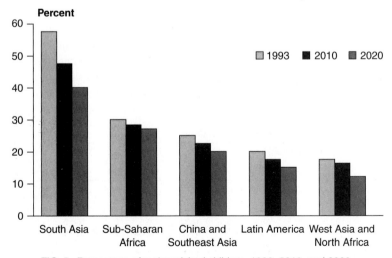

FIG. 3. Percentage of malnourished children, 1993, 2010, and 2020.

TABLE 3. Prevalence of vitamin A, iodine, and iron deficiencies by region

WHO region	Vitamin A deficiency Children (0–5 yr) with xerophthalmia (1991)		Iodine deficiency orders All people with goiter (1991)		Region	Anemia All women (15–49 yr) with low Hb (around 1988)	
	No. (millions)	Prevalence (%)	No. (millions)	Prevalence (%)		No. (millions)	Prevalence (%)
Africa	1.3	1.4	39	8.2	Africa	59.4	44
Eastern Asia	1.0	2.8	12	4.7		—	—
Latin America	0.1	0.2	30	7.0	Latin America	32.7	31
South-East Asia (Includes India)	10.0	4.2	100	5.9	Asia (includes India and China)	335.1	45
Western Pacific (Includes China)	1.4	1.3	30	2.3		—	—
Total	13.8	2.8	211	5.7		427	44

Pregnant <11 g/dl:nonpregnant <12 g/dl.
From WHO (13–15).

Iodine Deficiency

Iodine deficiency, resulting from a low intake of iodine in the diet, exists in most regions of the world. Up to 1990 it was estimated that about 40 million infants—one third of all babies born each year in the world—were at risk of mental impairment because of inadequate iodine in the maternal diet. The other consequences of iodine deficiency include goiter, increased rates of stillbirths and abortions, and infant deaths. Severe mental and neurologic impairment occurs in babies of iodine-deficient mothers. In 1997, because of the worldwide increase in the use of iodized salt, 12 million children were expected to be spared that risk. The number of babies born as cretins was expected to have fallen by more than half, from approximately 120,000 in 1990 to fewer than 55,000 worldwide (16).

Iron Deficiency

Iron deficiency, which is the most common nutritional disorder in the world, affects 1 billion people, particularly women of reproductive age and preschool children in the tropical and subtropical zones, and has a serious impact on school children. With dietary iron supply trends deteriorating in most regions, prevalence rates, particularly in Sub-Saharan Africa and south Asia, may be increasing and this is consistent with the decline in the dietary supply of iron (17). Intestinal helminth infections, especially from hookworm, which cause gastrointestinal blood loss, are one of the major causes of iron deficiency anemia. Other causes include malaria and other micronutrient deficiencies (*e.g.*, vitamin A deficiency). Data on anemia prevalence in children are inadequate and scattered in south Asia, where it is uniformly high. Studies show that severe anemia is found among 44% of Afghan children, 73% of preschoolers in Bangladesh, 67% of Indian preschool children, 78% of Nepalese children, and 65% to 78% of Pakistani children (18).

Vitamin A

Vitamin A deficiency is the one of the most common nutritional deficiency disorders in the world. WHO has estimated that more than 250 million children worldwide have deficient vitamin A stores. In 1991, WHO reported that nearly 14 million preschool children had eye damage caused by vitamin A deficiency and approximatley 10 million of these children live in Asia. Global progress is being made in combating the ocular effects of vitamin A deficiency, but the subclinical forms need to be fully controlled. Subclinical vitamin A deficiency is common in school children and adolescents in several settings in south Asia (18). Vitamin A deficiency in preschool children has marked implications for reduced growth and can lead to increased risk of mortality, morbidity, and blindness, although the immediate health consequences for school children and adolescents are not completely known (19).

Folic Acid Deficiency

Folic acid deficiency has been shown to incur risk of neural tube defects in industrialized and eastern European countries. However, information is sparse on the epidemiology of folic acid deficiency in developing countries. In rural Mexico, Black *et al.* (20) did not identify folic acid deficiency but identified vitamin B_{12} deficiency (21) among children, pregnant, and nursing women.

Zinc Deficiency

Zinc deficiency in mild and moderate forms, which is likely to be widespread, was largely overlooked until recently (22). It contributes to growth stunting in young children in many regions (23). Often protein-energy malnutrition, especially "low height for age," results from poor diet quality, including low levels of bioavailable zinc, rather than from an inadequate quantity of either protein or energy. Zinc deficiency may be a major cause of morbidity in young children, as shown by studies in India and elsewhere (24).

Obesity

An increasing number of nutritional problems have arisen from affluence, changing dietary habits, and changing lifestyles. Obesity in childhood merits attention in this regard.

Childhood obesity and its consequences are seen to be emerging as a global problem. Data from 79 developing countries and several industrialized countries suggest that approximately 22 million under-5 children are overweight by WHO standards (≥ 2 SD above the reference median weight for height). Obesity affects almost 10% of school children in industrialized countries and high rates are also emerging in the developing world.

In the United States, the prevalence of overweight (defined by the 85th centile of weight for height) among those 5 to 24 years of age from a biracial community of Louisiana showed an approximately twofold increase between 1973 and 1994. Similar trends were noted in Japan: the frequency of obese children aged 6 to 14 years increased from 5% to 10% between 1974 to 1993. Early obesity leads to an increased likelihood of obesity in later life, as well as an increased prevalence of obesity-related disorders (25).

In developing countries, increasing levels of childhood overweight and obesity indicate that these countries may be carrying a double burden in terms of nutritional problems into the next century. In Thailand, for instance, the prevalence of obesity among school children aged 6 to 12 years rose from 12.2% in 1991 to 15.6% in 1993 (26). In a recent study of Saudi Arabian children aged 6 to 18 years, the prevalence of obesity was found to be 15.8% (27).

Obesity is associated with various problems in children and adolescents, the most prevalent being the psychosocial consequences in adolescence and the persistence of obesity into adulthood, which in turn leads to a number of health consequences ranging from an increased risk of premature death to several nonfatal but debilitating complaints that affect the quality of life.

The wider implications of these trends in childhood malnutrition, which include the coexistence of undernutrition and overnutrition, especially in developing countries, may well be imagined, and an urgent call to address this burden awaits health professionals and workers.

REEMERGENCE AND EMERGENCE OF OLD AND NEW DISEASES

Despite an increasing coverage of immunization, which has been widely implemented through the WHO's expanded program on immunization since 1974, children are still slipping through the safety net, and this includes many of the world's poorest children, who are particularly vulnerable to disease. Sub-Saharan Africa fares the worst: each year almost half the children who should receive the necessary three doses of DPT vaccine to prevent diphtheria, pertussis, and tetanus do not receive them. Although coverage rates in the rest of the world are higher, the fact is that 26 million infants do not receive their three DPT shots (28).

Previously controlled diseases, including diphtheria, are noted to be reemerging, and measles continues to thrive in the cities of Africa and Asia, especially in deprived neighborhoods. Just 20 countries now account for 85% of measles deaths in children under 5: approximately 722,000 children die each year from measles, half of them in Africa, and 23,000 in India alone. Measles immunization coverage has remained static or slipped in 32 of the 44 poorest countries since 1990, including Burundi (25% decline in coverage), Papua New Guinea, Yemen (23%), Malawi (14%), Benin (13%), and Mali (12%) (28).

In India, with the national immunization program, measles, pertussis, and diphtheria deaths are now 80% less than preimmunization levels. But immunization coverage remains disparate, with up to 30% of children receiving no vaccination at all. The primary healthcare system continues to have difficulty in addressing health risks. Of all curative healthcare, 70% to 90% is delivered by the private sector. One of five children with acute respiratory infection receives no treatment. Of infant deaths, 15% to 20% are caused by lower respiratory tract infections. Although deaths from diarrheal dehydration have decreased, only 43% of mothers know about oral rehydration therapy, and only 26% report ever having used it (29).

Some of the poorest nations, Cambodia for example, have more than doubled their measles immunization rates, from 32% in 1990 to 72% in 1996. Guinea's coverage rate stands at 61%, compared with only 18% in 1990 (28). These are examples of political will in truly committed nations which should steer health actions toward addressing childhood diseases.

Rheumatic fever and rheumatic heart disease (the most common cardiovascular disease in children and young adults) are examples of how social and economic factors and subsequent improved health and medical care, have contributed to and then accelerated the decline of a disease that was once widely prevalent in developed countries. Currently, limited evidence suggests little decline in the occurrence of rheumatic heart disease in developing countries over the past few decades. Meningococcal meningitis is another childhood disease that occurs in all parts of the world. In the 1980s, an epidemic wave of meningococcal meningitis spread over Asia and Africa. In nonepidemic years, at least one million cases of bacterial meningitis are estimated to occur, which may double in epidemic years (1).

Although some of these common infectious diseases of childhood are coming under control through a combination of health promotion, prevention, and simplified standard treatment regimens, children are also threatened by another emerging new morbidity, the acquired immunodeficiency syndrome (AIDS). Globally, the new morbidity from AIDS is closely associated with behavioral problems and, therefore, is much more difficult to prevent than diseases that have been well known. AIDS presents a crucial challenge, with globally some 1,600 children under 15 years of age being infected with the human immunodeficiency virus (HIV) every day. The vast majority of these cases occur through mother-to-child transmission (30). WHO projects that with the present growing trends, by the year 2000 more than 13 million women will have been infected and 4 million will have died of AIDS. Their uninfected infants will comprise a growing group of potential orphans. By 2000, as many as 10 million children under age 10 may be orphaned as a result of maternal AIDS in Sub-Saharan Africa alone, and the projected deaths from AIDS may increase child mortality rates by as much as 50% in parts of Sub-Saharan Africa. Alarming trends are also noticed in South-East Asia.

With the increase of HIV infection, it seems that tuberculosis in children (especially pneumonia and meningitis) is not yet decreasing, even though immunization coverage with bacille Calmette–Guérin (BCG) is high (1). This new morbidity will certainly contribute to rapidly rising social and economic costs, both at the microeconomic level and at national levels, and it may even reverse the long-term effects of child health improvement initiatives.

On the whole, a need exists to bolster the health infrastructure, the inputs of workers, and the supply of affordable vaccines, and above all to maintain our technical and political structures. Governments need to assess priorities and closely view the true value of preventive strategies that can alleviate the global burden of disease in the long term.

MORTALITY OUTCOMES

The mortality caused by malnutrition and infection is the critical problem, the most vulnerable groups being developing fetuses and children up to the age of 3 years. Folate deficiency in expectant mothers can cause birth defects in infants (*e.g.*, such as spina bifida), all of which have serious implications for a child's quality of life. Vitamin A deficiency, even in its mild form, impairs the immune system, reducing children's resistance to diarrhea, which kills nearly 1 million children annually. New findings strongly suggest that vitamin A deficiency is a cause of maternal mortality as well, especially among women in impoverished regions (31). Vitamin A deficiency among preschool children in Nepal causes an estimated 14,000 to 20,000 Nepalese children to die of infections annually (32). Of nearly 12 million under-5 children who die each year in developing countries, mainly from preventable causes, the deaths of more than 6 million (54%) are either directly or indirectly attributable to malnutrition (Fig. 4) (33,34).

The nature of these deaths disguises the complex sequence of events leading to repetitive episodes of infection, which are accompanied by loss of appetite and decreased food intake, and the increased demands on the child's energy that the illness makes each time.

The burden of maternal mortality that looms large in Southeast Asia is another important area of concern. It is estimated that 585,000 maternal deaths occur in the world every year, and all but 6,000 are in the developing world. Southeast Asia alone contributes 40% of the world total. Women die from hemorrhage, infection, high blood pressure, obstructed labor, unsafe abortion, and a range of diseases that are aggravated by pregnancy (*e.g.*, malaria, hepatitis, and rheumatic heart disease) (7).

The maternal mortality rate in India is the second highest in the world, estimated to be between 385 and 487/100,000 live births (29). Contributory factors include poor nutrition and lack of general healthcare during pregnancy. Negative social practices still inhibit healthcare services and family planning education efforts. Women require the correct knowledge and confidence to take better care of themselves to ensure a better pregnancy outcome. In this regard, discrimination against women is seen as a major cause of malnutrition and mortality. For instance, striking disparities exist in the prevalence of maternal anemia, low birthweight incidence, weight gain during pregnancy, supplementary feeding practices, sanitation, and hygiene in south Asia as compared with Sub-Saharan Africa.

In India, some discernible relations exist between the survival of female children and the mother's characteristics. The female child of the young mother is at particu-

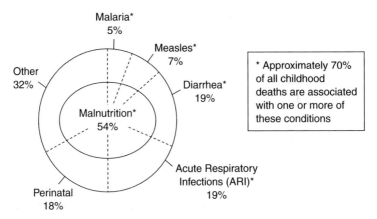

FIG. 4. Distribution of 11.6 million deaths among children aged less than 5 years in all developing countries, 1995.

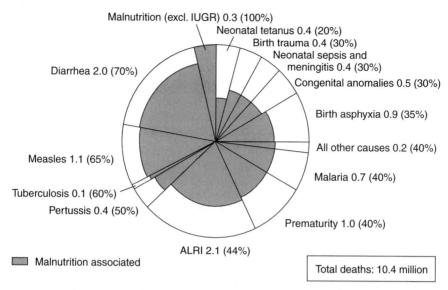

FIG. 5. Major causes of death among children aged less than 5 years in the developing world, 1995.

lar risk of death because young women are under the greatest pressure to produce sons, and the extent of this pressure is also related to women's economic status (35). Female education is also related strongly and inversely to infant mortality. Jain (36) established that female education and household economic status were important "household level" factors explaining mortality variations.

The mortality risks of child malnutrition are also influenced biologically by natural defenses and nutrition: the physical, microbial, social, and cultural environments. The living conditions of communities and societies, the prevalence and modes of transmission of infectious disease agents, and the nutritional status of the child are among the strongest immediate determinants that set different levels of under-5 mortality rates around the world. The decline in deaths among under-5s in developed countries since the late 1940s has been largely attributable to improvements in sanitation, water supply, housing, food supply and distribution, and general hygiene. However, in many countries (*e.g.*, Afghanistan, Guinea, Liberia, Malawi, Mali, Mozambique, Niger, Sierra Leone, and Somalia) that have been unable to make or sustain progress over the years, under-5 mortality rates are still above 200 (37); in others, the levels are declining only slowly, at a rate of no more than 1% to 2% per year.

In the developing world in 1995, approximately 7.5 million children died from one, or frequently more than one, of five conditions: malaria, malnutrition, measles, acute respiratory infections, and diarrhea. Seven target countries with infant deaths of 40% or more per 1,000 live births have been identified in Southeast Asia (7). Among these countries, Bangladesh, India, Indonesia, and Nepal account for approximately 40% of the global acute respiratory infection deaths. Poor access to health services, low utilization of government health facilities, and poor outreach of existing programs are major contributory factors to acute respiratory infection deaths. Malaria also exists as a major cause of child death in large areas of the world, taking a major toll on child growth and development. In parts of Africa where malaria is common, nearly one third of childhood malnutrition is caused by malaria. The major causes of death among under-5 children in developing countries (1) are shown in Figure 5.

NEONATAL DEATHS

Although the causes of nearly 4 million stillbirths occurring worldwide are difficult to assess, research shows that nearly half of all stillborn babies are the result of maternal complications during labor and delivery. WHO (1) shows that 2 million babies are either born dead or are born alive only to die within their first 28 days of life. The negative effects of maternal malnutrition in perinatal life and the risk of fetal mortality are higher among stunted populations who have poor pelvic development. Many stillbirths can be circumvented and result in perfectly normal infants if appropriate care is given at birth. More than two thirds of the nearly 4.8 million newborn deaths are among fully developed babies born at term and apparently well equipped for life; however, at least four of every five newborn deaths are caused by infection, birth asphyxia, congenital anomalies, birth injury, and problems linked to preterm birth (Fig. 6) (1).

In 1997, an estimated 275,000 neonatal tetanus deaths occurred, which from the 1980s had been drastically reduced in most countries, with Brazil, Vietnam, and

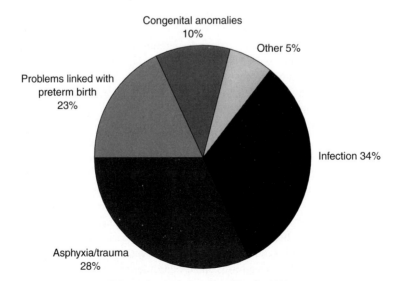

FIG. 6. Causes of neonatal death, 1995.

China recording greatest progress (1). However, in Nigeria deaths soared from 23,000 in 1990 to 37,000 in 1997 (up by 62%). Neonatal tetanus results from tetanus spores being introduced through poor hygiene during childbirth, often exacerbated by traditional childbirth practices, such as the use of clarified butter or even cattle dung to "heal" the umbilical stump.

Helping these babies to survive and grow up healthy does not require sophisticated equipment but calls for preventive measures and prompt additional care.

LOW BIRTHWEIGHT—A CONSEQUENCE OF POOR MATERNAL NUTRITION

In developing countries where large proportions of women are short and underweight, the number of low birthweight infants is particularly high (30% in south Asia, 10% to 20% in other regions) (38,39), with the incidence of low birthweight being highest in low income groups. A sex difference has also been noted in mean birthweights: female infants tend to weigh less than male infants (40).

Maternal prepregnancy nutrition affects intrauterine growth and birthweight, with anemia and low maternal hemoglobin concentration having distinct influences on birth and delivery outcomes and the quality of the offspring's life. Infants who start with the initial handicap of low birthweight, despite of their being full term, do not recover from their initial handicap and under these conditions of deprivation, a vicious cycle of malnutrition is set up.

LOW BIRTHWEIGHT AND THE DEVELOPMENT OF CHRONIC DISEASE

Valuable insights into the influence of intrauterine nutrition on the development of diet-related diseases in later life have emerged recently. Links are emerging between malnutrition in early life—including the period of fetal growth—and the development later in life of chronic conditions such as coronary heart disease, diabetes, and high blood pressure, giving the countries in which malnutrition is already a major problem new causes for concern (41).

Examination of fetal and placental size and the risk of hypertension in adult life has shown that the highest blood pressure levels occur in subjects who had been small babies with low birthweight but heavy placentas. Maternal dietary imbalances in critical periods of intrauterine life can trigger a redistribution of fetal resources, affecting a fetus's structure and metabolism in ways that predispose to later cardiovascular and endocrine diseases (42).

In terms of health and development, the low birthweight child is at a particular disadvantage because of the risk of malnutrition and infection. An additional risk to the infant may come from the fact that iron deficiency and anemia in the mother can also produce alterations in brain function and impair schooling later. The mortality rate of low birthweight infants is estimated to be 86/1,000 births (43). Those who survive have greater mortality rates and poorer neurologic development.

TABLE 4. *Global burden of disease and injury attributable to selected risk factors, 1990*

Risk factor	Deaths (thousands)	As % of total deaths	YLLs (thousands)	As % of total YLLs	YLDs (thousands)	As % of total YLDs	DALYs (thousands)	As % of total DALYs
Malnutrition	5,881	11.7	199,486	22.0	20,089	4.2	219,575	15.9
Poor water supply, sanitation, and, personal and domestic hygiene	2,668	5.3	85,520	9.4	7,872	1.7	93,392	6.8
Unsafe sex	1,095	2.2	27,602	3.0	21,100	4.5	48,702	3.5
Tobacco	3,038	6.0	26,217	2.9	9,965	2.1	36,182	2.6
Alcohol	774	1.5	19,287	2.1	28,400	6.0	47,687	3.5

YLD, years of life disabled; YLL, years of life lost; DALY, disability—adjusted life years.
From Murray C, Lopez A (45) and WHO (22).

DISEASE BURDEN OF MALNUTRITION

With the multitude of consequences arising from malnutrition and infection, the disease burden of malnutrition is indeed immense. The Global Burden of Disease (GBD) study, which began in 1992, has assessed the major risk factors using a time-based calculation of future potential years of life lost or lived with a disability, namely disability-adjusted life years (DALYs). In 1990, nearly 1.3 billion DALYs were reportedly lost as a result of new cases of disease and injury that year, almost 90% occurring in developing countries. Of the major risk factors evaluated, malnutrition was by far the leading contributor to DALYs worldwide, causing an estimated 16% of the global burden of disease in 1990 (18% in developing regions), with the contributions to disease burden being particularly evident in Sub-Saharan Africa (33%) and India (22%) (44).

Malnutrition (including protein-energy malnutrition, vitamin A deficiency, iodine deficiency, and anemia) is included among group I causes of death, accounting for 11.7% of total deaths, followed by poor water and sanitation as the next risk factor (Table 4) (45).

COSTS OF MALNUTRITION

The burden of childhood malnutrition and disease can lead to substantial loss of adult productivity. The ultimate cost of malnutrition in children can be divided into the well-known visible and the less well-known invisible costs. The visible part includes the cost of drugs, hospital admission, transportation, and food, plus the cost of treatment of non-nutritional diseases. The larger and invisible part is composed of loss of family income and national productivity as a result of one or both of the parents attending to the child; expenses incurred by hospital costs and the cost of pregnancy, childbirth, and lactation; the cost of food consumed by the child; clothing, education, and other related expenses; and the loss of a potential working population, lowered capacity to work, and, thus, a slower national economic growth. If this is translated into quantifiable terms of national losses of productivity, the burden at the global level can be immense.

REDUCED COGNITION, PHYSICAL WORK CAPACITY, AND PRODUCTIVITY

Malnourished children, unlike well-nourished children, not only have lifetime disabilities and weakened immune systems, but also lack the capacity for learning of their well-nourished peers. Undernutrition could also have a direct effect on the child's central nervous system. Stunted children reportedly have smaller heads than those who are not stunted, and head size was shown to be a stronger predictor of intelligence quotient at 7 years of age than other previous or current anthropometric measures (46). In young children, malnutrition dulls motivation and curiosity and reduces play and exploratory activities. These effects, in turn, impair mental and cognitive development. Such children grow up to be adults with fewer productive capacities.

Table 5 shows productivity losses of protein-energy malnutrition and iron deficiency in Asian countries, which are indicative of the impending burden (47).

In an expectant mother, malnutrition, especially iodine deficiency, can produce varying degrees of mental retardation in her infant. Even in populations known to be at risk of iodine deficiency disease where no evidence of cretinism is seen, a downward shift in the frequency distribution of IQ in school children has been noted, as has been documented in Italy and Spain (48). In Indonesia, 140 million IQ points were lost each year, owing to iodine deficiency, before the Ministry of Health started its current preventive campaign (49).

Of greatest concern, is that iodine deficiency in infants and children is associated with impaired physical and cognitive development. The mental and motor effects of iron deficiency or anemia have not been studied closely in infants in Asia, but studies elsewhere show that iron-deficient infants are at risk of long-term impairment in mental and motor development (50). Lower scores in IQ tests and poorer performance in school at a later age were seen to be associated with iron deficiency during infancy (51). Anemic preschool and school-aged children in India and Pakistan performed more poorly than children with normal hemoglobin levels in learning and se-

TABLE 5. *Productivity losses associated with malnutrition*

	Current losses (manual labor) (%)	Losses based on childhood malnutrition (cognitive) (%)
Protein-energy Malnutrition	2–6 (moderate stunting) 2–9 (severe stunting)	10
Iron deficiency	17 (heavy labor) 5 (blue-collar)	4

From ADB-UNICEF (47).

lected cognitive function tests (52,53). Earlier studies carried out in India and Pakistan (54,53) likewise revealed impaired ability among anemic preschool children to perform physical work.

Activity levels and frequency of children's play, which are important for long-term developmental and cognitive outcomes, have increased with zinc supplementation. Studies in India (55) and China (56) have shown positive effects of zinc supplementation on exploratory, neuromotor, and cognitive functions in children.

Deficits in cognitive performance in early life can, therefore, lead to cumulative deficits in school performance, resulting in higher school dropout rates and a high burden of illiteracy in our future populations. Reduced ability to engage in physical activity has implications in that it limits the child's scope for exploratory activities and does not allow optimal development of motor skills in such children. Growth deficits arising out of malnutrition, thus, invariably persist into adulthood, adversely affecting work performance and productivity, and additionally, for girls, increasing the risk of bearing infants with low birthweight.

THE NEED FOR INTEGRATED APPROACHES

To fight and succeed against malnutrition and infection, a range of preventive and practical actions is necessary, using integrated approaches.

The greatest preventive measures for combating child mortality include the combined inputs of immunization, improved maternal health, and family planning. As part of improved health and nutrition interventions, they serve to prevent or provide effective treatment for common childhood infectious diseases. An integrated management of childhood illnesses and rationalization of the task of health workers are mandatory. It is gratifying to note that many infectious disease control programs now include a major section on nutritional management. Diarrheal disease, acute respiratory infection (including measles), and AIDS all have vital nutritional components to management (1).

Empowerment of women and communities is ultimately crucial for nutritional improvement and for addressing disease concerns of both the women themselves and their children. Most countries in which nutrition has improved have employed integrated community-based programs using holistic participatory approaches in reaching the vulnerable groups. Self-reliance needs to be emphasized at the community level by developing need-based programs and furnishing support to strengthen the self-help capabilities of the disadvantaged, with a special focus on mothers and children (57).

This approach is based on the principle that community nutrition projects cannot be sustained if they are planned solely from the top, focus only on individuals, and are isolated from the entire community development process. Community involvement, being fundamental to solving local nutrition and related health problems, relies heavily on the participatory approach, which eventually leads to greater coverage of the target population, namely mothers and children. Certain key community-based nutrition program components are included (Fig. 7).

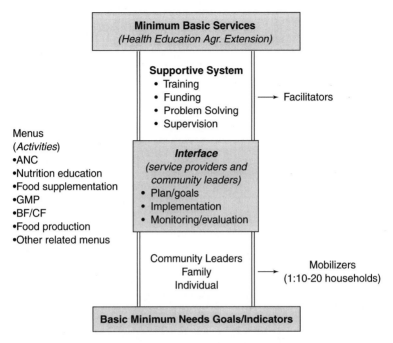

FIG. 7. Community-based nutrition program components.

For a community-based approach to have a chance of success, the objectives of each activity as well as for the program overall must be made clear to the implementing personnel in all major sectors, namely health, education, agriculture, and rural development, all of which impinge on the nutritional status of communities and, specifically, on children. This depends largely on participatory action in not only implementing the activities but also following up on recommended actions. Crucial to this is empowering facilitators and mobilizers with the knowledge and motivation to translate vital ideas into action. This is one of the reasons why it is so essential to integrate nutritional interventions both into primary healthcare activities and into overall community development initiatives that are being planned and managed at various levels. For example, between 1982 and 1991 Thailand dramatically reduced severe and moderate malnutrition, and almost eradicated it through an accelerated action program that focused on nutrition (58). Protein-energy malnutrition was identified as the most important nutritional problem, and a separate national plan for food and nutrition was included in the National Economic and Social Development Plan, with clear goals to eradicate all severe forms of protein-energy malnutrition and to reduce moderate forms by 50% and mild forms by 25%. Comprehensive nutritional surveillance was instituted through growth monitoring, and a program of nutrition education and communication was rigorously implemented throughout the country. Household and community food security was strengthened through home gardening, fruit trees, fish ponds, and prevention of epidemic diseases in poultry. School lunch programs were instituted in poor areas, and food fortification was introduced to iodize salt. Food and nutrition was integrated in the context of the poverty alleviation plan in Thailand, which enabled virtual eradication of severe and moderate malnutrition within a decade.

REFERENCES

1. The World Health Report. *Life in the 21st century, a vision for all*. Geneva: WHO; 1998.
2. Arrieta AC, Zaleska M, Stutman HR, et al. Vitamin A levels in children with measles in Long Beach, California. *J Pediatr* 1992; 121: 75–8.
3. Waterlow JC. *Protein-energy malnutrition*. London: Edward Arnold; 1992.
4. Tomkins A, Watson F. *Malnutrition and infection—a review*. ACC/SCN State-of-the-Art Series. Nutrition policy discussion paper No. 5, 1993.
5. Scrimshaw NS, Taylor CE, Gordon JE. *Interactions of nutrition and infections*. WHO monograph series No. 57. Geneva: WHO; 1968.
6. United Nations Children's Fund. *Strategy for improved nutrition of children and women in developing countries*. Policy review paper E/ICEF/1990/1.6. New York, UNICEF; 1990.
7. WHO SEAR (South East Asia Region). Regional health report. New Delhi; 1997.
8. United Nations Development Program. *Human development report*. New York: UNDP; 1994.
9. UNICEF. *The state of the world's children*. Oxford: Oxford University Press; 1996.
10. Food and Agricultural Organization. *The sixth world food survey*. Rome: FAO; 1996.
11. United Nations. *Update on the nutrition situation*. Summary of results for the 3rd report on the world nutrition situation. New York; 1996.
12. The International Food Policy Research Institute. *Food policy report*. Washington, DC: IFPR; 1997.
13. World Health Organization. *National strategies for overcoming micronutrient malnutrition*. 45th World Health Assembly provisional agenda, item 21. Geneva: WHO; 1992.
14. World Health Organization. *Infant and young child nutrition, progress and evaluation report*. 43rd World Health Assembly document agenda item 17. Geneva: WHO, 1990; 14.
15. World Health Organization. *The prevalence of anemia in women: a tabulation of available information*, 2nd ed (WHO/MCH/MSM92.2). Geneva: WHO; 1992.
16. UNICEF. *State of the world's children*. New York: UNICEF; 1998.
17. United Nations. *Focus on micronutrients*. New York: ACC/SCN, SCN News; 1993.
18. UNICEF. Regional Office for South Asia. *Malnutrition in South Asia: a regional profile*. Kathmandu, Nepal; 1997.
19. West K, Khatry SK, Katz J, et al. *Impact of weekly supplementation of women with vitamin A or beta carotene on fetal, infant and maternal mortality in Nepal* [Abstract]. Cairo: XVII IVACG Meeting, 22–26 September, 1997.
20. Black AK, Allen LH, Pelto GH, et al. Iron, vitamin B12 and folate status in Mexico: associated factors in men and women and during pregnancy and lactation. *J Nutr* 1994; 124: 1179–88.
21. Allen LH, Rosado J, Casterline JE, et al. Vitamin B12 deficiency and malabsorption are highly prevalent in rural Mexican communities. *Am J Clin Nutr* 1995; 62: 1013–9.
22. World Health Organization. *Indicators for assessing vitamin A deficiency and their application in monitoring and evaluating intervention programmes*. Micronutrient series. (WHO/NUT/96.10). Geneva: WHO; 1996.
23. Sandstead HH. Zinc deficiency. A public health problem? *Am J Dis Child* 1991; 145: 853–9.
24. Sazawal S, Bentley M, Black RE, et al. Effect of zinc supplementation on observed activity in low socio-economic Indian preschool children. *Pediatrics* 1996; 98: 1132–7.
25. World Health Organization. *Obesity—preventing and managing the global epidemic*. Report of a WHO Consultation on Obesity, Geneva: WHO; 3–5 June, 1997.
26. Mo-suwan LC, Junjana C, Puetpaiboon A. Increasing obesity in school children in a transitional society and the effect of the weight control program. *Southeast Asian J Trop Med Public Health* 1993; 24: 590–4.
27. al-Nuaim AR, Bamgboye EA, al-Herbish A. The pattern of growth and obesity in Saudi Arabian male school children. *Int J Obes Relat Metab Disord* 1996; 20: 1000–5.

28. Henderson RH. Immunization: going that extra mile. In: *Progress of nations*. New York: UNICEF, 1998: 13.
29. *UNICEF in India 1999–2000: challenges and opportunities*. New Delhi: UNICEF, India Country Office; 2000.
30. UNICEF. *Progress for children. Achieving the world summit for children goals in East Asia and the Pacific*. Bangkok: UNICEF East Asia and Pacific Regional Office; 1998.
31. UNICEF. *The state of the world's children*. New York: UNICEF; 1998.
32. Bloem MW, de Pee S, Darton-Hill I. Vitamin A deficiency in India, Bangladesh and Nepal, In: *Malnutrition in South Asia: a regional profile*. Kathmandu, Nepal: UNICEF Regional Office for South Asia; 1997.
33. Bailey K, de Onis M, Blossner M. Protein-energy malnutrition. In: Murray CJL, Lopez AD, eds. *Malnutrition and the burden of disease: the global epidemiology of protein-energy malnutrition, anemias and vitamin deficiencies*. Vol. 8. The Global Burden of Disease. Cambridge: Harvard University Press; 1996.
34. Pelletier DL, Forngillo EA, Habicht JP. Epidemiologic evidence for a potentiating effect of malnutrition on child mortality. *Am J Public Health* 1993; 83: 1130–3.
35. Bardhan PK. *On the economic geography of sex disparity in child survival in India: a note*. Berkeley: University of California at Berkeley; 1987 (mimeo).
36. Jain A. *Determinants of regional variations in infant mortality in India*. Working paper No 20. New York: Population Council, 1984.
37. UNICEF. *The state of the world's children—education*. New York: UNICEF; 1999.
38. ACC/SCN. *Second report on the world nutrition situation*. Vol. 1. Global and regional results. Geneva: ACC/SCN; 1993.
39. Malvankar DV, Gray RH, Trivedi CR, Parikh VC. Risk factors for small for gestational age births in Ahmedabad, India. *J Trop Pediatr* 1994; 40: 285–9.
40. National Institute of Nutrition (NIN). *Nutrition in India*. UN ACC/SCN country case study supported by UNICEF, prepared for the XV International Congress of Nutrition. Adelaide; 1993.
41. Hoet JJ. The role of fetal and infant growth and nutrition in the causality of diabetes and cardiovascular disease in later life. *SCN News* 1997; 14: 10–3.
42. Barker DJP, Bull AR, Osmond C, et al. Fetal and placental size and risk of hypertension in adult life. *BMJ* 1990; 301: 259–62.
43. Wynn A, Crawford M, Doyle W, Wynn S. Nutrition of women in anticipation of pregnancy. *Nutr Health* 1991; 7: 69–88.
44. Lopez A. Global burden of disease study. *SCN News* 1997; 14: 42–3.
45. Murray C, Lopez A, eds. *The global burden of disease*. Cambridge: Harvard School of Public Health, on behalf of the World Health Organization, Harvard School of Public Health, and the World Bank; 1996.
46. Grantham-McGregor SM, Fernald LC. Stunting and mental development. Paper prepared for the ACC/SCN Commission on Nutrition in the 21st Century. In: *Third report on the world nutrition situation, ACC/SCN*; December 1997: 9.
47. ADB-UNICEF Regional study on reducing child malnutrition in Asian countries; 1998.
48. Stanbury JB. The damaged brain of iodine deficiency: cognitive, behavioural, neuromotor, educative aspects. Cognizant Communication Corporation; 1993: 335.
49. ICCIDD. Indonesia battle against IDD. *ICCIDD Newsletter* 1996; 12: 56–8.
50. Lozoff B, Jimenez E, Wolf AW. Long term developmental outcome of infants with iron deficiency. *N Engl J Med* 1991; 325: 687–94.
51. Walter T, de Andraca I. Iron deficiency in infancy and its effects on psychological development at age 10 [Abstract]. *Nestlé Foundation Annual Report, 1995*; cf Gillepsie S. Draft paper on major issues in developing effective approaches for the prevention and control of iron deficiency—an overview, prepared for MI and UNICEF; 1996.
52. Seshadri S, Hirode K, Naik P, et al. Behavioural responses of young anemic Indian children to iron-folic acid supplements. *Br J Nutr* 1982; 48: 233–40.
53. Paracha P, Kirvin LK, Lindsay HA, Gretel HP, Holger H. Functional consequences of iron deficiency anemia. Impact of iron supplementation on pre-adolescent school girls in north west frontier province. Pakistan: *Abstracts of 6th Asian Congress, Malaysia*, 1992; 177.
54. Satyanarayana K, Raj Pradhan D, Ramnath T, et al. Anemia and physical fitness of school children of rural Hyderabad. *Indian Pediatr* 1990; 27: 715–21.

55. Sazawal S, Bentley M, Black RE, et al. Effect of zinc supplementation on observed activity in low socio-economic Indian preschool children. *Pediatrics* 1996; 98: 1132–7.
56. Penland JG, Sandstead HH, Alcock NW, et al. Preliminary report: effects of zinc and micronutrient repletion in growth and neurological function of urban Chinese children. *J Am Clin Nutr* 1997; 16: 268–72.
57. Tontisirin K, Kachodham Y, Winichagoon P. Trends in the development of Thailand's nutrition and health plans and programs. *Asia Pacific J Clin Nutr* 1992; 1: 231–8.
58. Tontisirin K, Attig G, Winichagoon P. An eight-stage process for national nutrition development. *Food Nutr Bull* 1995; 16: 8–16.

Nutrition, Immunity, and Infection in Infants and Children, edited by Robert M. Suskind and Kraisid Tontisirin. Nestlé Nutrition Workshop Series, Pediatric Program, Vol. 45. Nestec Ltd., Vevey/Lippincott Williams & Wilkins, Philadelphia ©2001.

The Malnourished Child

An Overview

Robert M. Suskind, Leslie Lewinter-Suskind, Krishna K. Murthy, David Suskind, Dana Suskind, and Donald Liu

Louisiana State University School of Medicine, New Orleans, Louisiana, USA

In 1980, approximately 39% of the world's preschool children, 141 million in all, suffered from some degree of malnutrition. Of these children, 59% lived in southeast Asia. It is estimated that in India alone 56 million and in Africa and the Middle East 18 to 20 million preschool children are less than 80% of their weight for age.

Although primary protein-energy malnutrition is not commonly seen in hospitals in the United States, physicians are becoming increasingly aware of malnutrition secondary to disease states such as the acquired immunodeficiency syndrome (1) and renal, hepatic, and cardiopulmonary disease. Secondary nutritional deficits must also be considered when evaluating the nutritional status of children throughout the world.

It is important to recognize that the child who is malnourished as a result of inadequate intake or recurrent infections has deficits in protein, energy, vitamin, and mineral stores. In recognition of this fact, it is proposed that the term "the malnourished child" replace the term "protein-calorie" or "protein-energy" malnutrition when referring to the undernourished child.

CLASSIFICATION OF PROTEIN-ENERGY MALNUTRITION

Weight and Height Criteria

Gomez *et al.* (2) in 1955 were among the first to define malnutrition in terms of deficits in weight for age. Using local standards, they defined first, second, and third degree malnutrition in terms of 75% to 90% of weight for age, 60% to 75% of weight for age, and less than 60% of weight for age, respectively. Today, the Gomez *et al.*

23

classification has been modified. Instead of using local standards as a basis for comparison, internationally accepted standards derived from the mean weights and heights of healthy children from North America or Europe (3) are used. Inasmuch as little or no evidence indicates that genetic differences affect growth potential during the early years of life (3), the norms of developed countries are applicable to communities where malnutrition is common.

Height for age and *weight for height* are often more useful tools for defining an individual's nutritional status than weight for age, which does not take into consideration the height deficit caused by chronic malnutrition (4). The child who has a decreased weight for height is acutely malnourished or wasted, whereas a child who has a decreased height for age is chronically malnourished or stunted. Children who are 80% to 90%, 70% to 80%, and less than 70% of weight for height are classified as having evidence of *acute malnutrition*, grades I, II, and III, respectively. Children who are 90% to 95%, 85% to 90%, and less than 85% of height for age are classified as having evidence of *chronic malnutrition*, grades I, II, and III, respectively. Studies from several developing countries have shown that both wasting and stunting are commonly seen in children between the ages of 1 and 2 years of age; however, by 3 to 4 years of age, children who may still be underweight for age are largely stunted rather than wasted (4). In other words, they have stopped growing linearly but are of normal weight for height.

Clinical Criteria

In 1959, Jelliffe (5) used the term "protein-calorie malnutrition" to include the whole spectrum of nutritional disorders, including marasmus, marasmic-kwashiorkor, and kwashiorkor. These three states of malnutrition can be differentiated most clearly on the basis of clinical findings.

Marasmus, which predominates in infancy, is clinically characterized by severe weight reduction, gross wasting of muscle and subcutaneous tissue, marked stunting, and no detectable edema (Fig. 1). Children often develop marasmus as a result of severe deprivation of protein, energy, vitamins, and minerals, which can happen in cases where a significant decrease or absence of breast-feeding exists. The hair and skin changes and hepatomegaly resulting from fatty infiltration of the liver, which are seen in kwashiorkor, are not usually found in marasmus. The marasmic child often is psychologically irritable and apathetic. The most striking characteristics found in the marasmic child are the marked deficit in weight relative to height and a significant degree of stunting.

The child with marasmic-kwashiorkor has clinical findings of both marasmus and kwashiorkor (Fig. 2). Characteristically, the child with marasmic-kwashiorkor has edema and gross wasting and is usually stunted. These children usually have mild hair and skin changes and a palpable fatty-infiltrated liver. The clinical findings associated with marasmus-kwashiorkor occur as a result of the combined effects of inadequate intake and infection.

Kwashiorkor, which is predominant in older infants and young children, results

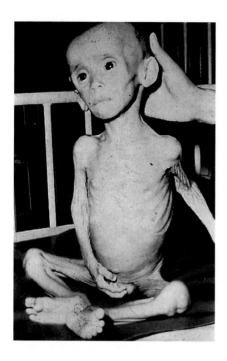

FIG. 1. Marasmic child (aged 2 years) with characteristic growth retardation, weight loss, muscular atrophy, and loss of subcutaneous tissue.

from a combination of a diet with an inadequate protein intake, with or without superimposed infection. The clinical picture is characterized by edema, skin lesions, hair changes, apathy, anorexia, a large fatty liver, and a decreased serum albumin (Fig. 3). The diet of the child with kwashiorkor is usually characterized by a decreased protein and increased carbohydrate intake. This has led to the term "sugar baby." The edema of kwashiorkor is explained by low serum albumin and other contributing factors, including increased cortisol and antidiuretic hormone levels.

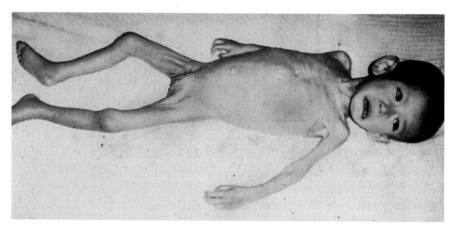

FIG. 2. Child with marasmic-kwashiorkor.

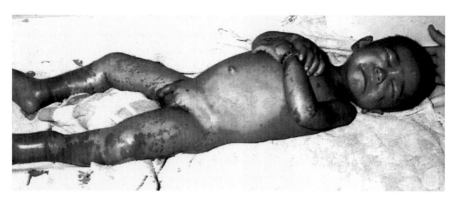

FIG. 3. Child with kwashiorkor (aged 2.5 years) with evidence of edema, skin lesions, muscular atrophy, and enlarged liver.

In addition, infection plays a major role in the pathophysiology of kwashiorkor. Production of cytokines including tumor necrosis factor (TNF) in response to infection leads to the production of acute phase reactants in place of visceral protein synthesis. Albumin, lipoproteins, and retinol-binding protein decrease; as a result of the decreased albumin synthesis, intravascular oncotic pressure decreases, which leads to edema. In addition, fatty infiltration of the liver occurs secondary to a decrease in lipoprotein synthesis.

PROGNOSIS AND MORTALITY

Mortality in severe protein-energy malnutrition is high and has been reported in some areas of the world to be more than 20%. Most deaths occur during the first days after hospital admission. Ramos Galvan and Calderon (6), after reviewing over 2,400 children with protein-energy malnutrition, concluded that the worst prognostic factors in malnourished children were infection and water and electrolyte disturbances. Garrow and Pike (7) found that decreased serum sodium and increased serum bilirubin were ominous prognostic signs. Waterlow *et al.* (8) found a high mortality rate among children with gross hepatomegaly. Kahn and Falcke (9) reported that hypothermia with a rectal temperature of less than 35°C carried a grave prognosis. Thus, factors that influence the prognosis in protein-energy malnutrition include infection, fluid and electrolyte imbalance, hepatomegaly, hypothermia, hypoglycemia, severe dermatosis, xerophthalmia, and raised concentrations of serum bilirubin and certain liver enzymes. Profound hypoglycemia accompanied by hypothermia requires immediate attention.

PATHOGENESIS OF PROTEIN-ENERGY MALNUTRITION

It is well established that the primary cause for marasmus is inadequate energy intake. Although Williams (10,11) was the first to describe the classic findings of kwashiorkor, not until after World War II was it recognized that kwashiorkor resulted from infection as well as from relative deficiency of dietary protein.

Reports from west Africa and other parts of the world showed that the distribution of kwashiorkor and marasmus varies according to dietary protein and energy intake. Clinical surveys indicated that kwashiorkor occurred almost exclusively in zones of low protein:energy ratios, whereas marasmus occurred in areas of high protein:energy ratios, but a deficit in total energy intake. Gopalan (12), however, claimed in 1968 that no essential difference existed between the protein:energy ratios in the diets of children with marasmus and those with kwashiorkor. He found that the two clinical syndromes could appear simultaneously in children for whom no demonstrable difference was found in dietary backgrounds. The factors that appeared to have the greatest impact on the development of both types of protein-energy malnutrition were the duration of breast-feeding and infection.

In 1968, Gopalan (12) coined the term "dysadaptation." He suggested that kwashiorkor was essentially a failure of adaptation that occurred when sufficient food was consumed for energy maintenance but where insufficient dietary protein was available for the synthesis of visceral proteins. As a result of infection and cytokine production, amino acids, for the most part, were shuttled into the production of acute phase reactants at the expense of visceral protein synthesis. As a result, the production of albumin and lipoproteins decreased, leading to the development of edema and fatty infiltration of the liver.

On the other hand, in children with marasmus, where both energy and protein are lacking, adaptation has taken place. Muscle provides the essential amino acids to maintain visceral protein synthesis, leading, in turn, to the production of adequate amounts of serum albumin and lipoprotein, which prevents the occurrence of edema or fatty infiltration of the liver.

With the superimposition of infection on these metabolic states, essential amino acids are diverted to the production of acute phase reactants rather than visceral proteins, with cortisol and growth hormone rather than insulin being the major contributors to the metabolic status of the patient. Growth hormone further contributes to the amino acid deficit by virtue of its action of driving amino acids into the lean body mass so that they are no longer available for visceral protein synthesis.

Scrimshaw and Behar (13) developed a schematic method of describing the evolution of a spectrum of protein-energy deficiency states (Fig. 4). Time is on the horizontal axis of a triangle, whereas the rapid development of metabolic disorders leading to edema and fatty infiltration of the liver seen in kwashiorkor is on the vertical axis, with the hypotenuse reflecting the overall slower process of wasting seen in marasmus. The typical patient falls somewhere in between.

It is well recognized that certain social customs in various parts of the world also affect the child's welfare and nutrition. As an example, some local customs in Africa promote the cessation of breast-feeding once a new pregnancy has started, for fear that the infant will poison the fetus through the breast milk. In addition, several societies have their taboos regarding what is and what is not edible, and belief is widespread that eggs can cause sterility in females. Broken homes also contribute to the problem of the child who is often separated from the mother or father as a result of divorce. Large families and birth order are also factors that can place children at

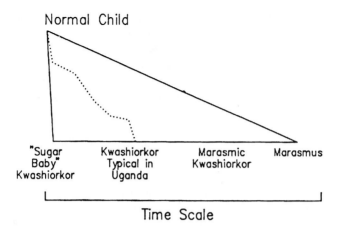

FIG. 4. The development of the protein-energy malnutrition spectrum of diseases. Adapted from Scrimshaw and Behar (13).

special risk. Morley *et al.* (14) found high incidence of kwashiorkor in Nigerian families with more than seven children. Gopalan (15) found that the prevalence of protein-energy malnutrition significantly increased when the family had more than three children.

More recently, poverty, as an underlying cause of protein-energy malnutrition, has begun to be recognized for the role it plays in childhood malnutrition. Poverty causes overcrowding and lack of food. Overcrowding leads to increased numbers of infants and children who are exposed to infection. This, in turn, leads to an increased food requirement and to the development of malnutrition.

INTERACTION OF INFECTION AND NUTRITION

The interrelationship between infection and body wasting is now well accepted. It has been clearly shown that the malnourished child is more susceptible to infection (16). Infection is one of the major factors contributing to the increased morbidity and mortality associated with protein-energy malnutrition. In 1973, Puffer and Serrano (17) showed that nutritional deficiency was an associated cause in 61% of the deaths from infectious diseases as compared with only 33% of deaths from other causes. The major infectious diseases with the greatest morbidity and mortality were diarrhea and measles (18).

The detrimental effects of infection on nutritional status are mediated by several factors. These include (*a*) anorexia; (*b*) the replacement of solid foods by a low energy, low protein diet; (*c*) decreased nutrient absorption as often occurs with diarrhea and intestinal parasites; and (*d*) increased urinary losses of nitrogen, potassium, magnesium, zinc, phosphate, sulfur, and vitamins A, C, and B_2 (19). Increased urinary nitrogen excretion is seen in even the mildest of infectious diseases. The increased excretion of nitrogen results mainly from an increased mobilization of amino acids from peripheral muscle for gluconeogenesis in the liver, with deamination and excretion of nitrogen in the form of urea. Unless dietary intake is increased, the loss of nitrogen will not be compensated for and a kwashiorkorlike syndrome will result. In addition, occurring with infection is sequestration or diversion of iron, copper, and zinc from normal metabolic pathways. Despite the mobilization of amino acids from peripheral muscle, whole blood amino acids decrease after exposure to an infectious agent (20).

In addition, there is an increased synthesis of acute phase reactants, including haptoglobin, C-reactive protein, α1-antitrypsin, and α2-macroglobulin, accompanied by a concomitant decrease in visceral protein synthesis (21). The metabolic consequence of severe gastroenteritis, measles, or one of several other communicable infectious diseases is often the development of marasmus-kwashiorkor or kwashiorkor (22). Gastroenteritis, in addition to being a seasonal infection, can occur as a result of weaning and the introduction of unclean bottle feeding practices (23). A major characteristic in the development of kwashiorkor is the decrease in serum albumin, which is closely associated with the appearance of infection. In chronic infections, anemia can occur as a result of defective hemoglobin synthesis accompanied by inadequate bone marrow stores of iron (24). Infection also affects the endocrine system. Changes in hormone levels occur simultaneously with infection and precede the changes in amino acids and serum albumin levels (24). With infection, is a decrease in serum albumin and insulin levels and an increase in cortisol, growth hormone, and antidiuretic hormone. These normal changes can occur as a result of the stress of infection stimulating the pituitary or the hypothalamus (24). Thus, a combination of increased cortisol levels and decreased food intake results in negative nitrogen balance secondary to increased tissue catabolism.

During infectious episodes, serum electrolytes also decrease because of diarrhea, resulting in a significant loss of potassium and magnesium in the stools (25). In addition urinary loss of electrolytes occurs as a result of increased muscle breakdown (26). Iron absorption and metabolism are affected by infection as well (24,27). Infections (*e.g.*, malaria and typhoid) can cause increased hemolysis and resultant acute hemolytic anemia. Thus, a continuous interaction occurs between infection and nutritional status.

NUTRITION AND IMMUNITY

Cellular Immune Response

It has been clearly established that malnourished children have an increased susceptibility to infection. Several host defense mechanisms have been shown to be altered in the malnourished child, including cellular and humoral immunity as well as polymorphonuclear leukocyte and complement activity.

It has been observed that the cell-mediated immune response is compromised in malnourished children. Its impact is illustrated by the fact that the measles mortality among malnourished children is four times that of well-nourished children (28). In addition, individuals given supplemental protein have a significantly lower incidence of tuberculosis than nonsupplemented, poorly nourished individuals (29).

Thymus atrophy was the first indication that malnutrition could affect cellular immunity in children who died from kwashiorkor (30). In addition to atrophy of the thymus, the lymph nodes, tonsils, and spleen also appeared to be smaller in malnourished children (31). In 1958, a significantly lower percentage of positive tuberculin skin tests was observed in children who were malnourished than among a well-nourished control population (32). Later, other investigators confined this defective skin test responsiveness to a variety of antigens such as *Monilia* (33), streptococcal antigen (34), trichophyton (35), and mumps virus (36). In 1971, Smythe *et al.* (37) conducted a comprehensive study of the effect of malnutrition on the cell-mediated immune response. The study showed considerably reduced tonsil size in malnourished children. In addition, the weight of the thymus and the spleen was reduced as well, more so in children with kwashiorkor than in those with marasmus. A correlation has also been shown between the degree of immunologic impairment and the degree of weight loss, with alterations in cellular immunity being normalized when the patient's nutritional status improved (38). Zinc deficiency and protein-energy malnutrition result in thymic atrophy (39), which in turn results in decreased production of thymic hormones, thus leading to the underlying T-cell deficiency (40) and increased susceptibility to infections normally contained by the cellular immune response (41).

To understand the alteration in the cellular immune response fully, Edelman *et al.* (42) performed a series of *in vivo* and *in vitro* experiments evaluating the inflammatory, sensitizing, and recall limbs of the cell-mediated immune system, as well as the responsiveness of isolated lymphocytes. To evaluate T-lymphocyte function *in vivo*, intact circulating thymus-derived T lymphocytes must be present that are capable of being sensitized to a foreign antigen. The lymphocytes that have been sensitized must also be able to identify that foreign antigen and respond with a release of lymphokines, which in turn will produce a localized inflammatory response. The initial study evaluated the inflammatory response of 30 children with protein-energy malnutrition. Dinitrofluorobenzene was applied to the forearms of these children. The result of the initial study indicated that only four of 30, or 13%, had positive inflammatory responses, and that children with protein-energy malnutrition were unable to develop a normal inflammatory response. Several investigators have found that isolated peripheral lymphocytes from malnourished children react poorly to stimulation with mitogens such as phytohemagglutinin (PHA) (35,37) and pokeweed mitogen (36). The depression in lymphocyte transformation improved with nutritional recovery (36,37). Sellmeyer *et al.* (43) also found a profound depression of lymphocyte transformation in children who had measles and gastroenteritis but who were well nourished. Decreased response to mitogen or antigen by T cells has been attributed to an increase in cell cycle duration (44), deficiency of a humoral factor required for optimal response of T cells (45), presence of an inhibitory substance in the serum (46), or to increased levels of α-fetoprotein (47). In addition to the depressed *in vitro* responsiveness of isolated lymphocytes to antigenic and mitogenic stimulation (48), circulating lymphocytes are numerically decreased in malnourished children (48), particularly the helper phenotype (49), with a proportionate increase in "null" lymphoid cells (49,50).

Natural Killer Cells

Natural killer (NK) cells are non-T, non-B large granular lymphoid cells that play a vital role in immune surveillance against virus-infected and cancer cells. Unlike cytotoxic T cells, which are antigen-specific and major histocompatibility complex restricted, NK cells act nonspecifically and in an unrestricted manner (51). Depressed NK cell activity was observed in children with protein-energy malnutrition, and renutrition resulted in a return to normal levels of NK cell activity (52). Addition of exogenous interferon, a potent stimulator of NK cells *in vitro*, had variable effects on NK activity, depending on the degree of malnutrition. In well-nourished and nutritionally recovered children, interferon enhanced NK activity but had no effect on cells from marasmic children and had a suppressive effect on cells from kwashiorkor patients.

Interleukins

Interleukins (IL) are a family of peptide or glycoprotein hormones or factors produced by activated leukocytes that act as auto or paracrine signals for activation, differentiation, and proliferation of a variety of cell types that participate in an immune response. Several of these factors with pluripotential biological activity have been studied extensively, and genes for some of them have been cloned. Recombinant products are undergoing different phases of clinical trials. The most extensively characterized interleukins are IL-1 and IL-2, products primarily of macrophages and T cells, respectively. In addition, macrophages also produce tumor necrosis factor or cachectin. IL-1 acts as an activation signal for T- and B-cell proliferation, as well as participating in inflammatory responses. On the other hand, IL-2 is synthesized and secreted by activated helper T cells with T4 or CD4 phenotype and acts as a potent stimulator of cytotoxic or suppressor T cells, NK cells, B cells, and lymphokine-activated killer cells. Helper T cells also produce interferon, which has potent stimulatory effects on macrophages and NK cells.

The effect of malnutrition on synthesis and secretion of these interleukins has not been evaluated extensively, and the available information is sparse. A significant decrease in IL-1 activity was observed following *in vitro* stimulation of macrophages from children with severe malnutrition (53). In addition, macrophages from children with kwashiorkor produced a suppressor factor that inhibited proliferation of murine thymocytes. The investigators suggest that a significant impairment of macrophage function can result in suppression of cell-mediated immunity in malnutrition. Zinc has been shown to enhance the activation and response of thymocytes to IL-1 (54). The addition of zinc to *in vitro* cultures of human peripheral blood T cells (55) or murine splenic T cells (56) resulted in the induction of interferon and IL-4 production, respectively. The other macrophage products, cachectin and tumor necrosis factor, originally isolated and identified independently by different investigators (57,58), have recently been shown to be identical molecules, based on their bioactivity, on immunologic studies, and on amino acid sequence homology (59–61). Increased serum cachectin has been reported in human patients with gram-negative septic shock (62), parasitism, and severe malnutrition (63,64). Cachectin also appears to play an important role in the pathogenesis of the cerebral form of murine malaria (65,66) and in the early stages of graft-versus-host disease (67).

Earlier studies suggested that severe malnutrition has a markedly suppressive and long-lasting effect on cell-mediated immunity, as reflected by defective T-cell functions. As T cells play a central role in regulating the duration and magnitude of the immune response, a wide ranging effect can be expected on different cell types participating in a protective immune response. In fact, two studies suggested that cell-mediated immunity may remain depressed for several years in small-for-gestational age, low birthweight infants (68,69). Paradoxically, overnutrition or obesity can also result in variable impairment of cell-mediated immune responses (70,71). Information on IL-2 levels in patients with malnutrition is not available to the best of our knowledge. However, deficiency of single nutrients such as vitamin A (72,73) or iron (74) has been shown to result in decreased T-cell proliferation and IL-2 production in animal model systems. Murthy *et al.* (72) evaluated the effect of vitamin A deficiency in rats on T-cell numbers and function. A decrease in the absolute number and percentage of T cells was observed, primarily reflecting the helper T-cell subset, which in turn resulted in altered T helper:T suppressor cell ratio. Furthermore, T cells from vitamin A-deficient rats had a significantly decreased proliferative response to PHA and produced decreased levels of IL-2 when compared with pair-fed and normal control rats. These observations have been extended to *in vitro* studies by Murthy *et al.* (Murthy KK, Bhandaru S, Pethe S, Sharma S. Effect of vitamin A analogs on interleukin-2 production by splenic T-lymphocytes; unpublished information). Rat splenic T cells were cultured with PHA, or a combination of PHA and various concentrations of retinoic acid, and the proliferative response and production of IL-2 by the T cells were evaluated. Retinoic acid enhanced the level of PHA-induced T-cell proliferation and IL-2 production. Severe iron deficiency in mice results in decreased proliferative response of T cells to concanavalin A as well as suppressed levels of IL-2 production, whereas mild to moderate iron deficiency does not appear to influence T-cell functions (74). These limited observations suggest that synthesis and secretion of various interleukins produced by macrophages and T cells are adversely affected by deficiency of several different single nutrients. Severe protein-energy malnutrition and associated deficiency of essential vitamins and minerals are most likely to result in defective T-cell functions and, in turn, poor cell-mediated immune response to infections and vaccines.

In addition to a diversion of nutrients for the production of acute phase reactants, consider the possibility that certain factors such as α1-globulin and C-reactive protein, which are increased in response to infection and in children with protein-energy malnutrition (37), can interfere with the *in vivo* and *in vitro* cell-mediated immune response in malnourished children. All these influences can play roles of varying importance in the depressed cell-mediated immunity, which often improves long before the malnourished child has completely recovered nutritionally (48).

Humoral Immune Response

The B lymphocyte is responsible for immunoglobulin production. To determine if the humoral immune system has been altered, various aspects of the humoral immune system—serum immunoglobulins, secretory immunoglobulins, the number of circulating B cells, and the antibody response to various antigens—can be measured.

In the malnourished child, the number of B cells is normal or increased, as are the circulating immunoglobulin levels (75). It has been postulated that the normal or raised levels are secondary either to a depressed suppressor T-cell population or to an increased exposure to various antigens (75). Although normal or increased levels of circulating immunoglobulins and B cells exist, competency of the humoral immune response to foreign antigens cannot be assumed. The antibody response to antigens appears to be selective in malnourished children, with the response being impaired to some antigens and adequate to others. It has been shown that the antibody response to antigens such as yellow fever (76) and typhoid vaccines (77) is markedly impaired, whereas the response to such antigens as measles, polio virus, tetanus, and diphtheria toxoid is adequate (78). In addition, decreased affinity of antibodies to tetanus toxoid and increased incidence of circulating immune complexes, have been observed in malnourished children (79,80). The response to an antigenic stimulus constitutes a much more sensitive and reliable evaluation of the humoral immune system than the level of circulating immunoglobulins. Although malnourished children have normal or increased immunoglobulin concentrations, the fact that their antibody responses to several vaccines are depressed suggests that their nutritional state does affect their humoral immune system.

Malnourished children tend to have an increased incidence of respiratory and gastrointestinal tract infections, which may reflect a deficient secretory IgA system. A significant decrease in secretory IgA (sIgA) and secretory component levels associated with malnutrition has been reported (81,82). Appropriate renutrition results in restoration of sIgA to normal levels. It is significant that, as the malnourished child's nutritional status improves, the antibody response to certain antigens also improves.

Polymorphonuclear Leukocyte Response

The polymorphonuclear leukocyte (neutrophil), which is important in controlling bacterial infections, derives its energy for the phagocytosis and killing of bacteria from glycolysis. It has been shown that malnourished and normally nourished children have the same total white cell count and the same proportion of neutrophils, but in malnourished children leukocyte metabolism is impaired (83), which affects the activity of key enzymes needed for the completion of bactericidal action of the leukocyte (84). However, no defect in the phagocytosing ability of neutrophil has been shown in the malnourished child, although the glycolytic activity of neutrophils, as judged by lactate production, is impaired (85,86). Neither does malnutrition appear to affect the opsonic activity of plasma (86). In addition, no apparent abnormality is seen either in vacuole formation or in degranulation after phagocytosis by neutrophils (87). Studies of bactericidal activity of neutrophils have produced conflicting results (88,89). The neutrophils in malnourished children respond appropriately to dermal injury; they are able to phagocytose bacteria adequately and kill bacteria adequately in most patients. Further, renutrition appears to restore neutrophil function completely to normal levels. Thus, the neutrophil appears to be the least affected component of the immune system in protein-energy malnutrition.

Complement System

Defects in the complement system have been associated with increased susceptibility to bacterial infections. Activation of the complement system leads to production of complement fragments. These are involved in viral neutralization; chemotaxis of neutrophil leukocytes, monocytes, and eosinophils; opsonization of fungi; endotoxin inactivation; lysis of virus infected cells; and bacteriolysis (90). Coovadia *et al.* (91) were the first to report reduced hemolytic activity in the serum of children with protein-energy malnutrition. Many of the children they studied had C3 and C4 on the surface of the red blood cell as a result of activation of the complement system. Other investigators who have studied the complement system in malnourished children have generally found decreased complement values when comparing them with well-nourished controls (92–94). Suskind *et al.* (94) found that the hemolytic complement activity of children with malnutrition was depressed, and a significant percentage of children had anticomplementary activity in their serum. With recovery, the hemolytic activity of the patients' serum improved, and the anticomplementary activity disappeared. In addition, 11 of 28 children were found, at the time of admission, to have circulating endotoxin which also disappeared with treatment (95).

As a result of the effect of malnutrition on the immune response, children with protein-energy malnutrition have an increased morbidity and mortality associated with infection. In addition, malnourished children have an increased susceptibility to infectious agents. It has been well established by several investigators that this increased susceptibility to infection is secondary to the effect of severe protein-energy malnutrition on the cell-mediated immune system, humoral immune system, and complement system. This severe depression is reversed when nutritional status improves. It is also clear from these studies that the neutrophil leukocyte system is relatively intact. Thus, the interaction that occurs as a result of the metabolic consequence of infection on the nutritional status of the child leads to a compromised immune system. It is critical, therefore, to intervene in terms not only of combating potentially lethal infections with antibiotic treatment, but of supporting the child nutritionally as well.

TREATMENT OF THE MALNOURISHED CHILD

Diagnostic Program

Because the newly admitted child with severe protein-energy malnutrition has multiple deficiencies, including protein, energy, vitamins, and minerals, it is important to document the deficiencies present at the outset. In addition, nearly all seriously malnourished children are infected. It is essential to determine the site, causative agent, and antibiotic sensitivities of any identified pathogens. In addition to a history and physical examination, each child requires a complete blood count and cultures of nasopharynx, throat, ear exudate, blood, urine (by suprapubic aspiration), and stool. Cerebrospinal fluid is usually obtained, if clinically indicated. An electrocardiogram and chest film are routine. Serum electrolytes and plasma proteins including serum albumin are measured on admission and throughout recovery where possible. Plasma vitamin A and E are measured on admission.

Many malnourished children are infected (96). Of greatest concern is the patient with life-threatening sepsis. Signs that have been helpful in diagnosing the septic patient include hypothermia (rectal temperature less than 36°C), hypotension (blood pressure below 60/40), leukocytosis with marked shift to the left, petechiae, and a positive blood culture.

Fluid and Electrolyte Treatment

Children with protein-energy malnutrition have a marked increase in total body water and a decrease in trace minerals (97). Normally, the patient presents with normal or low serum sodium, low potassium, and often depressed magnesium. The use of magnesium in the treatment of children with protein-energy malnutrition is based on the work of Caddell *et al.* in Thailand (98) and in east and west Africa (99).

Where possible, oral rehydration by nasogastric tube should be undertaken, using an oral rehydration solution containing 75 mmol sodium. Once rehydrated (within 8 hours), the child can be started on formula. If oral rehydration is impossible, intravenous rehydration is undertaken. The initial rehydrating fluid is 1/2 normal saline/5% glucose or a 1:2:3 solution of lactate:normal saline:glucose, with 50 ml of 50% dextrose/water (D/W) added to each 500 ml of either solution to make a 10% glucose solution. This solution supplies 75 mmol/l of sodium. A patient showing evidence of severe potassium depletion can be given up to 6 to 7 mmol/kg of potassium by oral supplementation. The intravenous solution can contain up to 40 mmol/l of potassium. Although these children have an increase in their total body water, they often show evidence of intravascular dehydration. This is especially true of those children with a history of severe diarrhea. If evidence is seen of intravascular dehydration, the water deficit is replaced in the first 8 to 12 hours of treatment. This means that a 5 kg child who is 10% dehydrated receives a total of 500 ml of fluid over the first 8 to 12 hours of treatment. A severely dehydrated child can be given as much as 20 ml/kg of intravenous solution (2% of body weight) during the first hour of treatment to increase the intravascular volume and,

TABLE 1. *Diet composition*

Macronutrient composition of formula (per kg body weight):

Energy	Protein	Fat	Carbohydrate
175	4	9.5	18.3

Vitamin supplementation:

Vitamin	Daily initial therapy intramuscularly or intravenously for 3 days beginning on day 2	Daily maintenance therapy from the 5th day until the end of week 10
Thiamine (mg)	5.0	0.7
Riboflavin (mg)	5.0	1.0
Pyridoxine (mg)	2.5	1.0
Nicotinamide (mg)	37.5	11.0
Pantothenate (mg)	5.0	5.0
Ascorbic acid (mg)	200	45.0
Folic acid (mg)	1.5	0.1
Vitamin $B_{12}O$	7.5	5.0
Vitamin A (IU)a	5,000	2,500
Vitamin D (IU)s	400	400
Vitamin E (IU)		50
Vitamin K μg	300	100

Mineral requirements/day (formula plus supplement):

Mineral	Dose
Na (mmol/kg)	2–3
K (mmol/kg)	5
Mg (mmol/kg)	0.7
Zn (mg/kg)	1–2
Fe (mg/kg)	6
Ca (mg)	800
P (mg)	800
F (mg)	0.5–1.5
Mn (mg)	1.0–1.5
Cu (mg)	1.0–1.5
Mo (mg)	0.05–0.1
Cr (mg)	0.02–0.08
Se (mg)	0.02–0.08
I (mg)	0.07

therefore, the renal blood flow. B complex vitamins are given parenterally for the first 3 days (Table 1). Once the child can tolerate oral intake, oral rehydration and feeding should be initiated.

Following the initial rehydration, the child is placed on maintenance intravenous therapy using ¼ normal saline/5% glucose or 1:2:6 lactate:normal saline:glucose solution with 50 ml of 50% D/W added to each 500 ml until oral therapy is initiated. Because of the marked decrease in total body potassium, the patient is given supplemental intravenous and oral potassium at a maintenance dose of 5 mmol/kg/d. Magnesium is given at a dose of 0.2 mmol/kg intramuscularly for 7 days followed by oral supplements in a dose of 0.7 mmol/kg/d. Once a patient has reached an oral intake of 175 kcal and 4 g/kg/d protein, the child's requirement for magnesium at doses of 0.7

mmol/kg/d and potassium at 5 mmol/kg/d is met by the formula alone. No further oral supplementation is usually required.

Therapeutic doses of the fat-soluble vitamins are given as indicated to combat overt deficiency disease.

Dietary Therapy

In cases in which feeding is not tolerated, the patient can be kept on a nothing by mouth regimen for 12 to 24 hours. Problems with hypoglycemia are kept at a minimum as long as the patient has 10% D/W running in the intravenous infusion. After the first 24 hours, the patient can be placed on gradually increasing protein and energy intakes. Graham *et al.* (100), Waterlow (101), and others have shown that the dietary intake required for optimal recovery from protein-energy malnutrition is 175 kcal and 2 to 4 g of protein/kg/d.

When children with protein-energy malnutrition are offered ad libitum solid food, they quickly reach an intake of 160 to 180 kcal/kg and 4 g/kg of protein by the second week of hospital treatment. This intake is maintained through the first 3 to 4 weeks, after which it gradually decreases to 140 to 150 kcal/kg. By discharge at 10 weeks, when the children have attained optimal weight for height, their energy intake has fallen to 110 to 120 kcal/kg. It is essential for the child to be treated in the hospital day care center until at least 90% of optimal weight for height has been attained.

In the early stages of malnutrition, it is easier to give the necessary energy and protein in a milk-based formula that can be given by tube feeding when necessary. Formula is initially more readily taken than solid food (102). Several observers have noted prolonged lactose intolerance in children with malnutrition. Some investigators have noted monosaccharide intolerance. However, a milk-based formula supplemented with dextromaltose and corn oil does not appear to be associated with prolonged diarrhea. When a milk-based formula is used, it is important to consider the addition of essential vitamins and minerals (Table 1).

One of several important minerals to consider in the treatment of malnutrition is iron. Lynch *et al.* (103) have shown that iron absorption is decreased in malnutrition. Most patients have decreased bone marrow iron stores on admission, which gradually disappear within 4 to 6 weeks without supplementation. With intramuscular iron, an immediate increase is seen in bone marrow stores. Because of the poor absorption of oral iron in protein-energy malnutrition, consider the use of elemental iron given either parenterally or orally in high doses in the range of 6 mg/kg/d. However, iron treatment should be initiated only if the patient is on antibiotics or has been in hospital for 1 to 2 weeks and the threat of infection has passed.

A second important mineral in the treatments of the malnourished child is zinc. Investigators in Chile found that supplementation of marasmic infants with 2 mg/kg of elemental zinc as zinc acetate had significant positive effects on weight gain and host defense mechanisms and therefore recommended zinc supplementation for optimal recovery (104).

TABLE 2. *Antibiotics used in treating the malnourished child*

Indications	Antibiotic	Dose (mg/kg/d)
Pneumonia or otitis media	Ampicillin	50–100
	Penicillin	50–100
	Bactrim (TMP-SMZ)	8–10 mg/k TMP
Staphylococcal pneumonia	Oxacillin	100–200
Genitourinary infection	Ampicillin	100
	Gantrisin	150–200
Sepsis	Systemic antibiotics:	
	1. Ampicillin or	200–300
	2. Ceftriaxone	75–150
	3. and Gentamycin	3–7.5
	Colistin (for aerobic organisms)	5–10
Gastrointestinal antisepsis	Metronidazole (Flagyl) (for anaerobic organisms)	35–50

TMP-SMZ, trimethoprim and sulfamethoxozole.

Antibiotic Therapy

One of the most serious problems facing the child with protein-energy malnutrition is infection. As aforementioned, several of the host defenses against infection are affected in children with malnutrition. With a malnourished child's immunologic defenses being compromised and the response to overwhelming infection being inadequate, it is critical for the physician to give priority to localizing and treating infection.

The appropriate use of antibiotics is an important factor in determining the morbidity and mortality associated with protein-energy malnutrition. This is especially true in the septic child, in whom large doses of broad-spectrum antibiotics are used. A potential antibiotic regimen is presented (Table 2). A child who is considered septic is placed on a regimen of ampicillin or of a cephalosporin, and gentamicin. Gentamicin is used because of the common occurrence of pseudomonas sepsis.

Because of the occurrence of small bowel bacterial overgrowth, drugs can be used for intestinal antisepsis against aerobic and anaerobic organisms (Table 2) (95,96). Small bowel overgrowth is one of the major sources of gram-negative sepsis and endotoxin production in the malnourished child. If the gastrointestinal tract is sterilized, a potential source of gram-negative sepsis and endotoxic shock can be eliminated for the few days needed to regenerate an intact gastrointestinal mucosa. Gastrointestinal antisepsis plus one broad-spectrum antibiotic is considerably less expensive than systemic antibiotics presently used for 7 to 10 days.

SUMMARY

Hospital admission in a clinical environment for an adequate period of time is the best method of treatment for the very ill child with protein-energy malnutrition. Outpatient management may be sufficient in those less critically ill. Careful diagnosis of the type of deficiency disease present, the extent of fluid and electrolyte imbalance, and the kind, site, and antibiotic sensitivity of the infecting organism is crucial for the initiation of proper treatment. Fluid and electrolyte therapy calculated to replace deficits is begun immediately; parenteral vitamin and antibiotic therapy follows within a few hours; and dietary treatment is planned to provide at least 4 g protein and 175 kcal/kg/d, with all the vitamins and minerals required for catch-up growth during the first 3 weeks, and slightly lower amounts thereafter for a 10-week period. Sepsis is an especially serious and challenging problem and must be treated with multiple antibiotics. With this regimen, the mortality rate can be as low as 35%. The follow-up of these patients after discharge indicates that most of them (80%) remain well and show continuing catch-up growth. Although an effective treatment program for the malnourished child has clearly been established, those working in the field of malnutrition recognize the need to focus on programs that prevent malnutrition as well.

REFERENCES

1. Warrier RP, Kuvibidila S, Wulfe K, et al. Nutritional evaluation of children with hemophilia. *Clin Res* 1988; 36: 62A.
2. Gomez F, Galvan RR, Frenk S, et al. Mortality in second and third degree malnutrition. *J Trop Pediatr* 1956; 2: 77–83.
3. Habicht JP. Height and weight standards for preschool children. How relevant are ethnic differences in growth potential? *Lancet* 1974; i: 611–4.
4. Waterlow JC. Note on the assessment and classification of protein-energy malnutrition in children. *Lancet* 1973; ii: 87–9.
5. Jelliffe DB. Protein-calorie malnutrition in tropical preschool children. *J Pediatr* 1959; 54: 227–56.
6. Ramos Galvan R, Miranda Calderon J. Deaths among children with third degree malnutrition: influence of the clinical type of the condition. *Am J Clin Nutr* 1965; 16: 351–5.
7. Garrow IS, Pike MC. The short term prognosis of severe primary infantile malnutrition. *Br J Nutr* 1967; 21: 155–65.
8. Waterlow JC, Cravioto J, Stephen JML. Protein malnutrition in man. *Adv Protein Chem* 1960; 15: 131–238.
9. Kahn E, Falcke HC. Syndrome simulating encephalitis affecting children recovering from malnutrition (kwashiorkor). *J Pediatr* 1956; 49: 37–45.
10. Williams CD. Kwashiorkor: council on food and nutrition. *JAMA* 1953; 153: 1280–5.
11. Williams CD. Kwashiorkor: nutritional disease of children associated with maize diet. *Lancet* 1935; ii: 1151–2.
12. Gopalan C. Kwashiorkor and marasmus: evolution and distinguishing features. In: McCance RA, Widdowson EM, eds. *Calorie deficiencies and protein deficiencies*. Boston: Little, Brown and Company, 1968: 49–58.
13. Scrimshaw NS, Behar M. Protein malnutrition in young children. *Science* 1961; 133: 2039–47.
14. Morley D, Bicknell J, Woodland M. Factors influencing the growth and nutritional status of infants and young children in a Nigerian village. *Trans R Soc Trop Med Hyg* 1967; 62: 164–99.
15. Gopalan C. In: van Muralt A, ed. *Protein calorie malnutrition*. Berlin: Springer–Verlag, 1969: 77.
16. Scrimshaw NS, Taylor CE, Gordon JE. Interaction of nutrition and infection. *World Health Organization Monograph Series*, No 57. Geneva: WHO; 1968.
17. Puffer RR, Serrano CV. Nutritional deficiency and mortality in childhood. *Bol Oficina Sanit Panam* 1973; 75: 1–30.
18. Coovadia HM, Parent MA, Loening WEK, et al. An evaluation of factors associated with the depression of immunity in malnutrition and in measles. *Am J Clin Nutr* 1974; 27: 665–9.
19. Beisel WR. Malnutrition as a consequence of stress. In: Suskind RM, ed. *Malnutrition and the immune response*. New York: Raven Press, 1977: 21–6.
20. Feigin RD, Klainer AS, Beisel WR, et al. Whole-blood amino acids in experimentally induced typhoid fever in man. *N Engl J Med* 1968; 278: 293–8.

21. Beisel WR, Cockerell GL, Janssen WA. Nutritional effects on the responsiveness of plasma acute phase reactant glycoproteins. In: Suskind RM, ed. *Malnutrition and the immune response*. New York: Raven Press, 1977: 395–402.

22. Morley DC. Measles in Nigeria. *Am J Dis Child* 1962; 103: 230–3.

23. Alleyne GAO, Hay RW, Picou DI, et al. In: *Protein-energy malnutrition*. London: Edward Arnold, 1977: 17.

24. Alleyne GAO, Hay RW, Picou DI, et al. Effect of infection on nutrition. In: *Protein-energy malnutrition*. London: Edward Arnold, 1977: 95–6.

25. Alleyne GAO. Study on total body potassium in malnourished infants. Factors affecting potassium repletion. *Br J Nutr* 1970; 24: 205–12.

26. Alleyne GAO, Millward DJ, Scullard GH. Total body potassium, muscle electrolytes, and glycogen in malnourished children. *J Pediatr* 1970; 76: 75–81.

27. Beresford, CH, Neale RJ, Brooke OG. Iron absorption and pyrexia. *Lancet* 1971; i: 568–72.

28. Gordon JE, Jansen AA, Ascoli W. Measles in rural Guatemala. *J Pediatr* 1965; 66: 779–86.

29. Leyton GI. Effects of slow starvation. *Lancet* 1946; ii: 73–9.

30. Vint FW. Post-mortem findings in natives of Kenya. *East Afr Med J* 1937; 13: 352.

31. Mugerwa JW. The lymphoreticular system in kwashiorkor. *J Pathol* 1971; 105: 105–9.

32. Jayalakshmi VT, Gopalan C. Nutrition and tuberculosis. I. An epidemiological study. *Indian J Med Res* 1958; 46: 87–92.

33. Feldman G, Gianantonio CA. Immunologic aspects of malnutrition in children. *Medicina* 1972; 32: 1–9.

34. Work TH, Infekwunigwe A, Jelliffe DB, et al. Tropical problems in nutrition. *Ann Intern Med* 1973; 79: 701–11.

35. Chandra RK Immunocompetence in undernutrition. *J Pediatr* 1972; 81: 1194–200.

36. Law DK, Kudrick SJ, Abdou NI. Immunocompetence of patients with protein-calorie malnutrition. The effects of nutritional repletion. *Ann Intern Med* 1973; 79: 545–50.

37. Smythe PM, Brereton-Stiles GG, Grace HJ, et al. Thymolymphatic deficiency and depression of cell-mediated immunity in protein-calorie malnutrition. *Lancet* 1971; ii: 939–43.

38. Abbassy AS, El-Din MK, Hassan A, et al. Studies of cell-mediated immunity and allergy in protein energy malnutrition. I. Cell-mediated delayed hypersensitivity. *J Trop Med Hyg* 1974; 77: 13–17.

39. Golden MH, Jackson AA, Golden BE. Effect of zinc on thymus of recently malnourished children. *Lancet* 1977; ii: 1057–9.

40. Chandra RK. Serum thymic hormone activity protein-energy malnutrition. *Clin Exp Immunol* 1979; 38: 228–30.

41. Purtillo DT, Conner DA. Fatal infections in protein-calorie malnourished children with thymolymphatic atrophy. *Arch Dis Child* 1975; 50: 149–52.

42. Edelman R, Suskind R, Olson RE, et al. Mechanisms of defective delayed cutaneous hypersensitivity in children with protein calorie malnutrition. *Lancet* 1973; i: 506–9.

43. Sellmeyer E, Bhettay E, Truswell AS, et al. Lymphocyte transformation in malnourished children. *Arch Dis Child* 1972; 47: 429–35.

44. Murthy PB, Rahiman MA, Tulpule PG. Lymphocyte proliferation kinetics in malnourished children measured by differential chromatoid staining. *Br J Nutr* 1982; 47: 445–50.

45. Beatty DW, Dowdle EB. The effects of kwashiorkor serum on lymphocyte transformation in vitro. *Clin Exp Immunol* 1978; 32: 134–43.

46. Salimonu LS, Johnson AO, Williams A, et al. The occurrence and properties of E-rosette inhibitory substance in the sera of malnourished children. *Clin Exp Immunol* 1982; 47: 626–34.

47. Chandra RK, Bhujwala MA. Elevated serum alpha-fetoprotein and impaired immune response in malnutrition. *Int Arch Allergy Immunol* 1977; 53: 180–5.

48. Kulapongs P, Suskind R, Vithayasai V, Olson RE. In vitro cell-mediated immune response in Thai children with protein-calorie malnutrition. In: Suskind RM, ed. *Malnutrition and the immune response*. New York: Raven Press, 1977: 99–104.

49. Chandra RK. T and B lymphocyte subpopulations and leukocyte terminal deoxynucleotidyltransferase in energy-protein undernutrition. *Acta Paediatr Scand* 1979; 68: 841–5.

50. Salimonu LS. Soluble immune complexes, acute phase proteins and E-rosette inhibitory substance in sera of malnourished children. *Ann Trop Pediatr* 1985; 5: 137–41.

51. Ritz J, Schmidt RE, Michan J, et al. Characterization of functional surface structures on human natural killer cells. *Adv Immunol* 1988; 42: 181–211.

52. Salimonu LS, Ojo-Amaize E, Johnson AO, et al. Depressed natural killer cell activity in children with protein-calorie malnutrition. II. Correction of the impaired activity after nutritional recovery. *Cell Immunol* 1983; 82: 210–5.

53. Bhaskaram P, Sivakurnar B. Interleukin-1 in malnutrition. *Arch Dis Child* 1986; 61: 182–5.
54. Winchurch R A. Activation of thymocyte responses to interleukin-1 by zinc. *Clin Immunol Immunopathol* 1988; 47: 174–80.
55. Salas M, Kirchner H. Induction of interferon gamma in human leukocyte cultures stimulated with Zn. *Clin Immunol Immunopathol* 1987; 45: 139–42.
56. Winchurch RA, Togo J, Adler WH. Supplemental zinc (Zn^{++}) restores antibody formation in cultures of aged spleen cells. II. Effects on mediator production. *Eur J Immunol* 1987; 17: 127–32.
57. Kawakami M, Cerami A. Studies of endotoxin-induced decrease in lipoprotein lipase activity. *J Exp Med* 1981; 154: 631–48.
58. Craswell EA, Old LJ, Kassel RL, et al. An endotoxin-induced serum factor that causes necrosis of tumors. *Proc Natl Acad Sci USA* 1975; 72: 3666–70.
59. Beutler B, Mahoney J, LeTrang N, et al. Purification of cachectin, a lipoprotein lipase-suppressing hormone secreted by endotoxin-induced RAW 264.7 cells. *J Exp Med* 1985; 161: 984–95.
60. Pennica D, Hayflick JS, Pzringman TS, et al. Cloning and expression in *Escherichia coli* of the cDNA for murine tumor necrosis factor. *Proc Natl Acad Sci USA* 1985; 82: 6060–4.
61. Caput D, Bentler B, Hanog K, et al. Identification of a common nucleotide sequence in the 3-untranslated region of mRNA molecules specifying inflammatory mediators. *Proc Natl Acad Sci USA* 1986; 83: 1670–4.
62. Waage A, Halstensen A, Espevik T. Association between tumor necrosis factor in serum and fatal outcome in patients with meningococcal disease. *Lancet* 1987; i: 355–7.
63. Scuderi P, Lam KS, Ryan KJ, et al. Raised serum levels of tumor necrosis factor in parasitic infections. *Lancet* 1986; ii: 1364–6.
64. Cerami A, Ikeda Y, LeTrang N, et al. Weight loss associated with an endotoxin-induced mediator from peritoneal macrophages: the role of cachectin (tumor necrosis factor). *Immunol Lett* 1985; 11: 173–5.
65. Clark IA, Cowden WB, Butcher GA, Hunt NH. Possible roles of tumor necrosis factor in the pathology of malaria. *Am J Pathol* 1987; 129: 192–9.
66. Grau GE, Fajardo LF, Piguet P-F, et al. Tumor necrosis factor cachectin as an essential mediator in murine cerebral malaria. *Science* 1987; 237: 1210–2.
67. Piguet PF, Grau G, Allet B, et al. Tumor necrosis factor/cachectin has an effect on skin and gut lesions of the acute phase of graft-vs-host disease. *Immunobiology* 1987; 175: 27–38.
68. Chandra RK. Interactions of nutrition, infection and immune response. Immunocompetence in nutritional deficiency: methodological considerations and intervention strategies. *Acta Paediatr Scand* 1979; 68: 137–44.
69. Xanthou M. Immunologic deficiencies in small-for-dates neonates. *Acta Paediatr Scand* 1985; 319: 143–9.
70. Chandra RK, Kutty KM. Immunocompetence in obesity. *Acta Paediatr Scand* 1980; 69: 25–30.
71. Chandra RK. Immune response in overnutrition. *Cancer Res* 1981; 41: 3795–801.
72. Murthy KK, Suskind SAL, Venkatash V, et al. Decreased T lymphocyte function and interleukin-2 production associated with vitamin A deficiency [Abstract]. Sixth International Congress of Immunology, 1986: 86.
73. Murthy KK, Suskind RM. Vitamin A deficiency and T-lymphocyte function [Abstract]. Eleventh Clinical Congress, American Society of Parenteral and Enteral Nutrition (ASPEN), New Orleans 1987: 339.
74. Kuvibidila S, Murthy KK, Suskind RM. Interleukin-2 production in iron deficiency anemia [Abstract]. *FASEB J* 1989; 3: A664.
75. Suskind RM, Sirisinha, S, Edelman R, et al. Immunoglobulins and antibody response in Thai children with protein calorie malnutrition. In: Suskind RM, ed. *Malnutrition and the immune response.* New York: Raven Press, 1977: 185–90.
76. Brown RE, Katz M. Failure of antibody production to yellow fever vaccine in children with kwashiorkor. *Tropical Geographic Medicine* 1966; 19: 125–8.
77. Jose DG, Welch JS, Doherty RL. Humoral and cellular immune responses to streptococci, influenza and other antigens in Australian Aboriginal school children. *Aust Paediatr J* 1970; 6: 192–202.
78. Brown RE, Katz M. Antigenic stimulation in undernourished children. *East Afr Med J* 1965; 42: 221–32.
79. Chandra RK, Chandra S, Gupta S. Antibody affinity and immune complexes after immunization with tetanus toxoid in protein-energy malnutrition. *Am J Clin Nutr* 1984; 40: 131–4.
80. Spurr GB, Reina JC, Barac-Nieto M. Marginal malnutrition in school-aged Colombian boys: anthropometry. *Am J Clin Nutr* 1984; 40: 131–4.
81. Sirisinha S, Suskind R, Edelman R, et al. Secretory and serum IgA in children with protein-calorie malnutrition. *Pediatrics* 1975; 55: 166–70.

82. Watson RR, McMurray DN, Martin P, et al. Effect of age, malnutrition and renutrition on free secretory component and IgA in secretions. *Am J Clin Nutr* 1985; 42: 281–8.
83. Selvaraj RJ, Bhat KS. Metabolic and bactericidal activities of leukocytes in protein-calorie malnutrition. *Am J Clin Nutr* 1972; 25: 166–74.
84. Selvaraj RJ, Bhat KS. Phagocytosis and leukocyte enzymes in protein-calorie malnutrition. *Biochem J* 1972; 127: 255–9.
85. Yosida T, Metcoffe J. Intermediary metabolites and adenine nucleotides in leucocytes of children with protein-calorie malnutrition. *Nature* 1967; 214: 525–6.
86. Seth V, Chandra RK. Opsonic activity, phagocytosis, and bactericidal capacity of polymorphs in undernutrition. *Arch Dis Child* 1972; 47: 282–4.
87. Douglas SD, Schopfer K. The phagocyte in protein-calorie malnutrition—a review. In: Suskind RM, ed. *Malnutrition and the immune response*. New York: Raven Press, 1977: 231–43.
88. Patrick J, Golden M. Leukocyte electrolytes and sodium transport in protein energy malnutrition. *Am J Clin Nutr* 1977; 30: 1478–81.
89. Tuck R, Burke V, Gracev M, et al. Defective *Candida* killing in childhood malnutrition. *Arch Dis Child* 1979; 54: 445–7.
90. Sirisinha S, Suskind R, Edelman R, et al. The complement system in protein-calorie malnutrition—a review. In: Suskind RM, ed. *Malnutrition and the immune response*. New York: Raven Press, 1977: 309–20.
91. Coovadia HM, Parent MA, Loening WE, et al. An evaluation of factors associated with the depression of immunity in malnutrition and in measles. *Am J Clin Nutr* 1974; 27: 665–9.
91. Neumann CG, Lawlor GJ, Stiehm ER, et al. Immunologic responses in malnourished children. *Am J Clin Nutr* 1975; 28: 89–104.
93. Sirisinha S. Edelman R, Suskind R, et al. Complement and C3-proactivator levels in children with protein-calorie malnutrition and effect of dietary treatment. *Lancet* 1973; i: 1016–20.
94. Suskind R, Edelman R, Kulapongs P, et al. Complement activity in children with protein-calorie malnutrition. *Am J Clin Nutr* 1976; 29: 1089–92.
95. Klein K, Suskind RM, Kulapongs P, et al. Endotoxemia, a possible cause of decreased complement activity in malnourished children. In: Suskind RM, ed. *Malnutrition and the immune response*. New York: Raven Press, 1977: 321–8.
96. Suskind R. The in-patient and out-patient treatment of the child with severe protein-calorie malnutrition. In: Olson RE, ed. *Protein-calorie malnutrition*. New York: Academic Press, 1975: 403–10.
97. Garrow JS, Smith R, Ward EE. *Electrolyte metabolism in severe infantile malnutrition*. Oxford: Pergamon Press, 1968.
98. Caddell JL, Suskind R, Sillup H, et al. Parenteral magnesium load evaluation of malnourished Thai children. *J Pediatr* 1973; 83: 129–35.
99. Caddell JL, Goddard DR. Studies in protein-calorie malnutrition. I. Chemical evidence for magnesium deficiency. *N Engl J Med* 1967; 276: 533–55.
100. Graham GG, Cordano A, Baertl JM. Studies on infantile malnutrition. II. Effect of protein and calorie intake on weight gain. *J Nutr* 1963; 81: 249–54.
101. Waterlow JC. The rate of recovery of malnourished infants in relation to the protein and calorie levels of the diet. *J Trop Pediatr* 1961; 7: 16–22.
102. Dean RFA, Swanne J. Abbreviated schedule of treatment for severe kwashiorkor. *J Trop Pediatr* 1963; 8: 97–8.
103. Lynch SR, Becker D, Seftel H, et al. Iron absorption in kwashiorkor. *Am J Clin Nutr* 1970; 23: 792–7.
104. Castillo-Duran C, Heresi G, Fisburg M, Uauy R. Controlled trial of zinc supplementation during recovery from malnutrition: effects on growth and immune function. *Am J Clin Nutr* 1987; 45: 602–8.

DISCUSSION

Dr. Valyasevi: It is important to understand things at a molecular level, but at the same time to be thinking about what is going on around us outside—if we stick to molecular matters and do not pay attention to other things on the planet, we will be in even more trouble. The Thailand approach that Dr. Tontisirin mentioned was obtained after the government had adopted a primary healthcare approach. Such an approach aims to correct malnutrition by the provision of food and, thus, involves cooperation among the agricultural sector, food scientists, and community development sectors as well as nutrition education and communication. The pictures Prof. Suskind showed us a few moments ago are not at present relevant to Thailand.

Dr. Chandra: I just want to make two brief comments. First so far as Prof. Tontisirin's presentation, I wholeheartedly support the concept that is summarized in one sentence in his summary: "A minimum package of essential basic services, integrated into community-based nutrition programs using participatory approaches, is required according to community situations and context." Although each of us may be interested in working in a particularly narrow field of nutrition, immunity, or infection, with each of us having a certain agenda for that reason, from the point of view of the community and for the prevention of both malnutrition and infection, it is of the greatest importance to have a comprehensive program, otherwise we will be touching only a part of the problem. Many models of such interventions have been published; we published our own in 1991, giving different quantitative weighting to different intervention strategies. For example, more weight was given to preservation and promotion of breast-feeding, effective immunization, and agricultural production, and relatively less to targeted supplements.

The second comment I have is on the excellent summary that Dr. Suskind presented. It was only 25 years ago that we found it very difficult to convince so-called scientists that immunology and nutrition were linked. It is very pleasing that with the efforts of many people, most of whom are present in this room, the science of nutritional immunology has come into being; not only are there important cellular and molecular mechanisms to be looked into, but also important applications are relevant to public health and to the prevention of both malnutrition and infection.

Dr. Zoppi: I would like to make a comment on Dr. Suskind's presentation. In 1982, our group did a study on immune responses in children in Italy, as an example of a developed country. We showed that malnutrition was possible in developed countries if the quality of protein is not adequate (1,2). We demonstrated that the response to normal vaccination against pertussis, polio, diphtheria, and tetanus was impaired if children were fed on low quality protein such as soy protein. We had similar results to those of Dr. Chandra, who showed that malnourished infants had an impaired response to vaccination against measles. The response to a soy-based formula is very impaired compared with that in infants fed human milk.

Dr. Cochran: I just want to emphasize the importance of malnutrition, not just in the developing world, but also in the developed world. In the United States, we too are not immune from the problems associated with malnutrition, and yet it frequently goes unrecognized, because we do not think about this all the time. Studies have shown that up to 30% of children in the pediatric intensive care units are suffering from malnutrition. So we too in the United States still have work to do to try to educate our colleagues to think about nutrition as we treat these children.

Dr. Valyasevi: I think this is probably due to a lack of awareness on the part of the physicians.

REFERENCES

1. Zoppi G, Gerosa F, Pezzini A, et al. Immnocompetence and dietary protein intake in early infancy. *J Pediatr Gastroenterol Nutr* 1982; 1: 175–82.
2. Zoppi G, Gasparini R, Mantovanelli F, et al. Diet and antibody response to vaccinations in healthy infants. *Lancet* 1983; 2: 11–4.

Nutrition, Immunity, and Infection in Infants and Children, edited by Robert M. Suskind and Kraisid Tontisirin. Nestlé Nutrition Workshop Series, Pediatric Program, Vol. 45. Nestec Ltd., Vevey/Lippincott Williams & Wilkins, Philadelphia ©2001.

Nutrition, Immunity, and Infectious Diseases in Infants and Children

An Overview

Gerald T. Keusch

Tufts University School of Medicine, and New England Medical Center, Boston, Massachusetts, USA

In 1959, Scrimshaw *et al.* published a landmark review of the interactions of nutrition and infection, including a critical evaluation of the vast literature from both animal and human studies (1). Although they concluded that "few areas of investigation are more replete with unsupported statements of opinion, impression and speculation" and noted that many older studies could be disregarded because they failed to meet acceptable standards of modern research methodology, their systematic and critical review led them to conclude that malnutrition and infection interacted in one of two manners: *synergistic* or *antagonistic* (Table 1). Most often, the interaction resulted in a heightened severity and worsened outcome of infection, a relationship they termed *synergistic*. However, in certain situations malnourished individuals appeared to be protected when infected with particular infectious agents, a relationship they termed *antagonistic*. Now, 40 years after the publication of the Scrimshaw *et al.* review, at this workshop we are asking how much have we learned since then and how has this knowledge affected clinical and public health practice. This chapter reviews the *big picture*, and the detailed investigations of different states of malnutrition will be presented in subsequent chapters.

MALNUTRITION WORSENS INFECTIOUS DISEASES

Scrimshaw *et al.* clearly stated that chronically undernourished children are at great risk of infection and that repeated infections could trigger the rapid deterioration of nutritional status. They pointed out that "children who are basically undernourished

TABLE 1. *The nature of malnutrition-infection interactions*

Synergism: The situation where a nutritional deficiency results in increased frequency or severity of an infection.

Antagonism: The situation where a nutritional deficiency results in decreased frequency or severity of an infection.

are an easier prey to many infections and may die. Further, stress of any kind is likely to be followed by the development of . . . the kwashiorkor syndrome," overt protein-energy malnutrition with edema, a clinical presentation known to be associated with high case fatality rates. In addressing the underlying mechanisms of this interaction they noted that whereas "kwashiorkor can originate in dietary deficiency alone, . . . most cases are the result of synergism between infection and protein malnutrition" (1). Although noting the particular impact of diarrheal disease, whooping cough, malaria, and acute respiratory tract infections, they also emphasized that socioeconomic stress of many types (*e.g.*, social changes in the family, loss of a job, the death of a parent, or separation of the family) could also precipitate this deterioration in nutritional status. The likely consequence of such noninfectious stress was a deterioration in socioeconomic status leading to a secondary impact on nutritional intake. However, the idea that social stress might be a factor in precipitating overt protein-energy malnutrition was a remarkably prescient perspective in view of the current interest in the potential role of the neuroendocrine system in modulating the functional capacity of the immune system (2).

These relationships have been re-examined many times with increasingly sophisticated epidemiologic or laboratory methods in the past two decades in both developing country settings and in hospitalized adult surgical and medical patients in the industrialized world. The results have been consistent—malnutrition predisposes to greater susceptibility to infections and significantly worsens their consequences. However, the classification of malnutrition has usually been based on clinical, rather than laboratory, criteria, resulting in the lumping together of patients differing considerably in individual nutrient status. Biochemical assessments of specific nutrients now allow further classification according to individual mineral and vitamin status (3), whereas the use of body composition analysis, made possible by methodologic and technical developments, gives promise of further subclassification of subjects according to the impact of nutrient levels on the major body metabolic compartments (4). These refinements allow greater correlations of nutritional status with the risk of adverse consequences and streamline the development of preventative and corrective strategies, especially in the resource-limited developing countries.

INFECTION WORSENS NUTRITIONAL STATUS

Scrimshaw *et al.* also noted that the deleterious effect of infection on nutritional status is "a fact insufficiently recognized" (1). Unfortunately, 40 years later we can still say that this relationship remains insufficiently recognized. Scrimshaw *et al.*

used metabolic balance methods to assess nitrogen metabolism during infection, and showed clearly that clinical infections (*e.g.*, chickenpox) or even the mild infection induced by the attenuated live yellow fever vaccine virus, led to a state of negative nitrogen balance (5,6). They observed that nitrogen loss "may begin during the prodromal period before fever . . . appears" or "continue long after fever subsides" (1). The source of the nitrogen loss was subsequently demonstrated to be muscle protein by measuring the excretion of 3-methyl histidine, which is selectively released following catabolism of muscle protein and excreted in the urine. The breakdown of muscle protein releases amino acids into plasma; however, circulating amino acid levels do not rise (except for non-reutilized amino acids) because they are rapidly reutilized for the accompanying increased protein biosynthesis (7,8). However, this new anabolic activity is not directed toward the same proteins made in the preinfectious state. Rather, a transcriptionally regulated major shift occurs in the priorities for protein synthesis away from structural and transport proteins (*e.g.*, albumen or transferrin) to acute phase response proteins (*e.g.*, C-reactive protein, mannose-binding protein, α1-acid glycoprotein, and others) (Table 2) and the proteins of host defense and immune response (*e.g.*, complement, immunoglobulins and others) (9).

Aside from the general biological survival rationale for the shift from the synthesis of maintenance proteins to the production of urgently needed defense proteins under the stress of infection, the significance of most other aspects of acute phase changes is not well understood. One important acute change is the alteration in metabolism toward the utilization of amino acids for energy, either through metabolism of branched chain amino acids in muscle or the production of glucose in the liver by a number of mechanisms not, as previously thought, limited to hepatic gluconeogenesis (10). Scrimshaw *et al.* noted that "loss of urinary nitrogen is partly from greater energy requirements imposed by higher body temperature, but mainly from toxic destruction of protein. Nitrogen loss may continue long after fever has subsided or may begin during the prodromal period before fever . . . appears" (1). This has been well demonstrated in experimental human volunteer studies in which a mild infection has been induced and nitrogen balance is measured before, during,

TABLE 2. *Acute phase proteins in the inflammatory response*

Acute phase protein	Postulated role in host defense
Marked increases in concentration	
C-reactive protein	Fixes complement, opsonizes
Mannose-binding protein	Fixes complement, opsonizes
α_1-acid glycoprotein	Transport protein
Serum amyloid A	? Immunosuppressive
Moderate increases in concentration	
α_1-proteinase inhibitors	Limit proteolytic damage
C3, factor B of complement system	Increase complement activity
Ceruloplasmin	Oxygen scavenger to limit damage
Fibrinogen	Coagulation
Fibronectin	Cell adherence, opsonization

and after the febrile acute illness (6). Such studies clearly show that nitrogen losses are cumulative and maximal at the point at which the fever disappears and clinicians and patients consider the convalescent period to have begun. However, it takes much longer to restore nitrogen stores than it does to cause the losses, requiring both an infection-free period and adequate intake of good quality protein for efficient correction of acquired deficits (10,11). Neither of these conditions is likely to be satisfied for children in the developing world, and the next infectious insult will most likely add to the residual nutritional deficit from the prior episode. Repeated infectious diseases then result in the downward cyclical interaction observed between infection and nutritional status in these children, leading ultimately to the acute condition, kwashiorkor (10).

Another facet of the acute phase response is a rapid reduction in the concentration of serum iron, zinc, and vitamin A at the onset of infection, which is caused by the enhanced synthesis of transport proteins for the intracellular uptake of these nutrients (12). An increase in serum copper is also observed as increased synthesis of the copper transport protein ceruloplasmin carries copper in the reverse direction from the intracellular to extracellular compartments. The reduction in iron and zinc has been interpreted by some to be a natural defense mechanism designed by nature to reduce the availability of these essential nutrients to invading microorganisms, an attributed host response termed "nutritional immunity" (13).

A number of reasons are seen to doubt this explanation. For example, in the case of iron, microbial pathogens actually use the reduced availability of free iron as a signal to upregulate their own iron acquisition mechanisms, including the rapid production of high affinity iron-binding acquisition and uptake proteins. These systems compete extremely well with mammalian host iron-binding proteins to ensure an adequate supply for the pathogen. Hypoferremia, therefore, does not deprive the organisms of the needed iron. In addition, many pathogens also use low free iron as a signal for transcriptional upregulation of virulence genes. This commonly occurs through an iron-responsive gene called *fur*. The product of this gene, the Fur protein, is an iron-binding protein that, in the presence of adequate iron, binds to a consensus sequence in the promoter region of iron-regulated genes, thereby blocking transcription. Iron-depleted Fur does not bind to its consensus sequence, allowing the transcription of the iron-regulated genes. Use of these mechanisms for low free iron as the regulatory signal for gene regulation is clearly counterproductive to any role hypoferremia might play in host defense.

On the other hand, the cellular uptake of iron, zinc, and vitamin A can have important direct and positive effects on host defense. For example, iron- and zinc-containing metalloenzymes are essential for the synthesis of DNA, which must precede cell replication. Therefore, uptake of iron and zinc by cells of the immune system will promote cell division, a necessary event to the expansion of cell populations involved in host defense responses to invading microorganisms. Diminished antigen-specific amplification of lymphocyte, lymphocytes, and phagocytic cells is likely to be the difference between an asymptomatic or mild infection and a severe or even fatal one. Furthermore, zinc metalloproteins produced by the thymus (*e.g.*, thymulin) are critical for the functional maturation of one T lymphocyte, which is not only involved in cell-mediated immunity but also provides help to B cells in the differentiation to antibody-producing plasma cells.

Vitamin A metabolites play important roles in the intracellular milieu where they serve as critical transcriptional regulators affecting, among other genes, many involved in immune function and host defense. Vitamin A plays a role as an antioxidant to limit tissue damage from oxidative processes initiated by host defense cells. For example, neutrophils and monocyte or macrophages produce oxidative metabolites to kill infectious microorganisms or virus-infected cells but these can initiate *bystander* damage as well unless contained. Thus, the acute shift of all three of these micronutrients directly enhances host defense mechanisms whether or not any indirect effect is exerted through the reduction in plasma levels of these micronutrients that results in a diminished capacity of invading organisms to multiply (14).

GENERAL HOST RESPONSES AND THEIR RELATION TO IMMUNE ACTIVATION

Infections are associated with a set of common clinical manifestations, including fever, chills, anorexia, myalgia, and fatigue. These events are initiated by small peptide cytokine mediators, including interleukin (IL)-1, IL-6, and tumor necrosis factor (TNF)-α, released from inflammatory cells activated by infection and acting on the temperature regulatory centers in the hypothalamus (15). Fever may have beneficial effects on host defense by enhancing the speed of metabolic reactions and inflammatory and immune cell function; however, increased temperature also significantly increases energy consumption. Chills are a manifestation of involuntary muscle contractions, initiated by neural pathways activated by cytokines to generate the heat required to raise body temperature. Anorexia, which results in a reduction in nutrient intake in the face of increased metabolic demands, means that an alternate source of nutrients is needed. This source is found in body stores—initially glycogen, stored in the liver—and once that is exhausted, in the conversion to glucose of amino acids derived from muscle catabolism (16). Myalgia is the physical manifestation of proteolysis (17). IL-1 also induces slow wave sleep by a central action in the brain, which accounts for the feeling of fatigue. This has the benefit of reducing energy needs and partially compensating for the reduced food intake caused by anorexia.

This is a remarkable coordination of host responses that, on the surface, appear to be unrelated clinical events. The coordination is even more striking, because these cytokines also are essential in the activation of the immune response (18). However, cytokine responses are impaired in the malnourished host (19,20), accounting for many of the altered immune responses in the malnourished host (21,22). We are at the beginning of our understanding of the mechanisms involved (23), but because of the remarkable increase in our knowledge of cytokine regulation of metabolism and immune responses, we are finally able to move from phenomenologic to mechanistic studies (24), as will be summarized in this symposium. These studies will provide the basis for future therapeutic interventions in malnourished hosts, leading to an improvement in both nutritional status and immune function (25).

SUMMARY

Nutrition–infection interactions are complex and bidirectional; they lead to progressive deterioration in both body composition and host defenses. Impaired host defenses condition the host to more frequent and more severe infections, thus increasing the spiral of nutritional deterioration. Over the past two decades, the remarkable intertwining of the metabolic and host defense responses to infection has been linked to mediator peptides released during the inflammatory response. The role of specific nutrient deficiencies, alone or in combination, can now be studied because of improved tools for defining nutritional status, better measures of host defense, and aids to assess the production and effect of cytokine mediators. Forty years after the landmark first review by Scrimshaw *et al.* we are on the brink of really understanding and then controlling the pathophysiology associated with infection and malnutrition.

REFERENCES

1. Scrimshaw NS, Taylor CE, Gordon JE. Interaction of nutrition and infection. *Am J Med Sci* 1959; 237: 367–403.
2. Reichlin S. Neuroendocrinology of infection and the innate immune system. *Recent Prog Horm Res* 1999; 54: 133–81.
3. Hensrud DD. Nutrition screening and assessment. *Med Clin North Am* 1999; 83: 1525–46.
4. Brodie DA, Stewart AD. Body composition measurement: a hierarchy of methods. *J Pediatr Endocrinol Metab* 1999; 12: 801–16.
5. Wilson D, Bresani R, Scrimshaw NS. Infection and nutritional status. I. The effect of chickenpox on nitrogen metabolism in children. *Am J Clin Nutr* 1961; 9: 154–8.
6. Gandra YR, Scrimshaw NS. Infection and nutritional status. II. Effect of mild virus infection induced by 17-D yellow fever vaccine on nitrogen metabolism in children. *Am J Clin Nutr* 1961; 9: 159–63.
7. Feigin RD, Klainer AS, Beisel WR, Hornick RB. Whole-blood amino acids in experimentally induced typhoid fever in man. *N Engl J Med* 1968; 278: 293–8.
8. Beisel WR. Metabolic response to infection. *Annu Rev Med* 1975; 26: 9–20.
9. Suffredini AF, Fantuzzi G, Badolato R, Oppenheim JJ, O'Grady NP. New insights into the biology of the acute phase response. *J Clin Immunol* 1999; 19: 203–14.
10. Keusch GT. Host defense mechanisms in protein energy malnutrition. *Adv Exp Med Biol* 1981; 135: 183–209.
11. Chevalier P, Sevilla R, Sejas E, Zalles I, Bellmonte G, Parent G. Immune recovery of malnourished children takes longer than nutritional recovery: implications for treatment and discharge. *J Trop Pediatr* 1998; 44: 304–7.
12. Thurnham DI. Impact of disease on markers of micronutrient status. *Proc Nutr Soc* 1997; 56: 192–7.
13. Weinberg ED. Nutritional immunity. Host's attempt to withhold iron from microbial invaders. *JAMA* 1975; 231: 39–41.
14. Keusch GT. Micronutrients and susceptibility to infection. *Ann NY Acad Sci* 1990; 587: 181–8.
15. Dinarello CA, Bunn PA Jr. Fever. *Semin Oncol* 1997; 24: 288–98.
16. Chang HR, Bistrian B. The role of cytokines in the catabolic consequences of infection and injury. *JPEN* 1998; 22: 156–66.
17. Cooney RN, Kimball SR, Vary TC. Regulation of skeletal muscle protein turnover during sepsis: mechanisms and mediators. *Shock* 1997; 7: 1–16.
18. Biron CA. Role of early cytokines, including alpha and beta interferons (IFN-alpha/beta), in innate and adaptive immune responses to viral infections. *Semin Immunol* 1998; 10: 383–90.

19. Beisel WR. Infection-induced malnutrition—from cholera to cytokines. *Am J Clin Nutr* 1995; 62: 813–9.
20. Sauerwein RW, Mulder JA, Mulder L, et al. Inflammatory mediators in children with protein-energy malnutrition. *Am J Clin Nutr* 1997: 65; 1534–9.
21. Morlese JF, Forrester T, Jahoor F. Acute phase protein response to infection in severe malnutrition. *Am J Physiol* 1998; 38: E112–7.
22. Woodward B. Protein, calories and immune defenses. *Nutr Rev* 1998; 56: S84–2.
23. Hardin TC. Cytokine mediators of malnutrition: clinical implications. *Nutr Clin Pract* 1993; 8: 55–9.
24. Klasing KC. Nutritional aspects of leukocytic cytokines. *J Nutr* 1988; 118: 1436–46.
25. Moldawer LL, Lowry SF. Interactions between cytokine production and inflammation: implications for therapies aimed at modulating the host defense to infection. In: Cunningham-Rundles S, ed. *Nutrient modulation of the immune response.* New York: Marcel Dekker, 1993: 511–23.

DISCUSSION

Dr. Suskind: One question I have relative to an area you previously touched on is the effect of the microbe on the host in terms of the cytokine response, leading to a change in the production of visceral proteins. Could you comment on that briefly?

Dr. Keusch: I specifically avoided dealing with cytokines in order to present the larger picture. However, I think we are going to hear a great deal about the role of cytokines as the intermediary between the organism and the host. We now understand cytokines to be a set of small peptides that have regulatory properties. We have yet to discover all the cytokines there are—every time you pick up a journal there is a new one. At our present level of sophistication, we now understand that cytokines constitute the intermediary between the organism and the host, both activating and regulating the immune response, as well as altering the priorities for metabolism, changing the transcriptional activation of genes that result in changes in the synthesis of some visceral proteins, and increasing the synthesis of some of the acute phase proteins. To fully understand the system in mechanistic terms and find targets for interventions, we need to be able to meddle in the inflammatory response. We would love to be able to enhance it when it is inadequate, or to suppress it when it is overactive. I believe the promise of being able to do that is just ahead of us, with the completion of the sequencing of the human genome. We are going to find an enormous number of genes for which there is no known function, and where there are no homologies that we can use in animals. The only way we are going to begin to understand those genes is to see when they are present and activated in clinical situations. Thus, we need clinical investigation to tell us when a gene may be related to a human disease, or to human health. Once a gene is identified and the gene product discovered, a wonderful opportunity exists for therapeutic advance. This is the future for the pharmaceutical industry—using genetics to identify specific targets among genes and gene products or receptors for gene products, and, therefore, to manipulate the host response. So you are right: cytokines are at the center of the scientific revolution, because they are at the center of the host response.

Dr. Klish: I was fascinated by your discussion of microbial utilization of iron. You are fully aware that this a very contentious area in the United States, as it relates to iron supplementation in infancy. You started your statement by saying that in theory one should maintain iron deficiency in these children, but I do not think that is what you were actually saying at the end of your paper, when you talked about the way organisms utilize iron. Could you say what you really meant?

Dr. Keusch: Thank you for pointing that out. I am not a fan of the nutritional immunity hypothesis that states that the acute phase reduction in serum iron is geared by nature to remove iron from microorganisms. The microorganism does not care. It has its own mechanisms stimulated by low free iron to activate the systems to acquire the iron it needs, and the low iron can also be used as a signal for the production of virulence factors. So from that perspective, it does not make any difference what the iron level is. On the other hand, iron deficiency in the host impairs the host's immune response. So iron deficiency needs to be dealt with in the same way as other nutritional deficiencies—we need to correct it in populations. The iron and immunity hypothesis proposes that situations of iron excess cause infection. This directs our attention toward iron availability, and the possibility that it might be a good thing for people to be iron deficient. That is a very unsophisticated view of the interaction between high iron and the host, which also impairs the host immune response. High iron results in membrane and DNA damage through oxidative mechanisms, and organisms that thrive under those circumstances are the ones that have failed to evolve an iron-obtaining mechanism. They actually require situations of high iron in order to be able to grow and, therefore, to be virulent. Thus, on the one hand I am not a proponent of keeping the world iron deficient because the consequences of iron deficiency are severe and highly prevalent and they need to be dealt with by public health measures. On the other hand, you do not want to give parenteral iron in the course of an acute infection in individuals who are poorly nourished and have very low levels of circulating iron-binding proteins. These relationships need to be fully understood from the prospective of the host, the microorganism, and the host response.

Dr. Chandra: I think if we were to believe in the iron nutritional immunity hypothesis, we should also have to extend it to most other micronutrients. The basis for the hypothesis is that as serum iron drops during infection, it must be good for the host. Could we not say the same thing about zinc or copper? Most micronutrient levels in the serum fall during infection, and on that basis I do not think we should necessarily accept that a fall in serum iron contributes to increased resistance to infection. Maybe it has some other value for the body. One other comment I want to make is that we also need to consider what form of iron we give, either in prevention or treatment. We know that different forms of iron can have different effects in the oxidative pathways. That could be a third factor in the equation between microorganisms and nutrients. Finally, we may have underestimated the binding between iron and iron-binding proteins in the body. We have always felt that microorganisms are superior in extracting iron from host proteins, but I think that will also need to be re-examined in the light of new observations.

Dr. Suskind: Dr. Keusch, you mentioned something about gastric peptides in the gastrointestinal tract. I am not aware of any such studies in children who are malnourished. Could you comment on whether they may be one of the factors, in addition to decreased gastric acidity, leading to small bowel overgrowth?

Dr. Keusch: I am not aware of any studies on this. It is an area that could be explored. These antimicrobial peptides are not only present in the human gastrointestinal tract, they also form one of the defenses used by amphibians, which have a much more primitive immune system. They are being identified, isolated, and studied as potential therapeutic agents. They are different from other antimicrobial agents that we know about, and relatively little is understood about their regulation in the gastrointestinal tract, or what role, if any, they play in regulating the normal flora. In particular, we do not know whether any deficits occur in the synthesis of these proteins in the presence of protein-energy malnutrition or other circumstances of nutritional deficit. This is another frontier area for us to work on into the next century.

Dr. Marini: I think we should differentiate between iron in the gastrointestinal tract and the iron in the blood, remembering especially that maternal milk contains a lot of lactoferrin, which binds iron in the gastrointestinal tract. Another matter is the question of free radicals. We blame free radicals for disease, and you showed data suggesting that low antioxidant diets in Cuba are associated with increased disease. But consider the model of the full term, normal neonate, wherein are increased free radicals because of *oxygen shock*. Under these circumstances, the free radicals are said to be good for the baby because they prime the immune system. On the other hand, we have proof that if you give a lot of vitamin E, which is an antioxidant, to preterm neonates, infection increases (1). So I think that an excess of free radicals can be wrong in certain cases. In normal individuals, however, if nature makes free radicals it probably has a good reason (2).

REFERENCES

1. Johnson L, Bowen F, Hermann N, et al. Relationship of prolonged pharmacologic serum levels of vitamin E to incidence of sepsis and necrotizing enerocolitis in infants with birth weight 1,500 grams or less. *Pediatrics* 1985; 75: 619–38.
2. Guerini RC, Longaretti A, Viani P., Marini A, Cestaro B. Lipid peroxide levels of healthy full term neonates. Role of lipid composition and the mode of delivery. *Developmental Physiopathology and Clinics* 1998; 8: 195–204.

Nutrition, Immunity, and Infection in Infants and Children, edited by Robert M. Suskind and Kraisid Tontisirin. Nestlé Nutrition Workshop Series, Pediatric Program, Vol. 45. Nestec Ltd., Vevey/Lippincott Williams & Wilkins, Philadelphia ©2001.

A Review of the Immune System

Methodology for Evaluating the Impact of Nutrition on Its Function

Ricardo U. Sorensen, Boyd Butler, and Lily E. Leiva

Louisiana State University Medical Center, New Orleans, Louisiana, USA

Clinical immunology has undergone impressive changes over the past decades, significantly increasing our ability to recognize immunologic abnormalities and permitting better diagnoses and treatment of many immunologic abnormalities. In this chapter, we review methods of studying some of the host defense mechanisms affected in primary and secondary immunodeficiencies and link some of these immune abnormalities to susceptibility to specific infections.

OVERVIEW OF HOST DEFENSES

Host defense involves nonspecific and specific mechanisms. Nonspecific mechanisms include the complement system and the phagocytic system, which develop independently of the presence of infections and are not specific for given infectious agents. Specific mechanisms include antibody-mediated and cell-mediated immunity. The interaction of these different defense mechanisms to prevent or clear infections is depicted in Figure 1 (1). The first mechanism to clear microorganisms breaking epithelial surface integrity is phagocytosis by polymorphonuclear cells (neutrophils) and mononuclear phagocytes (monocytes and macrophages) (Mϕ). In the initial absence of antibodies, bacterial surface polysaccharides activate the alternative pathway of complement, resulting in the attachment of C3b to the bacterial surface, which in turn activates the membrane attack components of complement (C5–C9), which lyse susceptible bacteria. For resistant, encapsulated bacteria, C3b provides the necessary opsonization for phagocytosis by neutrophils and Mos. Furthermore, complement-derived factors increase vascular permeability and attract ad-

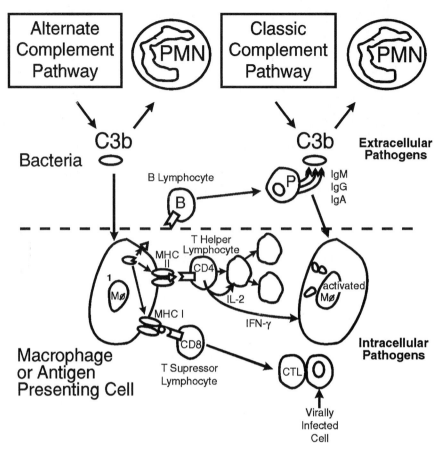

FIG. 1. Interactions of host defense mechanisms. AP, alternative pathway of complement activation; CP, classic pathway; Mo, monocytes-macrophages; B, B lymphocytes; P, plasma cells; CD4, T helper cells; CD8, T suppressor cells; CTL, cytotoxic T lymphocytes; IFN-γ, γ interferon.

ditional phagocytic cells to the site of infection. Minor bacterial infections are terminated by these mechanisms without the manifestation of disease, but such subclinical infections may be sufficient to trigger the development of protective antibodies or cell-mediated immunity.

Specific immunity develops after presentation of antigenic microbial components by antigen-presenting cells, usually Mφ or dendritic cells, to T and B lymphocytes. In response to stimulation by microbial antigens, T helper cells (CD4+ cells) proliferate and secrete lymphokines, for example interferon-γ (IFN-γ), which activates Mφ. This Mo activation is an essential step in clearing intracellular pathogens not eliminated after ingestion by nonactivated Mφ. On interaction with antigens, T suppressor cells (CD8+ cells) develop into cytotoxic cells capable of killing virally infected cells. This event contributes to the termination of a viral infection by exposing viruses liberated by lysed cells to the action of antibodies, complement, and phagocytic cells.

The binding of an antigen to B-cell surface immunoglobulins leads to cell division and differentiation into antibody producing plasma cells. The production of specific antibodies to many microbial antigens is dependent on the interaction with antigen-specific CD4$^+$ T helper cells. Secreted antibodies attach to surviving bacteria, producing further opsonization for phagocytosis by neutrophils and Mφs. Furthermore, immunoglobulins (Ig) M and G activate complement through the classic pathway, which also leads to lysis of susceptible bacteria and opsonization by C3b. Three to six days after the initial infection, specific antibodies direct and amplify the nonspecific host defense mechanisms, normally terminating infections that survive the early, nonspecific clearance mechanisms. If infections are not effectively cleared, the continued activation of phagocytic cells can cause tissue damage through the release of oxygen radicals, proteases, and other inflammatory mediators.

The relative importance and efficiency of these defense mechanisms against different infectious agents can be summarized as follows: phagocytosis, complement, and antibodies are effective against extracellular pathogens (*e.g.*, *Staphylococcus aureus*, *Haemophilus influenzae*, *Streptoccus pneumoniae*, *Neisseria meningitidis*) and viruses before intracellular infection occurs. Extracellular bacteria and fungi have surface polysaccharides that activate the alternative pathway of complement, leading to lysis of susceptible strains and opsonization and subsequent phagocytosis by neutrophils and Mφs. Viruses generally do not activate the alternative pathway of complement and will always cause disease in the unimmunized host. A viral infection is terminated only after the development of specific cytotoxic T cells capable of lysing virally infected cells. Protective immunity against viruses is established through the development of antibodies.

Cell-mediated immunity is essential against intracellular pathogens, including viruses, mycobacteria, salmonella, fungi (*e.g.*, *Pneumocystis carinii*), and protozoa (*e.g.*, *Toxoplasma gondii*). Intracellular pathogens are more resistant to intraphagocytic action and frequently survive within monocytes and macrophages. Cellular immunity with activation of monocytes and macrophages by T lymphocyte secreted lymphokines is the main mechanism of defense against these microorganisms.

In recent years, it has become clear that, although generalizations about host defense and susceptibility to infections are valid, specific components of host defense mechanisms appear essential for immunity against specific microorganisms. Therefore, recurrence of severe infections with some pathogens can point the way toward specific areas of possible immune deficiencies. New methods of evaluation have made it possible to identify some of these specific immune defects. This point will be illustrated through the analysis of deficiencies of cell-mediated immunity, with or without concomitant immunoglobulin or antibody deficiencies.

PHENOTYPIC ABNORMALITIES, MOLECULAR DEFECTS, AND GENE DEFECTS OF THE IMMUNE SYSTEM

A general trend in the development of immunologic evaluation methods has been driven by advances in our knowledge of primary immunodeficiencies (Fig. 2). Most

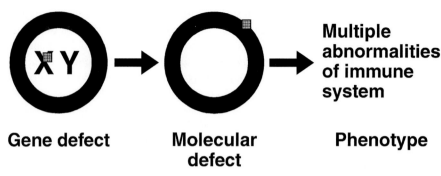

FIG. 2. Genotype, molecular defect, and phenotype of immunodeficiency diseases.

of these immunodeficiencies became known through their immunologic phenotypes, for example deficiencies in lymphocyte subpopulations or in circulating immunoglobulin concentrations. In many instances, it was then discovered that all these phenotypic abnormalities were caused by a single molecular defect affecting a lymphocyte surface molecule, an enzyme, or a cytokine key to the development of several components of the immune system. For many primary immunodeficiencies, a specific molecular defect has now been linked to a mutation in the gene coding for the affected protein.

Immunologic methods can be organized into those identifying (*a*) phenotypic abnormalities, (*b*) molecular defects, or (*c*) gene defects and errors in gene transcription (Table 1). These methods cannot always be clearly separated, as on some occasions the same general method (*e.g.*, flow cytometry) is used to describe a phenotype of an immunodeficiency with decreased lymphocyte subpopulations and also to identify a molecular defect responsible for a disease phenotype.

TABLE 1. *General diagnosis of immunodeficiencies*

Gene	Message	Protein molecular defect	Immune abnormalities
Direct			
Karyotype	Northern blot	Presence	Neutrophils
FISH (deletion)	PCR	Monoclonal antibodies	Complement
RFLP (Southern blot)		Western blot	Antibodies
DNA sequencing		Flow cytometry	T lymphocytes
Indirect		Function	Cytokines
X chromosome		Enzyme	
Inactivation		Ligand	
		Receptor	
		Cytokine	

FISH, fluorescence in situ hybridization; RFLP, restriction fragment length polymorphism; PCR, polymerase chain reaction.

METHODS FOR EVALUATING IMMUNOLOGIC PHENOTYPES

General

The initial evaluation of antibody and cell-mediated immunity in a patient with a suspected immunodeficiency should include the following screening tests (1–4), which are available in most diagnostic laboratories:

1. Complete blood cell count with differential cell analysis (neutrophil, lymphocyte, and platelet count)
2. Immunoglobulin (IgM, IgG, IgA, IgE) concentrations
3. Specific antibody concentrations against:
   a. protein antigens (antibodies to tetanus or diphtheria toxoids), and
   b. polysaccharide antigens (antibodies to serotypes in the 23-valent pneumococcal polysaccharide vaccine);
4. Delayed hypersensitivity skin testing in children more than 1 to 2 years of age)
5. Imaging of the thymus gland (posteroanterior and lateral chest radiograph)

Measurement of Immunoglobulin Concentrations

Antibodies are specific glycoproteins, known as immunoglobulins, found in blood and other body fluids, including tears, saliva, and colostrum. Of the five classes of immunoglobulins, IgG, IgM, and IgA are found mainly in serum. Measurement of these immunoglobulins in serum is essential for the diagnosis of primary and secondary immunodeficiency diseases.

The initial evaluation of antibody deficiencies includes the measurement of serum levels of IgM, IgG, and IgA. An Ig deficiency is diagnosed if levels are below the 95% confidence limits of age-matched controls. If clinical manifestations suggest an antibody deficiency, and yet IgM, IgG, and IgA levels are normal, IgG subclasses should also be measured.

The most commonly used assays for total IgM, IgG, IgA, or IgE are radial immunodiffusion and nephelometry. To measure each of the four IgG subclasses or the two IgA subclasses, radial immunodiffusion, enzyme-linked immunosorbent assay (ELISA), or nephelometric assays can be used. The use of age-related reference ranges is critical when evaluating immunoglobulin levels in children because concentrations change with age.

The measurement of total immunoglobulin concentrations allows the diagnosis of disorders characterized by decreased concentrations, ranging from complete absence of all classes of immunoglobulin to selective deficiencies of a single class or subclass (4–6). Selective IgA deficiency is the most common primary immunodeficiency disease, affecting 1 of 400 to 1 of 800 individuals (7,8). Raised serum concentrations of IgE are generally associated with allergies and parasitic infections, but levels are also significantly increased in hyper-IgE syndrome. The concentration of IgD, which is primarily a cell membrane immunoglobulin, accounts for less than 1% of the total immunoglobulin in plasma and has no direct clinical significance (6,7).

Measurement of Specific Antibodies

The most sensitive method for detecting antibody deficiencies is to assess the ability of an individual to produce specific antibodies against defined antigens. Antigens are classified as *thymus dependent*, usually proteins that require T cells to induce antibody responses, or *thymus independent*, usually polysaccharides, which can induce antibody production in the absence of T cells.

Measurement of specific antibody production after immunization with routine pediatric vaccines is the best way to evaluate B-cell function. Pediatric vaccines (*e.g.*, diphtheria, tetanus, pertussis, and the conjugate *Haemophilus influenzae* vaccine) are used to assess the ability to respond to protein antigens. Immunization with *H. influenzae* and pneumococcal polysaccharide vaccines, in children older than 2 years, is used to evaluate the ability to respond to polysaccharide antigens (4,5,9).

The most commonly used methods for measuring antigen-specific antibody levels are radioimmunoassay, a cumbersome method that uses intrinsically radiolabeled antigens, and ELISA, a widely used method that has been standardized for several protein antigens and more recently for several pneumococcal polysaccharide serotypes (10,11).

Unresponsiveness to pneumococcal polysaccharides after immunization is not unusual and can be found in patients with normal immunoglobulins and IgG subclasses (12,13). In our own and other clinics, this lack of response has been estimated to occur in approximately 5% to 10% of children referred for evaluation of recurrent infection (14,15). An association is also found between some IgG subclass deficiencies and different abnormalities in specific antibody development. Concomitant measurement of IgG subclasses and specific antibodies is important, because several studies have revealed that most of the response to pneumococcal polysaccharides can be found in IgG subclass 2 (16,17). Several associations with specific polysaccharide antibody production have been described, including responses to a restricted number of polysaccharides within the pneumococcal vaccine (18), poor immunologic memory with IgG antibody titers returning to preimmunization levels within 6 to 12 months (18), and lack of development of specific antibodies of the IgG2 isotype (19).

Delayed Hypersensitivity Skin Testing for Evaluating Cell-Mediated Immunity

Delayed hypersensitivity skin testing is used for *in vivo* evaluation of T-cell function after previous sensitization with microbial agents or vaccine antigens. For this test, a battery of recall antigens, usually mumps, Trychophyton, purified protein derivative (PPD), *Candida albicans*, and tetanus toxoid, is injected intradermally and the erythema and induration measured at 24 and 48 hours. The results of this test must be interpreted with caution because they can be negative in patients with T-cell immunodeficiencies, as well as in normal individuals with no previous exposure, and in patients receiving prolonged high dose steroid treatment (3). If these screening tests are normal (i.e., show a positive reaction), the possibility of a T-cell immunodeficiency can be excluded. If the clinical picture suggests a T-cell defect with decreased T-cell numbers or decreased T-cell function, a more extensive evaluation with confirmatory tests should follow.

Lymphocyte Subpopulations

Lymphocyte subpopulations are identified through the analysis of specific cell surface markers. This analysis is critical for the diagnosis of various primary and secondary immunodeficiency diseases. Lymphocyte enumeration is routinely performed in most laboratories by immunophenotyping using flow cytometry technology to detect antigens expressed on the surface of cells. Cells marked by antigen-specific monoclonal antibodies labeled with fluorochromes are analyzed with a flow cytometer, which categorizes the cells according to size, granularity, fluorochrome type, and intensity of fluorescence. The various surface markers used for immunophenotyping have been classified. The term *cluster of differentiation* (CD) with a specified number (*e.g.*, CD4, CD40, and so on) is used as the nomenclature to characterize antigens identified by monoclonal antibodies (20). The choice of immunophenotyping reagents or monoclonal antibody panel depends on the cells or the surface antigen studied. The Centers for Disease Control and Prevention have developed guidelines and proposed a monoclonal antibody panel for performing lymphocyte immunophenotyping in persons infected with the human immunodeficiency virus (21). The availability of multiple antibodies that identify the same cell subpopulation is a useful confirmatory control. For example, our laboratory uses two T-cell, two-B cell, and two natural killer cell markers to determine percentages and absolute numbers of lymphocyte subpopulations. In addition, CD3 combined with HLA-DR is used to detect activated T cells.

To ensure the validity of results, appropriate quality control and proficiency testing procedures must be strictly implemented in each laboratory. It is also important for laboratories performing these types of analyses to establish and use age-related reference ranges for the population being studied. The percentage and absolute numbers of lymphocytes, especially those of $CD3^+/CD4^+$ T cells, are significantly higher in children than in adults (3,4,22).

Examples of primary immunodeficiencies diagnosed by lymphocyte subpopulation analysis include (*a*) X-linked agammaglobulinemia, where B cells are absent; (*b*) severe combined immunodeficiency (SCID), characterized by absent or markedly decreased numbers of T cells; and (*c*) specific CD4 or CD8 deficiencies. Other conditions, including vitamin or other nutritional deficiencies and infections such as the acquired immunodeficiency syndrome, may also affect the number of lymphocyte subpopulations.

The evaluation of several specific surface molecules which define the molecular defect of an immunodeficiency is also performed by flow cytometry. Some examples will be described below in the section *Methods for Evaluating Molecular Defects*.

Normal lymphocyte counts do not rule out the diagnosis of a T-cell immunodeficiency. The next step is to find out if lymphocytes are able to function normally. *In vitro* assays testing the ability of lymphocytes to proliferate in response to mitogens or specific antigens are performed in more specialized laboratories.

Lymphocyte Proliferation Assay

The lymphocyte proliferation assay, an *in vitro* correlate of delayed hypersensitivity skin testing, is performed by measuring the incorporation of radioactive thymidine into lymphocytes stimulated with mitogens or specific antigens. Mitogens (*e.g.*, phytohemagglutinin, concanavalin A, and pokeweed mitogen) nonspecifically stimulate lymphocyte proliferation. Antigens such as PPD, *Candida albicans*, tetanus, and diphtheria toxoid are used to evaluate the specific response of T cells to recall antigens. A more recent method for assessing T-cell function without using radioisotopes is to use flow cytometry to detect activation markers such as CD69 on cells stimulated by mitogen or antigen. However, the limitation of this method is that CD69 induction does not necessarily correlate with cell division (23,24).

Detection of Cytokine Secretion

When lymphocytes are present but are not able to proliferate, it is important to find a possible cause by a systematic search for the cytokines required for lymphocyte blastogenic responses (25). This calls for other more specific functional assays to measure the ability of lymphocytes to produce cytokines or to express cytokine receptors and other surface molecules essential for a normal immune response.

T cells are the major regulatory components of the immune system. Their regulatory function is mediated by the highly regulated secretion of cytokines, which play a critical role in various biological activities. The identification of functionally distinct T helper cells, Th1 and Th2, through the cytokines they secrete has contributed to the understanding of the mechanisms by which polarized immune responses are induced during infection or allergies (26). Unstimulated peripheral blood T cells produce very low or undetectable levels of cytokines. Therefore, detection of cytokine production requires the *in vitro* stimulation of cells with mitogens or specific antigens.

Commercial kits based on an ELISA are commonly used to measure single cytokines in serum samples or in culture supernatants of stimulated cells.

Measurement of Intracellular Cytokines

To measure cytokines at the single cell level, more labor-intensive techniques are used, such as enzyme-linked immunospot assay, limiting dilution, or T-cell cloning (27). During the past several years, flow cytometry, in combination with cytokine-specific monoclonal antibody technology, has contributed to the understanding of the role of Th1 or Th2 regulatory mechanisms in several pathologic conditions (28,29). A recent, novel approach to studying antigen-specific T cells involves the use of multiparameter flow cytometric detection of one or more intracellular cytokines and the early activation marker, CD69, in combination with specific T-cell subset markers (28,29).

Measurement of Cytokine mRNA

Molecular biology techniques can also be used to measure cytokine-specific mRNA in stimulated cell cultures (30). These methods do not identify cytokine-producing cells unless purified cells are studied. However, it is possible to quantify the message for several cytokines produced in response to various mitogens and antigens by peripheral blood mononuclear cells isolated from small amounts of heparinized blood, making this method suitable for evaluation of infants and small children (31).

METHODS FOR EVALUATING MOLECULAR DEFECTS

Multiple identified molecular defects cause various phenotypic abnormalities of the immune system. Enzyme levels are measured by specific methods, whereas cell surface molecules are usually detected by flow cytometry. Classic examples are the measurement of adenosine deaminase (ADA) deficiency, which causes severe combined immune deficiency (SCID), or the detection of the surface molecule CD40 ligand (CD154, formerly CD40L) (32), deficiency, which causes the hyper-IgM syndrome.

Adenosine Deaminase Deficiency Detection by Enzyme Activity Determination

Adenosine deaminase is a monomeric zinc enzyme present in all cells and expressed in high levels in human thymocytes and T lymphoblasts. ADA deficiency causes lymphopenia because of the toxic effects of its substrates, particularly deoxyadenosine (33). Most patients with ADA deficiency develop classic features of early onset SCID during infancy (34). ADA can be measured directly in red cells or other cells from the patient. An indirect indication of abnormal ADA function is obtained by measuring nucleotides that increase in the absence of this enzyme.

CD154 (CD40L) Detection by Flow Cytometry

The CD154 molecule expressed on activated T cells is essential to switch B-cell immunoglobulin production from IgM to IgG. In its absence, mostly IgM is produced, which leads to a phenotype of hyper-IgM production with low IgG, IgA, and IgE concentrations. CD154 expression is detected by flow cytometry in phorbol-12-myristate-13-acetate (PMA) and ionomycin-stimulated T cells using a soluble CD40-Ig fusion protein (35) followed by fluorescein isothiocyanate (FITC) conjugated goat antihuman antibody or a directly conjugated monoclonal antibody specific to CD154.

METHODS FOR EVALUATING GENE ABNORMALITIES

Gene abnormalities can be detected indirectly by X-linked inactivation studies in X-linked diseases or linkage analysis, or directly by techniques such as restriction fragment length polymorphism (RFLP) analysis, single strand conformational polymorphism (SSCP) analysis, or gene sequencing.

Analysis of Patterns of X Chromosome Inactivation

According to Mary Lyon's hypothesis,* in normal females, one of each pair of X chromosomes is randomly inactivated early in development. Thus, most tissues are mosaics with approximately half the cells having maternally derived X as the active X and half having the paternally derived X as the active X. In instances where one X chromosome carries a gene defect detrimental to the maturation or survival of a particular cell lineage, all cells of the affected lineage have the nonmutant X as the active X. Therefore, nonrandom X chromosome inactivation will be found in that particular lineage in carriers of several X-linked immunodeficiencies: X-linked agammaglobulinemia, X-linked SCID, and the Wiskott–Aldrich syndrome. The finding of nonrandom X inactivation in a particular cell lineage is of help for the identification of X-linked inheritance in boys with no family history of disease and for family counseling.

Linkage Analysis by Restriction Fragment Length Polymorphism

Before the genes responsible for X-linked primary immunodeficiencies were discovered, genetic diagnosis was possible through the use of RFLP analyses of chromosome segments that were mapped and determined to be genetically linked to the affected loci. A limitation of this method is the large number of mutations leading to abnormalities in the same gene. Therefore, for each family, it is necessary to determine which RFLP markers are informative.

Mutation Detection by SSCP

The SSCP analysis is based on the observation that the two single stranded DNA molecules from each denatured polymerase chain reaction (PCR) product assume a three-dimensional conformation that is dependent on the primary sequence. If a sequence difference (mutation) exists between the wild type and mutant DNA, this may result in differential migration. As is the case with RFLP, this method does not identify the precise mutation that leads to the protein abnormality.

Mutation Detection by cDNA Analysis and Gene Sequencing

For all immunodeficiencies where the affected gene has been identified, it is now possible to use PCR and direct sequencing to analyze the cDNA size and gene se-

---

*For further information about this hypothesis, see Lyon MF. X-chromosome inactivation and developmental patterns in mammals. *Biol Reviews* 1972;47:1–35.

quence. Usually, the full-length cDNA is analyzed by reverse transcriptase PCR (RT-PCR), using flanking primers. PCR products are then subjected to polyacrylamide gel electrophoresis to determine size heterogeneity between healthy individuals and immunodeficient individuals. Abnormal exons can be analyzed individually by PCR amplification and subcloning into a sequencing vector (e.g, pCR2.1 [Invitrogen, San Diego, CA]). Sequencing is carried out using a modified dideoxy-chain termination sequencing protocol using commercial M13 and T7 as sequencing promoters.

INFECTIONS ASSOCIATED WITH GENERAL AND SPECIFIC IMMUNE DEFECTS

It has become clear in recent years that, although generalizations about host defense mechanisms and general susceptibility to groups of infections are valid, specific pathways and components of the immune response appear to be essential for immunity against specific microorganisms. The infections and immune defects listed in Table 2 are examples of these two types of association. They show that recurrence of more severe infections with some pathogens can point the way to specific areas of possible immune deficiencies. The methods of evaluation discussed in this chapter have made it possible to identify some of these specific immune defects.

TABLE 2. *Deficiencies of cell-mediated immunity and infections with intracellular pathogens*

Infections in primary or secondary CD4 deficiencies (AIDS, SCIDs)
  Extrapulmonary cryptococcosis
  Cryptosporidiosis or isosporiasis with chronic diarrhea
  Cytomegalovirus disease with onset after 1 month of age (site other than liver, spleen, or lymph nodes)
  Pneumocystis carinii pneumonia
  Disseminated histoplasmosis
  Disseminated or extrapulmonary *Mycobacterium tuberculosis* infection
  Disseminated *Mycobacterium avium intracellulare* or *Mycobacterium kansasii* infection
  Cerebral toxoplasmosis with onset after 1 month of age

Examples of infections associated with discrete defects in cell-mediated immunity

Specific defect	Associated infections (reference)
SLAM-associated protein deficiency (X-linked lymphoproliferative disease)	Severe Epstein–Barr virus infection (36)
IFN-γR deficiency, IL-12R deficiency, IL-12 p40 deficiency	BCGosis, infections with atypical mycobacteria, salmonellosis (37–39)
IL-2 deficiency	Cryptococcosis (25)
CD154 (CD40L) deficiency	Histoplasmosis (40)
	Pneumocystis carinii (41, 42)
	Toxoplasmosis (43)
Chronic mucocutaneous candidiasis	Persistent mucocutaneous candidiasis

AIDS, acquired immunodeficiency syndrome; SCIDs, severe combined immunodeficiency; SLAM, signaling lymphocyte activation molecule; IFN, interferon; BCC, bacillus Calmette–Guérin.

TABLE 3. *Differential diagnosis of primary immunodeficiencies, HIV infection, and malnutrition*

	Primary immunodeficiency	HIV infection	Malnutrition
Family history and risk factors	Sporadic, X-linked, autosomal recessive or dominant	Vertical transmission	Socioeconomic factors
Associated conditions	Various	Blood products Wasting	General and specific nutrient deficiencies
Infection	Specific organism	Encephalopathy Intracellular pathogens	Various
Immunoglobulins	Low or normal	Increased	
Cellular immunodeficiency	Often severe	Less severe, progressive	Less severe; response to nutrition
Specific gene or molecular defect	Present	None	None

HIV, human immunodeficiency virus.

DIFFERENTIAL DIAGNOSIS OF PRIMARY AND SECONDARY IMMUNODEFICIENCIES

We have highlighted the immune abnormalities observed mainly in primary immunodeficiencies. Although primary immunodeficiencies are increasingly recognized in different areas of the world (8), secondary immunodeficiencies caused by infection with the human immunodeficiency virus or malnutrition are much more common. A summary of how these forms of immunodeficiency can be differentiated both clinically and using immunologic methods is shown in Table 3.

New therapies are being developed for the treatment of different primary and secondary immunodeficiencies. Information gathered from the experiments of nature that are at the basis of each primary immunodeficiency should be helpful in making a better diagnosis and treating secondary immunodeficiencies also.

REFERENCES

1. Sorensen RU, Moore C. Immunology in the pediatrician's office. *Pediatr Clin North Am* 1994; 41: 691–714.
2. Buckley RH. Immunodeficiency diseases. *JAMA* 1992; 268: 2797–806.
3. Conley ME, Stiehm ER. Immunodeficiency disorders: general considerations. In: Stiehm ER, ed. *Immunologic disorders in infants and children*, 4th ed. Philadelphia: WB Saunders, 1996: 201–52.
4. Shearer WT, Paul ME, Smith CW, et al. Laboratory assessment of immune deficiency disorders. *Immunol Allergy Clin North Am* 1994; 14: 265–99.
5. Kumararatne DS, Bignall A, Joyce HJ, et al. Antibody deficiency disorders. In: Gooi HC, Chapel H, eds. *Clinical immunology. A practical approach.* New York: Oxford University Press, 1990: 1–22.
6. Turgeon ML. *Immunology and serology in laboratory medicine.* St. Louis: CV Mosby, 1990.
7. Ochs HD, Winkelstein J. Disorders of the B-cell system. In: Stiehm ER, ed. *Immunologic disorders in infants and children*, 4th ed. Philadelphia: WB Saunders, 1996: 296–338.
8. Zelazko M, Carneiro-Sampaio M, Cornejo de Luigi M, et al. Primary immunodeficiency diseases in Latin America: first report from eight countries participating in the LAGID. *J Clin Immunol* 1998; 18: 161–6.
9. Wasserman RL, Sorensen RU. Evaluating children with respiratory tract infections: the role of immunization with bacterial polysaccharide vaccine. *Pediatr Infect Dis J* 1999; 18: 157–63.
10. Quataert SACS, Kirch LJ, Quackenbush DC, et al. Assignment of weight-based antibody units to a human antipneumococcal standard reference serum, lot 89-S. *Clin Diagn Lab Immunol* 1995; 2: 590–2.

11. Sorensen RU, Leiva LE, Javier FC, et al. Influence of age on the response to *Streptococcus pneumoniae* vaccine in patients with recurrent infections and normal immunoglobulin concentrations. *J Allergy Clin Immunol* 1998; 102: 215–21.

12. Knutsen AP. Patients with IgG subclass and/or selective antibody deficiency to polysaccharide antigens: initiation of a controlled clinical trial of intravenous immune globulin. *J Allergy Clin Immunol* 1989; 84: 640–7.

13. Zora JA, Silk HJ, Tinkelman DG. Evaluation of postimmunization pneumococcal titers in children with recurrent infections and normal levels of immunoglobulin. *Ann Allergy* 1993; 70: 283–7.

14. Hidalgo H, Moore C, Leiva L, et al. Preimmunization and postimmunization pneumococcal antibody titers in children with recurrent infections. *Ann Allergy Asthma Immunol* 1996; 76: 341–6.

15. Epstein M, Gruskay F. Selective deficiency in pneumococcal antibody response in children with recurrent infections. *Ann Allergy Asthma Immunol* 1996; 75: 125–31.

16. Lim PL, Lau YL. Occurrence of IgG subclass antibodies to ovalbumin, avidin, and pneumococcal polysaccharide in children. *Int Arch Allergy Immunol* 1994; 104: 137–43.

17. Lortan JE, Kaniuk A, Monteil MA. Relationship of in vitro phagocytosis of serotype 14 *Streptococcus pneumoniae* to specific class and IgG subclass antibody levels in healthy adults. *Clin Exp Immunol* 1993; 91: 54–7.

18. Sorensen RU, Hidalgo H, Moore C, Leiva LE. Anti-pneumococcal antibody titers and IgG subclasses in children with recurrent respiratory infections. *Pediatr Pulmonol* 1996; 22: 167–73.

19. Sanders LA, Rijkers GT, Tenbergen-Meekes A-M, et al. Immunoglobulin isotype-specific antibody responses to pneumococcal polysaccharide vaccine in patients with recurrent bacterial respiratory tract infections. *Pediatr Res* 1995; 37: 812–19.

20. Fleisher TA. Immunophenotyping of lymphocytes by flow cytometry. *Immunol Allergy Clin North Am* 1994; 14: 225–240.

21. CDC. 1997 revised guidelines for performing CD4[+] T-cell determinations in persons infected with human immunodeficiency virus (HIV). *MMWR* 1997; 46: 1–29.

22. Erkeller-Yuksel FM, Deneys V, Yuksel B, et al. Age-related changes in human blood lymphocyte subpopulations. *J Pediatr* 1992; 120: 216–22.

23. Maino VC, Suni MA, Ruitenberg JJ. Rapid flow cytometric method for measuring lymphocyte subset activation. *Cytometry* 1995; 20: 127–33.

24. Leiva LE, Regueira O, Sorensen RU. Peripheral blood mononuclear cell sonicates as an alternative to irradiated allogeneic cells to stimulate a mixed lymphocyte reaction and to enumerate CD69[+] alloreactive T cells. *Hum Immunol* 1997; 56: 49–56.

25. Sorensen RU, Boehm K, Kaplan D, et al. Cryptococcal osteomyelitis and cellular immunodeficiency associated with interleukin-2 deficiency. *J Pediatr* 1992; 121: 873–9.

26. Muraille E, Leo O. Revisiting the Th1/Th2 paradigm. *Scand J Immunol* 1998; 47: 1–9.

27. Jooss J, Zanker B, Wagner H, et al. Quantitative assessment of interleukin-2-producing alloreactive human T cells by limiting dilution analysis. *J Immunol Methods* 1988; 112: 85–90.

28. Prussin C. Cytokine flow cytometry: understanding cytokine biology at the single-cell level. *J Clin Immunol* 1997; 17: 195–204.

29. Waldrop SL, Pitcher CJ, Peterson DM, et al. Determination of antigen-specific memory/effector CD4[+] T cell frequencies by flow cytometry. Evidence for a novel, antigen-specific homeostatic mechanism in HIV-associated immunodeficiency. *J Clin Invest* 1997; 99: 1739–50.

30. Carayol G, Bourhis JH, Guillard M, et al. Quantitative analysis of T helper 1, T helper 2, and infammatory cytokine expression in patients after allogeneic bone marrow transplantation. *Transplantation* 1997; 63: 1307–13.

31. Sorensen RU, Butler B, Ortigas A, et al. Upregulation of CD40 ligand and IL-4 mRNA expression, but not of IL-12 and IFN-γ mRNA after immunization with the 23-valent pneumococcal vaccine in children with recurrent respiratory infections [Abstract]. In: Pneumococcal vaccines for the world 1998 Conference. Washington, DC, 1998: 53.

32. Atkinson TP, Smith CA, Hsu Y-M, et al. Leukocyte transfusion-associated granulocyte responses in a patient with X-linked hyper-IgM syndrome. *J Clin Immunol* 1998; 18: 430–9.

33. Hershfield MS, Mitchell BS. Immunodeficiency diseases caused by adenosine deaminase deficiency and purine nucleoside phosphorylase deficiency. In: Scriver CR, Beaudet AL, Sly WS, Valle D, eds. *The molecular and metabolic basis of inherited diseases*, 7th ed. New York: McGraw-Hill,1994: 1725–68.

34. Hirschhorn R. Genetic deficiencies of adenosine deaminase and purine nucleoside phosphorylase: overview, genetic heterogeneity and therapy. In: Wedgwood RJ, Rosen FS, Paul NW, eds. *Primary immunodeficiency diseases*, New York: Alan R. Liss, Inc., 1983: 73–83.

35. Aruffo A, Farrington M, Hollenbaugh D, et al. The CD40 ligand, pg39, is defective in activated T cells from patients with X-linked hyper-IgM syndrome. *Cell* 1993; 72: 291–300.
36. Sayos J, Wu C, Morra M, et al. The X-linked lymphoproliferative-disease gene product SAP regulates signals induced through the co-receptor SLAM. *Nature* 1998; 395: 462–9.
37. Casanova J-L, Blanche S, Emile J-F, et al. Idiopathic disseminated bacillus Calmette–Guerin infection: a French national retrospective study. *Pediatrics* 1996; 98: 774–8.
38. Jouanguy E, Altare F, Lamhamedi S, et al. Interferon-γ-receptor deficiency in an infant with fatal bacille Calmette–Guerin infection. *N Engl J Med* 1996; 335: 1956–61.
39. Newport MJ, Huxley CM, Huston S, et al. A mutation in the interferon-γ-receptor gene and susceptibility to mycobacterial infection. *N Engl J Med* 1996; 335: 1941–9.
40. Hostoffer RW, Berger M, Clark HT, Schreiber J. Disseminated *Histoplasma capsulatum* in a patient with hyper IgM immunodeficiency. *Pediatrics* 1994; 94: 234–6.
41. Levy J, Espanol-Boren T, Thomas C, et al. Clinical spectrum of X-linked hyper-IgM syndrome. *J Pediatr* 1997; 131: 47–54.
42. Notarangelo LD, Duse M, Ugazio AG. Immunodeficiency with hyper-IgM (HIM). *Immunodeficiency Review* 1992; 3: 101–22.
43. Leiva LE, Junprasert J, Hollenbaugh D, et al. Central nervous system toxoplasmosis with an increased proportion of circulating T cells in a patient with hyper IgM syndrome. *J Clin Immunol* 1998; 18: 283–9.

DISCUSSION

Dr. Suskind: Bearing in mind the way you were able to dissect the very specific defect in these primary immunodeficiencies, would we be able to use the same technology to explore immune deficits in children who are malnourished? In dealing with these malnourished children could we be as sophisticated as you have been in dissecting the deficiencies in the primary immunodeficiency syndromes?

Dr. Sorensen: Certainly, I think what will happen. Studies of immune deficiency syndromes have provided us with the tools to measure the induction of cytokines under different conditions. I am sure that will be a fertile area for studies in nutrition. For example, when we studied the CD40 ligand message in response to pneumococcal immunization, we developed a probe because we wanted to diagnose CD40 ligand deficiency or mutation. It did not work because they are point mutations, so the message is not affected, but we then used the same probes to study the regulation of the immune response. We will now be able to use these probes to study the regulation of the response to Epstein–Barr virus.

Dr. Woodward: I have some concern about the extent to which one can use blood lymphocytes to get a picture of the entire lymphoid system.

Dr. Sorensen: I think we are always concerned that our sample of peripheral blood cells may not accurately reflect what goes on at the mucosal site or at the inflammation site. Again, the probes that are being developed can be used for *in situ* hybridization; that is a very fertile field, enabling the study of the presence of cytokine messages in different areas of the body. This can now also be applied using flow cytometry.

Dr. Zoppi: Is it possible to modify secondary immune deficiency by nutrition?

Dr. Sorensen: You ask about secondary immune deficiency, but let me turn the question round a little and tell you that even in primary immune deficiencies, nutrition is very important because it keeps the patient in better shape. If the patient is in good condition, we can use some of the many therapies that are becoming available, which include immunologic reconstitution through stem cells, gene therapy, and so on. These cannot be used if the primary defect is allowed to lead to infections and the infections to malnutrition, with the patient clinically deteriorating. Under those circumstances, almost nothing one can do will be effective. That is not exactly the answer you expected, I suppose, but it is the best I can do.

Nutrition, Immunity, and Infection in Infants and Children, edited by Robert M. Suskind and Kraisid Tontisirin. Nestlé Nutrition Workshop Series, Pediatric Program, Vol. 45. Nestec Ltd., Vevey/Lippincott Williams & Wilkins, Philadelphia ©2001.

The Molecular and Immunologic Evaluation of Nutritionally At-Risk Hosts

Jonathan Powell, Steven H. Yoshida, Judy Van de Water, and M. Eric Gershwin*

Division of Rheumatology, Allergy and Clinical Immunology, University of California at Davis School of Medicine, Davis, California, USA

Without proper nutrition, the immune system would be deprived of the components and mechanisms that are needed to generate an effective immune response. Some immunologic variables are often used as measures of the status of the immune system and its responsiveness to antigenic challenges, including leukocyte number and mobility, oxidant balance, protein activity, antibody production, and interleukin release. All of these immunologic indices, and more, are affected by nutrition. The effects of nutrition on these measurable characteristics also directly affect a person's health. The clinical outcomes of nutritional deficiencies that are of particular interest here involve those that compromise an individual's ability to resist infectious microorganisms. Decreased leukocyte proliferation and phagocytic activity could result in less clonal expansion of microbe-specific clones of lymphocytes and less vigorous microbial elimination. Shifts in oxidant balance will have repercussions on the cell cycle. Alterations in proteins could lead to immunologically important changes in transcription regulation (zinc-finger proteins) or antioxidant protection (selenium-glutathione peroxidase). Antibody synthesis is associated with virus neutralization, complement activation, and atopy. Nutritionally related changes in intercellular communication could have many effects on immune responsiveness and homeostasis through the disruption of cooperative leukocyte activity. Thus, the immune problems related to nutritional deficiencies could range from increased opportunistic infections to suboptimal responses to vaccinations, and perhaps to other immunologic disorders such as allergies.

---

*Correspondence to: megershwin@ucdavis.edu

Innate immune mechanisms, unlike acquired immune responses, are defined as those aspects of the immune response that do not appear to be either qualitatively or quantitatively affected by repeated contact with the same specific immunologic stimulus. Such responses are not customized for the offending stimulus, and no enhanced response occurs following another exposure with the stimulus because no immunologic memory exists of past contacts. Thus, innate immunity is considered a more primitive, basal, or constitutional form of defense. On this foundation, the more flexible acquired immune system developed.

PHAGOCYTES

Phagocytes are cells that consume other cells and particles and become important following breaches of physical barriers. As mentioned, phagocytosis was an early development in the evolution of the immune system and this activity is widely used in both innate and acquired immune responses. Neutrophils (polymorphonuclear cells) and macrophages—the two main phagocytes—are both produced in the bone marrow and released into blood. Mature neutrophils are characterized by a multilobed nucleus and a large reservoir of cytoplasmic granules that are used in the degradation of phagocytosed bacteria. Myeloperoxidase, defensins, bactericidal or permeability increasing factor, and cathepsin G are contained in the *primary azurophilic granules*, whereas lactoferrin, lysozyme, alkaline phosphatase, and cytochrome b558 are found in the secondary granules of neutrophils.

Macrophages circulate in the blood as monocytes (1) (normally 1% to 6% of circulating leukocytes) and then undergo further maturation to become tissue macrophages or histiocytes. They are widely distributed in the host and, in different tissues, attain distinct morphologic characteristics of separate nomenclature, such as Kupffer cells in liver or osteoclasts in bone. Macrophage granules differ from those in neutrophils as they are cytoplasmic bodies and contain acid hydrolases such as proteases, nucleases, and lipases. Importantly, unlike the polymorphonuclear cells, macrophages can recycle degraded antigen to the cell surface for antigen presentation to lymphocytes.

Phagocytes recognize bacteria in various ways ranging from nonspecific attachment through hydrophobicity to specific receptor-ligand interactions. In any case, particles larger than 100 nm in diameter activate intracellular contractile systems that trigger phagocytosis and fusion of the cytoplasmic granules with the particle-containing phagosome. Phagocytes also generate reactive oxygen molecules to kill microorganisms; this activity is called the respiratory, oxidative, or metabolic burst, owing to the characteristic increase in oxygen consumption (2). Cells are protected from their own toxic oxidative compounds by the sulfhydryl-containing tripeptide, reduced glutathione, or catalase, which enzymatically converts H_2O_2 to water and oxygen.

The longer lifespan of macrophages (months) compared with neutrophils (< 48 hours) is reflected by differences in their rate of degradation of engulfed materials. Phagocytosis by macrophages tends to be slower than by neutrophils, and the metabolic burst is less intense. Such a strategy provides both short- and long-term phagocytic function in the elimination of microbes and other particulate foreign materials. As with all circulating leukocytes, measurement of the frequency of neutrophils and monocytes is a useful indicator of immune status in an individual. This status can be assessed by the microscopic analysis and counting of cells in a blood film (blood count) or by using flow cytometry, which sorts cells based on their size, granularity, or specific cell surface antigens that are detected with fluorescent monoclonal antibodies. The flow cytometer uses a hydraulic system to pass single cells from a cell suspension before a laser source so that leukocytes can be individually phenotyped. Before analysis, cells are incubated with commercially available fluorescent monoclonal antibodies, allowing identification of different leukocyte subtypes or their degree of activation. Functional studies include the phagocytic activity, lysosomal activity, metabolic burst, and the resting and stimulated production of the macrophage cytokine interleukin 1 (3).

T LYMPHOCYTES

All leukocytes develop from a unique, self-renewing, pluripotential hematopoietic stem cell (4) and different developmental signals and tissue microenvironments give rise to the diversity of white blood cells. Much interest exists in the identification, purification, and nature of this stem cell as it may be ideal for bone marrow transplantation. Such a cell can reconstitute the full range of leukocytes without the hazards of graft-versus-host reaction that can occur following the implantation of more mature effector donor cells. In graft-versus-host disease, the donor immune system recognizes the host as foreign and initiates a reaction to recipient tissues. It is still unresolved whether the implantation of donor stem cells without also manipulating the tissue microenvironments, some of which change with age (e.g., the thymus), can fully reconstitute an entire immune system.

The T (thymic-dependent) lymphocytes develop from self-renewing progenitors, which migrate from the bone marrow to the thymic gland (5,6) where maturation occurs. Surface markers are commonly used in staging thymocytes; progenitors are initially $CD3^-CD4^- CD8^-$; however, following gene rearrangement in the thymic cortex, the T-cell receptor (TCR) is expressed ($CD3^+$). $\gamma\delta$ T cells remain $CD4^-CD8^-$, whereas $\alpha\beta$T cells convert to a $CD4^+CD8^+$ phenotype and mature to either $CD4^-CD8^+$ or $CD4^+CD8^-$ cells. Positive clonal selection results in T cells restricted to recognize host major histocompatibility complex (MHC). Finally, thymocytes migrate to the thymic medulla where clones recognizing self-antigen–MHC complexes are eliminated (negative selection) to minimize the potential for autoreactivity. Mature T cells are thus released into the peripheral circulation. Atrophy of the mammalian thymus begins during puberty, but T-cell development can shift to other tissues, in particular to the gastrointestinal tract (7,8).

Normally, T cells only recognize antigen that is presented to them by an antigen-presenting cell (APC) such as a macrophage or dendritic cell. APCs process and present antigen with either MHC class I or class II. Both MHC class I and II molecules are transmembrane heterodimers that contain structural domains formed by disulfide bridging. MHC class I heterodimers are composed of a nonpolymorphic β_2 microglobulin from chromosome 15 and a polymorphic α chain with three disulfide-linked domains. Class II antigens are formed by polymorphic α and β chains, each with two immunoglobulin domains. Both MHC molecules contain clefts that bind peptide antigens through noncovalent interactions. MHC class I is usually involved in the presentation of endogenous antigen, allowing the detection of abnormal cellular proteins that may arise, for example, from tumorigenesis or viral infections. In contrast, MHC class II presents protease-degraded exogenous antigen. In both cases interaction of the MHC-antigen complex and TCR are required for antigen recognition, although additional APC–T-cell interactions of co-stimulatory molecules are required to determine the magnitude and type of T-cell response.

The TCR, which is expressed with only a single antigenic specificity, is a heterodimer composed of disulfide-linked α and β chains (9,10) or γ and δ chains (11). The two isotypes ($\alpha\beta$ and $\gamma\delta$) are encoded by separate genes and show different antigen specificity, MHC restriction, effector functions, and anatomic location. The TCR includes a complex of nonpolymorphic accessory proteins (CD3) that are required for TCR expression and function. TCRs bind to the MHC presented peptide antigens through noncovalent molecular interactions such as electrostatic charges, hydrogen bonding, and Van der Waals forces.

A major feature of the adaptive immune system is immunologic memory, which reduces the probability of disease recurrence in normal individuals. Following initial contact with an immunogen, clonal selection of lymphocytes occurs, allowing rapid expansion of antigen-specific T and B cells on secondary antigenic exposure. Phenotypic and functional differences readily distinguish memory from naive lymphocytes. Memory T cells are more readily stimulated by succeeding contact with antigens, whereas alterations occur in the expression of various T-cell surface markers. Adhesion molecules increase and a change occurs in the isoform of the leukocyte common antigen, namely CD45, which is found in a high molecular weight form (CD45RA) on naive T cells and a low-molecular-weight form (CD45RO) on memory cells. Change from a CD45RA to CD45RO phenotype suggests T-cell activation, although in the absence of antigenic stimulation CD45RO+, cells can revert to the RA phenotype. Depending on local signaling and soluble mediators, activated T cells can differentiate into Th1 or Th2 type cells. The former favor inflammatory responses (*e.g.*, the activation of macrophages), whereas the latter activate humoral responses (*e.g.*, the B-cell production of antibody). Potentially activated T cells are also carefully audited by means of deletion, which is elimination of certain lymphocyte clones, or anergy, which renders T cells unresponsive (12). Several factors contribute to the selectivity of T cells for deletion or anergy, including maturity of the T cell, the type of APC involved in T cell–APC interaction, and the affinity of TCR-antigen-MHC binding. In particular, co-stimulatory receptor–ligand interactions and cytokine signaling dictate the selectivity of T cells. In the absence of such associated signals, TCR–MHC interactions tend to result in T-cell anergy rather than activation.

T-cell frequencies (*e.g.*, CD4$^+$ versus CD8$^+$) and their extent of activation can be determined by flow cytometry, which provides a useful indication of immune status in an individual. In addition, a clear feature of lymphocyte function is their ability to proliferate on activation. Thus, the extent of such proliferation following exposure to activation signals is often used as a measure of lymphocyte health. Purified lymphocytes are cultured in the presence and absence of T-cell mitogens that activate the cells in an antigen nonspecific (non-TCR) manner. Following a short period of culture ($\sim$ 3 days), cells are pulsed with ^{3}H-thymidine, which is incorporated into the *de novo* synthesized DNA of proliferating cells, allowing their quantitation by scintillation counting. Proliferation can also be induced by mixing leukocytes from genetically different sources. Such allogeneic activation is induced by TCR–MHC interactions, as cells from one source will recognize the other MHC as foreign. Both cell types can proliferate simultaneously and the selective measurement of proliferating cells from one source is achieved by γ-irradiating cells from the other source before mixing; γ-irradiated cells then serve solely as stimulators for the unirradiated cells and, again, proliferation is determined by ^{3}H-thymidine uptake. This test is used as one functional measure of MHC differences (histocompatibility) between individuals, and is considered an *in vitro* counterpart to tissue mixing (e.g., tissue grafts, bone marrow transplants).

Cytotoxic cells are required for the elimination of abnormal host cells. Mature $CD4^-CD8^+$, TCR^+ T cells are generally MHC class I restricted and traditionally fall into two major categories. Suppressor T cells inhibit the activation phase of immune responses, although reports vary regarding their MHC restricted interactions and expression of TCR, CD markers, and antigen specificity (13–15). Cytotoxic T cells are important in the killing of virally infected and tumor cells and their origins have been outlined above. Cytotoxic T cells can themselves act as effectors, killing infected cells directly (16), through recognition of target antigens by the TCR and the polarization and release of cytoplasmic granules in the vicinity of the target cell. Cytotoxicity is accomplished by apoptosis and lysis, whereas the release of γ-interferon reduces the spread of virus to neighboring host cells.

Elimination of abnormal host cells is the prime function of the natural killer (NK) cell (17). NK cells constitute approximately 15% of circulating lymphocytes and, morphologically, appear as large granular lymphocytes with low nucleus:cytoplasm ratios. They appear distinct from T- and B-lymphocyte lineages as certain immunodeficiency states are characterized by a lack of T and B cells but not NK cells. Nonetheless, NK cells share certain characteristics with cytotoxic T lymphocytes and $\gamma\delta$ T cells in terms of cytotoxic activities, target cell specificities, surface markers, and cytokine production. The binding of lectinlike NK receptors to carbohydrate ligands on target cells appears important in NK cell activity (18). Mice deficient in NK cells generally show an increased susceptibility to the metastatic spread of tumors, although NK cells do not eliminate all malignancies. Indeed, evidence indicates that the expression of MHC class I molecules on target cells is inversely related to their elimination. Immediately after NK–target cell interaction, cytotoxic granules are released by NK cells at the region of contact. The best characterized granule constituent, perforin or cytolysin, is structurally and functionally similar to the complement factor C9 and forms transmembrane pores. Apoptosis (programmed cell death) of the target cell follows shortly after. NK cells are protected from their own granules by the presence of chondroitin sulfate A, which is a protease-resistant, negatively charged proteoglycan that inhibits their autolysis.

Cytotoxicity assays are useful in determining the killing activity of cytotoxic T cells and NK cells. A genetically compatible source of indicator or target cells is used to determine cytotoxic activity of cytotoxic T cells as TCR–MHC interactions are required for this type of killing. In contrast, tumor cell lines are commonly used to measure NK cell function. In either case, target cells are loaded with ^{51}Cr, incubated with the effector lymphocytes, and release of the radiolabel is then used as a measure of target cell killing. Fluorescent markers that avoid the need for radioactivity have also been developed. Finally, DNA fragmentation is another possible outcome measure as target cell killing is mediated through apoptosis.

B CELLS AND IMMUNOGLOBULINS

Although the mammalian fetal liver is a source of B cells early in life, most B-cell production occurs in the bone marrow. The stages of B-cell lineage are noted by rearrangement and expression of antibody genes and cell surface markers such as CD5. It has been suggested that B2 cells (CD5$^-$) and $\alpha\beta$ TCR$^+$ T cells are recently evolved compared with B1 cells (CD5$^+$) and $\gamma\delta$ TCR$^+$ T cells (19). Although B cells may act as professional antigen-presenting cells, their unique role in the immune system is in the production of antigen neutralizing antibodies.

Antibodies to every possible foreign epitope cannot be constitutively produced, so antigen-specific lymphocyte clones are generated in response to antigen challenge. Each B lymphocyte synthesizes antibodies with one unique paratope characteristic and, therefore, one basic antigenic specificity (20). The host contains a large number of resting B-cell clones capable of responding to a range of immunogenic stimuli. In this way, bacteria, for example, expressing a finite quantity of antigenic epitopes, will encounter a large number of B lymphocytes of differing antigenic specificities. Microbial antigens will bind to the closest complementary B-cell receptors. On ligation, these B-cell clones are activated, and soluble antibodies with identical paratopes are released. The proliferation of activated cells ensures that the immune response is of sufficient magnitude to effectively neutralize the antigen. The B-cell antigen receptor is similar in structure to a secreted antibody (10). Indeed, the isotype and antigen specificity of the secreted and membrane-bound immunoglobulins (sIg and mIg, respectively), derived simultaneously from a B-cell clone, tend to be similar. However, important differences are seen between sIg and mIg, as mIg are always monomeric and form part of a hydrophobic transmembrane receptor.

Most immunoglobulins bind to native as opposed to denatured or degraded antigens and generally, therefore, recognize conformational epitopes that are formed by protein folding. The monomeric antibody molecule is a covalently linked complex of four polypeptide subunits, two smaller light chains and two larger heavy chains. Monomeric antibodies may covalently link to form dimeric or multimeric antibodies. All antibodies contain three major functional regions, namely a pair of clonally variable antigen binding sites, a constant *Fc* region that binds to Fc receptors present on the surfaces of many leukocytes, and between these ends, a portion of the antibody that activates the classical complement pathway. Thus, both Fc- and complement-activating regions are functions of the constant region, whereas antigen binding is a function of the variable region.

Five isotypes (classes) of antibodies exist, which are determined by the structure of the constant region of the heavy chain: IgM, IgG, IgA, IgE, and IgD. IgG and IgA are further divided by subclass (e.g., IgG1). Structural differences among heavy chain isotypes are limited to the constant regions and these influence the non–antigen-binding characteristics of antibodies. For example, secreted antibodies are not necessarily monomeric. IgM is released as a pentamer and IgA can be secreted, in mucosal secretions, as a dimer. Mast cells and basophils have Fc receptors for IgE (Fce) only, whereas neutrophils and macrophages express Fc receptors for IgG (Fcg). Effector mechanisms also combine humoral and cellular components in what is termed "antibody-dependent, cell-mediated cytotoxicity"(ADCC). Unlike opsonization, in which immune cells recognize antigen-bound antibodies through their FcRs, ADCC denotes the *arming* of leukocytes with antibodies through Fc–FcR interactions, which facilitates leukocyte binding to antigen. Both macrophages and NK cells possess FcRs that presumably can link with antigen-specific IgG. Cellular contact with antigens expressed on the surface of an infected cell then results in phagocytosis or cytotoxic killing of the target cell.

Quantification of circulating antibodies, their antigen specificity, and their isotypes are widely used in assessing immune status of an individual. Immunofluorescence and immunoblots are used, in addition to the widely applied enzyme-linked immunosorbent assay (ELISA). ELISAs are based on the binding of plasma or serum antibodies with defined antigens onto a solid phase, and using commercially available antibodies for detection. Standardized plastic plates are used for the assay and results are determined on commercially available readers.

Immunoblots are more useful for the detection of antibodies against ill-defined antigens. For example, antigens from a tissue homogenate can be separated by gel electrophoresis, transferred to blotting strips, and incubated with patient sera. Antigen-specific antibodies can then be detected by a color reaction. The location and intensity of the color changes provide information on relative amounts of antibody and the molecular mass of its ligand.

The enzyme-linked immunospot (ELISPOT) is used to quantitate antigen-specific B cells in a fashion similar to the ELISA. B cells are added to antigen-coated ELISA wells and nonspecifically activated to produce antibodies; B cells recognizing the antigen will then bind to the solid phase. The subsequent color reaction will be limited to those areas on the plate that captured the appropriate antibodies and produce a halo (spot) around the antigen-specific B cells. These spots are then counted visually and reasoned to represent individual B cells.

COMPLEMENT

Complement is a term for approximately 25 plasma proteins and protein fragments that are important in host defense (21). The functional roles of the complement system include the lysis of cells and enveloped viruses, facilitating phagocytosis, activating phagocytes, and aiding in their directed migration. Many of these proteins are zymogens or proenzymes that require proteolytic cleavage to become active. The complement cascade is a series of such cleavages mediated, in large part, by the complement proteins themselves. Unfortunately, the complement nomenclature, C1 to C9, is less than ideal as these designations are based on the order of their discovery and not on their order of reaction in the cascade. Two major cascade pathways exist: The innate *alternative* pathway and the antibody-dependent *classical* pathway have different initiation conditions, but eventually converge to a common series of reactions.

The most abundant and central complement component is C3. The slow, spontaneous removal of a C3 fragment, C3a, by water or enzyme results in the activation of a complement reactive intermediate, C3b. The accepted convention is to designate the smaller fragment "a" and the larger "b." In the presence of Mg^+, C3b complexes with factor B, and is cleaved by another plasma enzyme, factor D, to form C3 convertase. This convertase splits more C3 into fragments C3a and C3b. The potential positive feedback loop is controlled by the inherent instability of C3 convertase. Factor B can be displaced by factor H to form C3bH, which then reacts with the C3b inactivator, factor I. The inactive iC3b then undergoes proteolytic degradation.

In the presence of certain microorganisms, the C3 convertase is stabilized by the carbohydrate cell wall, which provides protection from factor H. Additional stability is derived from the binding of properdin to the convertase. The incorporation of another C3b component to the C3 convertase generates a C5 convertase. The cleavage of C5 leads to a soluble C5a fragment and a larger C5b portion that is loosely bound to C3b. The succeeding attachment of C6, C7, and C8 ultimately results in the insertion of the amphipathic component, C9, into the lipid membrane to form the membrane attack complex. This is followed by unrestricted water and salt flow through these transmembrane channels and cytolysis.

Aside from the formation of transmembrane pores, the complement cascade has other properties that are used in the antimicrobial response. Phagocytes have receptors for C3b and iC3b. These ligand–receptor interactions enhance the adherence and uptake of complement-coated bacteria by a process termed *opsonization*. In addition, C3a and C5a stimulate the respiratory burst of phagocytes, particularly neutrophils, and act as anaphylatoxins by signaling granulocytes such as mast cells and basophils to release their inflammatory mediators. C5a also attracts neutrophils to the site of C5a production (chemotaxis), induces vasodilatation, increases the permeability of capillary endothelial cells, and causes smooth muscle contraction. The regulation of C3a and C5a is achieved by a serum carboxypeptidase that removes their terminal arginines.

Unlike the alternate pathway, the classical pathway is initiated by secreted antibodies. The activation of C1q binding sites within the constant regions of aggregated IgG or a single IgM occurs following antigen binding. When two or more of its globular domains are bound by antibodies, the proteolytic function of C1q begins to cleave C4. This generates C4a, an anaphylatoxin similar to C3a and C5a, and C4b, which possesses weak opsonic activity. The complexing of C2 with C4b creates a C3 splitting enzyme similar to the C3 convertase of the alternate pathway. Subsequent reactions are identical to the alternate pathway and culminate in the formation of membrane attack complexes.

Owing to the presence of antigen-specific antibodies, phagocytosis of the foreign body is enhanced. Not only do antibodies act as opsonins, but *cross-linking* of Fc receptors occurs if more than one antibody is involved in this interaction. The binding of multiple antibody Fc regions by FcRs on phagocytes results in the transmission of cellular activation signals and heightened leukocyte activity.

CYTOKINES

Cytokines are molecules produced by virtually all nucleated cells, most of which have pleiotropic effects on hematopoietic and other cell types that are involved in host defense. Cytokines include lymphocyte-derived lymphokines, monocyte-derived monokines, hematopoietic colony-stimulating factors, and connective tissue growth factors (22). These factors differ from hormones in that they generally operate at short distances within a tissue as paracrine or autocrine communication vehicles. They also tend to be induced by infectious challenge or other stressors and, largely, are not constitutively released. Individual cytokines can also be synthesized and secreted by more than one cell type, and functional activity of a cytokine is mediated by typical ligand or receptor binding. The understanding of cytokine networks is complicated by the multiple cellular sources, targets, and the pleiotropic effects of most of the cytokines; and by the synergistic or antagonistic effects of cytokine mixtures and their ability to alter the production of other cytokines and their receptors.

Distinctions between the cytokine release profiles of type 1 and type 2 T-helper (Th1, Th2) cells are noteworthy (23). Although these helper cell types cannot be distinguished phenotypically, as they are both $CD4^+CD8^-$ T cells, they are separable based on the coordinated expression of distinct but overlapping sets of cytokines. Th1 cells are characterized by the release of γ-interferon, the induction of cell-mediated immune responses, and the facilitation of IgG2a production. Th2 cells, on the other hand, produce interleukin (IL)-4, IL-5, IL-6, and IL-10, and are primarily involved in the production of antibodies (other IgG, IgA, IgE). Interestingly, these cell types and the immune networks that they promote are antagonistic. For example, γ-interferon blocks the growth of Th2 cells, whereas IL-4 inhibits some functions of macrophages activated by γ-interferon. In addition, $CD5^+$ B-1 cells release IL-10 and themselves are activated by IL-5 (24).

Cytokines released by cells *in vitro* or present in plasma are commonly measured by ELISA or levels of cytokine mRNA in cells. Another method of potentially wide use is the intracellular detection of cytokines by anticytokine antibodies with detection by flow cytometry. Leukocytes, with membranes permeabilized by detergents, are incubated with anticytokine antibodies conjugated to fluorescent compounds. The intensity of fluorescence is then measured by flow cytometry.

HYPERSENSITIVITY

Hypersensitivity to exogenous antigens or allergens is a common problem in the human population. The strategy of avoiding contact with allergens in order to minimize the frequency or intensity of allergic reactions first requires the identification of these environmental agents. Skin tests are often used in this regard. Basically, samples of allergens are injected subcutaneously and a measure of reactivity is based on the size of the inflammatory skin reaction. Immediate hypersensitivities mediated by IgE (*e.g.*, pollen extract) will become evident in minutes. Delayed type hypersensitivity reactions (*e.g.*, the tuberculin test), which are caused by T-cell recruitment of phagocytes to the injection site, require 24 to 48 hours.

TIER SYSTEM

As nutritional deficits are often associated with societal disruptions, poverty, and a lack of public services, the materials and personnel needed to obtain and interpret immunologic information can be limiting. The types of immunologic studies and tests that can be done on selected individuals or populations depend on various factors (Table 1).

These factors include the ability to store and transport biological samples and test equipment, the location of test sites (a major city as opposed to an isolated village), and the expertise and personnel available. The conditions in which immunologic information must be obtained can vary widely. Desirable is a flexible system that can adapt to a variety of situations but still achieve the goal of obtaining useful immunologic information. A practical testing structure might include a tiered system that applies increasingly sophisticated examinations as the study materials or subjects move from provincial and isolated sites to metropolitan centers. One of us (SY) was a Peace Corps volunteer in west Africa for 2 years and another (MEG) helped run a rural hospital in Pakistan. Familiarity with conditions in the field, as

TABLE 1. *Hypothetical tiering system*

Tier	Characteristics	Methods
1	Absence of permanent public health facility	Dermatologic hypersensitivity tests Hematology (hematocrit, differential)
2	Rural medical clinic	Immunodiffusion, enzyme-linked immunosorbent assay and electrophoresis for immunochemical analysis Short-term cell culture for chemotaxis, phagocytosis, antibody production Immunofluorescent staining with fluorescent microscopy for cell phenotyping
3	Medical center	Flow cytometry for cytokines analysis, cell phenotyping, cell cycle analysis In situ hybridization and reverse transcription polymerase chain reaction for cytokine analysis Longer term cell culturing for cytotoxicity, proliferation, antigen presentation

well as the facilities that were available at a local American Baptist missionary hospital, provide a firsthand impression of the range of environments in which immunologic information can be gathered.

Tier 1

The first tier is embodied by a working situation in which a permanent health facility is not available. In this case, public health workers would travel into extremely rural or undeveloped regions. They might be required to perform their examinations from temporary quarters such as tents. The population being examined may reside in relatively permanent settlements (i.e., villages) or they may be potentially migratory and themselves live in impermanent shelters. Water comes from a well or neighboring stream, and electrical power should not be expected. As a result, these on-site tests should not require temperature-controlled or sterile environments, or a constant source of electricity (unless a portable generator is available).

Skin tests are appropriate for the first tier. These would include dermatologic testing for contact hypersensitivity to various immunologic stimuli, and tuberculin-type assays. The subjects could either have a history of known contact with immunogenic materials, or have received vaccinations. Subsequent skin testing could be used as an overall measure of the person's ability to generate an immunologic response. Immunodeficiencies may be evidenced by lower than normal or absent responses to antigenic challenges. The length of time needed for an observable skin reaction depends on the underlying immunologic mechanism in progress. Antibody (IgE) mediated *immediate hypersensitivity* (*e.g.*, pollen allergy) becomes evident in minutes. Measurable responses by cell-mediated delayed hypersensitivity (e.g., the tuberculin test) take about 2 days.

Blood smears may also be done in the field. Staining and microscopic analysis of blood cells for hematologic counts provide general information on the numbers of the various types of white blood cells. Concurrently, hematocrits could be obtained as a general measure of the concentration of red and white blood cells. Because hematocrit determination requires the centrifugation of capillary tubes, an electric generator is needed.

Tier 2

If blood samples taken in the field are transportable to a tier 2 facility, then the aforementioned hematologic tests could be done in a more controlled environment. Study of blood samples in a tier 2 facility would also allow the technician to gather information on additional immunologic variables.

The practicality of transportation would depend on various factors: distance and the condition of roads or airfields, temperature-controlled storage, and the ability to communicate and transmit information. For example, the aforementioned missionary hospital did have its own airfield and plane. However, the expense incurred for their use needs to be justified or compensated. The parties must also coordinate the arrival of samples with the readiness to deal with them.

The tier 2 scenario may be one of a clinic in a rural setting. Running water is present, although its quality may not be equal to that of a modern city in a developed country. Portable filtering devices and boiling are probably desirable. Electric power is fairly dependable but subject to occasional (maybe once a week) power cuts.

Other considerations limit the feasibility of some types of research and diagnostics work. For example, depending on the location and time of year, the ambient temperature may be higher than incubator temperature. An air conditioned workroom is an improbability (but not impossibility), but no ultracold ($-70°C$) freezers and no cold rooms are available for storage. Sterility for cell culturing may be problematic. This type of site would not have facilities for the responsible disposal of biohazardous or radioactive wastes as it is likely that in tier 2, and certainly in tier 1, waste disposal is highly unregulated.

On the other hand, equipment such as fluorescent microscopes and ELISA readers are conceivable in such a rural setting, assuming that the number of subjects to be studied is large enough to justify such procedures. These types of materials need not be permanent but could be brought into the clinic on a temporary basis when needed.

Various immunochemical tests are feasible in a tier 2 setting. Immunodiffusion assays are performed on agar-coated glass microscope slides. This is a relatively inexpensive and uncomplicated means of detecting the classes and subclasses and the antigen specificity of antibodies from peripheral blood. ELISAs that are more quantitative and sensitive than immunodiffusion tests are also appropriate for the second tier. The feasibility of these assays are limited by the ability to obtain the necessary materials including plasticware, ELISA reader, pipettors, and immunologic reagents. Except for the cost of buying these materials, no real obstacles exist to their safe storage or competent use in a rural setting.

The same may be said for other biochemical methods such as sodium dodecylsulfate-polyacrylamide gel electrophoresis. This method can be used in conjunction with more immunologically based techniques. For example, antigen-specific antibodies can be used to purify proteins before electrophoretic separation. Or, antibodies can be used to identify certain protein antigens after their electrophoretic separation. The materials for these analyses are easily stored and the temperature (ambient temperature, domestic refrigerator or freezers) and utility (electricity and water) requirements can be met by most rural clinics. Limits to autoradiography are primarily caused by the nature of restrictions on the disposal of radioactive wastes.

The activity and concentrations of complement proteins from patient sera are measurable by a variety of methods. Complement activity can be titrated by the hemolysis or sheep red blood cells. However, one limitation of this assay is the shelf life of these commercial sheep blood cells. Concentrations (but not activity) of serum complement proteins can be assayed by radial immunodiffusion or ELISA.

Short-term (hours to days) cell culturing could be done to measure certain cellular functions. The phagocytic activity of macrophages can be assessed through the incubation of cells with phagocytozable materials. Uptake of bacteria could be determined by the number of colonies recoverable from the culture medium (and therefore not phagocytozed). The uptake of plastic beads is quantified by microscopic examination and counting of beads.

The ability of leukocytes to migrate toward a chemotactic source is also a measure of immunologic responsiveness. One classic method is the use of a Boyden chamber. In this two compartment vial, cells are placed in one end and a chemotactic material is placed in the other. Migration is measured by the number of cells that cross the boundary between the two compartments. An alternative to measuring migration is the observation of morphologic changes that are believed to precede cell movement.

Quantification of antigen-specific B lymphocytes can be determined by the ELISPOT. B cells are incubated in the wells of ELISA plates precoated with the antigen of interest. Antibodies produced by antigen-specific B cells will bind to the antigens on the surface of the wells. The wells are then developed similarly to a standard ELISA. Antigen-specific B cells are quantified by counting the spots created by the antigen–antibody reactions.

Staining of cells with fluorescent antibodies and counting on a fluorescent microscope can be done to determine the relative numbers of different types of peripheral blood lymphocytes. Such visual counts do not permit the accurate quantitation of fluorescence intensity or the ability to segregate the fluorescence of multistained cells. However, this method can provide the technician with information regarding cells stained for a single marker. In this way, the ratios of T and B cells, or CD4 and CD8 T lymphocytes, may be measured.

Tier 3

The third tier envisions a modern medical center in a capital city. This facility provides the expertise and materials needed for more expensive, highly specialized, and probably less frequently done tests. When deemed necessary, biological samples could be sent to this centralized facility from tier 1 or 2 regions. But, as with the movement of samples from tier 1 to 2, transportation, communication, and storage are factors to consider.

The proliferative capacity of lymphocytes can be measured by various means. In the mixed leukocyte reaction, the stimulus is provided by allogeneic MHC complex molecules. Alternatively, mitogens (*e.g.*, bacterial lipopolysaccharide or concanavalin A) may be used. Such assays require incubation times of about a week. Proliferation is also measured by the incorporation of the radioactive isotope tritium. The cost and size of radiation counters, and the need for safe disposal of radioactive wastes, will probably preclude the use of these methods in tier 2 areas.

Studies on the cytotoxic capacity of peripheral blood T lymphocytes and natural killer cells are more appropriate for tier 3 than 2. The availability and disposal of radioactive isotopes are again a major consideration. The traditional means of measuring target cell killing is through the release of ^{51}Cr. Also, cytotoxicity must be demonstrated on live target cells. This will require facilities for the culturing of target cell lines and possibly the *in vitro* generation of target-specific cytotoxic T cells.

Natural killer cell cytotoxicity is typically determined by the killing of various transformed or lymphoblastic cell lines.

Monocyte–T-cell interactions during the process of antigen presentation are important for the generation of antigen-specific immune responses. Thus, the effects of nutrient deprivation on antigen presentation is likely to contribute to the immunodeficient status of the patient. Blood monocytes, T lymphocytes, and antigens are cultured together, and T-cell activation is monitored. The readouts are usually T-cell proliferation and cytokine production.

Flow cytometry is an indispensable tool for sophisticated immunologic diagnostics and research. A wide range of fluorescent probes is available for measuring the presence of cell surface markers (*e.g.*, CD4, adhesion molecules), intracellular molecules (cytoskeleton, DNA), and cellular processes (calcium release, cell cycle). The capacity to stain concurrently for more than one marker or process, and the ability to quantitate the intensity of fluorescence, gives the user the ability to monitor the status of specific cell types.

Measurement of cytokine synthesis and release by immune cells is probably not appropriate for tier 2 laboratories. Owing to the low levels or short half-lives of cytokines released by cells, detection by ELISA may be impractical. Northern blot analysis or the polymerase chain reaction is used to obtain measurements of the relative levels of cytokine mRNA within cells. Alternatively, intracellular cytokines are detectable by fluorescent anticytokine antibodies and quantifiable by flow cytometry.

REFERENCES

1. Gordon S, Clarke S, Greaves D, Doyle A. Molecular immunobiology of macrophages: recent progress. *Curr Opin Immunol* 1995; 7: 24–33.
2. Rosen GM, Pou S, Ramos CL, Cohen MS, Britigan BE. Free radicals and phagocytic cells. *FASEB J* 1995; 9: 200–9.
3. Lesourd BM, Meaume S. Cell mediated immunity changes in ageing, relative importance of cell subpopulation switches and of nutritional factors. *Immunol Lett* 1994; 40: 235–42.
4. Scott MA, Gordon MY. In search of the haemopoietic stem cell. *Br J Haematol* 1995; 90: 738–43.
5. Kisielow P, Von Boehmer H. Development and selection of T cells: facts and puzzles. *Adv Immunol* 1995; 58: 87–209.
6. Jameson SC, Hogquist KA, Bevan MJ. Positive selection of thymocytes. *Annu Rev Immunol* 1995; 13: 93–126.
7. Abo T. Extrathymic pathways of T-cell differentiation: a primitive and fundamental immune system. *Microbiol Immunol* 1993; 37: 247–58.
8. Franceschi C, Monti D, Sansoni P, Cossarizza A. The immunology of exceptional individuals: the lesson of centenarians. *Immunol Today* 1995; 13: 12–16.
9. Hein WR. Structural and functional evolution of the extracellular regions of T cell receptors. *Semin Immunol* 1994; 6: 361–72.
10. DeFranco AL. Transmembrane signaling by antigen receptors of B and T lymphocytes. *Curr Opin Cell Biol* 1995; 7: 163–75.
11. Havran WL, Boismenu R. Activation and function of gamma delta T cells. *Curr Opin Immunol* 1994; 6: 442–6.
12. LaSalle JM, Hafler DA. T cell anergy. *FASEB J* 1994; 8: 601–8.
13. Arnon R, Teitelbaum D. On the existence of suppressor cells. *Int Arch Allergy Immunol* 1993; 100: 2–7.
14. Kemeny DM, Noble A, Holmes BJ, Diaz-Sanchez D. Immune regulation: a new role for the CD8[+] T cell. *Immunol Today* 1994; 15: 107–10.

15. Le Gros G, Erard F. Non-cytotoxic, IL-4, IL-5, IL-10 producing CD8$^+$ T cells: their activation and effector functions. *Curr Opin Immunol* 1994; 6: 453–7.
16. Podack ER. Execution and suicide: cytotoxic lymphocytes enforce Draconian laws through separate molecular pathways. *Curr Opin Immunol* 1995; 7: 11–16.
17. Klein E, Mantovani A. Action of natural killer cells and macrophages in cancer. *Curr Opin Immunol* 1993; 5: 714–18.
18. Gumperz JE, Parham P. The enigma of the natural killer cell. *Nature* 1995; 378: 245–8.
19. Kantor AB, Herzenberg LA. Origin of murine B cell lineages. *Annu Rev Immunol* 1993; 11: 501–38.
20. Klinman NR. Selection in the expression of functionally distinct B-cell subsets. *Curr Opin Immunol* 1994; 6: 420–4.
21. Roitt I. *Essential immunology*, 8th ed. Oxford: Blackwell Scientific Publications, 1994.
22. Thompson AW, ed. *The cytokine handbook*. San Diego: Academic Press, 1994.
23. Anderson GP, Coyle AJ. TH2 and 'TH2-like' cells in allergy and asthma: pharmacological perspectives. *Trends Pharmacol Sci* 1994; 15: 324–32.
24. O'Garra A, Howard M. Cytokines and Ly-1 (B1) B cells. *Int Rev Immunol* 1992; 8: 219–34.

DISCUSSION

Dr. Suskind: Bearing in mind the specific entities that Dr. Sorensen was discussing, what can we do to dissect in a more effective way the observations that have been made at a superficial level? We can standardize the patient population in terms of nutritional status, but what can we do then to harness the methodologies that you and Dr. Sorensen and other immunologists have at your disposal that can give us a better evaluation of the immune system in the malnourished population?

Dr. Gershwin: In reality, people are outbred animals. Although we can genetically define point mutations using Sorensen's technology and that developed by others, for most people the situation is a more practical one. We are dealing not with an individual, but with a herd. Whatever methods are developed have to be applied to the herd. So how does the herd respond to infection? It has innate responses, it has the isoglutinins, it has natural antibodies, and it has a response to a specific pathogen. If I were involved in investigating a standardized population–a large number of subjects, age- and gender-matched, and environmentally matched as far as possible–I would first measure antibodies against the natural pathogens that are endemic in the area—bacteria, viruses, malaria, or whatever—and I would then challenge them with one or two different antigens and measure the immune response. If you do not do this in the field, you will have gone significantly further than doing tests of nonspecific immunity, such as responses to phytohemagglutinin, allergenic cells, skin tests, and so forth, because you will have asked what the host is capable of doing following vaccination, and what happens to those natural antibodies in people who have been involved in one of your nutritional supplement programs. That is how I would address it, though that is only the first tier.

Dr. Haschke: You touched very briefly on the intestinal flora and mentioned that we cannot influence it much—it is very stable no matter where you are living and under what conditions. Could you comment further?

Dr. Gershwin: What I was referring to is that we do acquire some natural flora that are resistant to change. We can dramatically modify the situation with antibiotics, and there may be ways we can improve it. For example, I am aware of some phenomenal strains of lactobacillus that have the potential to stimulate the immune system. They can remove a lot of proinflammatory material from the gut and I think these organisms do have major potential.

Dr. Haschke: In the infant, it would be very attractive to manipulate the gut flora to obtain a more bifidogenic flora. In the meantime, several groups have shown that you can induce a bifidogenic gut flora very close to that in the breast-fed infant with fructo-oligosaccharides;

however, the immunologic effects have not been defined, so it is not yet known whether this really changes the immune function. One recent study on otitis media seems to indicate that this is possible (1). In that study, xylitol seemed to inhibit the adhesion of bacteria that cause otitis media, and a decrease in specific infection was seen in a high risk group. This is a very interesting field for future research.

Dr. Gershwin: I think so. You also remind us that we should distinguish mucosal from systemic immunity. In fact, using organisms such as lactobacilli and other means, we may be able to influence the mucosal immune system and body secretions more than we can systemic immunity.

Dr. Kennedy: I think your tier system is quite pragmatic. Having run field studies in some unusual environments, it is nice to have a pragmatic approach to things. I am not a nutritionist nor an expert in epidemiology, but one of the difficulties I see in terms of focusing on whether or not nutritional supplements, or nutrition as a whole, play a role in modulating immune function is that we lack specific biomarkers of immune function and we do not know whether such biomarkers actually translate into some type of benefit. I think that performing tier 1 type studies—where you do broad-based population vaccination against antigens to see if an immune response occurs and whether various nutritional supplements induce an immune response or not—is not really getting at the specific question of whether a nutritional immunomodulating effect exists. I find it hard to believe that an epidemiologic study could show that a single marker of immune function can clearly define benefit *per se*.

Dr. Gershwin: With all respect, I would disagree. Although no guarantee is seen that a single outcome measure will reflect the ability of a herd to respond to an infection, on the other hand, I warrant that the outcome measure of natural immunity—that is, panels of antibodies against the pathogens in a particular area—plus the immune response to one or two antigens is about as cost-effective as you will get, given the resources available. And resources have to play a role in this equation. The human genome may ultimately become available, and as we begin to understand it, which will take years, we may develop other read-out patterns that could allow us to predict which individuals are more likely to have an adverse outcome to a challenge in a particular endemic area.

Dr. Sorensen: I would like to consider what kind of concrete results we could take home from this meeting. I would say that before even starting to discuss tiers 1, 2, and 3, it is essential to have a common format for clinical data collection. At a very similar meeting in 1994 in Santiago de Chile, where several people discussed immune deficiencies in Latin America, we decided right there that we needed to unify data collection. So we took everybody's clinical forms, unified them, and created a computerized program and distributed it to 12 participating countries, which all now collect data on the same standardized two page form, so that we can compare information obtained in Chile, Brazil, Mexico, and so on. I would say that if you really want to take advantage of this international group and compare all these issues (*e.g.*, the influence of the environment, nutrition, allergy, immunizations, and so on), it would be best to create a unified questionnaire in which the key issues are captured, so at least we are talking the same language, clinically speaking. We can then go on to decide how to collect information on DNA, RNA, immunoglobulins, and so forth. That is a second phase.

Dr. Gershwin: I agree the most important component of every physical examination is the history, but at some point we do have to get back to the bench.

Dr. Wasantwisut: I am very interested in your suggestions about immunologic monitoring in the public health system. This seems a very important issue. In the past, immunologic assays were unthinkable for many people in developing countries. Now you have shown that certain ways exist in which these can be used to answer questions related to public health programs. Can you and the other experts here suggest practical examples (*i.e.*, in this situation) in cases of such and such infections, that this is what to do and that these questions should be asked, using these kinds of indicators. I think that would be very useful.

Dr. Keusch: Dr. Sorensen's suggestion was a very important one, but it needs to go further than purely clinical descriptors. As Scrimshaw said 40 years ago, we need to define very carefully what we are talking about when we refer to "nutritional state." And when we deal with populations of humans who present with what we call protein-energy malnutrition or with a selective nutrient deficiency, it is very rare that one individual will be identical to another with respect to body composition and other markers. So, similarly to collecting the clinical information, we need to find a standardized way of collecting nutritional information, particularly on body composition, which I think is exceedingly important.

With respect to Dr. Suskind's comment at the beginning of the discussion, I was a little concerned that he was talking about methodology driving research. I think the research process has not changed; it is hypotheses and questions that drive research, and the methodologies are selected to be appropriate to the question. With respect to assessing the immune system, let us take the example of immunization. Most studies that we referred to this morning used immunization as a probe for the immune system: give an immunization and look 28 days later to see the response; give a second immunization and look again another 4 weeks later. In fact, the events that mediate what is going to happen occur very quickly, certainly within the first couple of days. In an old study we did at INCAP in Guatemala, we used diphtheria and tetanus toxoids and pertussis vaccine or typhoid immunization in young children who were recovering from protein-energy malnutrition as a model (Keusch GT, Chew F, McAdam K, Torun B, unpublished observations). We then looked at the cytokine and acute-phase response over the first 2 days and picked a couple of markers to follow. We found a very good correlation between the height of the immune response at 28 days and the nature of the cytokine response within the first 48 hours. So even with something such as immunization, we have to be very careful about what phase we are considering and what markers we wish to use.

My final comment is that even when we have selected those markers, they do not tell us what is happening phenotypically in humans living in particular circumstances, what their actual susceptibility to infection is, or what their response to contact with an infectious agent is going to be. So, as Scrimshaw said, we have to come back to the well-designed field study that can assess the importance of a particular immune response in a population with a defined nutritional deficiency, and really see that it makes an impact on something other than the *in vitro* test.

Dr. Wakelin: You mentioned that as part of your approach to assaying immune response you should use antigens for infections that were endemic in that area. Could you clarify that?

Dr. Gershwin: No. I said that as part of the initial screen for what might happen after a dietary intervention program, before and after quantitation could be done of antibodies to flaviviruses, arboviruses, and so on. Immunization is a second issue within that.

Dr. Wakelin: The problem seems to me that you have a circularity here. You are assaying, using the same test, immune competence, nutritional competence, and previous experience of those antigens or cross-reacting antigens. How do you separate out those three things?

Dr. Gershwin: That is the whole point of it. The nonspecific basal immune responses are the ones that are most likely to reflect what a host will do to a specific challenge. The ideal way would be not just to use serology, but to use cell-mediated responses as well. However, I do not think that is practical in the field. That is why we have selected the serologic responses. And that is why research has to go back to the initial field study, because what might be measured in Southeast Asia will be quite different from what will be measured in Sub-Saharan Africa.

Dr. Wakelin: But I thought you ruled out using responses to nonspecific tests such as mitogens in favor of specific tests?

Dr. Gershwin: Yes, it is a specific response to an antigen such as a virus, but it is not a response following an immunization. The response is really what is being measured. So maybe the problem is that the immunologist assesses the response to a direct challenge, as well as what the immune system will do serologically.

Dr. Wakelin: My point is: how do you eliminate the possibility of prior exposure being a variable?

Dr. Gershwin: You have to have large numbers of subjects in your groups. The ideal situation is that individuals have been exposed before and they do have basal titers. Of course, you are going to have variation and individuals are going to have repeated exposures to those agents in some cases. That is what innate immunity is about; that is what you want and why you need large groups—50 to 100, for example. This cannot be done on a group size of 6 to 8. That is why the panel has to include more than one agent, because people are outbred and there are individual differences.

Dr. Wakelin: I think there is probably confusion about what you mean by innate immunity and what I would understand by innate immunity.

Dr. Gershwin: Yes, I am not referring to immunity following an antigenic challenge; I'm talking about the basal responses that a host might have. Those responses could be as simple as antibodies to polysaccharides, or they could reflect the presence of antibodies that spontaneously exist in a population without being directly challenged with an organism.

Dr. Marini: I think the influence of the type of feeding is very important, for example breast milk and the presence of anti-idiopathic antibodies, not to mention antibodies received across the placenta. So if you are going to study native reactions, maybe these can be influenced by the history of the mother.

Dr. Gershwin: I think you are absolutely right. As soon as you bring the element of placental transmission of maternal antibodies into the equation, I do not think the approach I have suggested is going to work.

Dr. Woodward: In connection with your proposed tier system, I wonder if you could suggest some way to make it a bit more broadly based. If I understood your proposal correctly, you are suggesting using the antibody type of response as the basis and I think you indicated the reason for rejecting cell-mediated responses, no doubt for good pragmatic reasons. But my understanding is that cell-mediated immunity is more susceptible to modulation than the antibody response, and it is certainly more predictably modulated. I believe the antibody type of response has thus far proved to be highly variable in the way it is altered by dietary and other external influences.

Dr. Gershwin: Certainly, if we had an antigen-specific cell-mediated response that could be done in a practical tier 1 situation, that would be ideal. But even in the setting of the Johns Hopkins paradigm, it is extremely difficult to measure antigen-specific T-cell responses in the human host. You can do it as far as monilia is concerned, but that is not a reliable outcome measure for the pathogens we are discussing. With respect to serology, virtually all the data we heard about this morning looked at the levels of IgG or IgM or IgA, not at antibody-specific responses. I agree, I do not think that is an appropriate response, as it is looking primarily at whatever stimulation is taking place at the level of B cells; I doubt whether such responses are adequately reflective of a specific outcome measure in the field. I am trying to propose a system that is antigen specific, reflects natural immunity, is economical, and can be done on limited resources in the field, on a reasonable number of subjects. It is certainly not an answer to every nutritional problem in the world, but I think it offers a level of sophistication that goes beyond gross skin tests or serum immunoglobulin or complement or any other pathway we have heard about. Thus far, those are the variables that have been most widely used by nutritionists in the field.

Dr. Suskind: I appreciate what you have done in relation to tiering the evaluation of populations, but I also believe that we should look seriously at the population of individual patients to see the impact of nutritional deprivation or malnutrition using some of the more sophisticated studies to which you alluded today. Could you comment on that? It is a different approach.

Dr. Gershwin: I have taken the public health approach, which I think is the approach of the *herd*. You are absolutely right that individual approaches offer us a great deal of information. But I ran a missionary hospital in Pakistan about 25 years ago, and the nutritional problems there were so multifactorial that even if I had the sophisticated immunology that I do now, it would have been very hard to define the individual responses, because nutritional deprivations were so multifactorial and often came fairly late. Maybe this is the approach that should be taken in the mouse, where you could apply specific and single nutrient deficiencies. We should also go back earlier in development and look at human infants, before we end up with a situation that is too complicated to unravel.

REFERENCE

1. Uhari M, Kontiokari T, Niemela M. A novel use of xylitol sugar in preventing acute otitis media. *Pediatrics* 1998; 102: 879–84.

Nutrition, Immunity, and Infection in Infants and Children, edited by Robert M. Suskind and Kraisid Tontisirin. Nestlé Nutrition Workshop Series, Pediatric Program, Vol. 45. Nestec Ltd., Vevey/Lippincott Williams & Wilkins, Philadelphia ©2001.

The Effect of Protein-Energy Malnutrition on Immune Competence

Bill Woodward

Department of Human Biology and Nutritional Sciences, University of Guelph, Guelph, Ontario, Canada

The most common relationship between protein-energy malnutrition and infection is the synergism expressed in the concept of the malnutrition-infection cycle. Recently, this important concept has been developed further by an analysis showing that primary protein-energy malnutrition increases the risk of childhood mortality from infection in a potent multiplicative manner and with no threshold effect (1). The results pertaining to wasting disease were particularly clear cut, and the impact of all degrees of wasting was revealed to be greater than previously realized. A qualitatively similar impact of the stunting form of protein-energy malnutrition was also apparent (1).

Immunodepression is accepted as a determining factor in the infection-related morbidity and mortality of childhood protein-energy malnutrition. In an extension of this concept, immune competence may be a critical but under-recognized factor in the management of malnutrition, at least where primary malnutrition in childhood is concerned (2). Nutritional deficits typically depress diverse immunologic barriers simultaneously. This is fundamental to the impact of protein-energy malnutrition on a multitiered and tightly integrated physiologic system such as the immune system. Data on stunting malnutrition and immune defenses are scant but suggestive (3), whereas information relating wasting malnutrition to immunocompetence is abundant, although skewed toward grade 3 disease. Therefore, in this chapter the term *protein-energy malnutrition*, when used without qualification, refers to the acute forms of malnutrition.

The focus here is on the impact of protein-energy malnutrition on the physiologically labile immune system of the prepubescent individual. For this purpose, it is assumed that extrapolation from the study of adults requires caution, particularly where an immunologic impact of protein-energy malnutrition is unapparent in the adult. Recent progress of a descriptive nature includes aspects of both innate and adaptive defenses. It is important that our catalogue of descriptive information should continue to grow, but the goal is mechanistic knowledge that will permit rational, targeted interventions and dietary recommendations. Published reports on experimental animals are an invaluable source of insight for this purpose, and an objective here is to show the need to improve the relevance of animal systems to childhood protein-energy malnutrition in its various forms. Finally, the thesis is advanced that the physiologic (including immunologic) response to deficiency of dietary protein and energy is governed by endocrine-mediated metabolic priorities rather than by nonselective distribution of amino acids and energy simply in proportion to level of intake.

INNATE DEFENSES

Physical Barriers

Studies of rodents, albeit young adults, subjected to wasting protein deficiency provide formal evidence in support of the clinical observation that protein-energy malnutrition increases the risk of bacterial translocation (*i.e.*, gut origin septicemia) (4,5). Several characteristics of the gastrointestinal barrier in protein-energy malnutrition are likely contributors to this predisposition. Overgrowth of intestinal microorganisms including Gram-negative organisms is a consistent feature of malnutrition in childhood and in experimental animals (4,6). Stomach acid exerts control over enteric microbial ecology, and hypochlorhydria may be partly responsible for the disruption of the microfloral barrier in the malnourished state (6). In addition, the intestinal mucosa shows atrophy and disruption in childhood and experimental protein-energy malnutrition (4,6), and a particularly important aspect of this phenomenon appears to relate to the integrity of the mucus barrier (5). Early histologic impressions of reduced production of intestinal mucus have been supported more recently by quantitative chemical assays of material from rats, both adolescents subjected to severe stunting (7) and young adults subjected to wasting protein deficiency (5). The water-insoluble layer adherent to the epithelial surface was reported to be the component of intestinal mucus affected (5). Moreover, a malnutrition-associated reduction in the ability of this mucus fraction to bind coliform organisms *in vitro* was apparent (5). This outcome was interpreted as a protective adaptation because it correlated with a reduction in the numbers of mucosa-associated bacteria in the ileum and cecum (5). However, the distribution of bacteria between the mucus layer and the epithelial glycocalyx was not determined, nor was the impact of malnutrition on the adherence characteristics of the intestinal microflora evaluated. Consequently, the opposite interpretation is equally plausible—that is, that protein deficiency in this experimental system reduced the protective blocking action of intestinal mucus (both through a reduction in quantity and through an influence on chemical composition), thereby inducing a predisposition to bacterial translocation. The impact of protein-energy malnutrition on the quantity, composition, and function of epithelial mucus deserves systematic investigation.

Further to the subject of mucous secretions in protein-energy malnutrition, the quantity of saliva (rate of stimulated flow) was found to be reduced in childhood malnutrition, and its chemical composition was altered in a manner consistent with reduced antibacterial activity and a high risk of oral infections, including dental caries (8). These phenomena were identified in both wasting and stunting disease in their severe or even more moderate forms, and complementary findings are reported regarding the bacteria agglutinating glycoproteins of saliva in protein-deficient young adult rats (9). In another investigation, nasopharyngeal and buccal epithelial cells of marasmic children were reported to show an increased propensity to bind coliform bacteria (10). As the latter study involved washed epithelial cells, the results may reflect an impact of protein-energy malnutrition on expression of epithelial membrane glycoproteins rather than an influence on the chemistry or quantity of epithelial mucus.

The Professional Phagocytes: Cell Numbers

Studies on the neutrophil in protein-energy malnutrition are among the earliest contributions to the field of nutritional immunology. The blood neutrophil count is little affected by clinical or experimental malnutrition *per se* (11–13). Infection in malnourished individuals, however, produces neutropenia that has been attributed to involution of the bone marrow neutrophil pool on the indirect basis of the response of the blood neutrophil count to an injection of endotoxin (14). Recent results from a study of adult outbred mice subjected to wasting protein deficiency and sterile inflammation are instructive in this regard (12). Direct counts of femoral marrow cells revealed a modest decline in the size of the mature neutrophil pool, but inflammation-associated neutropenia in this experimental system appeared to result primarily from depressed mobilization of cells from this pool. It is fascinating that terminal differentiation was implicated in the depression of the neutrophil pool size in this experimental system, whereas early myeloid cell proliferation appeared substantially intact (12). In this connection, blood levels of granulocyte-macrophage colony-stimulating factor (GM-CSF) in children with overt infections are reported to be unaffected by protein-energy malnutrition (13) and were increased in a model of weanling murine protein deficiency (15). This type of information is easily overinterpreted in relation to paracrine functions such as a role in myeloid cell proliferation, but clearly these results warrant further investigation.

Late stage differentiation of mononuclear phagocytes is also implicated as a point of impact of protein-energy malnutrition in studies of protein-deficient mice, both young adults (12) and weanlings (15). In the latter system, the malnourished animals showed low blood monocyte counts and Kupffer cell numbers and reduced expression of hepatic M-CSF mRNA, but responded rapidly to exogenous M-CSF (despite continued wasting disease) with a large increase in cell numbers in both compartments. These results may provide the beginnings of an explanation for the long-standing observation (14,16,17) that malnutrition results in depressed numbers of fixed and free-floating macrophages in many species including primates. Low macrophage numbers are also apparent in prepubescent rodents subjected to only moderate degrees of malnutrition that permit weight gain (18).

Clear, quantitative information is lacking to describe the impact of protein-energy malnutrition on the production and turnover of myeloid cells. Although myeloid cell proliferation is probably depressed in malnutrition (15), a basis appears to exist for focusing attention on myeloid cell terminal differentiation as a point of impact of this disease.

Blood Clearance Activity and Phagocytosis

As reviewed briefly elsewhere (19), clearance of colloidal particles and bacteria from the blood is consistently depressed in experimental protein-energy malnutrition, and this has been interpreted to reflect depression in phagocytic activity by hepatic and splenic macrophages *in vivo*. In fact, clearance of colloidal particles from the blood is accomplished by pinocytosis and is a function mainly of cells other than macrophages (*e.g.*, hepatic endothelial and parenchymal cells) (20). Moreover, blood clearance can provide only an indirect measure of phagocytosis or pinocytosis because factors such as blood perfusion and cell numbers also influence clearance rate. In this connection, studies of animals, including primates, collectively indicate that blood clearance in protein-energy malnutrition could be limited by the numbers of reticuloendothelial cells including macrophages (14–17,21).

Where phagocytosis is the clearance mechanism (*e.g.*, in the case of bacteria), opsonizing activity is an additional variable to consider. The opsonizing activity of the blood plasma can be depressed in childhood malnutrition, but this phenomenon is detectable only in diluted samples (22,23), an important observation corroborated by studies of weanling rats (24). Therefore, it must be anticipated that an influence on plasma opsonizing activity is a minor factor in the malnutrition-associated depression of blood clearance. However, although this may apply to particles opsonized primarily by complement fragments (25) or immunoglobulins (22,26), studies with adult rats suggest that fibronectin-dependent opsonization may be more sensitive to malnutrition (19). Moreover, studies with diluted sera may be highly relevant to the opsonizing conditions outside the vascular compartment (14,22), about which no information pertinent to protein-energy malnutrition appears to exist.

The weight of evidence points to the preservation of phagocytic capability in protein-energy malnutrition in childhood and in experimental malnutrition (14,16,19,27). Most studies provide information relating either to phagocytic capacity or to the proportion of phagocytes showing phagocytic activity. Information regarding the influence of protein-energy malnutrition on phagocytic rate concurs (27) but is scant. It is instructive to examine reports indicating a malnutrition-associated depression of phagocytic activity (17,28–31). These relate to the macrophage. In particular, phagocytosis of nonopsonized particles by macrophages is susceptible to depression in protein-deficient rodents (17,28,29,31). Interestingly, this outcome correlates with reduced expression of the macrophage mannose receptor in one experimental system (17), and probably with depressed expression of similar receptors in other rodent systems (18,29). It is questionable whether such results predict phagocytic activity *in vivo*, where opsonization is inevitable. Moreover, depression of phagocytic activity is not predictive of an impact of wasting protein-energy malnutrition on microbicidal capacity (29,30).

The Professional Phagocytes: Microbicidal and Chemotactic Capabilities

Early studies established that a depressed ability to kill ingested bacteria and fungi is characteristic of neutrophils from children suffering from primary protein-energy malnutrition (14). This important phenomenon is reported even in the more moderate degrees of wasting disease (32) as well as in childhood stunting, albeit to a modest degree (3). Likewise, a large impact of malnutrition on the bactericidal activity of neutrophils from suckling rats has been reported (11). The latter results are of interest particularly because infection is unlikely to complicate their interpretation. Thus, protein-energy malnutrition *per se* can exert a large depressive influence on the bactericidal capacity of the neutrophil. Nevertheless, infection is an important confounding factor, as is made clear by the modest depression reported in neutrophil microbicidal activity in childhood malnutrition when overt infection is excluded (14,27). The neutropenia associated with infection in malnutrition is accompanied by disproportionately large numbers of band cells (14). Therefore, the depression reported in microbicidal activity of neutrophils from malnourished children with signs of infection may partly reflect the functional limitations of immature cells.

A reasonably consistent picture has emerged as to the impact of protein-energy malnutrition on the microbicidal (and phagocytic) capacity of the blood neutrophil when these functions are assessed *in vitro*. However, some caution is warranted in the interpretation of this information. Although the neutrophil is a terminally differentiated cell, studies conducted in isolation from inflammatory cytokines and endotoxin can yield false impressions of the functional capabilities of this cell at sites of infection (33).

The same caveat must apply to inconsistent reports on the influence of protein-energy malnutrition on the chemotactic responsiveness of neutrophils in diffusion chambers (14). Where a decrease in neutrophil chemotaxis has been observed in malnutrition, the effect appears to be related to overt infection (14), although aseptic stimuli (*e.g.*, endotoxemia and chronic activation of the complement system) have also been implicated in childhood malnutrition (34). The scant evidence suggests that the chemotactic capability of the neutrophil may be preserved in the more moderate forms of wasting disease (34), and that even grade 3 wasting disease fails to exert a consistent influence (14). The same conclusion must be drawn regarding the macrophage, in which innate chemotactic responsiveness is sometimes maintained (16,24) and sometimes depressed (28) in animal models of protein-energy malnutrition.

Information on the influence of malnutrition on the innate ability of the macrophage to kill bacteria and fungi is somewhat narrowly based on studies of weanling and young adult rats and mice. In systems involving weight loss through protein deficiency, usually no effect is seen on macrophage microbicidal activity when this is assessed directly (*i.e.*, not simply on the basis of related biochemical indices) (16,24,29) and studies of rats subjected to restricted food intake concur (16,30). In one study, the microbicidal activity of alveolar macrophages was assessed *in vivo* and found intact following inhalant bacterial challenge (29). A dissenting report should be acknowledged, in which wasting protein deficiency induced depression in the innate fungicidal activity of resident peritoneal macrophages (17). However, in this experimental system, reduced expression of the macrophage mannose receptor was found, together with reduced phagocytic uptake of the nonopsonized *Candida* organisms used to test microbicidal activity (17). Thus, in general, it appears that the innate microbicidal capability of the macrophage is preserved in the face of acute wasting malnutrition. These results differ from findings relating to the neutrophil, but may reflect the capacity of the macrophage for differentiation, for example in response to the aseptic endotoxemia that can occur in protein-energy malnutrition (14). Although T-cell–stimulated actions of the macrophage are depressed (*e.g.*, granuloma formation) (35), this is attributable to the T-cell component of the reaction system, whereas the macrophage retains responsiveness to lymphocyte-derived activation stimuli (35).

The Professional Phagocytes: the Respiratory Burst

It is instructive to examine reports regarding the influence of protein-energy malnutrition on the respiratory burst of the professional phagocytes. Eliciting stimuli have been delivered using phagocytosable particles, endotoxin, or phorbol myristate acetate, and biochemical indices used to assess this microbicide-related function include oxygen consumption, superoxide or hydrogen peroxide release, nitroblue tetrazolium reduction, fixation of iodine, and the activity of reduced nicotinamide adenine dinucleotide phosphate (NADPH) oxidase or the hexose monophosphate shunt.

The results obtained with neutrophils from children, which are similar to the results of direct measurement of microbicidal activity, implicate infection as a critical confounding factor and source of variable outcomes (14,27). An additional potential source of conflicting information is methodologic and relates to the inconstant application of stimuli to elicit a respiratory burst. For example, no malnutrition-related influence was apparent on nitroblue tetrazolium reduction by unstimulated neutrophils from children with edematous malnutrition, whereas neutrophils from the same subjects showed depressed iodination activity when subjected to a procedure involving stimulation of the respiratory burst (27). Nevertheless, the simplest interpretation of available information is that the primary biochemical basis of depression in neutrophil microbicidal capacity in protein-energy malnutrition is a reduction in the ability to activate NADPH oxidase in response to the stimulus of particle attachment and phagocytosis. A cogent proposal to the physiologic basis for such a phenomenon lies in the well-known hypercortisolemia of protein-energy malnutrition and the inhibitory action of the glucocorticoids on the activity of NADPH oxidase (14). Although this idea has not been tested in relation to the neutrophil, both adrenalectomy and intervention with a glucocorticoid receptor antagonist abolished the depression of superoxide anion production by macrophages in the protein-deficient young adult rat (36).

In contrast to the neutrophil, the macrophage has almost always shown depression in the numerous biochemical indices relating to the respiratory burst in protein-energy malnourished rats and mice (17,21,24,31,36,37), although a report indicating no effect must be noted (16), and little influence was apparent in a model allowing modest weight gain in weanling animals (18). Thus, although malnutrition exerts little impact on the innate ability of macrophages of rats and mice to kill bacteria and fungi, a depressive influence is generally apparent on closely related biochemical activities. Perhaps this reflects a degree of redundancy in the respiratory burst of the macrophage. However, a second possibility must be considered. In addition to the NADPH oxidase-initiated pathway and several oxygen radical-independent mechanisms, macrophages of rats and mice possess an inducible nitric oxide synthase that initiates production of microbicidal, nitrogen-containing radicals (38). The activity of this pathway is depressed in activated macrophages from protein-deficient young adult mice (35,39), but the influence of protein-energy malnutrition on the innate activity of this biochemical pathway in the macrophage remains to be determined.

At this juncture, an important species difference must be emphasized. The professional phagocytes of humans, unlike those of rats and mice, do not possess an inducible nitric oxide synthase and, consequently, do not use nitrogen-containing radicals in killing ingested microorganisms (38). Thus, information about the innate microbicidal activity of the macrophage in protein-energy malnutrition, based as it is on studies of the rat, cannot be extrapolated with confidence to humans. Inasmuch as the tissue macrophage is not easily accessible in human subjects, it will be important to study appropriate animal species (*e.g.*, the rabbit [38] or the guinea pig [35]) to understand the impact of malnutrition on the innate microbicidal activity of the macrophage. Presently no reason is found, on the basis of species peculiarities, for skepticism over the relevance to humans of information obtained from animal models on other functions of this cell in protein-energy malnutrition, for example phagocytosis, chemotaxis, synthesis and release of cytokines and eicosanoids, or antigen-processing and presentation.

The Complement System

Infection is a key factor connecting protein-energy malnutrition and the complement system. In fact, even the most severe forms of primary malnutrition appear to exert only a modest influence on the complement system of children in the absence of overt infection (40,41). In the face of infectious challenge, however, children with malnutrition appear unable to maintain or increase the blood complement protein (C3) concentration or serum complement-mediated lytic bioactivity (40,42). Inasmuch as infection usually accompanies protein-energy malnutrition in children, this phenomenon presumably underlies the low concentrations of blood complement proteins and reduced capacity of serum to support complement-mediated hemolysis (through either the classical or alternative pathways) that is characteristic of protein-energy malnutrition in childhood (14,40–43). By contrast, moderate degrees of wasting malnutrition in childhood have generally been reported to exert little or no influence on the complement system in terms of lytic activity and the blood concentration of C3 (41,43,44), although a dissenting report should be acknowledged (42). Likewise, the sparse information on stunting malnutrition indicates little impact on the complement system (42).

Studies on experimental animals are consistent with the reports on children, for example in regard to the modest impact of protein-energy malnutrition on the complement system in the absence of overt infection (45–51). Experimental studies include investigations of weanling and young adult animals (including rats, guinea pigs, and primates) subjected to weight loss through protein or energy deficit. Nevertheless, less information appears available in experimental malnutrition than in childhood malnutrition regarding blood concentrations of individual complement proteins, particularly of the alternative pathway. Importantly, the studies of animals provide evidence that protein-energy malnutrition attenuates the response of the complement system to infectious challenge (47,48), thereby supporting a key finding relating to malnutrition in childhood. It is noteworthy that reports both on children (41) and on rodents (45) indicate that the complement system is more resistant to malnutrition than is adaptive, cell-mediated immune competence. However, this important comparison has not been made in studies examining the capacity of the complement system to respond to infectious challenge, arguably the most discriminating index of the impact of protein-energy malnutrition on this component of innate defense.

The mechanism whereby protein-energy malnutrition exerts its influence on the complement system is unclear. Indirect evidence stemming from replenishment of blood levels in children during rehabilitation has been interpreted, logically, as indicating that malnutrition reduces the capacity to synthesize complement proteins (14). Nevertheless, adult rats subjected to wasting protein deficiency from prepubescence retained the ability, both in the presence and in the absence of infectious challenge, to synthesize a constellation of complement proteins detectable on the basis of affinity for an antigen–antibody complex (47). In a similar experimental system, the malnourished animals responded to pharmacologic stimulation by increasing the blood concentration of C3 (51), the level of serum complement-mediated lytic activity (51), and the ability of serum to opsonize particles with the C3 fragment, iC3b (25). In the light of these results, quantification of complement protein synthesis rates in malnourished prepubescents would be of great interest. This would require investigations that account for pool sizes of specific complement proteins and of the amino acids used as tracer compounds.

Other evidence suggests that protein-energy malnutrition may influence the complement system partly through enhanced turnover. Thus, early studies revealed a high prevalence of presumptive C3 activation fragments, as well as high concentrations of immunoconglutinin, in the blood of children suffering primary malnutrition (14,40). These observations were recorded in subjects not showing signs of overt infection. Therefore, the reasonable suggestion has emerged that a high rate of consumption of complement proteins is a feature of protein-energy malnutrition, and that this characteristic originates with the aseptic endotoxemia that has been reported in this disease (14). Thus, the well-known attenuation of the inflammatory response in protein-energy malnutrition (14) may result, in part, from a chain of events including hypochlorhydria, intestinal Gram-negative overgrowth, increased entry of endotoxins into the portal blood, reduced clearance of these potent molecules by Kupffer cells, and consequent activation-related losses of complement proteins.

The complement system was among the first components of immune defense to be studied in connection with protein-energy malnutrition, and a sound database was established. During the last 15 years, however, little interest has been seen in pursuing this subject and very little progress has been made. In particular, rigorous information is needed to describe quantitatively the impact of malnutrition and rehabilitation strategies on the synthesis and turnover of complement proteins, especially in the face of infectious challenge.

The Acute Phase Response

A triad of cytokines—tumor necrosis factor-α (TNF-α), interleukin (IL)-1, and IL-6—is produced by the macrophage as a cascade of hormones mediating the acute phase response, although other cytokines may also be involved and IL-6 may be the principal endocrine mediator of the group (52). Recent evidence shows a depression in release (and presumably synthesis) *in vitro* of TNF-α, IL-1, and IL-6 by endotoxin-stimulated monocytes from children with wasting malnutrition (53,54), of TNF-α by macrophages of protein-deficient guinea pigs following stimulation by mycobacterial products (35), and of IL-6 by endotoxin-stimulated macrophages of wasting, protein-deficient young adult rats (36). These results are based on immunoassays and, thus, significantly extend reports of attenuated production of macrophage cytokine bioactivities in comparable systems (55,56). A report must be noted that endotoxin elicited a normal increase in IL-6 production by peripheral blood mononuclear cells from a group of children in whom severe stunting was the prevalent form of protein-energy malnutrition (57). However, the weight of evidence is that malnutrition reduces the capacity of the mononuclear phagocyte to release the cytokines that mediate the acute phase response. A mechanistic clue in this regard derives from studies revealing increased levels of transforming growth factor-β (TGF-β) in the blood of protein-deficient guinea pigs (35). This cytokine can induce depression in TNF-α production by activated macrophages (35).

Despite the foregoing results, children with protein-energy malnutrition and overt infection are reported to sustain blood concentrations of IL-1 that are either normal or only modestly reduced (13), and a small sample of subclinically infected children with malnutrition showed blood levels of IL-6, TNF-α, and (antagonistic) soluble TNF receptors that did not differ from controls with similar laboratory evidence of infection (58). Results of experimental animal studies appear consistent with these findings. Thus, the blood concentration of IL-6 was raised in protein-deficient weanling mice (15), and did not differ from well-nourished controls (except for a modest delay in response) in protein-deficient young adult rats subjected to aseptic inflammatory challenges (59). Presuming blood IL-1, TNF-α, and IL-6 to be produced mainly by mononuclear phagocytes (52), the results suggest that reduced turnover compensates for the impact of malnutrition on the synthesis and release of these cytokines, thus maintaining their circulating concentrations during infectious challenge. The scant information base relating to blood concentrations of the acute phase cytokines and their antagonists in protein-energy malnutrition must be increased if more than a descriptive understanding of the acute phase response is to be achieved in relation to this disease.

Protein-energy malnutrition in children consistently attenuates both the febrile response (13,26) and infection-related neutrophilia (13,14), and studies with experimental animals concur (11,12,60,61). Likewise, an attenuated increase in blood concentrations of acute phase proteins is reported in childhood malnutrition during natural infection (62) or following vaccination (63), as well as in weanling rats subjected to protein deficiency or to food intake restriction together with a sterile inflammatory challenge (64,65). In the studies of malnourished rats, both stunting and wasting deficiencies exerted a measurable impact on the peak response using α2-macroglobulin as the indicator protein. Likewise, an attenuated acute phase protein response has been suggested even in mild childhood malnutrition without wasting (63). Despite these results, an important study of marasmic children emphasized their ability to mount a comprehensive acute phase protein response to infection at a level anticipated among comparable well-nourished subjects, albeit historical controls (66). Similarly, malnourished children with subclinical infections had high blood concentrations of C-reactive protein (58), and wasting protein deficiency did not affect the ability of young adult mice to maintain high blood concentrations of acute phase globulins in response to a sterile inflammation (12). Thus, a substantial increase in blood concentrations of acute phase proteins can be sustained even in the most severe forms of wasting protein-energy malnutrition (although this can be reduced relative to the response mounted by well-nourished subjects), whereas other components of the acute phase response appear to be more severely and consistently affected. It is important to note that the acute phase protein response to infection in childhood malnutrition is reported to be achieved through reduced turnover rather than, as in well-nourished subjects, through increased hepatic synthesis (66).

Collectively, the available information suggests that protein-energy malnutrition usually reduces the capacity of the macrophage to produce the triad of cytokines that regulates the acute phase response. Nevertheless, the ability to sustain high blood levels of these cytokines appears to be maintained in the malnourished state, presumably by way of an influence on turnover, although the database is scant and mechanistic evidence is lacking. The prediction follows that target cell responsiveness to the acute phase cytokines is depressed in protein-energy malnutrition. In this connection, protein-deficient guinea pigs responded to purified IL-1 with a reduction in serum iron and zinc concentrations, but showed neither neutrophilia nor a febrile response (61). In other work, protein-deficient rabbits had a normal fever response when injected with supernatants of activated monocytes (60). Thus, some responsiveness to acute phase cytokines appears to be retained in protein-energy malnutrition, and the level of responsiveness may be target specific. This proposition provides a framework within which to pursue findings such as the report implicating depressed mobilization of neutrophils from the bone marrow in response to inflammatory stimuli in malnutrition (12). Precise, quantitative information is needed as to the impact of protein-energy malnutrition, in its different degrees of severity and various metabolic forms, on the blood concentrations of acute phase cytokines and their soluble inhibitors, and on the response capacity of target cells.

The Natural Killer Cell

The natural killer (NK) cell is considered particularly important in defense against viral diseases, but also may be important in resistance to some prokaryotic intracellular parasites (67). Early findings of depressed NK-cell lytic activity in blood mononuclear cells of children with grade 3 protein-energy malnutrition (68) could not distinguish between an effect on cellular numbers and an effect on cellular activity. These results have been extended recently in a study of protein-deficient weanling mice (69). In this investigation, splenic NK-cell lytic activity declined on a per cell basis, and NK cell numbers declined in proportion with the atrophy of the splenic mononuclear cell compartment.

The mechanism of depression in NK-cell activity is unknown, although overproduction of prostaglandin E_2 (PGE_2) is reported in adolescent (16) and young adult (37) experimental animals subjected to wasting protein deficiency. In addition, the influence of protein-energy malnutrition on γ-interferon production by NK cells has not been investigated despite the probability that this function is a key initiator of the microbicidal action of macrophages and of the primary cell-mediated adaptive immune response (67). With regard to NK cell numbers, nothing is known of the impact of protein-energy malnutrition on NK-cell progenitor activity. Moreover, it remains unknown whether a redistribution of NK cells occurs in malnutrition away from sites such as the spleen wherein these cells are normally located.

A synthesis of evidence developed elsewhere (70) emphasizes the resistance of NK-cell activity to diverse nutritional deficiency conditions. Thus, NK-cell activity is reported to be preserved in stunted children (3). Moreover, adult mice subjected to stunting initiated at weaning showed preservation (71) or only modest depression (72) of splenic NK-cell lytic activity. Although depressed lytic activity of NK cells from children suffering grade 3 protein-energy malnutrition failed to respond to interferon *in vitro* (68) and NK cells of protein-deficient young adult mice likewise failed to respond to IL-2 *in vitro* (73), injections of a drug that generates interferon *in vivo* produced activation of splenic NK-cell lytic activity in stunted, energy-restricted mice (72). Systematic analysis is warranted regarding the responsiveness of NK cells to regulatory signals in protein-energy malnutrition.

ADAPTIVE DEFENSES

Systemic Immune Competence: Humoral and Cell-Mediated Responses

It is a longstanding and firmly established concept that childhood protein-energy malnutrition consistently reduces cell-mediated immune competence but exerts a less predictable impact on the systemic antibody response. As reviewed elsewhere (14,74,75), this is supported by a large weight of evidence that includes studies in which measurements of both humoral and cell-mediated immune competence were made concurrently in the same children or experimental animals. In clinical studies, such comparisons can be complicated by the influence of rehabilitation. This is because cell-mediated responses are commonly examined as delayed hypersensitivity reactions to recall antigens, whereas antibody production—commonly studied as the more slowly developing primary response—is usually examined only after a longer period of rehabilitation. This concern is reinforced by early studies showing more rapid recovery of humoral immunocompetence than of the capacity to generate a cytotoxic T-cell response during rehabilitation of mice from experimental protein-energy malnutrition (76). However, the concern appears to be addressed satisfactorily by several types of investigation, including population-based studies in which clinical intervention was not offered, investigations of experimental animals, and clinical studies in which both humoral and cell-mediated immune responses were assessed as primary reactions (14,74,75). Perhaps the most direct evidence that adaptive cell-mediated and humoral responses differ in sensitivity to protein-energy malnutrition derives from a study of weanling mice in which primary delayed hypersensitivity and antibody responses were each elicited by intraperitoneal administration of sheep red blood cells at the same stage in development of protein deficiency (75).

The delayed hypersensitivity skin test is a critical component of the database relating to cell-mediated immune competence in childhood protein-energy malnutrition. Both primary and recall responses are consistently depressed in this disease (14,26), even with only moderate degrees of wasting (77,78). By contrast, the recall response is reported to be unaffected by stunting (77,78), although other investigators do not concur with this (3) and the point clearly deserves further investigation. Infection has an important depressive influence on delayed cutaneous hypersensitivity in malnutrition (74), but carefully designed studies show that this response is depressed independently of overt infection in childhood malnutrition (77–79). In addition, concurrent infection is unlikely to be a factor in studies of experimental animals; yet primary and recall cutaneous delayed hypersensitivity responses are consistently depressed in diverse species, including primates, subjected to wasting malnutrition (14,45,49,80).

Interpretation of skin test results is also complicated by the depression of the cutaneous inflammatory response that often accompanies malnutrition (74). Thus, a depressed skin test response is not unambiguous evidence of an effect on adaptive cell-mediated immune competence. The same limitation must be recognized in relation to results showing depression in the skin allograft response in experimental protein-energy malnutrition (14,49,81). However, polyclonal mitogen tests in both clinical and experimental settings (14,74), as well as studies of antigen-driven proliferation of T cells from experimental animals (35,56,73,80), adoptive transfer experiments (35,74), and studies of the cytotoxic T-cell response *in vitro* (73,76), show a depressive impact of malnutrition on T-cell functions relating to cell-mediated immunity. In addition, the course of viral, mycobacterial, and protozoan infections in protein-energy malnutrition strongly suggests depression of cell-mediated immune competence through an influence on the T-cell system (74), and an important series of studies with tuberculous guinea pigs (35) has provided clear evidence of this. The latter experimental system has been used to show that effective antimycobacterial resistance, including the capacity to generate a granulomatous reaction, can be restored to protein-deficient animals by adoptive transfer of syngeneic immune T cells (35).

The best evidence pertaining to humoral immunocompetence in childhood malnutrition derives from studies of the serum antibody titer generated in response to vaccination procedures. Even in the most severe forms of wasting disease, outcomes range from depression through normal, and their most outstanding feature appears to be unpredictability (14,26,82). This point is illustrated with clarity in a recent summary of the T-cell–dependent response to tetanus toxoid in malnourished children (82). In this connection, coculture experiments using blood T and B cells from well-nourished and malnourished children indicate that, when this type of response is depressed in protein-energy malnutrition, the phenomenon relates to the competence of T cells rather than of B cells (83). Likewise, a predominant influence of protein-energy malnutrition on T cell help rather than on B cell competence is suggested by early experiments in which adoptive transfer of thymocytes improved the humoral immune competence of protein-deficient weanling mice (14). Thus, studies of humoral immune competence that pertain to regulatory T-cell activities have extended the substantial information base showing depression in both effector and regulatory T-cell actions in protein-energy malnutrition.

The T-cell–independent type of antibody response (e.g., to typhoid O antigen) is also often depressed in malnourished children (26). Although no clear evidence points to a cellular basis for this phenomenon, ontogeny is potentially a variable in the resistance of the B-cell system to the effects of murine protein-energy malnutrition (75,84). Antigen dose can also influence the impact of malnutrition on the antibody response. This was demonstrated in early studies of the T-cell–independent response of protein-deficient weanling rodents (85), and is a phenomenon that should be pursued in exploring the mechanisms of immune depression in protein-energy malnutrition. Concurrent infection often exerts a depressive influence on humoral immune competence in malnutrition (14), and may contribute to the unpredictability of the antibody response in this situation. However, numerous studies of experimental protein-energy malnutrition show depression of T-cell–dependent (84,86,87) and T-cell–independent (85,88) antibody responses, apart from the confounding influence of infection.

Blood concentrations of IgM, IgG, and IgA are generally unaffected or modestly increased in childhood protein-energy malnutrition (14,26). This appears to be the case even in the absence of overt infection, an observation supported by results obtained with weanling mice (89). Nevertheless, concurrent infection is clearly associated with high blood immunoglobulin levels in protein-energy malnutrition (14). In the case of IgG, this has been attributed to increased rates of synthesis in a study of patients with kwashiorkor syndrome (14), thereby providing evidence compatible with humoral immune competence despite the pathology of wasting protein-energy malnutrition.

It is important to note that blood IgM is a mainly polyreactive, low affinity (*natural*) antibody, probably produced by the B1 subset of B cells (90). This subset is also thought to release significant quantities of IgG and IgA class natural immunoglobulin in the absence of high dose antigen exposure, and so it is distinct from the conventional B2 subset that generates the classical high affinity, high specificity antibody response (90). Thus, the malnutrition-associated phenomenon of high or normal blood immunoglobulin levels despite low or normal antibody responses to specific immune challenge could occur if the conventional B2 subset were affected more severely than the B1 subset. In fact, B1 cells appear to participate in the primary antibody response (90), and longstanding reports indicate that malnutrition results in production of low affinity antibody to specific antigenic challenge (14). However, no information is available to address directly the proposition of a subset imbalance between B1 and B2 cells under these conditions.

Mucosal Humoral Immune Competence

Most information on the adaptive defenses in protein-energy malnutrition pertains to systemic responses, despite the fact that most infections in wasting disease are opportunistic mucosal infections. The mucosal secretory IgA antibody response has been widely accepted as more sensitive to wasting disease than systemic humoral immunity. The main reason for this is that IgA concentrations of diverse mucosal secretions, including those of the gastrointestinal tract, salivary glands, lacrimal glands, and nasopharynx, are almost always depressed in childhood malnutrition. This has been reviewed briefly elsewhere (14,89), and is an outcome with which studies of weanling rodents concur (89,91–94). Even grade 2 protein-energy malnutrition is reported to result in low secretory IgA levels in the lacrimal secretions of children (95), although occasional inconsistencies in published reports relating to grade 3 disease are important to acknowledge (95). In addition, the few studies reporting mucosal IgA responses to defined antigens in protein-energy malnutrition consistently demonstrate depression. These reports include only one study of children (96), but several studies of protein-deficient weanling rodents (91,93,97,98).

Nevertheless, the concept that systemic and mucosal antibody responses differ fundamentally in sensitivity to malnutrition deserves renewed attention (99). Recent investigations of weanling mice emphasize the resistance of both systemic and mucosal antibody-producing cellular compartments, even to profound protein deficiency (89). Thus, increases were recorded (per organ) in the numbers of IgG-containing splenic plasma cells and in the numbers of IgA-containing intestinal plasma cells, despite weight loss and atrophy of the inductive compartment of lymphocytes in the two anatomic sites. In addition, indirect evidence has suggested that isotype switching is substantially intact, both to IgG class immunoglobulins in the spleen and to IgA in the lamina propria in experimental weanling protein-energy malnutrition (89). As a further point of similarity between systemic and mucosal humoral competence, malnutrition-associated depression in the intestinal IgA response to oral immunization appears likely to reflect an impact on the action of regulatory T cells (93,98).

In studies of weanling mice subjected to wasting protein deficiency (100), or to a marasmus-like condition (94), expression of the hepatic polymeric immunoglobulin receptor (pIgR), the epithelial IgA-transporting protein, was depressed sufficiently to account for the low concentrations of secretory IgA found in intestinal secretions. These results extend reports that the concentration of free secretory component is low in tears of wasted children, although not in grades 1 and 2 stage disease (95), and in lacrimal secretions, saliva, bile, and intestinal washings of weanling rats and mice subjected to protein-energy malnutrition (92,94,100). Thus, an experimental basis is forming for the proposition that epithelial IgA transport is a focal point of the influence of malnutrition on mucosal immunity, and that immunoglobulin production responds similarly to malnutrition at systemic and mucosal sites. An implication with regard to mucosal defense is that clinical interventions should be aimed at the synthesis and function of the pIgR.

These recent studies relating to mucosal defenses highlight an issue regarding the use of animal models. According to present information, transport of IgA into intestinal mucus is primarily a function of the intestinal epithelium in humans, but is substantially a function of the liver in rats and mice (99). In view of evidence that control of pIgR synthesis differs among anatomic sites (101), these species differences are potentially critical. Consequently, the use of rats and mice may permit identification of the pIgR as a point of impact of protein-energy malnutrition on mucosal immunity, but is arguably unsuitable for mechanistic analyses relevant to the human intestine (99).

Mechanisms of Depression in Adaptive Immunocompetence: Lymphoid Involution

Lymphoid involution, as indicated by the size and cellularity of the thymus and secondary lymphoid organs, is characteristic of wasting malnutrition and is of such magnitude that it must contribute to depression of adaptive immunocompetence (99). The thymus is affected particularly severely, and loss of cortical thymocytes is the most obvious aspect in observational histology. The extent of thymic involution in protein-energy malnutrition has been used in studies suggesting that immunologic recovery from childhood malnutrition (assessed by the size of the thymic shadow) may require more time than recovery of the standard anthropometric indices (2). With regard to the periphery, an estimate of the size of the recirculating pool of lymphocytes in the protein-deficient weanling mouse indicates that secondary lymphoid organ size may yield an inflated impression of the extent of lymphoid involution in malnutrition (86). Likewise, peripheral lymphoid organs can show pronounced differences in the extent of cellular losses in malnutrition, as reported in the weanling mouse (102). Thus, compartment-specific complexities are emerging with regard to malnutrition-associated lymphoid involution, and our inability to predict such outcomes highlights a surprising dearth of mechanistic information. Indeed, a recent study of young adult mice (103) allows the speculation that at least some forms of malnutrition can increase the propensity of T cells to undergo apoptosis following engagement of the T-cell receptor. Depression of proliferative capacity is clearly a feature of lymphocytes in malnutrition (35) but is, logically, a less satisfactory basis than cell death on which to build an understanding of peripheral lymphoid involution. Early studies using adrenalectomized rodents implicated the high levels of glucocorticoids characteristic of protein-energy malnutrition in the involution of lymphoid organs in this disorder (14). It will be important to pursue these threads of evidence and their potential connection. As pointed out elsewhere (99), the thymocyte in malnutrition would be studied more profitably using a species such as the guinea pig rather than other rodents or rabbits. Guinea pigs, like humans and unlike rats, mice, or rabbits, possess cortical thymocytes with a high degree of resistance to glucocorticoid-mediated lysis.

Information from observational histology and blood leukocyte counts is widely interpreted as showing that malnutrition causes a greater reduction in T-cell numbers than in B-cell numbers (104). To the extent that the blood lymphocyte compartment is informative in this regard, more moderate forms of wasting disease in children may exert a similar disproportionate impact on the T-cell system (78), whereas this is not the case in stunted children (3). Despite a low blood T-cell count, lymphopenia is relatively rare in childhood malnutrition (14,26). This may be attributed, at least in part, to the large numbers of immature T-lineage cells that are found in the blood in this condition (14,26) and which have most recently been quantified by means of the surface marker, CD1a (105). It is of interest that *in vitro* exposure of blood mononuclear cells from malnourished children to thymic hormones, or to extracts containing such peptides, effects a rapid increase in the numbers of phenotypically mature T cells and a corresponding decrease in the numbers of immature cells (104,105). Thus, depression in adaptive immune competence in malnutrition may result, in part, from release of thymocytes that have received insufficient maturational stimuli. This concept may be extended to include the B-cell system on the basis of indirect phenotypic evidence suggesting premature release of B-lineage cells from the bone marrow of protein-deficient weanling rats (93).

Despite the potential importance of primary lymphoid organs in relation to the capacity of wasted subjects to respond to therapeutic interventions, little is known about lymphopoiesis in protein-energy malnutrition, and no information is available on the impact on the T-cell or B-cell repertoire. However, an immunohistochemical analysis produced evidence of depressed production of thymulin by the thymic epithelium in children suffering various forms of grade 3 wasting malnutrition but without overt infection (106). Even stunting malnutrition in children is reported to produce a modest depression in serum thymulin bioactivity (3), albeit much less marked than in wasted children and weanling rodents (104). Moreover, studies of weanling mice subjected to wasting through either protein or energy deficiencies revealed profound atrophy of the thymic epithelium, together with ultrastructural evidence of derangements in the secretory vacuolar apparatus of this tissue (104). The impact on the vacuolar apparatus was detectable sufficiently early in the progress of malnutrition to permit the proposition that the thymic epithelium is a primary point of impact of protein-energy malnutrition on adaptive immune competence (104).

Mechanisms of Depression in Adaptive Immunocompetence: T Cell Subset Imbalances

Imbalances between or among critical subsets of lymphocytes may also contribute to the initiation or the continuation of malnutrition-induced immunodepression. This important concept originates with the discovery of a low CD4:CD8 ratio in the blood of malnourished human subjects (99). The same phenomenon is reported in weanling mice (102) and has become widely accepted as a key factor in the depression of T-cell–dependent immunity in protein-energy malnutrition (99,104). In fact, however, a low blood CD4:CD8 ratio sometimes fails to develop in malnutrition, both in children (105) and in weanling rodents (102). Moreover, diverse rodent models of weanling malnutrition show profound depression of T-cell–dependent adaptive responses in the absence of a low CD4:CD8 ratio, either within the circulating surveillance pool of T cells or within the secondary lymphoid organs in which immune responses are initiated (86,87,102). Recent studies of tuberculous, protein-deficient guinea pigs reveal an extremely low CD4:CD8 ratio in the lymph nodes draining the infected lungs (35). However, this phenomenon appears to reflect an influx of CD8$^+$ (presumptive) effectors rather than a paucity of CD4$^+$ T cells. A low CD4:CD8 ratio, therefore, commonly occurs in the blood in protein-energy malnutrition but appears unnecessary and generally irrelevant to immunodepression. In fact, the CD4:CD8 ratio is not reliable as a helper-to-suppressor index, or even as a helper versus suppressor/cytotoxic index. Many recirculating suppressor T cells, for example, may show a CD4$^+$ phenotype (107). In addition, CD8$^+$ T cells are a major source of cytokines that serve in a helper capacity (108).

In this context is seen an important caveat relating to the interpretation of blood lymphocyte data. The blood is a small and unique lymphoid compartment in which disease-related disturbances among lymphocytes are often unrepresentative of events within the secondary lymphoid organs (109). Therefore, although the use of blood lymphocyte data in studies on human subjects is fully understandable, it is subject to overinterpretation, as has occurred in relation to the CD4:CD8 ratio.

An overabundance of the quiescent, CD45RA$^+$ (naive) phenotype has been identified recently within the involuted T-cell compartment of the blood and secondary lymphoid organs of weanling mice subjected to either energy restriction or protein deficiency (87,110). This naive shift was apparent in both CD4$^+$ and CD8$^+$ T-cell subsets, and similar results are reported in the blood of elderly humans with protein-energy malnutrition (111). At this stage, the phenomenon appears likely to contribute to immune depression only in the advanced stages of protein-energy malnutrition (110). In addition, information on this imbalance is confined to analysis of surface phenotype and, thus, relates only indirectly to cellular function. Nevertheless, the phenomenon is interesting in the light of the recent proposition that T cells of protein-deficient, tuberculous guinea pigs home preferentially to the lymph nodes draining the infected lungs (35). Such trafficking behavior would be expected of naive type T cells which show a migratory preference for lymphoid rather than nonlymphoid sites (112). Likewise, homing to the small intestine was depressed on the part of lymphoblasts adoptively transferred from protein-deficient rats, whereas localization within the associated mesenteric lymph nodes was not affected (113). Finally, it is noteworthy that experimental protein-energy malnutrition has occasionally been reported to impose immunodepression without affecting the ability of T cells to show antigen-driven proliferation (114,115). This is interesting because naive phenotype T cells are capable of matching memory phenotype cells in terms of proliferation if their stringent activation requirements are met (116). Thus, an understanding of the real significance of an overabundance of naive phenotype T cells in protein-energy malnutrition requires precise information on the cytokine and antigen presentation microenvironments within which these cells must function in this disease.

Mechanisms of Depression in Adaptive Immunocompetence: Antigen Processing and Presentation

The influence of protein-energy malnutrition on antigen processing and presentation has been studied only in rodent systems, and information is scant. One study has addressed the influence of malnutrition on antigen processing and presentation for the primary response (114). This is accomplished by the dendritic cell, which is uniquely capable of meeting the activation requirements of naive type T cells (117). Thus, the ability of spleen cells to stimulate a mixed leukocyte response, the classic assay of dendritic cell competence (117), was depressed in mice subjected to protein deficiency from weaning through young adulthood (114). The results did not distinguish between effects on cellular numbers and cellular function. However, a recent report shows that the numbers of mature splenic dendritic cells are much reduced in the advanced stages of weaning protein or energy deficiency in the mouse (118). Presently, no information is available on the impact of malnutrition on the functional capacity of dendritic cells. In addition, information about dendritic cells in malnutrition is at present confined to the spleen, an important limitation in view of the heterogeneity of these cells in diverse lymphoid sites (117). Studies of the development and function of dendritic cells in malnutrition are needed to improve our understanding of the primary adaptive immune response in this disorder.

Some information is available on antigen processing and presentation in the secondary response in protein-energy malnutrition. Thus, in a study of weanling mice subjected to energy restriction sufficient to produce stunting and modest lymphoid involution, splenic cellular suspensions containing the three professional antigen-presenting cells (B cells, macrophages, and dendritic cells) showed a reduced capacity to stimulate antigen-induced proliferation and production of γ-interferon by memory T cells (115). These results appear likely to reflect reduced function on a per cell basis. Comparable findings derive from a study of protein-deficient mice in which antigen-presenting cells—undoubtedly a mixture of macrophages, B cells, and dendritic cells—were recovered from the peritoneum (119). As in a report pertaining exclusively to dendritic cells (114), the latter study suggested that antigen presentation (rather than uptake and processing) is the main point of impact of malnutrition on the cellular functions that prepare antigen for recognition by T cells. Although reduced production of IL-1 has been implicated mechanistically (114), systematic analysis of the competence of antigen-presenting cells in malnutrition is lacking. In view of results showing that T cells from rodents subjected to either protein or energy deficiencies sometimes retain their capacity to respond to appropriately presented antigen, for example in terms of proliferative capacity (114,115), improved knowledge of antigen processing and presentation in malnutrition is important.

Mechanisms of Depression in Adaptive Immunocompetence: Cytokines

Early reports, summarized elsewhere (55), indicated depression in the production of several cytokine bioactivities—including macrophage migration inhibition factor, viral interferons, and leukocyte inhibition factor—by blood leukocytes in childhood malnutrition. More recent results showed that the production of IL-6 by mitogen-stimulated blood T cells was unaffected by malnutrition in children from a predominantly stunted population (57). In addition, severe protein-energy malnutrition, but not more moderate forms of the disease, caused depression in the capacity to produce IL-2 on the part of blood T cells of elderly human subjects (111). A scant and disperse literature, therefore, documents the impact of protein-energy malnutrition on cytokine production by lymphocytes in humans, and the results suggest that the degree and type of malnutrition is important to the outcome.

Current understanding of lymphocyte-derived cytokines in prepubescent malnutrition is based mainly on studies of experimental animals. Although not extensive, these results are clearly germane to the depression in various indices of cell-mediated immunocompetence that characterize protein-energy malnutrition, including reports of an inability to generate a granulomatous response to infection with facultative intracellular parasites (35,120). Thus, depressed production of IL-2 is reported in studies of mitogen- and antigen-stimulated blood and splenic T cells from protein-deficient guinea pigs (35,80) and adolescent rats (121). Together with evidence of reduced responsiveness to this cytokine in the protein-deficient guinea pig system (35,80), these findings initiate an explanation of the characteristically low T-cell proliferative capacity in malnutrition. Depressed γ-interferon production is also reported consistently in experimental protein-energy malnutrition. Thus, γ-interferon production was low in concanavalin A-stimulated splenic mononuclear cells from adolescent rats subjected to wasting protein deficiency (121). In this system, the mRNA level for γ-interferon was depressed in parallel with the level of functional protein assessed by bioassay, and γ-interferon was affected more severely than IL-2 in terms of both protein and transcript levels. In addition, modest energy restriction was sufficient to depress antigen-stimulated γ-interferon production by splenic mononuclear cells from nematode-infected weanling mice (115), and the level of mRNA for this cytokine was depressed in the lungs of protein-deficient young adult mice during the early stages of tuberculosis infection (120). In other work with mice subjected to protein deficiency from weaning to young adulthood, depression was noted both in production of macrophage migration inhibition factor by mitogen-stimulated splenic T cells and in responsiveness to this cytokine by peritoneal macrophages, although an impact on responsiveness could not be confirmed in studies of protein-deficient guinea pigs (35).

It is important to recognize that cytokines function in networks and show redundancy. Consequently, full appreciation of the involvement of these regulatory molecules in the immunopathology of protein-energy malnutrition requires that they be studied simultaneously as networks. Although this has not yet been done in the context of malnutrition, three examples of the study of abbreviated panels of T-cell cytokines in this disorder serve to illustrate the potential of such a research strategy. Thus, the ability of splenic T cells to produce IL-4, IL-5, and IL-10 in response to antigenic stimulation *in vitro* was unaffected by energy restriction of nematode-infected weanling mice, whereas production of γ-interferon was depressed (115). Likewise, a protein-deficiency protocol that produced depressed resistance to *Candida* in young adult mice also produced depression in the production of γ-interferon while exerting no effect on the production of IL-4 or IL-10 by mitogen-stimulated splenic T cells (39). These important outcomes are suggestive in relation to the sensitivity to malnutrition shown by cell-mediated immunocompetence relative to antibody responses. Similarly, recent results point to cytokine balance as a basis for understanding the enhancement in cell-mediated immunocompetence that occurs in some rodent models of stunting protein deficiency. In such an experimental system, the capacity of murine splenic T cells to release IL-2 and γ-interferon when stimulated with anti-CD3 *in vitro* was preserved or increased, whereas the capacity to release IL-4 was depressed (122).

Both cytokine production and the responsiveness of cytokine targets in protein-energy malnutrition deserve systematic investigation, with attention to the impact of malnutrition on the balance between Th1- and Th2-type cytokines. Proposals about the physiologic basis for altered cytokine production in malnutrition include a shift in eicosanoid metabolism favoring cyclo-oxygenase products (16) and glucocorticoid-mediated depression of the synthesis of numerous cytokines (99). In addition, an intriguing recent study reports increased bioactivity of the broadly immunosuppressive cytokine, TGF-β, in the blood of protein-deficient guinea pigs (35). This could downregulate the synthesis of numerous cytokines (123) and might underlie early reports (124) that blood plasma from children with protein-energy malnutrition shows a reduced capacity to support T-cell functions (*e.g.*, blastogenesis) *in vitro*. Knowledge relating to the control of cytokine activities in malnutrition requires much refinement to accommodate the complex variation in the effects on these regulatory proteins in different forms of malnutrition.

IMMUNODEPRESSION: A COMPONENT OF THE SYSTEMIC PATHOPHYSIOLOGY OF PROTEIN-ENERGY MALNUTRITION

It appears widely accepted that synthesis of proteins and other amino acid-containing compounds in protein-energy malnutrition is nonselectively depressed because of a general shortage of amino acid substrate or energy. This model is often invoked as underlying the malnutrition-induced depression of immunologic functions (*e.g.*, antibody or cytokine synthesis and antigen-driven clonal expansion of lymphocytes).

Fine control at the level of transcription, however, has been reported in relation to hepatic protein synthesis when wasting protein deficiency was imposed on weanling rodents (125). Thus, transcript levels were low relative to total cellular RNA for some proteins (*e.g.*, albumin), but were either unaffected or even increased for others (*e.g.*, ubiquitin). A similar effect is seen in the control of leukotriene (LT) synthesis in kwashiorkor. Although amino acids and glutathione are in limited supply in this condition, leukotriene synthesis has been reported to shift from LTB_4 toward the synthesis of the cysteinyl compounds LTC_4 and LTE_4 (126). Thus, the classical model connecting low intake of amino acids and energy directly to a generalized reduction in protein synthesis does not accommodate available information on malnutrition in childhood or on experimental protein-energy malnutrition. This point has occasionally been made elsewhere (12,99).

The physiologic response to malnutrition is orchestrated by endocrine hormones that govern the systemic distribution of substrates and energy (99). Thus, it is critical that the immunobiology of protein-energy malnutrition is understood in the context of the hormonally mediated reorganization of metabolism in this disorder (99,104), and much current interest focuses on the glucocorticoids. For example, depressed synthesis of IL-6 and of the superoxide radical by macrophages is prevented by either adrenalectomy or the administration of a glucocorticoid receptor antagonist in a model of protein-deficient young adult mice that features the high blood glucocorticoid concentrations characteristic of protein-energy malnutrition (36). As a second example, in systems of either protein- or energy-deficient weanling mice, administration of triiodothyronine can prevent the development of depression of primary adaptive immunocompetence (81) as well as depression of splenic NK-cell lytic activity (69). In the cited examples, the hormonal interventions achieved immunomodulation in the presence of unabated weight loss and profound lymphoid atrophy. Some experimental evidence, therefore, points to the concept that the endocrine microenvironment is likely to define the limits of immunocompetence in protein-energy malnutrition. Recent evidence, including results from studies of short-term murine starvation, implicates leptin as an endocrine link between nutritional status and immune competence (127). Perhaps this new clue will stimulate research leading to a cohesive knowledge of the immune-endocrine nexus in protein-energy malnutrition.

KEY FEATURES OF DESIGN IN STUDIES OF EXPERIMENTAL PROTEIN-ENERGY MALNUTRITION

An urgent need exists to establish criteria and standards for assessing the nutritional status of animals in studies of experimental protein-energy malnutrition. At present, it is difficult to assign most experimental animal systems to any particular category of human malnutrition, and this problem limits the relevance of experimental studies to the human disease. Two critical variables are stage of life and the nature of the diet-induced disease (*i.e.*, whether the form of protein-energy malnutrition imposed is stunting or wasting and whether it should be classified as moderate or severe). These points have been discussed elsewhere (99).

Stage of life appears to have a critical influence on the impact of both wasting and stunting forms of protein-energy malnutrition on immune function (99). For example, the rejection response to a completely MHC disparate skin allograft was profoundly depressed in wasting protein-deficient weanling mice (81). This reflects a depression in the competence of naive T cells of both $CD4^+$ and $CD8^+$ phenotypes. In contrast, a comparable primary one-way mixed leukocyte reaction revealed functional sufficiency on the part of naive $CD4^+$ and $CD8^+$ T cells from wasted, protein-deficient adult mice (56). Also in connection with adaptive immunity, the ability of murine macrophages (in a preparation probably also containing dendritic cells) to present antigen *in vitro* to memory T cells was unaffected even by severe wasting protein deficiency when imposed at the adult stage of life (56), an outcome contrasting with results of similar studies of antigen presentation in weanling protein-energy malnutrition (115,119). In relation to innate defenses, the capacity of macrophages to synthesize and release IL-1 and TNF-α bioactivities was preserved in young adult mice subjected to nonedematous (*i.e.*, marasmic type) protein-energy malnutrition (128), and comparable findings are reported relating to the production of IL-1, IL-6, and TNF-α by monocytes from elderly human subjects with nonedematous protein-energy malnutrition secondary to a variety of noninfectious, nonmalignant conditions (129). These results contrast with the depressive influence of marasmus on the production of these cytokines by monocytes from children (53,54).

Apart from the factor of physiologic age, diet composition is a critical point of misunderstanding and misinterpretation relating to studies of experimental protein-energy malnutrition. It is important to duplicate the critical features that characterize a human pathology, but less important to reproduce the details of the human diet that produced the pathology. Currently, much skepticism as to the value of studies with experimental animals centers on the details of dietary composition. However, it is not surprising that species differences exist relating to the details of the diet required to produce a particular pathology. For example, it is reasonable to expect that a lower dietary protein content would be required to produce the signs of kwashiorkor in a coprophagous animal such as a rodent than in children. As a separate but related point, it is desirable that growth and physiologic indices should be applied as rigorously in studies of animals as they are in studies of children. However, to render this possible, it is necessary to establish standards that can be used to connect experimental models with specific categories of wasting and stunting malnutrition in childhood. Currently, this essential information base is entirely lacking.

A third point regarding experimental design relates to the need for a zero-time control group in order to identify diet-induced immunologic change unambiguously. This design feature is rare, but is particularly important where diet-related influences can be confounded by ontogeny. For example, in a recent study of protein-deficient weanling mice (89), comparison with an age-matched control group emphasized the small sizes of both the splenic IgG-containing cell compartment and the intestinal IgA-containing cell compartment in the deficient animals. It would be easy to interpret these results as reflecting compartmental atrophy. Comparison with a zero-time control group, however, revealed a malnutrition-associated attenuation of the ontogenetic expansion in splenic and intestinal plasma cell numbers. This feature of design, thus, provided an important additional perspective by highlighting the remarkable resistance of both mucosal and systemic antibody-producing effector compartments to wasting disease, even in the weanling animal.

CONCLUDING PERSPECTIVE

A substantial catalogue of clinical and experimental information documents the influence of protein-energy malnutrition on immune defenses in the young. This body of immunologic knowledge must continue to grow, particularly in relation to stunting disease and the more moderate forms of wasting malnutrition. Research directions with a mechanistic focus have also emerged. These activities include research into cellular and molecular mechanisms and, at least as importantly, investigations aimed at a metabolically integrated understanding of malnutrition-associated immune depression as a component of the systemic, endocrine-mediated attempt to adapt to dietary deprivation. Thus, even in wasting malnutrition, it is probable that the associated immunodepression has adaptive value, although it imposes an unacceptable cost in terms of risk of opportunistic infection (104). A key factor limiting opportunities to develop depth of knowledge on immunocompetence in protein-energy malnutrition is the paucity of thoroughly characterized experimental animal models and the complete absence of growth and physiologic standards that would allow animal systems to be clearly related to established categories of childhood malnutrition. Finally, although research on the immunologic response to protein-energy malnutrition must continue, recent evidence suggests that microorganisms may also respond to the nutritional status of the malnourished host (130). Thus, a diet-induced compromise of antioxidant defenses can promote mutation to pathogenicity on the part of normally avirulent microorganisms. As antioxidant status appears to be compromised in some forms of protein-energy malnutrition, a new dimension may be emerging in the host–microbe interaction in this disease.

REFERENCES

1. Pelletier DL. The relationship between child anthropometry and mortality in developing countries: implications for policy, programs and future research. *J Nutr* 1994; 124: 2047–81S.
2. Chevalier P, Sevilla R, Sejas E, et al. Immune recovery of malnourished children takes longer than nutritional recovery: implications for treatment and discharge. *J Trop Pediatr* 1998; 44: 304–7.
3. Chandra RK, Sarchielli P. Body size and immune responses. *Nutr Res* 1996; 16: 1813–19.
4. Deitch EA, Ma W-J, Ma L, et al. Protein malnutrition predisposes to inflammatory-induced gut-origin septic states. *Ann Surg* 1990; 211: 560–7.
5. Katayama M, Xu D, Specian RD, et al. Role of bacterial adherence and the mucus barrier on bacterial translocation: effects of protein malnutrition and endotoxin in rats. *Ann Surg* 1997; 225: 317–26.
6. Brunser O, Araya M, Espinoza J. Gastrointestinal tract changes in the malnourished child. In: Suskind RM, Lewinter-Suskind L, eds. *The malnourished child.* Nestlé Nutrition Workshop Series, No. 19. New York: Raven Press, 1990: 261–72.
7. Sherman P, Forstner J, Roomi N, et al. Mucin depletion in the intestine of malnourished rats. *Am J Physiol* 1985; 248: G418–23.
8. Johansson I, Saellstrom A-K, Rajan BP, et al. Salivary flow and dental caries in Indian children suffering from chronic malnutrition. *Caries Res* 1992; 26: 38–43.

9. Johansson I, Ericson T. Biosynthesis of salivary bacteria-agglutinating glycoprotein in the rat during protein deficiency. *Caries Res* 1987; 21: 7–14.
10. Chandra RK, Gupta SP. Increased bacterial adherence to respiratory and buccal epithelial cells in protein-energy malnutrition. *Immunol Infect Dis* 1991; 1: 55–7.
11. Nwankwo MU, Schuit KE, Glew RH. Effects of maternal protein deprivation on the nutritional status and neutrophil function of suckling neonatal rats. *J Infect Dis* 1985; 151: 23–32.
12. Borelli P, Mariano M, Borojevic R. Protein malnutrition: effect on myeloid cell production and mobilization into inflammatory reactions in mice. *Nutr Res* 1995; 15: 1477–85.
13. Aslan Y, Erduran E, Gedik Y, et al. Serum interleukin-1 and granulocyte-macrophage colony stimulating factor levels in protein malnourished patients during acute infection. *Cent Afr J Med* 1996; 42: 179–84.
14. Gross RL, Newberne PM. Role of nutrition in immunologic function. *Physiol Rev* 1980; 60: 188–302.
15. Honda Y, Takahashi K, Naito M, Fujiyama S. The role of macrophage colony-stimulating factor in the differentiation and proliferation of Kupffer cells in the liver of protein-deprived mice. *Lab Invest* 1995; 72: 3696–706.
16. Skerrett SJ, Henderson WR, Martin TR. Alveolar macrophage function in rats with severe protein calorie malnutrition. *J Immunol* 1992; 144: 1052–61.
17. Redmond PH, Leon P, Lieberman MD, et al. Impaired macrophage function in severe protein-energy malnutrition. *Arch Surg* 1991; 126: 192–6.
18. Papadimitriou JM, van Bruggen I. The effects of malnutrition on murine peritoneal macrophages. *Exp Mol Pathol* 1988; 49: 161–70.
19. Dillon BC, Saba TM, Cho E, et al. Opsonic fibronectin deficiency in the etiology of starvation-induced reticuloendothelial phagocytic dysfunction. *Exp Mol Pathol* 1982; 36: 177–92.
20. Praaning-van Dalen DP, Brouwer A, Knook DL. Clearance capacity of rat liver Kupffer, endothelial and parenchymal cells. *Gastroenterology* 1981; 81: 1036–44.
21. Reynolds JV, Redmond HP, Ueno N, et al. Impairment of macrophage activation and granuloma formation by protein deprivation in mice. *Cell Immunol* 1992; 139: 493–504.
22. Keusch GT, Urrutia JJ, Guerrero O, et al. Serum opsonic activity in acute protein-energy malnutrition. *Bull World Health Organ* 1981; 59: 923–9.
23. Keusch GT, Torun B, Johnston RB, et al. Impairment of hemolytic complement activation by both classical and alternative pathways in serum from patients with kwashiorkor. *J Pediatr* 1984; 105: 434–6.
24. Keusch GT, Douglas SD, Hammer G, et al. Antibacterial functions of macrophages in experimental protein-calorie malnutrition. II. Cellular and humoral factors for chemotaxis, phagocytosis, and intracellular bactericidal activity. *J Infect Dis* 1978; 138: 134–42.
25. Sakamoto M, Nishioka K. Complement system in nutritional deficiency. *World Rev Nutr Diet* 1992; 67: 114–39.
26. Keusch GT. Malnutrition, infection, and immune function. In: Suskind RM, Lewinter-Suskind L, eds. *The malnourished child.* Nestlé Nutrition Series No 19. New York: Raven Press, 1990: 37–55.
27. Salimonu LS, Johnson AOK, Williams AIO, et al. Phagocyte function in protein-calorie malnutrition. *Nutr Res* 1982; 2: 445–54.
28. Weeks B. Effects of age and nutrition on macrophage function. *Journal of the Reticuloendothelial Society* 1979; 26: 459–62.
29. Jakab GJ, Warr GA, Astry CL. Alterations of pulmonary defense mechanisms by protein depletion diet. *Infect Immun* 1981; 34: 610–22.
30. Shennib H, Chiu RC-J, Mulder DS, et al. Depression and delayed recovery of alveolar macrophage function during starvation and refeeding. *Surg Gynecol Obstet* 1984; 158: 535–40.
31. Machaiah JP. Effects of protein restriction on functional properties of rat peritoneal macrophages. *Indian J Exp Biol* 1991; 29: 468–73.
32. Tuck R, Burke V, Gracey A, et al. Defective *Candida* killing in childhood malnutrition. *Arch Dis Child* 1979; 54: 445–7.
33. Surette ME, Dallaire N, Jean N, et al. Mechanisms of the priming effect of lipopolysaccharides on the biosynthesis of leukotriene B4 in chemotactic peptide-stimulated human neutrophils. *FASEB J* 1998; 12: 1521–31.
34. Anderson DC, Krishna GS, Hughes BJ, et al. Impaired polymorphonuclear leukocyte motility in malnourished infants: relationship to functional abnormalities of cell adherence. *J Lab Clin Med* 1983; 101: 881–95.

35. McMurray DN. Impact of nutritional deficiencies on resistance to experimental pulmonary tuberculosis. *Nutr Rev* 1998; 56: S147–52.
36. Hill ADK, Naama HA, Gallagher HJ, et al. Glucocorticoids mediate macrophage dysfunction in protein-calorie malnutrition. *Surgery* 1995; 118: 130–7.
37. Redmond HP, Shou J, Kelly CJ, et al. Immunosuppressive mechanisms in protein-calorie malnutrition. *Surgery* 1991; 110: 311–17.
38. Schneemann M, Schoedon G, Hofer S, et al. Nitric oxide synthase is not a constituent of the antimicrobial armature of human mononuclear phagocytes. *J Infect Dis* 1993; 167: 1358–63.
39. Hill ADK, Naama H, Shou J, et al. Antimicrobial effects of granulocyte-macrophage colony-stimulating factor in protein-energy malnutrition. *Arch Surg* 1995; 130: 1273–8.
40. Chandra RK. Serum complement and immunoconglutinin in malnutrition. *Arch Dis Child* 1975; 50: 225–9.
41. Sakamoto M. The sequence of recovery of the complement systems and phytohemagglutinin skin reactivity in malnutrition. *Nutr Res* 1982; 2: 137–45.
42. Kielmann AA, Curcio LM. Complement (C3), nutrition, and infection. *Bull World Health Organ* 1979; 57: 113–21.
43. Jagadeesan V, Reddy V. Serum complement levels in malnourished children. *Indian J Med Res* 1979; 70: 745–9.
44. Reyes MA, Saravia NG, Watson RR, et al. Effect of moderate malnutrition on immediate hypersensitivity and immunoglobulin E levels in asthmatic children. *J Allergy Clin Immunol* 1982; 70: 94–100.
45. Sakamoto M, Nishioka K, Shimada K. Effect of malnutrition and nutritional rehabilitation on tuberculin reactivity and complement level in rats. *Immunology* 1979; 38: 413–20.
46. Petersen BH, Watson RR, Holmes DH. Protein malnutrition and complement activity in guinea pigs, germ-free and conventional rats. *J Nutr* 1980; 110: 2159–65.
47. Sakamoto M, Ishii S, Nishioka K, et al. Incorporation of [^{14}C]-leucine into complement in experimental infection of rats in malnourished stages. *Am J Clin Nutr* 1981; 34: 2127–32.
48. Sakamoto M, Ishii S, Nishioka K, et al. Level of complement activity and components C1, C4, C2, and C3 in complement response to bacterial challenge in malnourished rats. *Infect Immun* 1981; 32: 553–6.
49. Qazzaz ST, Mamattah JHK, Ashcroft T, et al. The development and nature of immune deficit in primates in response to malnutrition. *Br J Exp Pathol* 1981; 62: 452–60.
50. Lanza-Jacoby S, Skibber J, Miller E, et al. Effect of protein malnutrition and tumor growth on serum total complement, C3, and IgG levels during *E. coli* infection in the rat. *Nutr Res* 1982; 2: 277–87.
51. Sakamoto M, Ishii S, Nishioka K. Heightened resistance against *Listeria monocytogenes* injection in malnourished rats after lentinan treatment: correlation with C3 levels. *Nutr Res* 1983; 3: 705–18.
52. Moldawar LL, Lowry SF. Interactions between cytokine production and inflammation: implications for therapies aimed at modulating the host defence to infection. In: Cunningham-Rundles S, ed. *Nutrient modulation of the immune response*. New York: Marcel Dekker, 1993: 511–23.
53. Doherty JF, Golden MHN, Remick DG, Griffin GE. Production of interleukin-6 and tumor necrosis factorα in vitro is reduced in whole blood of severely malnourished children. *Clin Sci* 1994; 86: 347–51.
54. Munoz C, Arevalo MT, Lopez M, et al. Impaired interleukin-1 and tumor necrosis factor production in protein-calorie malnutrition. *Nutr Res* 1994; 14: 347–52.
55. Woodward WD. Morphometric and functional studies of the thymus and production of cytokines in protein-energy malnutrition. In: Young KW, Cha LY, Yull LK, Soon JJ, He KS, eds. *Proceedings of XIV International Congress of Nutrition*, Vol 1. Seoul, 1989: 281–4.
56. Redmond HP, Gallagher HJ, Shou J, et al. Antigen presentation in protein-energy malnutrition. *Cell Immunol* 1995; 163: 80–7.
57. Malave I, Vethencourt MA, Chacon R, et al. Production of interleukin-6 in cultures of peripheral blood mononuclear cells from children with primary protein-calorie malnutrition and from eutrophic controls. *Ann Nutr Metab* 1998; 42: 266–73.
58. Sauerwein RW, Mulder JA, Mulder L, et al. Inflammatory mediators in children with protein-energy malnutrition. *Am J Clin Nutr* 1997; 65: 1534–9.
59. Lyoumi S, Tamion F, Petit J, et al. Induction and modulation of acute-phase response by protein malnutrition in rats: comparative effect of systemic and localized inflammation on interleukin-6 and acute-phase protein synthesis. *J Nutr* 1998; 128: 166–74.

60. Hoffman-Goetz L, Kluger MJ. Protein deprivation: its effects on fever and plasma iron during bacterial infection in rabbits. *J Physiol* (Lond) 1979; 295: 419–25.
61. Drabik MD, Schnure FC, Mok KT, et al. Effect of protein depletion and short-term parenteral refeeding on the host response to interleukin 1 administration. *J Lab Clin Med* 1987; 109: 509–16.
62. Duran-Chavez C, Sanchez-Herrera G, Canedo-Solares I, et al. C-reactive protein in severely malnourished children. *Nutr Res* 1994; 14: 967–75.
63. Doherty JF, Golden MHN, Raynes JG, et al. Acute-phase protein response is impaired in severely malnourished children. *Clin Sci* 1993; 84: 169–75.
64. Jennings G, Bourgeois C, Elia M. The magnitude of the acute phase protein response is attenuated by protein deficiency in rats. *J Nutr* 1992; 122: 1325–31.
65. Jennings G, Elia M. Effect of dietary restriction on the response of 2-macroglobulin during an acute phase response. *JPEN* 1994; 18: 510–5.
66. Morlese JF, Forrester T, Jahoor F. Acute-phase protein response to infection in severe malnutrition. *Am J Physiol* 1998; 38: E112–7.
67. Scott P, Trinchieri G. The role of natural killer cells in host-parasite interactions. *Curr Opin Immunol* 1995; 7: 34–40.
68. Salimonu LS, Ojo-Amaize E, Williams AIO, et al. Depressed natural killer cell activity in children with protein-calorie malnutrition. *Clin Immunol Immunopathol* 1982; 24: 1–7.
69. Ingram KG, Crouch DG, Douez DL, et al. Effects of triiodothyronine supplements on splenic natural killer cells in malnourished weanling mice. *Int J Immunopharmacol* 1995; 17: 21–32.
70. Ingram KG, Croy BA, Woodward BD. Splenic natural killer cell activity in wasted, protein-energy malnourished weanling mice. *Nutr Res* 1995; 15: 231–43.
71. Petro TM, Schwartz KM, Schmid MJ. Natural and immune anti-tumor interleukin production and lymphocyte cytotoxicity during the course of dietary protein deficiency or excess. *Nutr Res* 1991; 11: 679–86.
72. Weindruch R, Devens BH, Raff HV, et al. Influence of dietary restriction and aging on natural killer cell activity in mice. *J Immunol* 1983; 130: 993–6.
73. Lieberman MD, Reynolds J, Goldfine J, et al. Protein-calorie malnutrition inhibits antitumor response to interleukin-2 immunotherapy. *Surgery* 1990; 108: 452–9.
74. Edelman R. Cell-mediated immune response in protein-calorie malnutrition—a review. In: Suskind RM, ed. *Malnutrition and the immune response*. New York: Raven Press 1977: 47–75.
75. Woodward BD, Woods JW, Crouch DA. Direct evidence that primary acquired cell mediated immunity is less resistant than is primary thymus-dependent humoral immunity to the depressive influence of wasting protein-energy malnutrition in weanling mice. *Am J Clin Nutr* 1992; 55: 1180–5.
76. Good RA, Jose D, Cooper WC, Fernandes G, Kramer T, Yunis E. Influence of nutrition on antibody production and cellular immune responses in man, rats, mice, and guinea pigs. In: Suskind RM, ed. *Malnutrition and the immune response*. New York: Raven Press, 1977:169–83.
77. Shell-Duncan B. Evaluation of infection and nutritional status as determinants of cellular immunosuppression. *American Journal of Human Biology* 1997; 9: 381–90.
78. Rivera J, Habicht J-P, Torres N, et al. Decreased cellular immune response in wasted but not in stunted children. *Nutr Res* 1986; 6: 1161–70.
79. Mishra OP, Agrawal S, Ali Z. Adenosine deaminase activity in protein-energy malnutrition. *Acta Paediatr* 1998; 87: 1116–19.
80. McMurray DN, Mintzer CL, Bartow RA, et al. Dietary protein deficiency and *Mycobacterium bovis* BCG affect interleukin-2 activity in experimental pulmonary tuberculosis. *Infect Immun* 1989; 57: 2606–11.
81. Woods JW, Woodward BD. Enhancement of primary systemic acquired immunity by exogenous triiodothyronine in wasted, protein-energy malnourished weanling mice. *J Nutr* 1991; 121: 1425–32.
82. Dietz V, Galazka A, van Loon F, et al. Factors affecting the immunogenicity and potency of tetanus toxoid: implications for the elimination of neonatal and non-neonatal tetanus as public health problems. *Bull World Health Organ* 1997; 75: 81–93.
83. Chandra RK. Numerical and functional deficiency in T helper cells in protein-energy malnutrition. *Clin Exp Immunol* 1983; 51: 126–32.
84. Pocino M, Malave I. Affinity and distribution of subpopulations of antibody-producing cells in protein-restricted C57BL/6 mice. *Cell Immunol* 1984; 89: 169–85.
85. Price P. Responses to polyvinyl pyrrolidone and pneumococcal polysaccharide in protein-deficient mice. *Immunology* 1978; 34: 87–96.

86. Woodward B, Miller RG. Depression of thymus-dependent immunity in wasting protein-energy malnutrition does not depend on an altered ratio of helper (CD4[+]) to suppressor (CD8[+]) T cells or on a disproportionately large atrophy of the T-cell relative to the B-cell pool. *Am J Clin Nutr* 1991; 53: 1329–35.

87. Woodward BD, Bezanson KD, Hillyer LM, et al. The CD45RA+ (quiescent) phenotype is over-abundant relative to the CD45RA- phenotype within the involuted splenic T cell population of weanling mice subjected to wasting protein-energy malnutrition. *J Nutr* 1995; 125: 2471–82.

88. Carlomagno MA, Alito AE, Almiron DI, Gimeno A. T and B lymphocyte function in response to a protein-free diet. *Infect Immun* 1982; 38: 195–200.

89. Ha C-L, Paulino-Racine LE, Woodward BD. Expansion of the humoral effector cell compartment of both systemic and mucosal immune systems in a weanling murine model which duplicates critical features of human protein-energy malnutrition. *Br J Nutr* 1996; 75: 445–60.

90. Lydyard PM, Youinou PY. Human CD5[+] (B1) B cells in health and disease. *Fundamental and Clinical Immunology* 1995; 2: 9–25.

91. McGee DW, McMurray DN. The effect of protein malnutrition on the IgA immune response in mice. *Immunology* 1988; 63: 25–9.

92. Sullivan DA, Vaerman J-P, Soo C. Influence of severe protein malnutrition on rat lacrimal, salivary and gastrointestinal immune expression during development, adulthood and ageing. *Immunology* 1993; 78: 308–17.

93. Flo J, Roux ME, Massouh E. Deficient induction of the immune response to oral immunization with cholera toxin in malnourished rats during suckling. *Infect Immun* 1994; 62: 4948–54.

94. Ha C-L, Woodward B. Depression in the quantity of intestinal secretory IgA and in the expression of the polymeric immunoglobulin receptor in caloric deficiency of the weanling mouse. *Lab Invest* 1998; 78: 1255–66.

95. Watson RR, McMurray DN, Martin P, et al. Effect of age, malnutrition and nutrition on free secretory component and IgA in secretions. *Am J Clin Nutr* 1985; 42: 281–8.

96. Chandra RK. Reduced secretory antibody response to live attenuated measles and polio virus vaccines in malnourished children. *BMJ* 1975; ii: 583–5.

97. Koster F, Pierce NF. Effect of protein deprivation on immunoregulatory cells in the rat mucosal immune response. *Clin Exp Immunol* 1985; 60: 217–24.

98. McGee DW, McMurray DN. Protein malnutrition reduces the IgA immune response to oral antigen by altering B-cell and suppressor T-cell functions. *Immunology* 1988; 64: 697–702.

99. Woodward B. Protein, calories and immune defenses. *Nutr Rev* 1998; 56: S84–92.

100. Ha C-L, Woodward, B. Reduction in the quantity of the polymeric immunoglobulin receptor is sufficient to account for the low concentration of intestinal secretory immunoglobulin A in a weanling mouse model of wasting protein-energy malnutrition. *J Nutr* 1997; 127: 427–35.

101. Lambert RW, Kelleher RS, Wickham LA, et al. Neuroendocrinimmune modulation of secretory component production by rat lacrimal, salivary and intestinal epithelial cells. *Optom Vis Sci* 1994; 35: 1192–201.

102. Lee W-H, Woodward BD. The CD4/CD8 ratio in the blood does not reflect the response of this index in secondary lymphoid organs of weanling mice in models of protein-energy malnutrition known to depress thymus-dependent immunity. *J Nutr* 1996; 126: 849–59.

103. Lepage LM, Giesbrecht JC, Taylor CG. Expression of T lymphocyte p56[lck], a zinc-finger signal transduction protein, is elevated by dietary zinc deficiency and diet restriction in mice. *J Nutr* 1999;129:620–627.

104. Woodward B. Influence of wasting protein-energy malnutrition on apparent thymic T cell inductive capacity and on recirculating lymphocyte pool sizes in the weanling mouse. In: Chandra RK, ed. *Nutrition and immunology*. St John's, Newfoundland: ARTS Biomedical Publishers and Distributors, 1992: 163–77.

105. Parent G, Chevalier P, Zalles L, et al. In vitro lymphocyte-differentiating effects of thymulin (Zn-FTS) on lymphocyte subpopulations of severely malnourished children. *Am J Clin Nutr* 1994; 60: 274–8.

106. Jambon B, Ziegler O, Maire B, et al. Thymulin (facteur thymique sérique) and zinc content of the thymus glands of malnourished children. *Am J Clin Nutr* 1988; 48: 335–42.

107. Weiner HL. Oral tolerance: immune mechanisms and treatment of autoimmune diseases. *Immunol Today* 1997; 18: 335–43.

108. Conlon K, Osborne J, Morimoto C, et al. Comparison of lymphokine secretion and mRNA expression in the CD45RA[+] and CD45RO[+] subsets of human peripheral blood CD4[+] and CD8[+] lymphocytes. *Eur J Immunol* 1995; 25: 644–8.

109. Westermann J, Pabst R. Lymphocyte subsets in the blood: a diagnostic window on the lymphoid system? *Immunol Today* 1990; 11: 406–10.
110. Woodward B, Hillyer L, Hunt K. T cells with a quiescent phenotype (CD45RA⁺) are overabundant in the blood and involuted lymphoid tissues in wasting protein and energy deficiencies. *Immunology* 1999;96:246–253.
111. Lesourd BM, Mazari L, Ferry M. The role of nutrition in immunity in the aged. *Nutr Rev* 1998; 56: S113–25.
112. Westermann J, Pabst R. How organ-specific is the migration of 'naive' and 'memory' T cells? *Immunol Today* 1996; 17: 278–82.
113. McDermott MR, Mark DA, Befus AD, et al. Impaired intestinal localization of mesenteric lymphoblasts associated with vitamin A deficiency and protein-calorie malnutrition. *Immunology* 1982; 45: 1–5.
114. Conzen SD, Janeway CA. Defective antigen presentation in chronically protein-deprived mice. *Immunology* 1988; 63: 683–9.
115. Shi HN, Scott ME, Stevenson MM, et al. Energy restriction and zinc deficiency impair the functions of murine T cells and antigen-presenting cells during gastrointestinal nematode infection. *J Nutr* 1998; 128: 20–7.
116. Horgan KJ, van Seventer GA, Shimizu Y, et al. Hyporesponsiveness of "naive" (CD45RA⁺) human T cells to multiple receptor-mediated stimuli but augmentation of responses by co-stimuli. *Eur J Immunol* 1990; 20: 1111–8.
117. Banchereau J, Steinman RM. Dendritic cells and the control of immunity. *Nature* 1998; 392: 245–52.
118. Konyer J, Woodward B. Time kinetics of involution of splenic dendritic cell subpopulations in weanling murine protein-energy malnutrition [Abstract]. *Can Fed Biol Soc* 1998; 41: 252.
119. Rose AH, Holt PG, Turner KJ. The effect of a low protein diet on the immunogenic activity of murine peritoneal macrophages. *Int Arch Allergy Appl Immunol* 1982; 67: 356–61.
120. Chan J, Tian Y, Tanaka KE, et al. Effects of protein calorie malnutrition on tuberculosis in mice. *Proc Natl Acad Sci USA* 1996; 93: 14857–61.
121. Mengheri E, Nobili F, Crocchioni G, et al. Protein starvation impairs the ability of activated lymphocytes to produce interferon-γ. *J Interferon Res* 1992; 12: 17–21.
122. Zhang S, Petro TM. The effect of moderate protein malnutrition on murine T cell cytokine production. *Nutr Res* 1997; 17: 51–64.
123. Letterio JJ, Roberts AB. Regulation of immune responses by TGF-Beta. *Annu Rev Immunol* 1998; 16: 137–61.
124. Hoffman-Goetz L. Lymphokines and monokines in protein-energy malnutrition. In: Chandra RK, ed. *Nutrition and immunology*. New York: Alan R Liss, 1988: 9–23.
125. Straus DS, Marten NW, Hayden JM, et al. Protein restriction specifically decreases the abundance of serum albumin and transthyretin nuclear transcripts in rat liver. *J Nutr* 1994; 124: 1041–51.
126. Mayatepek E, Becker K, Gana L, et al. Leukotrienes in the pathophysiology of kwashiorkor. *Lancet* 1993; 342: 958–60.
127. Lord GM, Matarese G, Howard JK, et al. Leptin modulates the T-cell immune response and reverses starvation-induced immunosuppression. *Nature* 1998; 394: 897–901.
128. Filteau SM, Hall NRS. Increased production of tumor necrosis factor and interleukin 1 by peritoneal macrophages from severely undernourished mice: lack of correlation with serum corticosterone. *Nutr Res* 1991; 11: 1001–11.
129. Cederholm T, Wretlind B, Hellstrom K, et al. Enhanced generation of interleukins 1 and 6 may contribute to the cachexia of chronic disease. *Am J Clin Nutr* 1997; 65: 876–82.
130. Beck MA. Increased virulence of coxsackievirus B3 in mice due to vitamin E or selenium deficiency. *J Nutr* 1997; 127: 966–70S.

DISCUSSION

Dr. Chandra: I would emphasize the age of the subject—whether human or an animal model, because obviously there are differences between immune responses at baseline and during nutritional stress. In addition to that, I think it would be useful to know the severity and the speed of induction of nutritional deprivation, both in animals and in humans. For instance, adults who are subjected to acute energy deprivation over 5 to 7 days of complete fasting have a very different immunologic profile from a more chronic energy deprivation. Finally, I think that replenishing malnourished animals or humans with appropriate nutrients and looking at the immunologic profile afterward should also be done. It is only then that you can say that the results are truly related to the nutritional insult.

You raised the issue of what animal model might be most appropriate. For obvious reasons, subhuman primates are ideal, but they are very expensive and it is often difficult to get ethics approval to do experiments on them.

My final comment is that we also need to look more deeply into the question of movement of cells. We have all looked at blood cells, some have looked at tissue cells, but how cells or their components traffic from one site to another may also be important. From the limited information that is available, both for protein-energy malnutrition and perhaps for vitamin A deficiency, the cell surface proteins of lymphocytes are changed in a way that suggests they traffic differently to different sites, particularly to the gastrointestinal tract. I think that needs to be looked at in greater depth.

Dr. Woodward: Dr. Chandra's point on trafficking is an interesting one. I think you may be referring to the work of McDermott and Bienenstock on the mouse (1), showing that adoptive transfer of lymphocytes from malnourished into well-nourished animals resulted in failure of these cells to distribute in normal ways; in particular, they did not home in on the gut, where you would have anticipated they would go. Likewise, McMurray (2), who uses a very relevant model of the protein-deficient tuberculous guinea pig, has recently shown that CD8$^+$, antigen-specific T cells in this system appear to home in on the lymph nodes draining the infected lungs, but cannot get into the lungs and hence cannot interact with the macrophages in the lungs; this provides some basis for an understanding of the inability of malnourished individuals to generate a granulomatous response. I see a real parallel between those results and what we have found in our own system with regard to an overabundance of naive phenotype, quiescent T cells, which one would expect to do exactly what McMurray found—that is, they would home in on lymph nodes but not on the nonlymphoid sites where infections are occurring, because that is how naive-type cells recirculate. So I suspect there really are, as Dr. Chandra has just said, some very important changes in the trafficking of T cells (and I am sure the changes are not limited to the T cells) that are induced by various forms of malnutrition.

Dr. Suskind: Some years ago, we did some studies where we put normal lymphocytes into media where one specific nutrient was deficient. We made up a series of media, leaving out a different nutrient in each experiment, then adding it back to give a dose-response curve (unpublished data). Interestingly, every single nutrient affected the cellular immune response. So, with the lymphocyte, we have a very sensitive cell that needs all those nutrients to function effectively. I think that was an important observation. I would be interested in your comments.

Dr. Woodward: I agree, I think that is an important observation and I doubt whether it is confined to the T cell. I would suspect that would be the case for any cell that might be cultured, immunologic or otherwise. The traditional nutritionist's perspective on any nutrient deficiency condition in an intact animal or human, let alone in tissue culture, would be that there is no such thing as a simple nutritional deficiency. So, for example, the idea that the nutritional deficiency produced with zinc deficiency or vitamin A deficiency is somehow a simpler condition than the one produced with protein-energy malnutrition, I think, is mistaken. In the tissue culture work you referred to, you may come closer than you can in an intact animal to seeing what a simple nutritional deficiency condition can produce, but I doubt that there is such a thing in the intact animal. That is the principal reason why I think in terms of the hormonal microenvironment within which cells have to operate as being the underlying physiologic determinant of the immunologic changes we see, rather than the availability of any particular nutrient. I believe that the idea that there is a generalized decrease in protein synthesis in response to decreased intake, and that this is responsible for the immune depression, is now untenable. The metabolism of the malnourished is every bit as complex and every bit as well-controlled as the metabolism of the well-nourished; it is just different. Different metabolic priorities are established, I am sure, by endocrine hormonal means, so what we are doing is studying an immune system that has come off the metabolic priority list.

Dr. Ashworth: In commenting on the diets fed to animals, you drew attention to the very low protein of your laboratory diet. It would also have been helpful to bring out the fact that the animals have complete mineral and vitamin supplements. That is in contrast to the reality of malnourished children, whose diets are low in micronutrients. I would support your emphasis on protein-energy malnutrition being a very complex entity; we need always to bear in mind that this is a multideficiency state.

Dr. Woodward: We did some work in the mid-1980s where we doubled and tripled the micronutrient package that we include in our experimental diets. This never made any difference. Regardless, for example, of the level of dietary zinc that we included, serum zinc levels were always profoundly depressed. We can put as much as 200 μg/g of zinc in the diet and it just does not touch serum zinc levels at all (3). I think there is a sense in which the protein-energy malnourished animal, and I suspect human too, is not formally deficient in micronutrients. That is not to say that they are in an admirable nutritional state, but I do not think they can respond to micronutrient supplements in the way that you and I can, because their metabolic priorities are different. So, giving a protein-energy malnourished animal a supplement of zinc is not going to do anything immunologically. In human populations where there appears to have been a response to zinc supplements, I think you will find the subjects were stunted, not wasted.

Dr. Cochran: Older studies have shown that if you subject rodents to malnutrition during pregnancy, the offspring are smaller, and it takes several generations for them to come back to the normal size, although they are well nourished. Has anybody looked at the effects on the immune system in that kind of a setting?

Dr. Woodward: There are studies of an intergenerational nature like that. The first one of which I am aware was done by Dr. Chandra, and then Lucille Hurley's group picked up on that in the early 1980s (4,5). In the United Kingdom, Barker's work on the impact of *fetal malnutrition* (although I think that is a term many would dispute) and its long-term impact on the ability of the endocrine system to develop properly (6), is a rather *broad paintbrush* view of what I suspect is the underlying mechanism. What we are seeing are long-term impacts on endocrine development, on the development of the heart and the pancreas and on the immune system as well. I suspect that the impact on reproductive hormones, whatever it may be, is such as to carry over and influence the development of other organ systems in the F2 and even the F3 generation.

Dr. Gershwin: In the early 1980s, we fed animals on diets deficient in zinc and we saw abnormal responses for the second and even the third generation, although the abnormality decreased significantly. We went back to those studies some years later, and found if the animals were housed in pathogen-free environments we did not see those multigenerational effects (5,7). So, although we never explained the mechanism, we felt that it had a lot to do with the flora and whatever organisms the animals happened to carry.

Dr. Griffin: In relation to early priming effects on development, some very interesting studies are coming from the Medical Research Council unit in Gambia. In that region, there is cyclical malnutrition in the dry season followed by good nutrition in the wet season. When children born in the dry, malnutrition season and in the wet, good nutrition season were followed for 20 years, there was a profound increase in death from infection in the children born in the malnutrition season (8,9). The mechanisms are not known, but clearly some very early priming goes on which results in a relatively deficient immune system in later life.

Dr. Keusch: It does not necessarily make sense to me to take cells from a deficient environment in the host and put them into a nutritionally complete medium in the *in vitro* setting, but we will continue to need culture experiments to dissect out aspects of the immune response—we cannot do it on cells as they are removed immediately from the host. The environment in the host is not medium 199 or some other artificial mixture; in fact it is serum or plasma. So, from a standardization point of view, should we not be using autologous plasma for the cultivation of the cells? Analogous to many kinds of experimental situation where we are trying to standardize results across geographic regions and between laboratories, should we not establish reagent repositories of standardized reagents, and perhaps in this case standardized plasma? You asked for challenges for the next century. I put this challenge to Nestlé, to take on the development of a reagent repository that people could use in their own laboratories, so that they can compare autologous plasma with a reference sample in different situations. When we are able to characterize the nature of malnutrition using a standardized protocol to collect clinical information and to define the nutritional state of the host, I think we will make a lot of progress in understanding what we are talking about.

Dr. Kennedy: We looked at that issue in a lot of our experiments. We were puzzled by published reports on experiments in which lymphocytes or blood were placed in Roswell Park Memorial Institute (RPMI) or various types of media and still showed the biological effects under study. We felt that if these effects were related to micronutrient deficiency they should be reversed in RPMI media. We found that it did not matter whether we used autologous plasma or whether we supplemented with RPMI media, and this led us to believe that in our studies at least the nutritional deficiency may not be playing the primary role in modulating the immune response. I am not saying that it plays no role at all, but perhaps the nutritional deficiency sets up a series of neuroendocrine changes that are what really affects the immune cell, and that repleting nutrition as a single entity is probably not going to alter the immune deficit.

Dr. Woodward: Some old studies have indicated that unidentified serum factors (still unidentified in fact) in malnutrition can exert influences such as reduced T-cell blastogenesis, whereas serum from otherwise comparable, well-nourished controls does not exert such suppressive influences. I am quite taken by the idea of using autologous serum as part of an experimental design. At the same time, there clearly are hormonal influences that program cells, so that once you take them out of the environment in which they have been programmed, they continue to function as if they were still in the old environment.

Dr. Tontisirin: Can you summarize the intercellular communications in malnutrition? What are the hormonal or endocrine mechanisms?

Dr. Woodward: There have been a number of suggestions of what might influence down-regulation of cytokine production on the part of T cells. One is glucocorticoids. High levels of cortisol can be downregulatory for many cytokines (IL-1 to 6, IL-11, TNF-α, GM-CSF, and so on). I am sure there would be individual dose-response curves that we would need to sort out for each of those. Another really interesting suggestion is that the eicosanoid metabolism of the malnourished is shifted toward prostaglandin synthesis, and everybody focuses on PGE$_2$, which will do some specific things such as reducing the ability to produce IL-2. Thirdly, an interesting possibility has come out of McMurray's work at Texas A&M, in which he found in his model of low protein tuberculous guinea pigs a high level of transforming growth factor-β in the blood (2). That is a broadly immunosuppressive, although not uniformly immunosuppressive, cytokine; in fact, I even wonder if it might be a contributor to the longstanding observations of what autologous serum from the malnourished can do to blast cell transformation. So, several possibilities exist.

Dr. Suskind: I think we forget that a number of years ago the real emphasis was on the influence of nutrition on the endocrine system. I wonder if somehow we could bring together all that information and gain new insights into those changes that occur in the immune system that can be modulated by nutrition, or by nutrition via the endocrine system.

Dr. Woodward: The amount of experimental work directly demonstrating that you can influence immune function by intervening with a hormone or by removing a hormone is really quite slight. It is one thing to say that A results in B, and B results in C, but you cannot then say A causes C. That is why I would say the information base we have right now is sufficient for hypothesis generation but nothing more.

Dr. Chandra: In relation to the possible role of sex hormones in modulating the immune response in nutritionally deprived individuals, some studies show that antibody affinity and phagocytic abilities, when tested in protein-deficient or amino acid-deficient mice, show different results in males and females. As the rest of the protocol is similar, there is an obvious need to investigate this further to explore the role of the sex hormones.

REFERENCES

1. McDermott MR, Mark DA, Befus AD, et al. Impaired intestinal localization of mesenteric lymphoblasts associated with vitamin A deficiency and protein-calorie malnutrition. *Immunology* 1982; 45: 1–5.
2. McMurray DN. Impact of nutritional deficiencies on resistance to experimental pulmonary tuberculosis. *Nutr Rev* 1998;56:S147–52.
3. Filteau SM, Woodward B. The effect of severe protein deficiency on serum zinc concentration of mice fed a requirement level or a very high level of dietary zinc. *J Nutr* 1982; 112: 1974–7.
4. Chandra RK. Antibody formation in first and second generation offspring of nutritionally deprived rats. *Science* 1975; 190: 289–90.
5. Beach RS, Gershwin ME, Hurley LS. Gestational zinc deprivation in mice: persistence of immunodeficiency for three generations. *Science* 1982; 218: 469–71.
6. Barker DJ, Gluckman PD, Godfrey KM, et al. Fetal nutrition and cardiovascular disease in adult life. *Lancet* 1993; 341: 938–41.
7. Vruwink K, Gershwin ME, Keen CL. Effects of gestational zinc deficiency in mice on growth and immune function. *Journal Nutritional Immunology* 1994; 2: 24–41.
8. Ceesay SM, Prentice AM, Cole TJ, et al. Effects on birth weight and prenatal mortality of maternal dietary supplements in rural Gambia: 5 year randomized controlled trial. *BMJ* 1997; 315: 786–90.
9. Moore SE, Cole TJ, Poskitt EM, et al. Season of birth predicts mortality in rural Gambia. *Nature* 1997; 388: 434.

Nutrition, Immunity, and Infection in Infants and Children, edited by Robert M. Suskind and Kraisid Tontisirin. Nestlé Nutrition Workshop Series, Pediatric Program, Vol. 45. Nestec Ltd., Vevey/Lippincott Williams & Wilkins, Philadelphia ©2001.

Low Birthweight Infants, Infection, and Immunity

Ann Ashworth

Public Health Nutrition Unit, London School of Hygiene & Tropical Medicine, London, UK

In this chapter, I will examine whether infants of low birthweight (LBW) are more susceptible to infection and to death from infection, than infants of adequate birthweight (ABW), and briefly compare their immunocompetence. As more than 90% of LBW infants are born in developing countries, the focus is on diarrheal and respiratory infections, measles, and malaria, which are major causes of childhood illness and death in these populations. LBW infants are estimated to comprise 16% of global births, so any increased susceptibility to illness or death among them is of public health relevance.

HETEROGENEITY OF LOW BIRTHWEIGHT INFANTS

The definition of LBW is a weight less than 2,500 g at birth and embraces newborns who differ in their maturity, body proportions, and composition, and in their physiologic and metabolic make-up. LBW infants can be divided into two broad subgroups: those born preterm (< 37 weeks' gestation) and those who are growth retarded *in utero* and are born small-for-gestational age (SGA). In developed countries, most LBW infants are the result of a preterm delivery and are appropriately grown. In contrast, in low-income populations with high prevalences of LBW, intrauterine growth retardation (IUGR) is the major cause.

Visible differences in body size and body proportions are clearly evident among IUGR newborns. Fetal linear growth occurs mainly in the first 28 weeks of gestation (1), and chronic undernutrition and other adverse influences in early fetal life result in proportionate reductions in skeletal and soft tissues. Such infants are typically stunted at birth, but are not wasted. As the immune system starts to develop in early fetal life, and as an adverse fetal environment can permanently alter gene expression, organ structure, cell number, and hormonal responses (2), a differential impact of

121

LBW on immune function can be expected, depending on the causation, timing, and severity of fetal growth impairment. Thus, it is plausible that stunted LBW infants will be more susceptible to infectious disease than wasted or preterm LBW infants, and that any differential susceptibility may extend not only into childhood, but also into adulthood. In this chapter, in addition to comparing the relative risk of infection in LBW and ABW infants, I shall also explore evidence for a differential susceptibility among LBW infants.

LOW BIRTHWEIGHT AND INFECTION IN INFANCY AND EARLY CHILDHOOD

Risk of Death

Large population-based studies of birthweight-specific mortality consistently show an increased risk of neonatal and postneonatal mortality for both preterm and term LBW infants (3). Such studies are facilitated by computerized systems of linked birth and death records, which are rarely feasible in low income countries. For specific causes of death, few data sources disaggregate by birthweight and those that do tend to be small, community-based studies. Table 1 presents the relative mortality risks in LBW infants compared with ABW infants for diarrhea (three studies), respiratory infections (four studies), infections other than respiratory or diarrhea (two studies), and all infections combined (one study) (4–17). Predominant among *other* infections were meningitis, sepsis, and measles. Studies of all-cause mortality have been included if infections were reported to comprise a large proportion of deaths (seven studies).

Although in only two studies were confounding variables controlled (4,13), the data are consistent with an increased risk of death from diarrheal, respiratory, and other infections during the first year of life in LBW infants. The data also suggest that this increased risk continues into early childhood. No disaggregated data by birthweight were located for measles or malaria, but in the Gambia, where malaria is the main cause of childhood mortality, deaths from malaria are not greater among *hungry season* births (the season with a high prevalence of LBW births). This suggests that LBW infants are not more susceptible than ABW infants to malaria (18).

Risk of Hospital Admission

During the first 2 years of life, low birthweight is associated with an increased risk of hospital admission for infection. This has been shown for diarrhea and dehydration (19–22), and pneumonia (20,22,23). For diarrhea, the risk may extend beyond 2 years (24). In southern Brazil, after controlling for family income, IUGR children were at almost twice the risk of being admitted to the hospital for diarrhea as ABW infants, but preterm children experienced only a slightly increased risk. In contrast, for pneumonia, both IUGR and preterm children had similar increased risks (22). In northeast Brazil, after controlling for confounding variables, LBW term infants had a fourfold

TABLE 1. *Low birthweight and risk of mortality*

Country (reference)	Design	Gestation	Age (months)	Sample size (deaths)	Birthweight (g)	Risk ratio (95% CI)	Outcome
Brazil (4)	Cohort	Term	0–6	393 (12)	3,000–3,499	1.0	All causes
					1,500–2,499	10.2 (2.2–46.7)	
						6.6* (1.4–31.2)	
India (5)	Cohort	Term	0–11	4,590 (213)	≥2,500	1.0	All causes
					2,000–2,499	2.6	
India (6)	Cohort	Term	0–11	4,220 (362)	≥2,500	1.0	All causes
					<2,500	1.7	
Guatemala (7,8)	Cohort	Term	0–11	385 (24)	≥2,500	1.0	All causes
					<2,500	1.7	
Indonesia (9)	Cohort	Term + preterm	12–47	(39)		1.8	
			0–11	687 (83)	≥2,500	1.0	All causes
					<2,500	3.4	
Nigeria (10)	Cohort	Term + preterm	0–11	4,334 (133)	>2,500	1.0	All causes
					≤2,500	5.8	
Brazil (11,12)	Cohort	Term + preterm	0–11	5,914 (215)	≥2,500	1.0	All causes
					<2,500	11.0 (8.7–14.4)	ARI
						6.7 (3.0–14.9)	Diarrhea
						2.5 (0.9–6.7)	Other infections
						2.9 (1.0–8.3)	All causes
						3.3	
Brazil (13)	Case-control	Term + preterm	12–59	(29)	≥2,500	1.0	ARI
			0.25–11	1,070 (357)	1,500–2,499	1.9* (1.1–3.6)†	Diarrhea
						2.0* (1.1–3.6)†	Other infections
						5.0* (1.3–18.6)†	All infections
						2.3*(1.6–3.4)†	
India (14)	Cohort	Term + preterm	0–11	659 (19)	≥2,500	1.0	ARI
					<2,500	8.0	
United Kingdom (15)	Cohort	Term + preterm	1–50	5,522 (40)	≥2,500	1.0	Bronchitis + pneumonia
					<2,500	3.6	
United States (16)	Cohort	Term + preterm	1–11	51,931 (371)	≥2,500	1.0	Infectious disease
			12–84	(258)	1,500–2,499	2.4 (1.4–4.0)	
United States (17)	Cohort	Term + preterm	1–11	193,733 (93)	≥2,500	2.5 (1.3–4.5)	Diarrhea
					<2,500	1.0	
						7.1	

*Adjusted for confounders; †90% confidence intervals.
CI, confidence interval; ARI, Acute respiratory infections.

higher rate of hospital admission in the first 6 months than ABW infants (4). The main causes were diarrhea and respiratory infections. In Norway, SGA infants had twice the risk of hospital admission for respiratory infections as ABW infants, although the prevalence of respiratory infections was similar in both groups (25). This suggests that when SGA infants become infected, their illness may be more severe than in ABW infants.

Risk of Morbidity

Table 2 shows the association between birth weight and morbidity (4,14,15,26–31). Three studies report diarrhea morbidity, of which two controlled for socioeconomic and maternal confounders (4,29). In these two studies, from northeast Brazil and Papua New Guinea, LBW infants experienced significantly more days with diarrhea (33% and 60%) than ABW infants. An increased risk of diarrhea morbidity among LBW infants has also been reported from Guatemala (8) and India (32), but the data do not permit calculation of relative risk. Seven studies have reported morbidity for respiratory infections, but only two are adjusted for confounding factors (4,30). For one of these, no association was found between LBW and the prevalence of cough, or cough with fever (4). In the other, also from northeast Brazil, only infants weighing less than 2,000 g were at significant risk of pneumonia (30). No studies were located of birthweight and risk of malaria infection, and only one of measles morbidity. LBW infants were no more likely than ABW infants to contract measles (15).

   Low birthweight infants may be disadvantaged in more ways than just their birthweight. For example, in our study of term LBW and ABW infants in northeast Brazil, where only low income families were recruited, the LBW group still had poorer household environments, fewer resources, and mothers with less education than the ABW controls (4). Therefore, potential exists for bias in studies that fail to take possible confounders into account. Bearing in mind such limitations in most studies, nevertheless there is strong evidence from Tables 1 and 2 of a significantly increased susceptibility to diarrhea, at least in term LBW infants, and of pneumonia in infants weighing less than 2,000 g. There is also strong evidence of an increased risk of hospital admission and death from diarrhea and pneumonia, which may reflect increased susceptibility to attack and/or increased severity or duration of infection episodes. There is some indirect evidence of an increased risk of death from measles, but a decreased susceptibility to malaria.

DIFFERENTIAL SUSCEPTIBILITY TO INFECTION

Among term IUGR infants in Guatemala, diarrheal rates in the first 2 months of life were negatively associated with ponderal index (33). Because a higher ponderal index in IUGR infers a symmetric (stunted) infant, these data can be interpreted as indicating a higher risk in stunted than in wasted LBW infants. In Norway, the risk of hospital admission during infancy in symmetric (stunted) SGA term infants was

TABLE 2. Low birthweight and risk of morbidity

Country (reference)	Design	Gestation	Age (months)	Sample size	Birthweight (g)	Risk ratio (95% CI)	Outcome
Ethiopia (26)	Cohort	Term	3–40	201	≥2,500	1.0	All infections
				393	<2,500	1.5 (1.1–2.1)	
Brazil (4)	Cohort	Term	0–6		3,000–3,499	1.0	Diarrhea
India (27)	Cohort	Term	0–3	152	1,500–2,499	1.3* (1.1–1.6)	
					≥2,500	1.0	Diarrhea
					1,500–2,499	2.4	ALRI
						3.6	Mostly sepsis and ALRI
Guatemala (28)	Cohort	Term	2 days–3 months	267	≥2,500	1.0	
					<2,500	3.0	
Papua New Guinea (29)	Cohort	Term + preterm	0–17	400	≥2,500	1.0	Diarrhea
			18–35		<2,500	1.7 *(1.4–2.1)	
			36–59			1.4 *(1.0–1.9)	
						1.2 *(0.5–1.8)	
Brazil (30)	Case-control	Term + preterm	0–23	1,300	≥2,500	1.0	Pneumonia
					2,000–2,499	1.4	
					<2,000	3.2 *(1.1 to 8.9)	
India (14)	Cohort	Term + preterm	0–11	659	≥2,500	1.0	ARI
					<2,500	1.2	
Uruguay (31)	Cohort	Term + preterm	0–35	166	≥2,500	1.0	ARI
					<2,500	0.9 (0.7–1.2)	
United Kingdom (15)	Cohort	Term + preterm	0–23	690	≥2,500	1.0	ALRI
					2,300–2,499	1.2	
					2,000–2,299	1.6	
					<2,000	3.5	

*Adjusted for confounders.
ARI, acute respiratory tract infection; CI, confidence interval; ALRI, acute lower respiratory tract infection.

twice that of ABW infants (odds ratio 2.0, 95% confidence interval 1.2–3.3), but no such risk was evident for asymmetric (wasted) infants (25). When the symmetric babies were further disaggregated, the increased risk was confined to the infants whose mothers smoked daily in early gestation. The major cause of hospital admission was for respiratory infections. Whether the increased risk is caused by the effect of periconceptional smoking on fetal immune function or to postnatal exposure to passive smoking, is not made clear.

LOW BIRTHWEIGHT AND INFECTION IN ADULTHOOD

Novel findings from the Gambia indicate that *hungry season* births have a tenfold greater risk of premature death in young adulthood than infants born in other months, with a predominance of infectious deaths (40%) and maternal deaths (15%) (34). A permanent reprogramming of the immune system during fetal life as a result of nutritional stresses is considered a likely cause, and particular emphasis is given to the vulnerability of the thymus to damage, owing to its complex structure, diverse cellular content, and its specialized function in thymopoiesis (18,34,35).

MECHANISMS FOR INCREASED SUSCEPTIBILITY TO INFECTION

Fetal and Postnatal Programming

The concept of *programming*, in which a stimulus applied at a sensitive period of development has lifelong effects, is now well established (36). As several components of the immune system mature during fetal life (37), with functional lymphocytes appearing by 10 to 12 weeks' gestation, this system is vulnerable to maternal undernutrition and to possible reprogramming (2,18), and animal studies clearly show a sustained effect of fetal undernutrition on immune function (38,39), even lasting into the F2 and F3 generations (40).

In late gestation, a rapid increase occurs in fetal plasma cortisol levels with an associated switching of the cell cycle from proliferation to differentiation (41). This stimulus to maturation is thought to reset the hypothalamic-pituitary-adrenal (HPA) axis in order to prepare the fetus for extrauterine life. In maternal undernutrition and other conditions associated with fetal growth retardation, the fetal HPA axis is activated earlier and fetal cortisol levels remain raised for a longer period before delivery (41). This reduces the period available for cell proliferation and may reduce cell number permanently. Raised plasma cortisol is known to be associated with thymic atrophy (42), and in animal experiments, maternal zinc deficiency is also associated with raised cortisol levels (42). This may be one mechanism whereby maternal undernutrition permanently impairs immune function.

Prentice *et al.* (18) point to toxic exposure as a further possibility for fetal nutritional programming of immunity. For example, transplacental transfer of aflatoxin occurs in proportion to maternal exposure, and aflatoxin is a potent immunosuppressant.

Micronutrient Deficiencies

Not only may immune function be adversely affected *in utero* as a result of maternal undernutrition or toxic exposure, but once born, LBW infants are at increased risk of nutrient deficiencies. For example, preterm infants are born with much less zinc, copper, and iron than term babies because approximately 50% of the transfer from mother to fetus occurs in the last 6 to 8 weeks of gestation (43). Fetal liver retinol stores double between 25 and 37 weeks' gestation (44), and low plasma retinol has been reported in preterm infants at delivery (45). Preterm infants seem to be particularly susceptible to postnatal depletion of liver vitamin A reserves, with a 50% reduction in mean hepatic concentration in the first 2 months of life, in contrast to term infants who show no reduction (46).

Also, less zinc, copper, iron, and vitamin A are found in IUGR term babies than in ABW infants because their liver size is 30% to 40% smaller (47). About half the newborn's body copper content is in the liver, and a quarter of the zinc. Term neonates with small livers also have lower hepatic concentrations of copper and zinc than larger babies (48,49). As micronutrients play a pivotal role in immune function (38,39), these differences in micronutrient reserves are likely to affect preterm infants adversely in the short term and IUGR infants in the long term. Preterm neonates supplemented with zinc recovered their cell-mediated immunity more quickly than controls (39). In term LBW infants, zinc supplementation for 8 weeks was associated with a 28% reduction in diarrhea prevalence in the first 6 months of life, but no significant reduction in the prevalence of respiratory infections (50).

Reduced Breast-Feeding

A lower prevalence of breast-feeding is often reported for LBW infants compared with ABW infants, and this can be expected to increase their risk of infection, particularly to sepsis, diarrheal diseases, and otitis media. In our morbidity studies in northeast Brazil, the median durations of breast-feeding in LBW and ABW infants were 2.8 and 3.4 months, respectively. Although in the sample as a whole, feeding mode was strongly related to the rate of onset of diarrhea, inclusion of feeding mode in the multiple regression analyses had no impact on the estimated effects of birthweight on morbidity outcomes (4).

THE IMMUNE SYSTEM

This complex and vital defense system is described in detail elsewhere in this volume. In summary, the two principal response types are (*a*) adaptive or antigen-specific mechanisms, of which the two main components are the immunoglobulin-antibody system and cell-mediated immunity; and (*b*) innate or nonspecific responses, which include the complement system, phagocytes, lysozyme, interferon and other humoral factors, and the physical barriers of skin and mucous membranes.

Development of the immune system begins around the sixth week of gestation, and responses to mitogens and natural killer cell activity are detectable by 10 weeks. Maturation occurs predominantly *in utero* (51). When the intrauterine environment is disturbed, as in IUGR or preterm births, cell-mediated immunity is the main component affected.

Specific Immunity

Immunoglobulins

Little immunoglobulin G (IgG) is transferred from mother to fetus before 32 weeks' gestation and babies delivering before this time have very low serum IgG concentrations, which decline further during the first weeks of life. Hypoimmunoglobulinemia is thought to contribute to the high frequency of sepsis (52,53) and respiratory and meningeal infections in preterm LBW neonates (54). Giving intravenous immune globulin to neonates with sepsis improves their survival sixfold, and when given prophylactically has a small but demonstrable benefit in reducing the incidence of infection (52,55).

Term SGA neonates have lower serum concentrations of IgG than ABW neonates, and this has been ascribed to smaller placental surface area in the former, which limits fetal transfer (32,56). IgM concentrations in SGA neonates did not differ from ABW infants in these studies, but conflicting findings were reported for IgA. Neither IgA nor IgM is acquired transplacentally.

Antibodies

Active neutralizing antibody responses in IUGR infants following vaccination to bacille Calmette–Guérin vaccine (57), hepatitis B (58), and polio virus vaccines (59) are reported to be similar to the responses in ABW infants.

Cell-mediated Immunity

The lymphoid tissues (thymus, spleen, and lymph nodes) of the fetus are more severely affected by maternal undernutrition than other tissues and organs (39). These are the key sites for the production and processing of T lymphocytes, and hence for mounting cell-mediated responses to infection. Term SGA and preterm LBW newborns have fewer T lymphocytes than ABW infants (32,39,60), but by 3 months preterm infants have normal levels, whereas SGA infants continue to have reduced numbers for several months or even years (39,61). Within the T-cell subpopulation, the helper $CD4^+$ cells are reduced in number, and the $CD4^+$:$CD8^+$ helper:suppressor ratio is significantly lower in term SGA than in ABW infants (56).

Reduced lymphocyte stimulation response to phytohemagglutinin (PHA) at birth has been reported in both preterm and term SGA neonates, the extent of the reduction paralleling the reduction in T-lymphocyte count (61). This reduction persists only in SGA infants and is associated with lower serum thymic hormone activity. Moscatelli *et al.* (62) found normal responses to PHA in most term SGA infants at birth, and the remainder normalized by 3 weeks. In Brazil, term LBW infants tested at 6 months had normal responses to PHA (50).

Nonspecific Immunity

Complement

Cord blood C3 levels are significantly lower in preterm and term SGA neonates compared with ABW term newborns (32,56). As placental transfer occurs in the last trimester, and fetal C3 synthesis occurs predominantly in the liver, it is plausible for both preterm and IUGR newborns to be adversely affected, but by different routes. By 6 months, serum C3 concentrations are similar (32).

Polymorphonuclear Leukocytes

Phagocytosis, intracellular bacterial killing capacity, and chemotaxis of polymorphonuclear leukocytes are deficient in preterm newborns. By 2 weeks of age, phagocytosis becomes normal, and this can be achieved in 5 days by giving vitamin E (63), but other functions remain deficient.

FUTURE RESEARCH

Methodologically robust studies with sufficient sample size are needed to clarify whether term LBW infants have an increased risk of respiratory infections. As preterm infants weighing less than 2,000 g have impaired lung function until at least 7 years of age, future incidence studies should have sufficient sample size to allow disaggregation of preterm and term LBW infants.

Comparative studies of the susceptibility of LBW and ABW infants to malaria, measles, and the human immunodeficiency virus are warranted. These studies should include sensitive measures of immune function.

Little is known about infection rates and immune function in LBW term infants who differ in their body proportions at birth (stunted vs wasted). This is an area that could provide useful insights into the functional consequences of sensitive periods of development.

Given the significance to public health of the likely association between birthweight and infection in adulthood, the long-term consequences of LBW should be a priority area for further research.

Further nutritional interventions, in which both morbidity and immune function are outcomes, could help elucidate important causal factors for increased susceptibility to infection and guide effective public health strategies.

Acknowledgment: I thank Melissa Dan for contributing to this review.

REFERENCES

1. Falkner F, Holzgreve W, Schloo RH. Prenatal influences on postnatal growth: overview and pointers for needed research. *Eur J Clin Nutr* 1994; 48 (Suppl. 1): S15–24.
2. Barker DJP. In: *Mothers, babies, and disease in later life*. London: BMJ Publishing Group, 1994.
3. Ashworth A. Effects of intrauterine growth retardation on mortality and morbidity in infants and young children. *Eur J Clin Nutr* 1998; 52: S34–42.
4. Lira PIC, Ashworth A, Morris SS. Low birth weight and morbidity from diarrhea and respiratory infection in northeast Brazil. *J Pediatr* 1996; 128: 497–504.
5. Ghosh S, Ramanujacharyulu TKTS, Hooja V, et al. Mortality patterns in an urban birth cohort. *Indian J Med Res* 1979; 69: 616–23.
6. Rao PSSS, Inbaraj SG. A prospective study of infant mortality and congenital malformations in relation to intra-uterine growth rates in south India. *Indian J Med Res* 1978; 67: 245–54.
7. Mata LJ. Malnutrition-infection interactions in the tropics. *Am J Trop Med Hyg* 1975; 24: 564–73.
8. Mata LJ. In: *The children of Santa Maria Cauque: a prospective field study of health and growth*. Cambridge: MIT Press, 1978.
9. Kusin JA, Kardjati S, de With C. Infant mortality in Madura, Indonesia. Implications for action. *J Trop Pediatr* 1989; 35: 129–32.
10. Ayeni O, Oduntan SO. The effects of sex, birthweight, birth order and maternal age on infant mortality in a Nigerian community. *Ann Human Biol* 1978; 5: 353–8.
11. Barros FC, Victora CG, Vaughan JP, et al. Infant mortality in southern Brazil: a population based study of causes of death. *Arch Dis Child* 1987; 62: 487–90.
12. Victora CG, Barros FC, Huttly SRA, et al. Early childhood mortality in a Brazilian cohort: the roles of birthweight and socioeconomic status. *Int J Epidemiol* 1992; 21: 911–15.
13. Victora CG, Smith PG, Vaughan JP, et al. Influence of birth weight on mortality from infectious diseases: a case-control study. *Pediatrics* 1988; 81: 807–11.
14. Datta N, Kumar V, Kumar L, et al. Application of case management to the control of acute respiratory infections in low-birth-weight infants: a feasibility study. *Bull World Health Organ* 1987; 65: 77–82.
15. Douglas JWB, Mogford C. Health of premature children from birth to four years. *BMJ* 1953; i: 748–54.
16. Read JS, Clemens JD, Klebanoff MA. Moderate low birth weight and infectious disease mortality during infancy and childhood. *Am J Epidemiol* 1994; 140: 721–33.
17. Gibson JJ, Alexander GR. Correlates of infant death from infectious diarrhea in the southeastern United States. *South Med J* 1985; 78: 26–30.
18. Prentice AM, Cole TJ, Moore SE, et al. Programming the adult immune response. In: O'Brien PMS, Wheeler T, Barker DJP, eds. *Fetal programming: influences on development and disease in later life*. London. RCOG Press 1999; 399–413.
19. Victora CG, Fuchs SC, Kirkwood BR, et al. Breast-feeding, nutritional status, and other prognostic factors for dehydration among young children with diarrhoea in Brazil. *Bull World Health Organ* 1992; 70: 467–75.
20. Victora CG, Barros FC, Kirkwood BR, et al. Pneumonia, diarrhea, and growth in the first 4 years of life: a longitudinal study of 5914 Brazilian children. *Am J Clin Nutr* 1990; 52: 391–6.
21. Ittiravivongs A, Songchitratna K, Ratthapalo S, et al. Effect of low birth weight on severe childhood diarrhea. *Southeast Asian J Trop Med Public Health* 1991; 22: 557–62.
22. Barros FC, Huttly SRA, Victora CG, et al. Comparison of the causes and consequences of prematurity and intrauterine growth retardation: a longitudinal study in southern Brazil. *Pediatrics* 1992; 90: 238–44.
23. Victora CG, Fuchs SC, Flores JAC, et al. Risk factors for pneumonia among children in a Brazilian metropolitan area. *Pediatrics* 1994; 93: 977–85.
24. Mertens TE, Cousens SN, Feachem RG. Evidence of a prolonged association between low birthweight and paediatric diarrhoea in Sri Lanka. *Trans R Soc Trop Med Hyg* 1987; 81: 196.
25. Vik T, Vatten L, Markestad T, et al. Morbidity during the first year of life in small for gestational age infants. *Arch Dis Child* 1996; 75: F33–7.
26. Kebede A, Larson C. The health consequences of intrauterine growth retardation in southwestern Ethiopia. *Trop Doct* 1994; 24: 64–9.
27. Das BK, Mishra RN, Mishra OP, et al. Comparative outcome of low birth weight babies. *Indian Pediatr* 1993; 30: 15–21.

28. Bartlett AV, de Bocaletti MEP, Bocaletti MA. Neonatal and early postneonatal morbidity and mortality in a rural Guatemalan community: the importance of infectious diseases and their management. *Pediatr Infect Dis J* 1991; 10: 752–7.

29. Bukenya GB, Barnes T, Nwokolo N. Low birthweight and acute childhood diarrhoea: evidence of their association in an urban settlement of Papua New Guinea. *Ann Trop Paediatr* 1991; 11: 357–62.

30. Fonseca W, Kirkwood BR, Victora CG, et al. Risk factors for childhood pneumonia among the urban poor in Fortaleza, Brazil: a case-control study. *Bull World Health Organ* 1996; 74: 199–208.

31. Hortal M, Benitez A, Contera M, et al. A community-based study of acute respiratory tract infections in children in Uruguay. *Rev Infect Dis* 1990; 12: S966–73.

32. Saha K, Kaur P, Srivastava G, et al. A six-months' follow-up study of growth, morbidity and functional immunity in low birth weight neonates with special reference to intrauterine growth retardation in small-for-gestational-age infants. *J Trop Pediatr* 1983; 29: 278–82.

33. Villar J, Smeriglio V, Martorell R, et al. Heterogeneous growth and mental development of intrauterine growth-retarded infants during the first 3 years of life. *Pediatrics* 1984; 74: 783–91.

34. Moore SE, Cole TJ, Poskitt EME, et al. Season of birth predicts mortality in rural Gambia. *Nature* 1997; 388: 434.

35. Moore SE. Nutrition, immunity and the fetal and infant origins of disease hypothesis in developing countries. *Proc Nutr Soc* 1998; 57: 241–7.

36. Lucas A. Role of nutritional programming in determining adult morbidity. *Arch Dis Child* 1994; 71: 288–90.

37. Whitelaw A, Parkin J. Development of immunity. *Br Med Bull* 1988; 44: 1037–51.

38. Scrimshaw NS, SanGiovanni JP. Synergism of nutrition, infection, and immunity: an overview. *Am J Clin Nutr* 1997; 66: 464–77S.

39. Chandra RK. 1990 McCollum Award lecture. Nutrition and immunity: lessons from the past and new insights into the future. *Am J Clin Nutr* 1991; 53: 1087–101.

40. Chandra RK. Antibody formation in first and second generation offspring of nutritionally deprived rats. *Science* 1975; 190: 289–90.

41. Fowden AL, Li J, Forhead AJ. Glucocorticoids and the preparation for life after birth: are there long-term consequences of the life insurance? *Proc Nutr Soc* 1998; 57: 113–22.

42. Shankar AH, Prasad AS. Zinc and immune function: the biological basis of altered resistance to infection. *Am J Clin Nutr* 1998; 68: 447–63S.

43. Widdowson EM, Dauncey J, Shaw JCL. Trace elements in foetal and early postnatal development. *Proc Nutr Soc* 1974; 33: 275–84.

44. Farrell PM, Zachman RD, Gutcher GR. Fat soluble vitamins A, E and K in the premature infant. In: Tsang RC, ed. *Vitamin and mineral requirements in preterm infants.* New York: Marcel Dekker,1985: 63–98.

45. Powers HJ. Micronutrient deficiencies in the preterm neonate. *Proc Nutr Soc* 1993; 52: 285–91.

46. Olson JA, Gunning DB, Tilton RA. Liver concentrations of vitamin A and carotenoids, as a function of age and other parameters, of American children who died of various causes. *Am J Clin Nutr* 1984; 39: 903–10.

47. Usher RH, McLean FH. Normal fetal growth and the significance of fetal growth retardation. In Davis JA, Dobbing J, eds. *Scientific foundations of pediatrics.* London: Heinemann, 1974: 69–80.

48. Dorea JG, Brito M, Araujo MOG. Concentration of copper and zinc in liver of fetuses and infants. *J Am Coll Nutr* 1987; 6: 491–5.

49. Dorea JG, de Araujo MOG. Zinc and vitamin A in liver of foetuses and infants. *Acta Paediatr Scand* 1988; 77: 85–8.

50. Lira PIC, Ashworth A, Morris SS. Effect of zinc supplementation on the morbidity, immune function and growth of low-birth-weight, full-term infants in northeast Brazil. *Am J Clin Nutr* 1998; 68: 418–24S.

51. Chandra RK, Newborne PM. In: *Nutrition, immunity and infection: mechanisms of interactions.* London: Plenum Press, 1977.

52. Jenson HB, Pollock BH. Meta-analyses of the effectiveness of intravenous immune globulin for prevention and treatment of neonatal sepsis. *Pediatrics* 1997; 99: E2.

53. Baker CJ, Rench MA, Noya FJ, et al. Role of intravenous immunoglobulin in prevention of late-onset infection in low-birth-weight neonates. The Neonatal IVIG Study Group. *Rev Infect Dis* 1990; 12: S463–8.

54. Amato M, Huppi P, Imbach P, et al. Immunoglobulin subclass concentration in preterm infants treated prophylactically with different intravenous immunoglobulins. *Am J Perinatol* 1995; 12: 306–9.

55. Baker CJ, Melish ME, Hall RT, et al. Intravenous immune globulin for the prevention of nosocomial infection in low-birth-weight neonates. The Multicenter Group for the Study of Immune Globulin in Neonates. *N Engl J Med* 1992; 327: 213–19.
56. Chatrath R, Saili A, Jain M, et al. Immune status of full-term small-for-gestational age neonates in India. *J Trop Pediatr* 1997; 43: 345–8.
57. Mussi-Pinhata MM, Goncalves AL, Foss NT. BCG vaccination of full-term infants with chronic intrauterine malnutrition: influence of immunization age on development of post vaccination, delayed tuberculin hypersensitivity. *Bull World Health Organ* 1993; 71: 41–8.
58. Huang FY, Lee PI, Lee CY, et al. Hepatitis B vaccination in preterm infants. *Arch Dis Child* 1997; 77: F135–8.
59. Adenyi-Jones SC, Faden H, Ferdon MB, et al. Systemic and local immune responses to enhanced-potency inactivated poliovirus vaccine in premature and term infants. *J Pediatr* 1992; 120: 686–9.
60. Ferguson AC. Prolonged impairment of cellular immunity in children with intrauterine growth retardation. *J Pediatr* 1978; 93: 52–6.
61. Chandra RK. Serum thymic hormone activity and cell-mediated immunity in healthy neonates, preterm infants, and small-for-gestational age infants. *Pediatrics* 1981; 67: 407–11.
62. Moscatelli P, Bricarelli FD, Piccinini A, et al. Defective immunocompetence in foetal undernutrition. *Helv Paediatr Acta* 1976; 31: 241–7.
63. Chirico G, Marconi M, Colombo A, et al. Deficiency of neutrophil phagocytosis in premature infants: effect of vitamin E supplementation. *Acta Pediatr Scand* 1983; 72: 521–4.

DISCUSSION

Dr. Wasantwisut: I found the Brazil zinc supplementation trial very interesting. What was the iron and vitamin A status of these infants? You mentioned before that these low birthweight infants are susceptible to other deficiencies besides zinc. Secondly, could you comment on the failure to restore serum zinc to normal after zinc supplementation? I think other studies have found the same thing. Could this be caused by infection or an inflammatory response? In populations where inflammation is widespread, it is very difficult to bring the serum zinc back into the normal range.

Dr. Ashworth: One of the discussions that we had in designing the study was whether we should give a cocktail of all three nutrients. In the end we decided just to go with zinc. There is good reason to believe that the vitamin A and iron status would not be particularly good, for the same reasons as for zinc. However, I cannot say what the actual status was; we just focused on zinc. In relation to infection and its effect on serum zinc, the analyses of serum zinc and thymulin were very kindly done by Dr. Chandra. The question of infection was raised by him when the serum zinc values came out low. We, therefore, looked particularly at the infection status before the blood was taken, but were unable to explain the low values on that basis.

Dr. Suskind: In your review of the literature on the low birthweight infant, did you ever come across any studies which looked at supplementing low birthweight infants with more than just zinc? Based on our experience with children who have malnutrition after birth, we found in Thailand, as others have found, that the requirement for catch-up may be as high as 150% of the recommended daily allowance in energy, i.e., 180 kcal/kg protein at 4 g/kg, and 150% of the RDA for vitamins and minerals. I wonder if anyone has ever intervened in low birthweight children with that sort of regimen, looking not only at growth but also at immune status.

Dr. Ashworth: I am not aware of any community-based study. I would be very interested in that, too.

Dr. Marini: It is very important to measure the length of the baby in intrauterine growth retardation. Having measured the length of the baby, the ponderal index can be calculated and the category of growth retardation defined. The likelihood of growth recovery is strongly related to the ponderal index. My second comment is about the distinction you made between industrialized countries and developing countries. In fact, similar babies are to be found even in the industrialized countries. I am referring particularly to babies who receive betamethasone *in utero* to enhance pulmonary maturation. These babies have depressed immune function and often die of sepsis.

Dr. Ashworth: We weighed the children and measured their length at birth, 4, 8, 12, 17, and 26 weeks and at one year. You are quite right that if you classify the children by ponderal index and length for age, those children in the Brazilian setting with a low ponderal index had very rapid growth in the first 8 weeks, and then they maintained that Z-score, before drifting down a little. Although the stunted ones start off at exactly the same standard deviation score in terms of weight for age, they diverge completely from the wasted ones. They improve in their Z-score only a little, and from about 8 weeks they maintain their Z-score in parallel with the wasted group but on a lower track (1). It is certainly very important to characterize these children in terms of their length for age at birth, their ponderal index, and their gestational age.

Dr. Woodward: Has anybody produced any measurements of endotoxin in the blood of low birthweight infants in the way that Dr. Suskind was suggesting this morning with regard to postweaning malnutrition?

Dr. Ashworth: I am not aware of any.

Dr. Marini: There are data on endotoxin levels in very low birthweight infants without bacteremia (2), which was considered to be one of the causes of necrotizing enterocolitis.

Dr. Woodward: The reason I asked the question was that I would have thought it might at least provide the beginnings of an understanding of a low serum zinc measurement.

Dr. Coovadia: We did a study some years ago on anti-endotoxin antibodies. It was a randomized, controlled trial on newborn babies to check their endotoxin levels (3). The aim was to use antibody against endotoxins. Not surprisingly, many of these babies had endotoxin but were culture negative. Our results showed that anti-endotoxin antibodies had no effect whatsoever.

Dr. Tantibhedhayangkul: There is an interaction between zinc and copper, and even between zinc and iron. We gave zinc to malnourished children at a dose of 1 mg/kg bodyweight and found a fall in serum copper together with a fall in ceruloplasmin. Do you know what happened to the other micronutrients in your study?

Dr. Ashworth: These interactions are very important, and we were aware of them when we were starting the study. I think that this level of dosage (5 mg/d for 8 weeks) was probably not sufficient to interact adversely with iron. We did not measure serum copper.

Dr. Wakelin: A theory to explain the present increase in atopy and asthma in developed countries is reduced exposure to infectious organisms in early life. Your review shows that low birthweight infants have an increased exposure, or at least an increased susceptibility to infections. Pathogens are not passive agents. Many of them can polarize or program the immune response in one direction or another. Have you any views on the long-term consequences of such an increased exposure to infection in low birthweight infants in later life, other than mortality?

Dr. Ashworth: I cannot answer that. It is outside my area of expertise. Maybe someone else can comment?

Dr. Calder: Some data may be relevant to that question. A study from Southampton, United Kingdom (4) found a positive correlation in cases where head circumference at birth was related to circulating IgE in adulthood; in other words, the larger the head, the higher the circulating IgE at approximately 60 years of age. I think the odds ratio of having elevated serum IgE in adulthood was about 4.5 in the group with the largest head circumference at birth. A second study (5) was a related one, where birthweight was related to the occurrence of allergy, asthma, and atopy at 16 years of age. That showed a curious biphasic response of birthweight to the incidence of those diseases.

Dr. Chandra: In relation to autoimmune diseases and low birthweight, there are no prospective studies that I know of. However, in looking at patients with rheumatoid arthritis and control them for other variables, they are more likely to have been of low birthweight. Thus there may be an increased risk of autoimmune disease, especially rheumatoid arthritis, in low birthweight individuals. My second point is about low birthweight and atopy. Some evidence indicates that the incidence of atopy varies in low birthweight infants, depending on whether the infant is preterm or small for gestation, and whether or not there is a family history. Some studies indicate that given a positive family history, preterm babies have nearly a 30% to 35% higher risk of eczema at about 3 to 5 years of age, whereas this is less true for small gestational age infants. So, some interaction may exist between rates of infection, family history, and the incidence of atopic disease.

Dr. Marini: I would like to stress that allergy is not only the consequence of a preterm birth, but could be the cause as well. Several studies (6) show an increased likelihood of an allergic history in mothers delivering preterm babies. This is probably related to increased prostaglandin production or altered cytokine production during intercurrent infectious disease. Thus, allergy can be viewed as both a cause of and a consequence of preterm birth.

Dr. Wakelin: As this workshop is concerned with the interaction between nutrition, infection, and immunity, the point I wanted to emphasize was that several studies now show that nutritional disturbances can have immunologic consequences. These may be related to specific activities of the pathogen. Dr. Woodward showed how mice infected with a parasite had a polarized cytokine response. That was presumably a consequence of nutrition affecting immunity to the pathogen and influencing the immune response. I think this might be an important factor to bear in mind when looking at population studies, particularly where the population is exposed to a lot of infectious disease.

Dr. Keusch: Pursuing the issue of the relation with low birthweight and the outcomes you described, Leonardo Mata, of the Institute of Nutrition of Central America and Panama (INCAP) in Guatemala, used to talk about maternal care in a generalized sense as *maternal technology*—that is, the understanding of what you need to do to keep young infants growing and healthy. This is learned and not innate; it is learned in part by lessons from other women who have had babies, and it is learned in the course of having multiple babies. I suspect that most low birthweight babies in your study were firstborns, but I wonder about your adequate weight babies—whether those were subsequent children and whether some of the explanation for differences may lie in the maternal technology component of taking care of young infants.

Dr. Ashworth: There was no significant difference in parity (7). In relation to your question about maternal care, we did collect a lot of information about the environment and the maternal histories. Although some of these variables can be controlled for in the regression analysis, the subtle aspects of maternal care are difficult to measure and control for, so I think that is an important point you raised.

Dr. Cochran: Could you clarify the effects you were seeing? Do you think they were purely related to the nutritional insult that the children suffered *in utero*, or were those same children still having nutritional deficiencies throughout the study period?

Dr. Ashworth: It is very difficult to answer that without doing a randomized, controlled trial. I think that fetal undernutrition might be having an effect on immune function through programming, but even if that was not the case, there could be differences in micronutrient reserves because of their much smaller liver size. We did look at diet between the two groups from 0 to 6 months and we did not see any difference between the low birthweight and the adequate birthweight groups on a cross-sectional basis in terms of the types of food they were eating.

Dr. Suskind: Does the literature show any more extensive characterizations of the immune system in low birthweight infants versus appropriate for gestational age infants other than the cellular immune response?

Dr. Ashworth: Yes, studies have shown an impairment. Dr. Chandra may want to comment on his studies.

Dr. Chandra: We published some data in the mid-1970s. We found no problems with phagocytosis or ingestion of bacteria, but did find a modest reduction in intracellular killing of bacteria. There was also a reduction in complement levels, particularly C3, in the small for gestational as well as preterm babies. We followed the infants for more than one year, and most of the abnormalities disappeared within 3 to 6 months, in contrast to cell-mediated immunity, which continued to show some depression in most infants. This prolonged even intergenerational effect has also been shown in controlled animal experiments.

Dr. Farthing: Have you considered any controlled interventions during pregnancy? At what point in pregnancy do you think you would have to intervene?

Dr. Ashworth: In terms of preventing low birthweight, several possible interventions exist (8). Improving maternal nutrition with micronutrient or balanced protein and energy supplementation are two possibilities; others are malaria prophylaxis and not smoking. I think those are probably the top four.

Dr. Farthing: Have any of these been formally tested in the population that you were studying?

Dr. Ashworth: Not in that part of Brazil, but randomized, controlled trials on prevention of low birthweight have been done in other countries.

Dr. Tontisirin: With a colleague, I recently prepared a paper about a community-based program to reduce low birthweight. The key thing is to obtain the cooperation of pregnant women and persuade them to attend for antenatal care. We propose to create a *social mobilization* mechanism to link with the antenatal care services and increase coverage from 35% or 50% to more than 85%. Second, we aim for at least four or five antenatal care visits. This regimen has been successfully used in Thailand during the last 15 or 20 years. At the antenatal care visits, the woman has a high-risk checkup, health and nutrition education especially relating to food taboos and food beliefs and the importance of an adequate diet. In addition, she receives advice to stop smoking and drinking alcohol. She also gets multivitamin and iron supplements from the start, to be continued throughout pregnancy. We have shown that by these means we can increase birthweight in marginalized populations. For high risk pregnancy, a referral system is required. One other point I would like to make is that several studies in India have shown that low birthweight is associated with severe anemia during the pregnancy.

Dr. Fawzi: We carried out a trial in Tanzania among pregnant women who were human immunodeficiency virus positive. We found that micronutrients, mainly multivitamin supplements, resulted in nearly a 40% reduction in low birthweight, among other improvements in pregnancy outcome (9).

REFERENCES

1. Ashworth A, Morris SS, Lira PLC. Postnatal growth patterns of full-term low birthweight infants in northeast Brazil are related to socioeconomic status. *J Nutr* 1997; 127: 1950–6.
2. Caplan MS, Hsveh W. Necrotizing enterocolitis: role of platelet activating factor, endotoxin and tumor necrosis factor. *J Pediatr* 1990; 117: 47–51.

3. Adhikari M, Coovadia HM, Gaffin SL, et al. Septicaemic low birth weight neonates treated with human antibodies to endotoxin. *Arch Dis Child* 1985; 60: 382–4.
4. Godfrey KM, Barker DJP, Osmond C. Disproportionate fetal growth and raised IgE concentration in adult life. *Clin Exp Allergy* 1994: 24; 641–8.
5. Fergusson DM, Crane J, Beasley R, et al. Perinatal factors and atopic disease in childhood. *Clin Exp Allergy* 1997; 27: 1394–1401.
6. Lucas A, Brooke OG, Morley R, et al. Early diet of preterm infants and development of allergic or atopic disease: randomised prospective study. *BMJ* 1990; 300: 837–40.
7. Lira PI, Ashworth A, Morris SS. Low birth weight and morbidity from diarrhea and respiratory infection in north east Brazil. *J Pediatr* 1996; 128: 497–504.
8. de Onis M, Villar J, Gülmezoglu M. Nutritional interventions to prevent intrauterine growth retardation: evidence from randomized controlled trials. *Eur J Clin Nutr* 1998; 52 (Suppl. 1); S83–93.
9. Fawzi WW, Msamanga GI, Spiegelman D, et al, for the Tanzania Vitamin and HIV infection Trial Team. Randomized trial of effects of vitamin supplements on pregnancy outcomes and T cell counts in HIV-1-infected women in Tanzania. *Lancet* 1998; 351: 1477–1482.

Nutrition, Immunity, and Infection in Infants and Children, edited by Robert M. Suskind and Kraisid Tontisirin. Nestlé Nutrition Workshop Series, Pediatric Program, Vol. 45. Nestec Ltd., Vevey/Lippincott Williams & Wilkins, Philadelphia ©2001.

The Effect of Dietary Fatty Acids on the Immune Response and Susceptibility to Infection

P. C. Calder

Institute of Human Nutrition, University of Southampton, Southampton, UK

All mammals can synthesize fatty acids *de novo* from acetyl coenzyme A. The end product of the fatty acid synthetase enzyme is palmitic acid (16:0), which can be elongated to stearic acid (18:0). Little need is seen for the synthesis of saturated fatty acids in individuals in the Western world as the diet normally supplies adequate amounts. However, cell membranes require unsaturated fatty acids to maintain their structure, fluidity, and function. Therefore, a mechanism, termed *desaturation*, exists for the introduction of double bonds into acetyl chains. The introduction of a single double bond between carbon atoms 9 and 10 is catalyzed by the enzyme Δ^9-desaturase, which is universally present in both plants and animals. This enzyme results in the conversion of stearic acid to oleic acid (18:1*n*-9). Plants, unlike animals, can insert additional double bonds into oleic acid between the existing double bond at the 9-position and the methyl terminus of the carbon chain; a Δ^{12}-desaturase converts oleic acid into linoleic acid (18:2*n*-6), whereas a Δ^{15}-desaturase converts linoleic acid into α-linolenic acid (18:3*n*-3). Using the pathway outlined in Figure 1, animal cells can convert dietary α-linolenic acid into eicosapentaenoic acid (EPA; 20:5*n*-3) and docosahexaenoic acid (DHA; 22:6*n*-3); by a similar series of reactions dietary linoleic acid is converted via γ-linolenic (18:3*n*-6) and dihomo-γ-linolenic (20:3*n*-6) acids to arachidonic acid (20:4*n*-6). Because their tissues do not contain the Δ^{12}- or Δ^{15}-desaturases, animals are unable to interconvert the *n*-9, *n*-6, and *n*-3 families of polyunsaturated fatty acids (PUFA). Many marine plants, especially the unicellular algae in phytoplankton, also carry out chain elongation and further desaturation of α-linolenic acid to yield the long chain *n*-3 PUFA EPA and DHA. It is the formation of these long chain *n*-3 PUFA by marine algae and their transfer through the food chain to fish that accounts for

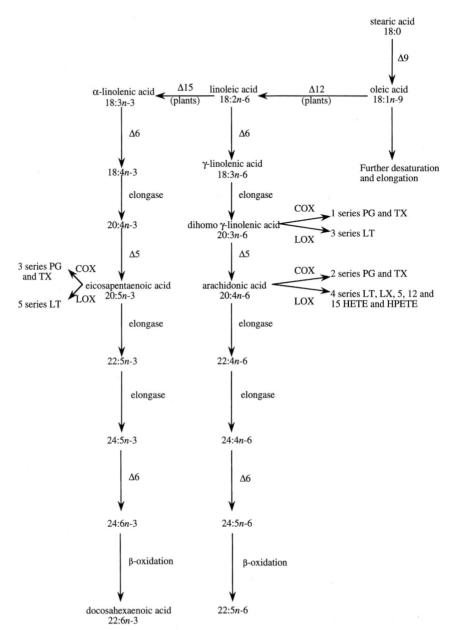

FIG. 1. Metabolism of polyunsaturated fatty acids. Δ^5, Δ^6, Δ^9, Δ^{12}, and Δ^{15}, desaturase enzymes; COX, cyclo-oxygenase; LOX, lipoxygenase enzymes; PG, prostaglandins; LT, leukotrienes; TX, thromboxanes; LX, lipoxins; HETE, hydroxyeicosatetraenoic acids; HPETE, hydroperoxyeicosatetraenoic acids.

TABLE 1. *Principal fatty acids in various dietary fats and oils*

Fat or oil	Principal fatty acids
Lard	Palmitic (16:0) comprises 20% to 35% of fatty acids
	Oleic (18:1n-9) comprises 35% to 65% of fatty acids
Beef tallow	Palmitic comprises 20% to 37% of fatty acids
	Oleic comprises 25% to 50% of fatty acids
Coconut oil	Medium chain saturated [capric (10:0), lauric (12:0), myristic (14:0)] comprise 65% to 80% of fatty acids
Palm oil	Palmitic comprises 40% to 50% of fatty acids
	Oleic comprises 35% to 45% of fatty acids
Olive oil	Oleic comprises 55% to 85% of fatty acids
Maize oil	Linoleic (18:2n-6) comprises 40% to 65% of fatty acids
Sunflower oil	Linoleic comprises 50% to 75% of fatty acids
Safflower oil	Linoleic comprises 65% to 85% of fatty acids
Soybean oil	Linoleic comprises 50% to 60% of fatty acids; α-linolenic (18:3n-3) comprises 5% to 10% of fatty acids
Evening primrose oil	Linoleic comprises 70% of fatty acids; γ-linolenic (18:3n-6 comprises 5% to 10% of fatty acids
Flaxseed oil	α-Linolenic comprises 35 to 65% of fatty acids
Fish (e.g., menhaden) oil	EPA (20:5n-3) comprises 10% to 15% of fatty acids
	DHA (22:6n-3) comprises 5% to 12% of fatty acids

EPA, elcosapentaenoic acid; DHA, docosahaxaeuoic acid.

their abundance in some marine fish oils. Table 1 lists the principal fatty acids found in various fats and oils that have been used experimentally.

Interest in the effects of fatty acids and dietary lipids on the immune system dates back many years, as reviewed by Meade and Mertin (1), but this interest has intensified with the elucidation of the roles of eicosanoids derived from arachidonic acid in modulating inflammation and immunity (2,3) and with the knowledge that the metabolism of arachidonic acid to yield these mediators can be inhibited by EPA and DHA (4,5). Despite its long history, the field remains a controversial one. Many cell culture and animal feeding experiments have been performed but relatively few good studies have been done in humans. Nevertheless, some key points have emerged:

- Essential fatty acid deficiency impairs cell-mediated immunity
- Cell-mediated immunity decreases as the fat content of the diet increases
- Within a high fat diet, different fatty acids can exert different effects

Various aspects of lipids and immunity have been reviewed (5–21) and this chapter will focus on more recent studies involving mononuclear cells (monocytes, macrophages, lymphocytes) and their functions *ex vivo* and *in vivo*. It will not cover in detail *in vitro* studies involving culture of isolated cells with purified fatty acids or fatty acid-containing lipids; these have been covered extensively elsewhere (7,9–11,16,20,21). Likewise, it will not deal with possible mechanisms of action of fatty acids in detail; these have also been discussed elsewhere (11,17,19).

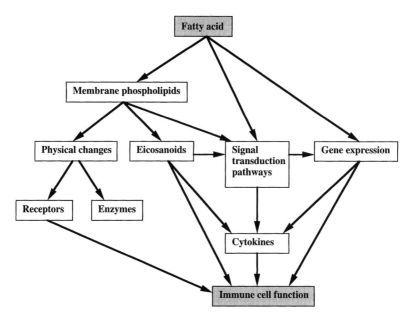

FIG. 2. Mechanisms by which fatty acids could influence immune cell function.

WHY SHOULD FATTY ACIDS EXERT EFFECTS WITHIN THE IMMUNE SYSTEM?

Various reasons are found to expect that different fatty acids might exert different effects within the immune system (Fig. 2). First, the fatty acid composition of membrane phospholipids changes according to the fatty acid composition of the diet, with some evidence indicating that this can alter the physical characteristics of the membrane (*e.g.*, its fluidity). This, in turn, can affect the functioning of some of the proteins within the membranes (*e.g.*, receptors, ion channels, and enzymes) that will alter the ability of the cell to respond to stimuli. Second, the phospholipids of the cell membrane are used to generate certain signaling molecules when an immune cell is stimulated and evidence suggests that altering the fatty acid composition of the phospholipids can alter the concentration and biological potency of these second messengers. Third, these signaling molecules include some such as prostaglandins and leukotrienes that are formed directly from arachidonic acid in the cell membrane; thus, lowering the concentration of this fatty acid, as happens when the level of *n*-3 PUFA in the diet is increased, will decrease the capacity to form these important immunoregulatory molecules. Fourth, it is now suspected that particular fatty acids act directly as signaling molecules within cells and so can directly influence their function. Finally, incorporation of PUFA into cells can alter the cellular redox status, so affecting cell function.

IMMUNE CELL FATTY ACID COMPOSITION AND EICOSANOID PRODUCTION

Modification of the fatty acid composition of immune cells such as macrophages and lymphocytes is readily achieved in culture simply by changing the fatty acid composition of the medium. Culture of these cells with n-3 PUFA results in replacement of arachidonic acid in phospholipids by the n-3 PUFA provided (22,23). Changing the fatty acid composition of the diet also results in significant modification of the fatty acid composition of macrophages (24,25) and lymphocytes (25–27). Again, one key change is the replacement of arachidonic acid by n-3 PUFA provided in the diet (Table 2).

Eicosanoids are a family of oxygenated derivatives of dihomo-γ-linolenic, arachidonic, and eicosapentaenoic acids. Eicosanoids include prostaglandins (PG), thromboxanes, leukotrienes (LT), lipoxins, hydroperoxy-eicosatetraenoic acids, and hydroxyeicosatetraenoic acids. In most conditions, the principal precursor for these compounds is arachidonic acid (Fig. 1). Prostaglandins (PG) are involved in modulating the intensity and duration of inflammatory and immune responses. PGE_2 has various proinflammatory effects: inducing fever and erythema; increasing vascular permeability and vasodilatation; and enhancing pain and edema caused by other agents such as bradykinin and histamine. In chronic inflammatory conditions, increased rates of PGE_2 production are observed and increased PGE_2 production has been observed in patients suffering from infections, burns, sepsis, and other traumas. Some leukotrienes act as chemoattractants, promoting movement of leukocytes to sites of inflammatory or immune activity, whereas others are involved in causing smooth muscle contraction and so have been implicated in diseases such as asthma where there is severe constriction of the airways.

TABLE 2. *Fatty acid composition of spleen leukocytes taken from rats fed diets containing different levels of long chain PUFA**

Fatty acid	Diet				
	Control	GLA	ARA	EPA	DHA
16:0	24.8 ± 1.7	29.6 ± 1.1	26.6 ± 1.6	29.4 ± 0.5	27.1 ± 1.8
18:0	15.8 ± 1.4	18.3 ± 0.9	18.5 ± 1.0	18.1 ± 0.5	18.2 ± 1.0
18:1n-9	10.9 ± 0.3	12.1 ± 0.2	11.1 ± 0.7	12.5 ± 0.3	12.2 ± 0.7
18:2n-6	11.9 ± 0.8	10.7 ± 0.1	7.9 ± 0.2	14.6 ± 1.7	16.4 ± 1.2
20:3n-6	0.8 ± 0.1	2.3 ± 0.1	0.7 ± 0.1	0.9 ± 0.1	0.4 ± 0.1
20:4n-6	16.2 ± 0.5	18.7 ± 0.7	23.5 ± 1.0	11.6 ± 0.5	12.8 ± 0.4
20:5n-3	0.20 ± 0.06	0.8 ± 0.5	0.26 ± 0.01	2.9 ± 0.2	0.32 ± 0.04
22:6n-3	0.7 ± 0.1	0.4 ± 0.1	0.4 ± 0.1	1.3 ± 0.4	3.8 ± 0.3

* Rats were fed for 6 weeks on a control diet (178 g fat/kg containing 31 g linoleic acid and 4.4 g α-linolenic acid/100 g total fatty acids) or on diets that replaced 4.4 g of linoleic acid with either γ-linolenic acid (GLA) or arachidonic acid (ARA) or which replaced 4.4 g α-linolenic acid with eicosapentaenoic acid (EPA) or docosahexaenoic acid (DHA). Spleen leukocytes were prepared and their fatty acid composition determined. Data are mean ± SEM.
PUFA, polyunsaturated fatty acids.
From Peterson LD et al. (27).

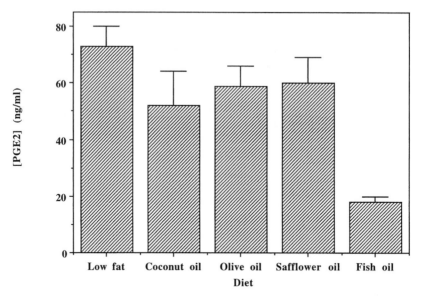

FIG. 3. Effects of dietary lipids on PGE_2 production. Mice were fed on a low fat (25 g/kg maize oil) diet or on diets containing 200 g/kg of either hydrogenated coconut oil, olive oil, safflower oil, or fish oil. Thioglycollate-elicited peritoneal macrophages were prepared and cultured with lipopolysaccharide (10 μg/ml) for 24 hours. PGE_2 concentrations were determined by enzyme-linked immunosorbent assay. Data are means; error bars = SEM. From Yaqoob P, Calder PC (30).

Not only do EPA and DHA replace arachidonic acid in cell membranes (Table 2), but they can competitively inhibit the oxygenation of arachidonic acid by cyclo-oxygenase. Thus, ingestion of n-3 PUFA results in a decreased capacity of cells to synthesize eicosanoids from arachidonic acid (24,25,27–31) (Fig. 3). In addition, EPA (but not DHA) is able to act as a substrate for both cyclo-oxygenase and 5-lipoxygenase (Fig. 1). Thus, the suppression of the production of arachidonic acid-derived eicosanoids is mirrored by an increase in the production of EPA-derived eicosanoids (32), such as the 3-series prostaglandins and thromboxanes and the 5-series leukotrienes. The eicosanoids produced from EPA are often less biologically potent than the analogues synthesized from arachidonic acid. For example, LTB_5 is 10 times less potent than LTB_4 as a neutrophil chemoattractant and PGE_3 is less proinflammatory than PGE_2. Thus, fish oil consumption is accompanied by a move toward the production of less inflammatory eicosanoids than those produced from arachidonic acid.

CHEMOTAXIS, PHAGOCYTOSIS, AND THE PRODUCTION OF REACTIVE OXYGEN AND NITROGEN SPECIES

Chemotaxis

Chemotaxis of blood monocytes toward the chemoattractants LTB_4 and formylmethionyl leucylphenylalanine was suppressed following supplementation of the human diet with approximately 5.5 g EPA plus DHA for 6 weeks (28,29,33). A recent study reported no effect of a lower dose of *n*-3 PUFA (0.65 g/d for 12 weeks) on monocyte chemotaxis toward pooled human serum (34).

Phagocytosis

It is likely that the process of phagocytosis will be influenced by membrane structure, in particular by the fluidity of the membrane; the latter property can be influenced by the fatty acid composition of membrane phospholipids. The phagocytic capacity of macrophages and monocytes is altered by the fatty acid composition of the medium in which they are cultured (21,22,35). A positive correlation is found between phagocytosis and percent PUFA, the ratio of unsaturated to saturated fatty acids, and the index of unsaturation of the cellular phospholipids (22).

Reports have shown that dietary fish oil does not affect phagocytosis of sheep erythrocytes or yeast particles by murine thioglycollate-elicited macrophages (36), or of latex beads by porcine alveolar macrophages (37). However, Eicher and McVey (38) found that fish oil feeding reduced the ability of murine Kupffer cells to phagocytose *Salmonella typhimurium*, although this was not associated with a reduced capacity of the cells to kill the bacteria. If the Kupffer cells were taken from mice infected with *S. typhimurium*, no apparent effect was seen of previous diet on either phagocytosis or bacterial killing. These observations contrast with those of D'Ambola *et al.* (39), who showed that fish oil given by gastric tube significantly diminished the ability of neonatal rabbits to clear a challenge of *Staphylococcus aureus*. A recent human study indicated no effect of 3.8 g EPA or DHA daily for 7 weeks on phagocytosis of opsonized or unopsonized *Escherichia coli* by human monocytes (40).

Production of Reactive Oxygen Species and Nitric Oxide

The enzymes that result in the synthesis of superoxide, hydrogen peroxide, and nitric oxide are regulated by eicosanoids, cytokines, and protein kinase C. As *n*-3 PUFA affect the production of eicosanoids (see above) and cytokines (see below) and might modulate protein kinase C activity (19), they might affect the production of reactive oxygen species and nitric oxide by macrophages and so regulate the cytotoxic activities of these cells. However, investigations of the effects of diets rich in *n*-3 PUFA on the production of hydrogen peroxide, superoxide, and nitric oxide have yielded contradictory results. Studies have reported that production of one or more of these mediators is enhanced, diminished, or not affected following fish oil feeding to laboratory animals (21). Likewise *n*-3 PUFA supplementation of the human diet has been reported to decrease zymosan-induced superoxide production by monocytes (41) but not to affect that induced by *E. coli* (40). The reasons for such significantly different experimental observations might include the different species of origin of the cells studied, the anatomic site of origin of the cells, the state of cellular differentiation, the state of activation of the cell, the stimulus used to elicit mediator production, the nature of the culture conditions used (presence or absence of serum, serum source, time of culture), the level of *n*-3 PUFA in the diet, the duration of feeding, the level of antioxidants in the diet, and so on.

EXPRESSION OF SURFACE MARKERS

Major Histocompatibility Antigens

Incubation with DHA inhibited interleukin (IL)-4- or γ-interferon–induced cell surface expression of major histocompatibility class II antigen (MHC II; in the mouse, these antigens are termed Ia) on mouse peritoneal macrophages (42); DHA was more inhibitory than EPA and other 20-carbon fatty acids and acted by inhibiting the increase in Ia mRNA, which occurs after stimulation of macrophages with cytokines (42). Hughes *et al.* (43) examined the effect of incubation of purified human monocytes with either EPA or DHA on expression of MHC II, which is termed *human leukocyte antigen* (HLA): both EPA and DHA reduced the proportion of HLA-DR or HLA-DP positive monocytes following incubation with γ-interferon and the level of expression of these molecules on the monocyte surface (43). In accordance with this, the ability of monocytes cultured with EPA and DHA to present antigen (tetanus toxoid) to autologous lymphocytes was diminished (44).

Inclusion of EPA plus DHA in the diet of mice or rats results in a diminished percentage of peritoneal exudate cells bearing MHC II antigens on their surface and level of MHC II expression on positive cells (45). Feeding fish oil to rats decreased the level of MHC II expression on thioglycollate-elicited peritoneal macrophages (46) and on dendritic cells obtained by cannulation of the thoracic duct (47). In accordance with these animal studies, supplementation of the diet of human volunteers with 1.6 g EPA plus DHA for 3 weeks resulted in a decreased level of MHC II (HLA-DP, HLA-DQ, and HLA-DR) expression on the surface of peripheral blood monocytes (48).

These observations suggest that diets rich in fish oil will result in diminished antigen presentation. Indeed, feeding mice the ethyl ester of EPA for a period of 4 to 5 weeks resulted in diminished *ex vivo* presentation of antigen (keyhole limpet hemacyanin; KLH) by spleen cells (49). Compared with feeding a low fat diet or a diet containing 200 g/kg safflower oil, feeding rats a diet containing 200 g/kg fish oil significantly diminished *ex vivo* KLH presentation by dendritic cells obtained by cannulation of the thoracic duct to KLH-sensitized spleen lymphocytes (47).

Adhesion Molecules

Incubation of human lymphocytes with EPA or DHA decreased the level of expression of various adhesion molecules, including leukocyte function associated molecule-1 (LFA-1) and L-selectin, without affecting expression of very late antigen 1; arachidonic acid did not influence surface expression of these molecules (50). In accordance with the effects on expression of some cell surface adhesion molecules, incubation of human lymphocytes with EPA or DHA reduced adhesion between the lymphocytes and untreated endothelial cells or endothelial cells stimulated by cytokine or bacterial lipopolysaccharide (LPS) (50). The proportion of purified human monocytes expressing intercellular adhesion molecule-1 (ICAM-1) and the level of ICAM-1 expression were reduced by incubation with EPA; DHA did not affect ICAM-1 or LFA-1 expression on resting monocytes (43). Both EPA and DHA reduced the proportion of ICAM-1 positive monocytes and the level of ICAM-1 expression following incubation with γ-interferon (43). DHA also reduced the expression of LFA-1 on γ-interferon–stimulated monocytes.

Feeding rats a fish oil rich diet caused a 30% reduction in the level of expression of CD18 (the β chain of LFA-1) on thioglycollate-elicited peritoneal macrophages (46), and significantly reduced levels of expression of CD2, CD11a, ICAM-1, CD18, CD44, and L-selectin on the surface of lymphocytes in various states of activation (51–53). Diets rich in evening primrose oil or olive oil also decreased the expression of some lymphocyte adhesion molecules (51–53). The fish oil or olive oil diets decreased the adhesion of both freshly prepared and concanavalin A-stimulated lymphocytes to macrophage monolayers or untreated endothelial cells (53). Furthermore, the fish oil diet resulted in a 50% reduction in concanavalin A-stimulated lymphocyte adhesion to endothelial cells stimulated by tumor necrosis factor-α (TNF-α) (53). Supplementation of the human diet with 1.6 g EPA plus DHA daily resulted in significantly lower levels of expression of ICAM-1 and LFA-1 on peripheral blood monocytes (48). These studies show that dietary lipids affect the expression of functionally important adhesion molecules on the surface of various cells of the immune system (and also on endothelial cells) (54). Furthermore, the study of Sanderson and Calder (53) suggests that such diet-induced effects on adhesion molecule expression alter the ability of leukocytes to bind to one another and suggests that fish oil feeding will affect the movement of leukocytes between body compartments and perhaps into sites of inflammatory or immune activity.

In accordance with the effect of olive oil feeding to rats, Yaqoob *et al.* (55) have shown that increasing the proportion of oleic acid in the human diet, at the expense of saturated fatty acids, significantly decreased (by 20%) the proportion of blood mononuclear cells expressing ICAM-1; the proportion of mononuclear cells expressing CD11b also declined but this was not statistically significant.

Cytokine Receptors

Feeding rats high fat diets rich in olive oil, evening primrose oil, or fish oil decreased the proportion of lymphocytes bearing the interleukin-2 (IL-2) receptor following concanavalin A stimulation (56) and lowered the level of IL-2 receptor on these cells (51). Jolly *et al.* (57) recently showed that feeding mice a diet rich in EPA or DHA significantly decreased the appearance of mRNA for the alpha subunit of the IL-2 receptor following concanavalin A stimulation, suggesting that these fatty acids regulate expression of the IL-2 receptor gene. Supplementation of the diet of patients with psoriasis or atopic dermatitis with 6 g EPA plus DHA ethyl esters daily caused a significant reduction in the percentage of IL-2 receptor-positive blood lymphocytes following phytohemagglutinin stimulation; the level of expression of the IL-2 receptor on the positive cells was also significantly reduced (58).

EFFECTS OF AMOUNT AND TYPE OF FAT IN THE DIET ON LYMPHOCYTE PROLIFERATION

Amount of Fat in the Diet

Many studies have compared the effects of feeding laboratory animals low and high fat diets on lymphocyte proliferation (7,9,16,20). Such studies have often found that high fat diets result in diminished *ex vivo* lymphocyte proliferation compared with low fat diets, but the precise effect depends on the level of fat used in the high fat diet and its source. A reduction in total dietary fat intake (from 40% to 25% of total energy) resulted in greatly enhanced human blood lymphocyte proliferation in response to concanavalin A or phytohemagglutinin (59,60), suggesting that high fat diets suppress human lymphocyte proliferation.

Saturated Fatty Acids

High fat diets using lard, beef tallow, palm oil, or hydrogenated coconut oil as the source of fat have been used in many animal studies of lymphocyte proliferation; in some studies, the high saturated fat diet has been compared, along with other high fat diets, to a low fat control, whereas in other studies the high saturated fat diet appears to serve as a high fat control to which the effects of PUFA-rich diets were compared (7,9,16,20). As a result, the precise nature of the effects of high saturated fat diets is difficult to gauge. Some studies have revealed that high saturated fat diets do not affect lymphocyte proliferation compared with feeding low fat diets, whereas others have shown that they are suppressive but less so than PUFA-rich diets. A third series of studies in which saturated fatty acids are used as a comparison with PUFA-rich diets simply shows that they have different effects from the PUFA-rich diets; whether one diet is without effect and the other inhibits the lymphocyte response or whether one is without effect and the other enhances the lymphocyte response is often unclear (7,9,16,20).

Only one study has compared the effects of different individual saturated fatty acids on lymphocyte proliferation (61). In this study, diets containing 178 g/kg fat were fed to rats; the diets differed according to the principal saturated fatty acids they contained (medium chain, lauric, palmitic, or stearic) and according to the position of the palmitic acid on the dietary triacylglycerols (sn-1(3) or sn-2) but the levels of total saturated, oleic, polyunsaturated, linoleic, and α-linolenic acids were identical. Spleen lymphocyte proliferation in response to concanavalin A was enhanced if the animals were fed the diet with palmitic acid at the sn-2 position of dietary triacylglycerols compared with feeding the other diets (61).

Oleic Acid

Berger *et al.* (62) reported that a 100 g/kg olive oil diet did not affect concanavalin A-stimulated proliferation of spleen lymphocytes; that study cultured the lymphocytes in fetal calf serum. In contrast, feeding rats a 200 g/kg olive oil diet resulted in diminished *ex vivo* lymphocyte proliferation when the cells were cultured in autologous serum (but not when they were cultured in fetal calf serum) (56), a finding confirmed using a 200 g/kg oleic acid rich sunflower oil diet (63). A significant inverse relationship was found between the proliferation of spleen lymphocytes in response to concanavalin A and the ratio of oleic acid to linoleic acid in the diet (64). One study of the effect of dietary intervention with oleic acid on human lymphocyte proliferation has been performed (55); after 2 months, a trend developed toward reduced proliferative responses to concanavalin A of whole blood cultures and of isolated blood lymphocytes, but the effect of diet was not statistically significant.

Linoleic Acid-Rich Oils

Several studies have reported lower concanavalin A- or phytohemagglutinin-stimulated T-lymphocyte proliferation following the feeding of diets rich in maize or safflower oils to laboratory rodents, compared with feeding diets rich in saturated fatty acids (7,9,16,20). In contrast, some studies have reported no effect of feeding linoleic acid rich diets on rodent T-lymphocyte proliferation (7,9,16,20). However, it is now apparent that the outcome of such measures of lymphocyte function is strongly influenced by the conditions used to culture the cells *ex vivo* (26,56) and this may account for the discrepancies in the literature. No difference was observed in the responses to T-cell mitogens of human blood lymphocytes from volunteers consuming low fat diets that were rich (12.9% of energy) or poor (3.5% of energy) in *n*-6 PUFA (59,60); the cells were cultured in fetal calf serum.

γ-Linolenic Acid

Rat lymph node and spleen lymphocyte proliferation in response to concanavalin A was decreased following the feeding of a diet rich in evening primrose oil, which provided approximately 7 g γ-linolenic acid/100 g total fatty acids (51,56). Inclusion of 4.4 g γ-linolenic acid/100 g fatty acids in the rat diet did not significantly affect concanavalin A-stimulated spleen lymphocyte proliferation (27).

α-Linolenic Acid

Feeding rats diets containing large amounts of flaxseed oil (rich in α-linolenic acid) suppressed spleen T-lymphocyte proliferation compared with feeding diets rich in hydrogenated coconut oil (65) or sunflower oil (66). Similarly, feeding chickens a flaxseed oil-rich diet suppressed spleen lymphocyte proliferation compared with feeding diets rich in canola or maize oils or lard (67). In a recent study, rats were fed diets containing 178 g fat/kg but differing in PUFA content (17.5 or 35 g/100 g fatty acids) and linoleic acid to α-linolenic acid ratio (ratios of 100,20,10,5,1 were used); the PUFA content was altered by replacing a proportion of palmitic acid with linoleic and α-linolenic acids (68). Lymphocyte proliferation decreased as the linoleic acid to α-linolenic acid ratio of the *low* PUFA diet decreased; the linoleic acid to α-linolenic acid ratio of the *high* PUFA did not significantly affect lymphocyte proliferation (68). This study indicates that both linoleic and α-linolenic acids reduce lymphocyte proliferation, that the effect of the latter is dependent on the total PUFA content of the diet, and that α-linolenic acid is more potent than linoleic acid. Wu *et al.* (69) fed monkeys for 14 weeks on diets containing 3.5% or 5.3% of energy as α-linolenic acid (PUFA comprised 28 g/100 g total fatty acids and the *n*-6:*n*-3 PUFA ratios of the two diets were 1.0 and 0.5). Blood lymphocyte proliferation in response to concanavalin A or phytohemagglutinin was unaffected compared with the basal diet, which had an *n*-6:*n*-3 PUFA ratio of 36. The observations of Wu *et al.* (69) and Jeffery *et al.* (68) are in agreement: both studies indicate that replacing a proportion of linoleic acid with α-linolenic acid in a *high* PUFA diet has minimal effect on lymphocyte proliferation.

Arachidonic Acid

Feeding mice a diet containing 20 g safflower oil plus 10 g arachidonic acid/kg did not affect concanavalin A-stimulated spleen lymphocyte proliferation compared with feeding a diet containing safflower oil (30 g/kg) (70). Inclusion of 4.4 g arachidonic acid/100 g fatty acids in the rat diet did not significantly affect concanavalin A-stimulated spleen lymphocyte proliferation (27). These observations agree with the outcome of the first study of dietary arachidonic acid and human lymphocyte function: 1.5 g arachidonic acid daily for 50 days did not affect the proliferative response of blood lymphocytes to concanavalin A, phytohemagglutinin, or pokeweed mitogen (71).

Eicosapentaenoic and Docosahexaenoic Acids

Feeding diets rich in fish oil to rabbits, chickens, rats, or mice results in suppressed proliferation of T (and in some studies B) lymphocytes compared with feeding hydrogenated coconut, safflower, maize, or flaxseed oils or lard (51,56,67,72–74). A recent study indicates that inclusion of EPA plus DHA in the rat diet at levels of 4.4 or 6.6 g/100 g total fatty acids is sufficient to significantly reduce spleen lymphocyte proliferation in response to concanavalin A (by ∼30%) (75). Supplementation of the diets of healthy women (51 to 68 years of age) with encapsulated EPA plus DHA (∼2.4 g/d) resulted in a lowered mitogenic response of blood lymphocytes to phytohemagglutinin (76); the mitogenic response of lymphocytes from young women (21 to 33 years of age) supplemented with this level of EPA plus DHA was unaffected. More recently, a decreased response of blood lymphocytes to concanavalin A and phytohemagglutinin following supplementation of the diet of volunteers on a low fat, low cholesterol diet with 1.23 g EPA plus DHA/d was reported (77).

These studies do not indicate whether the suppressive effect of fish oil feeding on lymphocyte proliferation is caused by EPA or DHA, or both; nor is there any indication of the level of long chain *n*-3 PUFA required to affect lymphocyte proliferation. These questions have recently been addressed (27,70,78). Feeding mice diets containing 20 g safflower oil plus 10 g of either EPA or DHA/kg reduced concanavalin A-stimulated spleen lymphocyte proliferation compared with feeding a diet containing 30 g/kg safflower oil (70); both *n*-3 PUFA were equipotent and reduced proliferation by approximately 80%. Peterson *et al.* (27) fed rats diets containing 178 g/kg fat and replaced α-linolenic acid (4.4 g/100 g fatty acids) with either EPA or DHA while keeping the total PUFA content and *n*-6:*n*-3 PUFA ratio of the diet constant. Both EPA and DHA reduced lymphocyte proliferation to the same extent (~30% to 35%) compared with the diet containing α-linolenic acid. Thus, these studies suggest that both EPA and DHA result in inhibition of lymphocyte proliferation and that relatively low levels are able to exert this effect, compared with the levels present in fish oil. Possible reasons for the quantitative differences in the effects between these studies are discussed elsewhere (27). Kelley *et al.* (78) reported that supplementation of the human diet with 6 g DHA daily for 90 days did not affect blood lymphocyte proliferation in response to concanavalin A or phytohemagglutinin. This observation suggests that DHA is less potent in humans than in rodents and that the effects of fish oil supplementation in humans (76,77) might result mainly from EPA.

Monkeys were fed for 14 weeks on diets containing 1.3% or 3.3% of energy as EPA plus DHA (PUFA comprised 30 g/100 g total fatty acids and the *n*-6:*n*-3 PUFA ratios of the two diets were 4.4 and 1.1): the proliferative response of blood lymphocytes to concanavalin A or phytohemagglutinin was enhanced (69). This observation is contradictory to previous observations in experimental animals (see earlier) and to previous observations in humans (76,77). The authors provide some evidence that this discrepancy is the result of better maintained levels of vitamin E in comparison with previous studies, thereby suggesting that long chain *n*-3 PUFA inhibit lymphocyte proliferation through a process which vitamin E protects against.

EFFECTS OF AMOUNT AND TYPE OF FAT IN THE DIET ON CYTOTOXIC ACTIONS OF LYMPHOCYTES

Cytotoxic T-Lymphocyte Activity

Cytotoxic T-lymphocyte activity is more reduced by feeding laboratory animals high fat diets rich in safflower oil, soybean oil, flaxseed oil, or fish oil than by feeding low fat diets or high fat diets rich in lard or hydrogenated coconut oil; fish oil appears to cause the greatest reduction in cytotoxic T-lymphocyte activity (7,9,16,20).

Natural Killer Cell Activity

A reduced fat intake (to less than 30% or 22% of total energy, respectively) is associated with a significant increase in natural killer (NK) cell activity of human blood lymphocytes (79,80), suggesting that high fat consumption suppresses NK cell activity in humans. Subsequent supplementation of the diet with 15 g coconut or safflower oil daily for 2 months reduced NK-cell activity to the prestudy level, both oils being equally effective (79).

Several early studies suggest little effect of high saturated fat or linoleic acid-rich diets on rodent NK-cell activity (7,9,16,20). Feeding a flaxseed oil-rich diet decreased rat spleen lymphocyte NK-cell activity compared with feeding a sunflower oil-rich diet (66). A high evening primrose oil diet also decreased NK-cell activity (51,81). Various studies have shown that feeding rats or mice on fish oil-rich diets results in suppressed spleen lymphocyte NK-cell activity compared with feeding low fat diets or high fat diets rich in saturated fat or *n*-6 PUFA (52,62,81,82); fish oil appears to be more suppressive than flaxseed oil (83). Although one study reports no effect of an olive oil-rich diet on *ex vivo* rat spleen NK-cell activity (62), diets containing 200 g/kg of olive oil or oleic acid-rich sunflower oil were found to significantly reduce this activity (52,63,81).

Recent animal studies have endeavored to establish the effects of particular discrete changes in dietary fatty acid composition on NK-cell activity. The type of saturated fatty acid in the rat diet has been reported to influence spleen NK-cell activity, which was greater if the animals had been fed a diet containing palmitic acid as the principal saturated fatty acid than if they had consumed diets rich in medium chain, lauric, or stearic acids (61). Another study reported a significant inverse linear correlation between the level of oleic acid or the ratio of oleic acid to linoleic acid in the rat diet and spleen lymphocyte NK-cell activity (64). One study of the effect of dietary intervention with oleic acid on human NK-cell activity has been performed (55). After 2 months of increased oleic acid intake at the expense of saturated fatty acids, a trend developed toward reduced NK- cell activity, but the effect of diet was not statistically significant (55). In another study, rats were fed diets containing 178 g/kg fat but differing in PUFA content (17.5 or 35 g/100 g fatty acids) and linoleic acid to α-linolenic acid ratio (ratios of 100,20,10,5,1 were used); the PUFA content was altered by replacing a proportion of palmitic acid with linoleic and α-linolenic acids (68). NK-cell activity decreased as the linoleic acid to α-linolenic acid ratio of the *low* PUFA diet decreased; the linoleic acid to α-linolenic acid ratio of the *high* PUFA had less impact on NK-cell activity (68). This study indicates that dietary α-linolenic acid reduces NK-cell activity but that its effect is dependent on the total PUFA content of the diet and its level relative to that of linoleic acid. Inclusion of 4.4 g arachidonic acid/100 g fatty acids in the rat diet did not affect NK-cell activity of spleen lymphocytes (27). Similarly, Kelley *et al.* (71) reported that 1.5 g arachidonic acid daily for 50 days did not affect the human NK-cell activity. Replacing α-linolenic acid (4.4 g/100 g fatty acids) with EPA in a high fat diet (with the total PUFA content and *n*-6:*n*-3 PUFA ratio of the diet kept constant) reduced rat spleen NK-cell activity, whereas replacing α-linolenic acid with DHA did not affect NK-cell activity (27). An intravenous injection of a triacylglycerol containing EPA into healthy human volunteers resulted in suppression of peripheral blood NK-cell activity 24 hours later (84). These observations suggest that the effects of fish oil on NK-cell activity might be caused mainly by EPA.

ANTIBODY PRODUCTION

Studies in Experimental Animals

Essential fatty acid deficiency impaired the ability of mice to produce IgG and IgM in response to sheep red blood cells (85); this response was restored by feeding diets containing 130, 500, or 700 g/kg maize oil (85). In contrast to this apparent enhancing effect of linoleic acid on antibody production, dietary linoleic acid was found to reduce the production of antibodies, including IgG and IgM, following antigenic challenges, compared with feeding low fat or high saturated fat diets (beef tallow, coconut oil) (86,87). Enhanced production of IgE to ovalbumin was reported in rats fed a diet high in fish oil compared with those fed a saturated fat diet (88). Total serum IgG and IgM levels were increased (two- and threefold, respectively) in mice fed fish oil compared with those fed maize oil (89).

Studies in Humans and Other Primates

Feeding cebus or squirrel monkeys on diets containing 143 g/kg coconut or maize oil for several years did not result in different antibody responses to measles vaccine (90). Kelley *et al.* (59,60) reported no effect on circulating IgM, IgG, IgE, or IgA levels of reducing total fat intake (from 40% to 25–30% of total energy) or of varying the amount of PUFA (3.5% or 12.9% of energy) in the human diet. Including flaxseed oil or salmon in the diet did not alter circulating antibody levels (91,92). Feeding healthy volunteers a diet containing 1.5 g arachidonic acid/d for 60 days did not alter serum antibody titers against three strains of the influenza virus (93).

CYTOKINE PRODUCTION

As cytokine production by macrophages is regulated by eicosanoids and as dietary lipids affect eicosanoid production (see earlier), it might be expected that dietary lipids, especially those containing *n*-3 PUFA, will affect cytokine production.

TNF, IL-1, and IL-6: Animal Studies

Several animal studies have investigated the effect of dietary lipids on *ex vivo* production of macrophage-derived cytokines, including TNF, IL-1, and IL-6. These studies have been reviewed in detail elsewhere (21). Several studies have reported that feeding rodents with *n*-3 PUFA-containing oils results in enhanced production of TNF by macrophages *ex vivo*, although decreased production or no effect following fish or flaxseed oil feeding has been reported (21). These differences between studies appear not to relate to species, duration of feeding, or type or amount of *n*-3 PUFA in the diet. However, some relationship may exist with the state of activation of the macrophages used. All studies that have used murine resident peritoneal macrophages, one study using rat resident alveolar macrophages and one study using rat resident peritoneal macrophages report an enhancing effect of *n*-3 PUFA on TNF production (21); only one study that used rat resident peritoneal macrophages has reported reduced TNF production following fish oil feeding (21). The effect of dietary *n*-3 PUFA on TNF production by thioglycollate-elicited peritoneal macrophages is unclear, with studies reporting no effect, reduction, or enhancement (21). Comparison of the outcome of these studies is complicated by the different procedures used for *ex vivo* culture of the cells (21). The only animal study that has investigated TNF production by peripheral blood mononuclear cells showed decreased production following the infusion of a 10% (vol/vol) fish oil emulsion (94); this is an interesting observation because it agrees with the findings of several studies using human blood mononuclear cells (see below). Fish oil feeding also significantly reduced TNF-α production by cultures of murine splenocytes stimulated with LPS (89). In addition to studies measuring TNF production *ex vivo*, it was reported that feeding mice *n*-3 PUFA-rich diets resulted in reduced ability of elicited peritoneal macrophages to kill L929 cells (31,95); L929 cells are killed by TNF and so the reduced cytotoxicity of macrophages toward these cells suggests a reduced ability to produce TNF.

Some studies have investigated the effects of dietary lipids on circulating TNF levels that would reflect *in vivo* production of the cytokine. TNF levels were significantly higher in the plasma of LPS-injected mice fed diets containing 100 g/kg perilla oil than in the plasma of those fed 100 g/kg safflower oil (96). Similarly, higher serum TNF levels following intraperitoneal injection of LPS were reported in fish oil fed mice compared with those fed coconut or maize oil (97,98). In contrast, compared with safflower oil, coconut or fish oil feeding both reduced peak plasma TNF-α concentrations after intraperitoneal injection of LPS in mice (99). Furthermore, parenteral nutrition supplemented with fish oil reduced serum TNF-α concentrations in burned rats compared with *n*-6 PUFA rich parenteral nutrition (100).

All studies that have used thioglycollate-elicited peritoneal macrophages and the only study to use Kupffer cells report that dietary fish oil results in decreased *ex vivo* production of IL-1 (30,101,102). Furthermore, fish oil feeding significantly reduced IL-1β production by cultures of murine splenocytes stimulated with LPS (89). Compared with safflower oil, coconut or fish oil feeding both reduced peak plasma IL-1β concentrations after intraperitoneal injection of LPS in mice (99). In contrast, one study reported that fish oil enhances IL-1 production by murine resident macrophages (103), whereas Blok *et al.* (104) report no difference in the concentrations of IL-1α or IL-1β in the medium of LPS-stimulated resident peritoneal macrophages taken from mice fed palm, maize, or fish oils. Ertel *et al.* (105) also showed no difference in IL-1 production by resident peritoneal macrophages taken from mice fed diets rich in maize, safflower, or fish oil.

No studies report the effect of dietary fatty acids on IL-6 production by resident peritoneal macrophages. One study using murine thioglycollate-elicited peritoneal macrophages showed a significant reduction in LPS-stimulated IL-6 production following fish oil feeding (30); production following stimulation of the cells with TNF was also significantly reduced (Yaqoob P and Calder PC, 1995, unpublished observations). Rat blood mononuclear cells showed reduced IL-6 production following fish oil infusion for 4 days (94). Compared with safflower oil, coconut or fish oil feeding both reduced peak plasma IL-6 concentrations after intraperitoneal injection of LPS in mice (99). These studies are supported by the *in vitro* observation that EPA and DHA inhibit IL-6 production by rat thioglycollate-elicited peritoneal macrophages (106).

Despite the apparent contradictions in published reports regarding the effects on proinflammatory cytokine production of feeding animals with *n*-3 PUFA rich diets, some patterns do emerge. It appears that fish oil feeding enhances, or does not affect, TNF and IL-1 production by resident macrophages. In contrast, fish oil feeding reduces TNF, IL-1, and IL-6 production by thioglycollate-elicited macrophages and blood mononuclear cells. Fish oil feeding to mice lowered TNF-α mRNA levels in LPS-stimulated, thioglycollate-elicited murine macrophages (95), completely abolished the appearance of mRNA for IL-1β, IL-6, and TNF-α in the kidneys of autoimmune disease-prone mice (107), and significantly diminished IL-1β mRNA production by LPS or phorbol ester-stimulated spleen lmphocytes (108); the lower IL-1β mRNA level was not caused by accelerated degradation but by impaired synthesis. These studies suggest that *n*-3 PUFA affect proinflammatory cytokine production by control at the transcriptional level.

Infection with human immunodeficiency virus (HIV) alters cytokine profiles, increasing TNF and IL-1; TNF-α and IL-1β can stimulate HIV expression in infected cells and a correlation between the progression of acquired immunodeficiency syndrome (AIDS) and serum TNF concentration was observed in one study (89). Murine AIDS is also associated with increased production of TNF and IL-1 (89). Feeding fish oil to mice infected with murine AIDS significantly reduced TNF-α and IL-1β production by LPS-stimulated splenocytes compared with feeding maize oil (89). Fish oil was shown to increase survival of mice infected with murine AIDS significantly compared with maize oil (109).

IL-2, IL-4, γ-Interferon, and IL-10: Animal Studies

In contrast with the large number of studies of the effects of dietary lipids, especially fish oils, on the *ex vivo* production of macrophage-derived cytokines, relatively few studies have been done on lymphocyte-derived cytokines. Fish oil and flaxseed oil have been shown to reduce IL-2 production by pig alveolar lymphocytes (37). Feeding mice diets rich in either EPA or DHA diminished *ex vivo* IL-2 production by concanavalin A-stimulated spleen lymphocytes (70) by altering the kinetics of the appearance of mRNA for IL-2 (57). In contrast, inclusion of fish oil in the diet of autoimmune disease-prone mice resulted in raised levels of mRNA for IL-2, IL-4, and transforming growth factor-β in the spleen (110). One animal study that compared the effects of dietary lipids on the production of both Th1- (IL-2, γ-interferon) and Th2-derived cytokines (IL-4, IL-10) showed little effect of dietary lipids, including fish oil, in mice (74). This was confirmed recently by the lack of effect of fish oil compared with maize oil on IL-2 and γ-interferon production by murine splenocytes (89). In the study of Wu *et al.* in monkeys described earlier (69), IL-2 production was increased in the groups fed diets enriched with EPA plus DHA. Although this observation is contradictory to some studies in animals and humans (see below), the investigators suggest that the difference reflects the level of vitamin E included in the monkey diets. Together, these studies suggest that different effects may be observed in different animal species and in different strains within a species, that fish oil might exert different effects on lymphocytes in healthy or diseased animals, and that an interaction may exist between fish oil and antioxidant vitamins.

Human Studies

A number of studies have shown that supplementation of the diet of healthy humans with between 1.1 and 5 g EPA plus DHA daily for several weeks (up to 24) leads to a significant reduction in *ex vivo* production of TNF (29,76,77,111,112), IL-1 (29,76,77,111–114), IL-6 (76,113,114), IL-2 (76,77,111,115), and γ-interferon (111) by blood mononuclear cells. A controlled study of fish oil-supplemented parenteral nutrition following major surgery was recently reported (116); the characteristic postoperative rises in the plasma concentrations of TNF-α and IL-6 that occurred in the control group who received a soya bean oil-rich emulsion were significantly blunted in the group receiving fish oil. Supplementation of the diet of healthy subjects with 0.65 g EPA plus DHA daily for 12 weeks did not affect *ex vivo* production of TNF-α, IL-1β, or IL-6 by blood mononuclear cells (34).

The effects of dietary α-linolenic acid on IL-1β and TNF-α production by human cells have been reported: subjects consumed a sunflower oil-rich diet (similar to their typical diet) or a diet rich in α-linolenic acid provided by flaxseed oil capsules and flaxseed oil-based spreads and cooking oils (112). In this way, the flaxseed oil consumption increased to a mean of 13.7 g/d. *Ex vivo* production of both IL-1β and TNF-α by blood mononuclear cells was decreased by the flaxseed oil diet (112). When the subjects then supplemented their diet with encapsulated EPA plus DHA, production of both cytokines was further decreased (112). These investigators showed an inverse correlation between mononuclear cell EPA content and production of IL-1β and TNF-α (112).

Arachidonic acid (1.5 g/d for 60 days) did not alter TNF-α, IL-1β, IL-6, or IL-2 production by human mononuclear cells (93).

IN VIVO MEASURES OF INFLAMMATION AND CELL-MEDIATED IMMUNITY

The studies outlined above have most often investigated the effects of dietary manipulations on *ex vivo* functions of isolated cell populations. Although various consistent patterns have emerged from these studies, contradictory reports were also made and it is evident that the outcome of such *ex vivo* measures is strongly influenced by the experimental conditions used. Furthermore, *in vivo* cells exist as part of a network being influenced by other cell types; often such interactions are disturbed by the purification of the particular cell types to be studied. Therefore, it is important to investigate the effect of dietary fats on the intact, fully functioning system in which all normal cellular interactions are in place. The ability to make *in vivo* measures of inflammation and of cell-mediated immunity offers the prospect of investigating the effects of dietary manipulations on the overall responses of these systems.

Acute Inflammatory Responses

Arachidonic acid-derived eicosanoids are involved in mediating inflammatory responses. As n-3 PUFA diminish the production of these mediators following an inflammatory challenge (117,118), they should exert anti-inflammatory activities. The changes in the pattern of inflammatory eicosanoid production after intraperitoneal injection of zymosan in rodents were accompanied by a decreased influx of neutrophils into the peritoneal cavity (118). Furthermore, feeding rats 100 g/kg cod liver oil for 10 weeks significantly lowered (by 40%) the inflammatory response to carrageenan injection into the footpad compared with feeding coconut oil or groundnut oil (119). In accordance with that observation, feeding rats high fat diets containing 20 g/kg of ethyl esters of EPA or DHA resulted in a 50% reduction in footpad swelling in response to carrageenan injection compared with feeding safflower oil (120); EPA and DHA were equally effective.

In vivo Response to Endotoxin and Cytokines

Two 24-hour intravenous infusions of a 10% (vol/vol) lipid emulsion rich in fish oil into guinea pigs significantly enhanced survival after intraperitoneally injected LPS compared with infusion of a 10% (vol/vol) safflower oil emulsion (121); the total amount of lipid infused was 13 g/animal. The same authors later showed that feeding a 145 g/kg fish oil diet to guinea pigs for 6 weeks significantly increased survival after an intraperitoneal injection of LPS compared with animals fed a 150 g/kg safflower oil diet (122). In accordance with the diminished susceptibility to the lethal effects of endotoxin in experimental animals, feeding weanling rats a 100 g/kg fish oil diet for 8 weeks significantly decreased several responses to intraperitoneal TNF-α: the rises in liver zinc and plasma C3 concentrations, the fall in plasma albumin concentration, and the increases in liver, kidney, and lung protein synthesis rates were all prevented by the fish oil diet (123). Fish oil feeding to rats or guinea pigs also diminished the pyrogenic (124, 125) and anorexic effects (123,126) of IL-1 and TNF-α compared with feeding linoleic acid-containing oils.

Delayed Type Hypersensitivity

The delayed type hypersensitivity (DTH) reaction is the result of a cell-mediated response to challenge with an antigen to which the individual has already been primed.

Essential fatty acid deficiency impaired the murine DTH response, which was restored by addition of maize oil (130 or 500 g/kg), to the diet (127). The DTH response in rats or guinea pigs is reduced by feeding high fat diets compared with feeding low fat diets (86,128); linoleic acid-rich diets are more suppressive than high saturated fat diets. Dietary fish oil reduces the DTH response in mice compared with n-6 PUFA rich or olive oil-rich diets (117), whereas the addition of ethyl esters of either EPA or DHA to the diet of mice consuming a safflower oil diet reduced the DTH response (129); EPA and DHA were equally effective. The DTH response to sheep red blood cells in mice was diminished following tail vein injections of emulsions of triacyl-glycerols rich in EPA or DHA (130). Feeding beagle dogs a diet with an *n*-6:*n*-3 PUFA ratio of 1.4 resulted in a reduced DTH response to intradermal KLH compared with diets with *n*-6 to *n*-3 PUFA ratios of 31 or 5.4 (131); the increased *n*-3 PUFA content was brought about by replacing linoleic acid with EPA plus DHA. These observations are consistent with many of the reported effects of dietary *n*-3 PUFA on *ex vivo* lymphocyte responses (*e.g.*, decreased proliferation and IL-2 production).

A 40-day reduction in fat intake (from 40% to 25–30% of energy) by healthy human volunteers did not alter the DTH responses to seven recall antigens (60); these responses were also unaffected by differences in the PUFA level of the diet (3.2% or 9.1% of energy) (60) or by consuming a salmon rich diet (500 g/d for 40 days) (92). Feeding a flaxseed oil rich diet to healthy human volunteers for 8 weeks lowered the DTH response to seven recall antigens, although this reduction was not statistically significant (91). Arachidonic acid (1.5 g arachidonic acid/d) did not affect the DTH response to seven recall antigens applied intradermally (71). Supplementation of the diet of volunteers consuming a low fat, low cholesterol diet with 1.25 g EPA plus DHA daily, diminished the DTH responses to seven recall antigens (77). Recently, Kelley *et al.* (78) reported that 6 g DHA/d for 90 days did not alter the DTH response to intradermal application of seven recall antigens.

Graft Versus Host and Host Versus Graft Responses

The so-called *popliteal lymph node assay* provides a useful experimental model in rodents for measuring graft *versus* host (GvH) and host *versus* graft (HvG) responses elicited by injection of allogeneic cells into the footpad of the host. The GvH response primarily involves the polyclonal activation and subsequent proliferation of host B cells, although NK cells can also be involved in the host defense. In contrast, the HvG reaction is a T-cell–mediated response, in which cytotoxic lymphocytes of the host recognize MHC antigens on the injected cells. In both cases, the enlargement in popliteal lymph node size is caused largely by proliferation of activated host cells; most of these originate within the popliteal lymph node, although some recruitment of cells also comes from the bloodstream. Using this assay, Mertin *et al.* (132) reported that both the GvH and HvG responses were suppressed following a single administration of fish oil concentrate (750 mg/kg body weight) by esophageal catheter to mice before or immediately after the inoculation with allogeneic cells. A suppressed HvG response was observed in mice fed a 160 g/kg fish oil diet compared with those fed a standard chow diet (133); lower levels of fish oil (25,50,100 g/kg) did not significantly affect the response. Diminished GvH and HvG responses (by 34% and 20%, respectively) were observed in rats fed 200 g/kg fish oil compared with those fed a low fat diet or diets containing 200 g/kg coconut, olive, safflower, or evening primrose oils (52). Such observations accord with the finding of significantly diminished *ex vivo* T-lymphocyte proliferation, NK-cell activity, and cytotoxic lymphocyte activity following fish oil feeding. The fish oil diet resulted in less IL-2 receptor-positive cells and $CD16^+/CD3^-$ cells in the popliteal lymph nodes following the GvH response (52), indicating an inhibition of lymphocyte activation and a decrease in the proportion of NK cells, respectively. A dose-dependent effect of flaxseed oil compared with sunflower oil on the GvH response in rats was reported (66); the level of fat in the diet was 200 g/kg. Replacing α-linolenic acid (4.4 g/100 g fatty acids) with EPA was observed to significantly decrease (by 15% to 20%) the GvH in rats (27); replacement of α-linolenic acid with DHA was without effect.

Animal Models of Inflammatory and Autoimmune Diseases

Dietary fish oil has been shown to have significantly beneficial clinical, immunologic, and biochemical effects in various animal disease models. These effects include increased survival and decreased proteinuria and anti-DNA antibodies in mice with autoimmune glomerulonephritis, a model for systemic lupus erythematosus, decreased joint inflammation in rodents with collagen-induced arthritis, and less inflammation in rats with various models of ulcerative colitis (16). These observations suggest that diets enriched in EPA plus DHA might be of some therapeutic benefit in these diseases in humans (see below).

Animal Models of Organ Transplantation

Linoleic acid given subcutaneously, intraperitoneally, or orally prolonged the survival of skin allografts in mice or rats (134). Renal or cardiac transplants have been shown to survive longer if recipient rats are fed oleic, linoleic, or eicosapentaenoic acids or fish oil (16). Greater prolongation of cardiac survival in rats receiving an infusion of fish oil after transplantation compared with those receiving soybean oil infusion has been reported (135,136); in turn, soybean oil enhanced survival compared with saline infusion. Oral fish oil (4.5 g/d) has also been shown to prolong the survival of islets of Langerhans grafts in mice (137). These observations are in accordance with the reduced lymphocyte responses observed following fish oil feeding in particular, and they indicate that intervention with *n*-3 PUFA may be useful before and following organ transplantation in humans (see below).

USE IN CHRONIC INFLAMMATORY DISEASES AND PANCREATIC CANCER

Various human diseases are characterized by dysregulation of the immune system. Several of these diseases involve inappropriate production of proinflammatory cytokines (*e.g.*, TNF-α) and so are termed *chronic inflammatory diseases*. Many cancers, including pancreatic cancer, and AIDS are also characterized by raised levels of proinflammatory cytokines in the circulation. Studies in healthy animals and humans reveal that fish oil decreases the ability of cells to produce proinflammatory cytokines (see above), suggesting that increasing the amount of long chain *n*-3 PUFA in the diet of patients with various diseases could be beneficial. This idea is supported by the fish oil-induced amelioration of symptoms observed in animal models of chronic inflammatory diseases (see earlier), which in some cases resulted in increased lifespan (*e.g.*, in mice carrying the murine AIDS virus (89,109), and in tumor-bearing mice (138). Thus, fish oil has been provided to patients with chronic inflammatory and autoimmune diseases, pancreatic cancer, and AIDS. It is beyond the scope of this article to review the effectiveness of this treatment in these diseases. However, reviews have been done of the use of long chain *n*-3 PUFA in rheumatoid arthritis (139–141), psoriasis (142), ulcerative colitis (143), Crohn's disease (144), IgA nephropathy (145), and pancreatic cancer (146). Generally, these studies show biochemical changes such as enrichment of plasma or mononuclear cells with EPA and DHA, decreased production of arachidonic acid-derived eicosanoids, and in some studies decreased production of proinflammatory cytokines. In addition, several of these studies show improvement in clinical symptoms and in some cases decreased use of drug treatment (139–146).

USE FOLLOWING ORGAN TRANSPLANTATION IN HUMANS

The animal studies described above indicate that PUFA, particularly long chain *n*-3 PUFA, could be used to prolong the survival of organ transplants. Recipients of kidney transplants who received 9 g fish oil/d for 1 year after transplantation (in conjunction with cyclosporin A and prednisolone) had significantly improved glomerular filtration rate and significantly diminished cyclosporin A nephrotoxicity, although no effect was seen on graft survival (147). A similar finding was made by van der Heide *et al.* (148). These investigators reported that renal transplant patients who received fish oil (6 g/d for the first postoperative year) in combination with cyclosporin A had better kidney function and fewer rejection episodes over 1 year compared with patients who received coconut oil and cyclosporin A. Better kidney function was reported in kidney graft recipients who consumed fish oil (8 g/d for 1 year after transplantation), although no reduction was seen in rejection episodes compared with controls (149). Bennett *et al.* (150) reported no rejection incidents in a group of kidney transplant recipients who received 9 or 18 g EPA/d for 16 weeks after transplantation; cyclosporin nephrotoxicity did not occur in this group but did occur in the control group who supplemented their diet with maize oil.

DO DIETARY LIPIDS DIMINISH HOST DEFENSE?

The diminished cellular responses observed after feeding diets rich in *n*-3 PUFA result in suppressed cell-mediated immune responses (see above), suggesting that these fatty acids could affect the host response to infection. Some animal studies support this suggestion. Mice fed a diet containing 200 g fish oil/kg showed lower survival over 15 days (48%) to orally administered *Salmonella typhimurium* than those fed maize oil (62.5%), coconut oil (87.5%), or a low fat diet (88%) (152); spleens from the fish oil-fed animals had a greater number of bacteria than those from animals fed the other diets. Similarly, a study of experimental tuberculosis in guinea pigs reported an increased number of bacteria in the spleen of fish oil-fed animals and it was concluded that this represented persistence of the experimental infection (152). Compared with safflower oil, fish oil decreased the clearance of bacteria (inspired *Staphylococcus aureus*) in neonatal rabbits (39). Recently, it was reported that 170 g/kg fish oil decreased survival of mice to an intraperitoneal injection of *Listeria monocytogenes* compared with feeding 200 g/kg of lard, but not compared with feeding 200 g/kg of soybean oil, which also resulted in lower survival (153). The spleens from the fish oil-fed mice contained significantly more bacteria than those from the other two groups (153). As the response to microbial infections is predominantly a Th1-mediated response, the reduced survival of rodents fed large amounts of fish oil to bacterial challenges suggests that fish oil suppresses the Th1 response; this is consistent with many of the observed effects of fish oil on cytokine (IL-2, γ-interferon) and antibody production. In contrast to these observations, some studies show that fish oil feeding does not affect resistance of laboratory rodents to bacterial (*L. monocytogenes*, *Pseudomonas aeruginosa*) and viral (murine cytomegalovirus) challenges (154,155). Furthermore, some studies have shown that dietary fish oil enhances survival during some infections. For example, Blok *et al.* (104) reported increased survival of fish oil-fed mice challenged by intramuscular injection with *Klebsiella pneumoniae*; 90% of fish oil-fed mice survived, compared with 30%, 40%, and 0 in groups fed maize oil, palm oil, or chow, respectively. Furthermore, cerebral malaria induced by intraperitoneal injection of erythrocytes infected with *Plasmodium berghei* occurred in only 23% of fish oil-fed mice compared with 61%, 81%, and 78% of mice fed maize oil, palm oil, or chow, respectively (104).

No reports have been made of compromised immunity in humans supplementing their diet with *n*-3 PUFA. In contrast, one study has reported decreased numbers of respiratory infections, decreased days of fever, and reduced absence from school in children 3 to 4 years of age who supplemented their diet with linoleic and α-linolenic acids (600 plus 855 mg/d) for 4 months over winter compared with children who used a placebo (156).

OUTSTANDING QUESTIONS

Given the potential for clinical use of fish oil-derived *n*-3 PUFA (see above) and the speculation that the ratio of *n*-6 to *n*-3 PUFA in the diet might be a predisposing factor in some diseases with an immunologic basis (157), it is surprising that so little is still known about the immunologic impact of these fatty acids. Several key questions remain unresolved:

- Are both EPA and DHA active within the immune system or are the effects of fish oil principally caused by one of these fatty acids? Recent animal experiments suggest that both fatty acids alter rodent lymphocyte proliferation but that NK-cell activity is influenced only by EPA (27). Another recent study indicates that even a large amount of DHA (6 g/d for 60 days) has very little immunologic impact in healthy humans (78). As some studies have reported marked effects of fish oil supplementation providing as little as 1.5 g EPA plus DHA daily, this finding suggests that most of the effects of fish oil in humans are caused by EPA. However, no study has been done of the dietary effects of EPA alone on immune function in healthy humans.

- What is the level of fish oil required to exert immunomodulatory effects? Related to this is the question of whether some immune functions (e.g., production of proinflammatory cytokines) are more sensitive to *n*-3 PUFA than others (e.g., lymphocyte proliferation). Surprisingly, no studies have been published on dose-response to fish oil or its component fatty acids with respect to their impact on human immune function. Again, recent animal studies suggest that EPA (alone or in combination with DHA) is effective at influencing lymphocyte functions at levels far below those provided in fish oil-rich diets and at levels which can be achieved by supplementation of the human-diet (27,75).
- Is the ratio of EPA to DHA an important factor in determining their potency?
- What is the *equivalence* of α-linolenic acid to EPA with respect to immunomodulation? This is an important issue to some because α-linolenic acid is more readily incorporated into foodstuffs than its long chain derivatives.
- Are there age, sex, or ethnic group related sensitivities to fish oil supplementation? Meydani *et al.* (76) showed more potent effects in older women than younger, but few if any other studies have made such comparisons, and no studies have determined whether the immune systems of men or women are equally sensitive to fish oil.
- What is the immunologic influence of the relation between the levels of *n*-3 PUFA and α-tocopherol in the diet? The study of Wu *et al.* (69) in monkeys highlights this as a key area of uncertainty.
- Is the immune response *in vivo* altered by the levels of *n*-3 PUFA that can be provided to humans, and how does this relate to effects on individual components of that response that can be examined *ex vivo*?
- Are the effects of *n*-3 PUFA the same in healthy and diseased subjects?

Another issue worth highlighting is that few good human studies have been performed: many of the studies of fish oil supplementation have not been controlled or blinded and most have used small numbers of subjects.

It seems important to address each of the above questions in well-controlled animal and human studies. Only then will the true immunologic impact of *n*-3 PUFA be known.

CONCLUSION

It seems likely that a significant reduction in fat consumption will enhance cell-mediated immune functions. Within the current Western style diet, it is unlikely that small to moderate changes in the amounts of saturated, monounsaturated, or linoleic acids consumed will alter immunity, although the ratios between these types of fatty acids and between these and the n-3 PUFA might have a hitherto little appreciated importance. Perhaps, surprisingly, recent animal and human studies indicate that even large amounts of arachidonic acid in the diet do not affect immunity. Thus, among the fatty acids, it is the n-3 PUFA that possess immunomodulatory activity, and among the n-3 PUFA those from fish oil (EPA and DHA) are more biologically potent than α-linolenic acid (notwithstanding the questions outlined above). The production of macrophage-derived proinflammatory eicosanoids such as PGE_2 is markedly reduced by feeding diets rich in n-3 PUFA. Furthermore, inclusion in the diet of high levels of EPA plus DHA significantly reduces the movement of human monocytes toward chemotactic agents and the production of proinflammatory cytokines by human mononuclear cells. Several contradictory observations can be made regarding the effects of dietary n-3 PUFA on production of proinflammatory cytokines by animal macrophages and lymphocytes; these most likely relate to the different experimental models and protocols used. EPA and DHA also appear to reduce adhesion molecule expression and, thus, might influence the movement of leukocytes between body compartments. Several studies indicate a reduction of MHC II expression on antigen presenting cells following fish oil feeding; this would suggest a diminished ability to present antigen. No clear consensus is found regarding the effects of n-3 PUFA consumption on the generation of reactive oxygen and nitrogen species and on macrophage-mediated phagocytosis. Inclusion in the diet of high levels of n-3 PUFA markedly alters the functions of lymphocytes subsequently tested *ex vivo*. Components of both natural and acquired immunity are affected. Recent studies have sought to identify the effects of lower levels of particular fatty acids in the diet; these studies reveal complex interactions between fatty acids. *In vivo* tests are perhaps the most appropriate approach for determining the effect of different dietary fatty acids on immune function. Several studies indicate that diets rich in EPA plus DHA are anti-inflammatory and immunosuppressive *in vivo*, although relatively few studies have been done in humans. Although some of the effects of n-3 PUFA may be brought about by modulation of the amount and types of eicosanoids made, it is possible that these fatty acids might elicit some of their effects by eicosanoid-independent mechanisms, including actions on intracellular signaling pathways and transcription factor activity (11,17,19). Such n-3 PUFA-induced effects may be of use as treatment for acute and chronic inflammation, disorders that involve an inappropriately activated immune response, and the enhancement of graft survival.

REFERENCES

1. Meade CJ, Mertin J. Fatty acids and immunity. *Adv Lipid Res* 1978; 16: 127–65.
2. Goodwin JS, Cueppens J. Regulation of the immune response by prostaglandins. *J Clin Immunol* 1983; 3: 295–315.
3. Roper RL, Phipps RP. Prostaglandin E_2 regulation of the immune response. *Advances in Prostaglandin, Thromboxane and Leukotriene Research* 1994; 22: 101–11.
4. Hwang D. Essential fatty acids and the immune response. *FASEB J* 1989; 3: 2052–61.

5. Kinsella JE, Lokesh B, Broughton S, Whelan J. Dietary polyunsaturated fatty acids and eicosanoids: potential effects on the modulation of inflammatory and immune cells: an overview. *Nutrition* 1990; 6: 24–44.

6. Kelly DS, Daudu PA. Fat intake and immune response. *Prog Food Nutr Sci* 1993; 17: 41–63.

7. Calder PC. Fatty acids, dietary lipids and lymphocyte functions. *Biochem Soc Trans* 1995; 23: 302–9.

8. Peck MD. Interactions of lipids with immune function. II: Experimental and clinical studies of lipids and immunity. *Journal of Nutritional Biochemistry* 1994; 5: 514–21.

9. Calder PC. Effects of fatty acids and dietary lipids on cells of the immune system. *Proc Nutr Soc* 1996; 55: 127–50.

10. Calder PC. Can n-3 polyunsaturated fatty acids be used as immunomodulatory agents? *Biochem Soc Trans* 1996; 24: 211–20.

11. Calder PC. Immunomodulatory and anti-inflammatory effects of n-3 polyunsaturated fatty acids. *Proc Nutr Soc* 1996; 55: 737–74.

12. Blok WL, Katan MB, van der Meer JWM. Modulation of inflammation and cytokine production by dietary (n-3) fatty acids. *J Nutr* 1996; 126: 1515–33.

13. Meydani SN. Effect of (n-3) polyunsaturated fatty acids on cytokine production and their biologic function. *Nutrition* 1996; 12: S8–14.

14. Endres S, von Schacky C. n-3 Polyunsaturated fatty acids and human cytokine synthesis. *Curr Opin Lipidol* 1996; 7: 48–52.

15. Calder PC. N-3 polyunsaturated fatty acids and cytokine production in health and disease. *Ann Nutr Metab* 1997; 41: 203–34.

16. Calder PC. Dietary fatty acids and the immune system. *Nutr Rev* 1998; 56: S70–83.

17. Yaqoob P. Lipids and the immune response. *Current Opinion in Clinical Nutrition and Metabolic Care* 1998; 1: 153–61.

18. Alexander JW. Immunonutrition: the role of o-3 fatty acids. *Nutrition* 1998; 14: 627–33.

19. Miles EA, Calder PC. Modulation of immune function by dietary fatty acids. *Proc Nutr Soc* 1998; 57: 277–92.

20. Calder PC. Dietary fatty acids and lymphocyte functions. *Proc Nutr Soc* 1998; 57: 487–502.

21. Calder PC. n-3 Polyunsaturated fatty acids and mononuclear phagocyte function. In: Kremer J, ed. *Medicinal fatty acids in inflammation*. Basel: Birkhauser Verlag, 1998: 1–27.

22. Calder PC, Bond JA, Harvey DJ, Gordon S, Newsholme EA. Uptake of saturated and unsaturated fatty acids into macrophage lipids and their effect upon macrophage adhesion and phagocytosis. *Biochem J* 1990; 269: 807–14.

23. Calder PC, Yaqoob P, Harvey DJ, Watts A, Newsholme EA. The incorporation of fatty acids by lymphocytes and the effect on fatty acid composition and membrane fluidity. *Biochem J* 1994; 300: 509–18.

24. Lokesh BR, Hsieh HL, Kinsella JE. Peritoneal macrophages from mice fed dietary (n-3) polyunsaturated fatty acids secrete low levels of prostaglandins. *J Nutr* 1986; 116: 2547–52.

25. Brouard C, Pascaud M. Effects of moderate dietary supplementations with n-3 fatty acids on macrophage and lymphocyte phospholipids and macrophage eicosanoid synthesis in the rat. *Biochim Biophys Acta* 1990; 1047: 19–28.

26. Yaqoob P, Newsholme EA, Calder PC. Influence of cell culture conditions on diet-induced changes in lymphocyte fatty acid composition. *Biochim Biophys Acta* 1995; 1255: 333–40.

27. Peterson LD, Jeffery NM, Thies F, Sanderson P, Newsholme EA, Calder PC. Eicosapentaenoic and docosahexaenoic acids alter rat spleen leukocyte fatty acid composition and prostaglandin E_2 production but have different effects on lymphocyte functions and cell-mediated immunity. *Lipids* 1998; 33: 171–80.

28. Lee TH, Hoover RL, Williams JD, et al. Effects of dietary enrichment with EPA and DHA on in vitro neutrophil and monocyte leukotriene generation and neutrophil function. *N Engl J Med* 1985; 312: 1217–24.

29. Endres S, Ghorbani R, Kelley VE, et al. The effect of dietary supplementation with n-3 polyunsaturated fatty acids on the synthesis of interleukin-1 and tumor necrosis factor by mononuclear cells. *N Engl J Med* 1989; 320: 265–71.

30. Yaqoob P, Calder PC. Effects of dietary lipid manipulation upon inflammatory mediator production by murine macrophages. *Cell Immunol* 1995; 163: 120–8.

31. Black JM, Kinsella JE. Dietary n-3 fatty acids alter mouse peritoneal macrophage cytotoxicity. *Ann Nutr Metab* 1993; 37: 110–20.

32. Chapkin RS, Hubbard NE, Erickson KL. 5-Series peptido-leukotriene synthesis in mouse peritoneal macrophages: modulation by dietary n-3 fatty acids. *Biochem Biophys Res Commun* 1990; 171: 764–9.

33. Schmidt EB, Varming K, Pederson JO, et al. Long term supplementation with n-3 fatty acids. II. Effect on neutrophil and monocyte chemotaxis. *Scand J Clin Lab Invest* 1992; 52: 229–36.

34. Schmidt EB, Varming K, Moller JM, Bulow Pederson I, Madsen P, Dyerberg J. No effect of a very low dose of n-3 fatty acids on monocyte function in healthy humans. *Scand J Clin Invest* 1996; 56: 87–92

35. Davidson J, Kerr A, Guy K, Rotondo D. Prostaglandin and fatty acid modulation of *Escherichia coli* 0157 phagocytosis by human monocytic cells. *Immunology* 1998; 94: 228–34.

36. Hubbard NE, Somers SD, Erickson KL. Effect of dietary fish oil on development and selected functions of murine inflammatory macrophages. *J Leukoc Biol* 1991; 49: 592–8.

37. Turek JJ, Schoenlein IA, Clark LK, van Alstine WG. Dietary polyunsaturated fatty acids effects on immune cells of the porcine lung. *J Leukoc Biol* 1994; 56: 599–604.

38. Eicher SD, McVey DS. Dietary modulation of Kupffer cell and splenocyte function during a *Salmonella typhimurium* challenge in mice. *J Leukoc Biol* 1995; 58: 32–9.

39. D'Ambola JB, Aeberhard EE, Trang N, Gaffar S, Barrett CT, Sherman MP. Effect of dietary (n-3) and (n-6) fatty acids on in vivo pulmonary bacterial clearance by neonatal rabbits. *J Nutr* 1991; 121: 1262–9.

40. Halvorsen DA, Hansen J-B, Grimsgaard S, Bonaa KH, Kierulf P, Nordoy A. The effect of highly purified eicosapentaenoic and docosahexaenoic acids on monocyte phagocytosis in man. *Lipids* 1997; 32: 935–42.

41. Fisher M, Levine PH, Weiner BH, et al. Dietary n-3 fatty acid supplementation reduces superoxide production and chemiluminescence in a monocyte-enriched preparation of leukocytes. *Am J Clin Nutr* 1990; 51: 804–8.

42. Khair-El-Din TA, Sicher SC, Vazquez MA, Wright WJ, Lu CY. Docosahexaenoic acid, a major constituent of fetal serum and fish oil diets, inhibits IFNγ-induced Ia-expression by murine macrophages in vitro. *J Immunol* 1995; 154: 1296–306.

43. Hughes DA, Southon S, Pinder AC. (n-3) Polyunsaturated fatty acids modulate the expression of functionally associated molecules on human monocytes in vitro. *J Nutr* 1996; 126: 603–10.

44. Hughes DA, Pinder AC. N-3 polyunsaturated fatty acids modulate the expression of functionally associated molecules on human monocytes and inhibit antigen presentation in vitro. *Clin Exp Immunol* 1997; 110: 516–23.

45. Huang S-C, Misfeldt ML, Fritsche KL. Dietary fat influences Ia antigen expression and immune cell populations in the murine peritoneum and spleen. *J Nutr* 1992; 122: 1219–31.

46. Sherrington EJ, Sanderson P, Calder PC. The effect of dietary lipid manipulation on macrophage cell surface molecule expression. *Biochemical Society Transactions* 1995; 23: 272S.

47. Sanderson P, MacPherson GG, Jenkins CH, Calder PC. Dietary fish oil diminishes antigen presentation activity by rat dendritic cells. *J Leukoc Biol* 1997; 62: 771–7.

48. Hughes DA, Pinder AC, Piper Z, Johnson IT, Lund EK. Fish oil supplementation inhibits the expression of major histocompatibility complex class II molecules and adhesion molecules on human monocytes. *Am J Clin Nutr* 1996; 63: 267–72.

49. Fujikawa M, Yamashita N, Yamazaki K, Sugiyama E, Suzuki H, Hamazaki T. Eiciosapentaenoic acid inhibits antigen-presenting cell function of murine splenocytes. *Immunology* 1992; 75: 330–5.

50. Khalfoun B, Thibault G, Bardos P, Lebranchu Y. Docosahexaenoic and eicosapentaenoic acids inhibit in vitro human lymphocyte-endothelial cell adhesion. *Transplantation* 1996; 62: 1649–57.

51. Sanderson P, Yaqoob P, Calder PC. Effects of dietary lipid manipulation upon rat spleen lymphocyte functions and the expression of lymphocyte surface molecules. *J Nutr Environ Med* 1995; 5: 119–32.

52. Sanderson P, Yaqoob P, Calder PC. Effects of dietary lipid manipulation upon graft vs. host and host vs. graft responses in the rat. *Cell Immunol* 1995; 164: 240–7.

53. Sanderson P, Calder PC. Dietary fish oil diminishes lymphocyte adhesion to macrophage and endothelial cell monolayers. *Immunology* 1998; 94: 79–87.

54. de Caterina R, Cybulsky MA, Clinton SK, Gimbrone MA, Libby P. Omega-3 fatty acids and endothelial leukocyte adhesion molecules. *Prostaglandins Leukot Essent Fatty Acids* 1995; 52: 191–5.

55. Yaqoob P, Knapper J, Webb D, Williams C, Newsholme EA, Calder PC. Effect of olive oil on immune function in middle-aged men. *Am J Clin Nutr* 1998; 67: 129–35.

56. Yaqoob P, Newsholme EA, Calder PC. The effect of dietary lipid manipulation on rat lymphocyte subsets and proliferation. *Immunology* 1994; 82: 603–10.
57. Jolly CA, McMurray DN, Chapkin RS. Effect of dietary n-3 fatty acids on interleukin-2 and inter-leukin-2 receptor α expression in activated murine lymphocytes. *Prostaglandins Leukot Essent Fatty Acids* 1998; 58: 289–93.
58. Soyland E, Lea T, Sandstad B, Drevon CA. Dietary supplementation with very long chain n-3 fatty acids in man decreases expression of the interleukin-2 receptor (CD25) on mitogen-stimulated lym-phocytes from patients with inflammatory skin diseases. *Eur J Clin Invest* 1994; 24: 236–42.
59. Kelley DS, Branch LB, Iacono JM. Nutritional modulation of human immune status. *Nutr Res* 1989; 9: 965–75.
60. Kelley DS, Dougherty RM, Branch LB, Taylor PC, Iacono JM. Concentration of dietary n-6 polyun-saturated fatty acids and human immune status. *Clin Immunol Immunopathol* 1992; 62: 240–4.
61. Jeffery NM, Sanderson P, Newsholme EA, Calder PC. Effects of varying the type of saturated fatty acid in the rat diet upon serum lipid levels and spleen lymphocyte functions. *Biochim Biophys Acta* 1997; 1345: 23–36.
62. Berger A, German JB, Chiang BL, et al. Influence of feeding unsaturated fats on growth and immune status of mice. *J Nutr* 1993; 23: 25–33.
63. Jeffery NM, Yaqoob P, Newsholme EA, Calder PC. The effects of olive oil upon rat serum lipid lev-els and lymphocyte functions appear to be due to oleic acid. *Ann Nutr Metab* 1996; 40: 71–80.
64. Jeffery NM, Cortina M, Newsholme EA, Calder PC. Effects of variations in the proportions of sat-urated, monounsaturated and polyunsaturated fatty acids in the rat diet on spleen lymphocyte func-tions. *Br J Nutr* 1997; 77: 805–23.
65. Marshall LA, Johnston PV. The influence of dietary essential fatty acids on rat immunocompetent cell prostaglandin synthesis and mitogen-induced blastogenesis. *J Nutr* 1985; 115: 1572–80.
66. Jeffery NM, Sanderson P, Sherrington EJ, Newsholme EA, Calder PC. The ratio of n-6 to n-3 polyunsaturated fatty acids in the rat diet alters serum lipid levels and lymphocyte functions. *Lipids* 1996; 31: 737–45.
67. Fritsche KL, Cassity NA, Huang S-C. Effect of dietary fat source on antibody production and lym-phocyte proliferation in chickens. *Poult Sci* 1991; 70: 611–17.
68. Jeffery NM, Newsholme EA, Calder PC. The level of polyunsaturated fatty acids and the n-6 to n-3 polyunsaturated fatty acid ratio in the rat diet both affect serum lipid levels and lymphocyte func-tions. *Prostaglandins Leukot Essent Fatty Acids* 1997; 57: 149–60.
69. Wu D, Meydani SN, Meydani M, Hayek MG, Huth P, Nicolosi RJ. Immunologic effects of marine- and plant-derived n-3 polyunsaturated fatty acids in nonhuman primates. *Am J Clin Nutr* 1996; 63: 273–80.
70. Jolly CA, Jiang Y-H, Chapkin RS, McMurray DN. Dietary (n-3) polyunsaturated fatty acids sup-press murine lymphoproliferation, interleukin-2 secretion and the formation of diacylglycerol and ceramide. *J Nutr* 1997; 127: 37–43.
71. Kelley DS, Taylor PC, Nelson GJ, Schmidt PC, Mackey BE, Kyle D. Effects of dietary arachidonic acid on human immune response. *Lipids* 1997; 32: 449–56.
72. Alexander NJ, Smythe NL. Dietary modulation of in vitro lymphocyte function. *Ann Nutr Metab* 1988; 32: 192–9.
73. Kelley DS, Nelson GJ, Serrato CM, Schmidt PC, Branch LB. Effects of type of dietary fat on indices of immune status of rabbits. *J Nutr* 1988; 118: 1376–84.
74. Yaqoob P, Calder PC. The effects of dietary lipid manipulation on the production of murine T-cell-derived cytokines. *Cytokine* 1995; 7: 548–53.
75. Peterson LD, Thies F, Sanderson P, Newsholme EA, Calder PC. Low levels of eicosapentaenoic and docosahexaenoic acids mimic the effects of fish oil upon rat lymphocytes. *Life Sci* 1998; 62: 2209–17.
76. Meydani SN, Endres S, Woods MM, et al. Oral (n-3) fatty acid supplementation suppresses cytokine production and lymphocyte proliferation: comparison between young and older women. *J Nutr* 1991; 121: 547–55.
77. Meydani SN, Lichtenstein AH, Cornwall S, et al. Immunologic effects of national cholesterol edu-cation panel step-2 diets with and without fish-derived n-3 fatty acid enrichment. *J Clin Invest* 1993; 92: 105–13.
78. Kelley DS, Taylor PC, Nelson GJ, Mackey BE. Dietary docosahexaenoic acid and immunocompe-tence in young healthy men. *Lipids* 1998; 33: 559–66.

79. Barone J, Hebert JR, Reddy MM. Dietary fat and natural killer cell activity. *Am J Clin Nutr* 1989; 50: 861–7.
80. Hebert JR, Barone J, Reddy MM, Backlund JY. Natural killer cell activity in a longitudinal dietary fat intervention trial. *Clin Immunol Immunopathol* 1990; 54: 103–16.
81. Yaqoob P, Newsholme EA, Calder PC. Inhibition of natural killer cell activity by dietary lipids. *Immunol Lett* 1994; 41: 241–7.
82. Meydani SN, Yogeeswaran G, Liu S, Baskar S, Meydani M. Fish oil and tocopherol-induced changes in natural killer cell-mediated cytotoxicity and PGE_2 synthesis in young and old mice. *J Nutr* 1988; 118: 1245–52.
83. Fritsche KL, Johnston PV. Modulation of eicosanoid production and cell-mediated cytotoxicity by dietary alpha-linolenic acid in BALB/c mice. *Lipids* 1979; 24: 305–11.
84. Yamashita N, Maruyama M, Yamazaki K, Hamazaki T, Yano S. Effect of eicosapentaenoic and docosahexaenoic acid on natural killer cell activity in human peripheral blood lymphocytes. *Clin Immunol Immunopathol* 1991; 59: 335–45.
85. DeWille JW, Fraker PJ, Romsos DR. Effects of essential fatty acid deficiency and various levels of dietary polyunsaturated fatty acids on humoral immunity in mice. *J Nutr* 1989; 109: 1018–22.
86. Friend JV, Lock SO, Gurr MI, Parish WE. Effect of different dietary lipids on the immune responses of Hartley strain guinea pigs. *International Archives of Allergy and Applied Immunology* 1980; 62: 292–301.
87. Erickson KL, Adams DA, Scibienski RJ. Dietary fatty acid modulation of murine B-cell responsiveness. *J Nutr* 1986; 116: 1830–40.
88. Prickett JD, Robinson DR, Bloch KJ. Enhanced production of IgE and IgG antibodies associated with a diet enriched in eicosapentaenoic acid. *Immunology* 1982; 46: 819–26.
89. Xi S, Cohen D, Chen LH. Effects of fish oil on cytokines and immune functions of mice with murine AIDS. *J Lipid Res* 1998; 39: 1677–87.
90. Meydani SN, Nicolosi RJ, Hayes KC. Effect of long-term feeding of corn oil or coconut oil diets on immune response and prostaglandin E_2 synthesis of squirrel and cebus monkeys. *Nutr Res* 1985; 5: 993–1002.
91. Kelley DS, Branch LB, Love JE, Taylor PC, Rivera YM, Iacono JM. Dietary alpha-linolenic acid and immunocompetence in humans. *Am J Clin Nutr* 1991; 53: 40–6.
92. Kelley DS, Nelson GJ, Branch LB, Taylor PC, Rivera YM, Schmidt PC. Salmon diet and human immune status. *Eur J Clin Nutr* 1992; 46: 397–404.
93. Kelley DS, Taylor PC, Nelson GJ, Mackey BE. Arachidonic acid supplementation enhances synthesis of eicosanoids without suppressing immune functions in young healthy men. *Lipids* 1998; 33: 125–30.
94. Grimm H, Tibell A, Norrlind B, Blecher C, Wilker S, Schwemmle K. Immunoregulation by parenteral lipids: impact of the n-3 to n-6 fatty acid ratio. *JPEN* 1994; 18: 417–21.
95. Renier G, Skamene E, de Sanctis J, Radzioch D. Dietary n-3 polyunsaturated fatty acids prevent the development of atherosclerotic lesions in mice: modulation of macrophage secretory activities. *Arterioscler Thromb Vasc Biol* 1993; 13: 1515–24.
96. Watanabe S, Hayashi H, Onozaki K, Okuyama H. Effect of dietary αlinolenate/linoleate balance on lipopolysaccharide-induced tumor necrosis factor production in mouse macrophages. *Life Sci* 1991; 48: 2013–20.
97. Chang HR, Arsenijevic D, Pechere JC, et al. Dietary supplementation with fish oil enhances in vivo synthesis of tumor necrosis factor. *Immunol Lett* 1992; 34: 13–18.
98. Blok WL, de Bruijn MFTR, Leenan PJM, et al. Dietary n-3 fatty acids increase spleen size and postendotoxin circulating TNF in mice; role of macrophages, macrophage precursors, and colony-stimulating-factor-1. *J Immunol* 1996; 157: 5569–73.
99. Sadeghi S, Wallace FA, Calder PC. Dietary lipids modify the cytokine response to bacterial lipopolysaccharide in mice. *Immunology* 1999; 96: 404–10.
100. Tashiro T, Yamamori H, Takagi K, Hayashi N, Furukawa K, Nakajima N. n-3 Versus n-6 polyunsaturated fatty acids in critical illness. *Nutrition* 1998; 14: 551–3.
101. Tappia PS, Grimble RF. Complex modulation of cytokine induction by endotoxin and tumour necrosis factor from peritoneal macrophages of rats by diets containing fats of different saturated, monounsaturated and polyunsaturated fatty acid composition. *Clin Sci* 1994; 87: 173–8.
102. Billiar T, Bankey P, Svingen B, et al. Fatty acid uptake and Kupffer cell function: fish oil alters eicosanoid and monokine production to endotoxin stimulation. *Surgery* 1988; 104: 343–9.
103. Lokesh BR, Sayers TJ, Kinsella JE. Interleukin-1 and tumor necrosis factor synthesis by mouse peritoneal macrophages is enhanced by dietary n-3 polyunsaturated fatty acids. *Immunol Lett* 1990; 23: 281–6.

104. Blok WL, Vogels MTE, Curfs JHAJ, Eling WMC, Buurmann WA, van der Meer JMW. Dietary fish oil supplementation in experimental gram-negative infection and in cerebral malaria in mice. *J Infect Dis* 1992; 165: 898–903.

105. Ertel W, Morrison MH, Ayala A, Chaudry IH. Modulation of macrophage membrane phospholipids by n-3 polyunsaturated fatty acids increases interleukin 1 release and prevents suppression of cellular immunity following hemorrhagic shock. *Arch Surg* 1993; 128: 15–21.

106. Tappia PS, Man WJ, Grimble RF. Influence of unsaturated fatty acids on the production of tumour necrosis factor and interleukin-6 by rat peritoneal macrophages. *Mol Cell Biochem* 1995; 143: 89–98.

107. Chandrasekar B, Fernandes G. Decreased pro-inflammatory cytokines and increased antioxidant enzyme gene expression by o3 lipids in murine lupus nephritis. *Biochem Biophys Res Commun* 1994; 200: 893–8.

108. Robinson DR, Urakaze M, Huang R, et al. Dietary marine lipids suppress continuous expression of interleukin-1β gene expression. *Lipids* 1996; 31: S23–S31.

109. Fernandes G, Tomar V, Venkatraman MN, Venkatraman JT. Potential of diet therapy in murine AIDS. *J Nutr* 1992; 122: 716–22.

110. Fernandes G, Bysani C, Venkatraman JT, Tomar V, Zhao W. Increased TGF-β and decreased oncogene expression by o-3 fatty acids in the spleen delays onset of autoimmune disease in B/W mice. *J Immunol* 1994; 152: 5979–87.

111. Gallai V, Sarchielli P, Trequattrini A, et al. Cytokine secretion and eicosanoid production in the peripheral blood mononuclear cells of MS patients undergoing dietary supplementation with n-3 polyunsaturated fatty acids. *J Neuroimmunol* 1993; 56: 143–53.

112. Caughey GE, Mantzioris E, Gibson RA, Cleland LG, James MJ. The effect on human tumor necrosis factor α and interleukin 1 β production of diets enriched in n-3 fatty acids from vegetable oil or fish oil. *Am J Clin Nutr* 1996; 63: 116–22.

113. Molvig J, Pociot F, Worsaae H, et al. Dietary supplementation with o-3 polyunsaturated fatty acids decreases mononuclear cell proliferation and interleukin-1β content but not monokine secretion in healthy and insulin-dependent diabetic individuals. *Scand J Immunol* 1991; 34: 399–410.

114. Cooper AL, Gibbons L, Horan MA, Little RA, Rothwell NJ. Effect of dietary fish oil supplementation on fever and cytokine production in human volunteers. *Clin Nutr* 1993; 12: 321–8.

115. Endres S, Meydani SN, Ghorbani R, Schindler R, Dinarello CA. Dietary supplementation with n-3 fatty acids suppresses interleukin-2 production and mononuclear cell proliferation. *J Leukoc Biol* 1993; 54: 599–603.

116. Wachtler P, Konig W, Senkal M, Kemen M, Koller M. Influence of a total parenteral nutrition enriched with o-3 fatty acids on leukotriene synthesis of peripheral leukocytes and systemic cytokine levels in patients with major surgery. *J Trauma* 1997; 42: 191–8.

117. Yoshino S, Ellis EF. Effect of a fish oil-supplemented diet on inflammation and immunological processes in rats. *International Archives of Allergy and Applied Immunology* 1987; 84: 233–40.

118. Lefkowith JB, Morrison A, Lee V, Rogers M. Manipulation of the acute inflammatory response by dietary polyunsaturated fatty acid modulation. *J Immunol* 1990; 145: 1523–9.

119. Reddy ACB, Lokesh BR. Studies on anti-inflammatory activity of spice principles and dietary n-3 polyunsaturated fatty acids on carrageenan-induced inflammation in rats. *Ann Nutr Metab* 1994; 38: 349–58.

120. Nakamura N, Hamazaki T, Kobayashi M, Yazawa K. The effect of oral administration of eicosapentaenoic and docosahexaenoic acids on acute inflammation and fatty acid composition in rats. *J Nutr Sci Vitaminol* (Tokyo) 1990; 40: 161–70.

121. Mascioli EA, Leader L, Flores E, Trimbo S, Bistrian B, Blackburn G. Enhanced survival to endotoxin in guinea pigs fed iv fish oil emulsion. *Lipids* 1988; 23: 623–5.

122. Mascioli EA, Iwasa Y, Trimbo S, Leader L, Bistrian BR, Blackburn GL. Endotoxin challenge after menhaden oil diet: effects on survival of guinea pigs. *Am J Clin Nutr* 1989; 49: 277–82.

123. Mulrooney HM, Grimble RF. Influence of butter and of corn, coconut and fish oils on the effects of recombinant human tumour necrosis factor-α in rats. *Clin Sci* 1993; 84: 105–12.

124. Pomposelli J, Mascioli EA, Bistrian BR, Flores SM. Attenuation of the febrile response in guinea pigs by fish oil enriched diets. *JPEN* 1990; 13: 136–140.

125. Cooper AL, Rothwell NJ. Inhibition of the thermogenic and pyrogenic responses to interleukin-1 beta in the rat by dietary n-3 fatty acid supplementation. *Prostaglandins Leukot Essent Fatty Acids* 1993; 49: 615–26.

126. Hellerstein MK, Meydani SN, Meydani M, Wu K, Dinarello CA. Interleukin-1-induced anorexia in the rat: influence of prostaglandins. *J Clin Invest* 1989; 84: 228–35.

127. DeWille JW, Fraker PJ, Romsos DR. Effects of dietary fatty acids on delayed-type hypersensitivity in mice. *J Nutr* 1981; 111: 2039–43.

128. Crevel RWR, Friend JV, Goodwin BFJ, Parish WE. High fat diets and the immune response of C57 Bl mice. *Br J Nutr* 1992; 67: 17–26.

129. Fowler KH, Chapkin RS, McMurray DN. Effects of purified dietary n-3 ethyl esters on murine T lymphocyte function. *J Immunol* 1993; 151: 5186–97.

130. Taki H, Morinaga S-I, Yamazaki K, Hamazaki T, Suzuki H, Nakamura N. Reduction of delayed-type hypersensitivity by the injection of n-3 polyunsaturated fatty acids in mice. *Transplantation* 1992; 54: 511–14.

131. Wander RC, Hall JA, Gradin JL, Du S-H, Jewell DE. The ratio of dietary (n-6) to (n-3) fatty acids influences immune system function, eicosanoid metabolism, lipid peroxidation and vitamin E status in aged dogs. *J Nutr* 1997; 127: 1198–205.

132. Mertin J, Stackspoole A, Shumway S. Nutrition and immunity: the immunoregulatory effect of n-6 essential fatty acids is mediated through prostaglandin E. *International Archives of Allergy and Applied Immunology* 1985; 77: 390–5.

133. Hinds A, Sanders TAB. The effect of increasing levels of dietary fish oil rich in eicosapentaenoic and docosahexaenoic acids on lymphocyte phospholipid fatty acid composition and cell-mediated immunity in the mouse. *Br J Nutr* 1993; 69: 423–9.

134. Ring J, Serfeit J, Mertin J, Brendel W. Prolongation of skin allografts in rats treated with linoleic acid. *Lancet* 1974; ii: 1331.

135. Grimm H, Tibell A, Norrlind B, Schott J, Bohle RA. Nutrition and allorejection impact of lipids. *Transplant Immunol* 1995; 3: 62–7.

136. Grimminger F, Grimm H, Fuhrer D, et al. Omega 3 lipid infusion in a heart allotransplant model: shift in fatty acid and lipid mediator profiles and prolongation of transplant survival. *Circulation* 1996; 93: 365–71.

137. Linn K, Lux W, Woehrle M, et al. Fish oil diet prevents insulitis in transplanted islets of Langerhans. *Transplant Proc* 1990; 22: 871–2.

138. Calder PC, Davis J, Yaqoob P, Pala H, Thies F, Newsholme EA. Dietary fish oil suppresses human colon tumour growth in athymic mice. *Clin Sci* 1998; 94: 303–11.

139. Geusens PP. n-3 Fatty acids in the treatment of rheumatoid arthritis. In: Kremer J, ed. *Medicinal fatty acids in inflammation*. Basel: Birkhauser Verlag, 1998: 111–23.

140. Volker D, Garg M. Dietary n-3 fatty acid supplementation in rheumatoid arthritis—mechanisms, clinical outcomes, controversies, and future directions. *J Clin Biochem Nutr* 1996; 20: 83–97.

141. James MJ, Cleland LG. Dietary n-3 fatty acids and therapy for rheumatoid arthritis. *Semin Arthritis Rheum* 1997; 27: 85–97.

142. Ziboh VA. The role of n-3 fatty acids in psoriasis. In: Kremer J, ed. *Medicinal fatty acids in inflammation*. Basel: Birkhauser Verlag, 1998: 45–53.

143. Rodgers JB. n-3 Fatty acids in the treatment of ulcerative colitis. In: Kremer J, ed. *Medicinal fatty acids in inflammation*. Basel: Birkhauser Verlag, 1998: 103–9.

144. Belluzzi A, Miglio F. n-3 Fatty acids in the treatment of Crohn's disease. In: Kremer J, ed. *Medicinal fatty acids in inflammation*. Basel: Birkhauser Verlag, 1998: 91–101.

145. Grande JP, Donadio JV. n-3 Polyunsaturated fatty acids in the treatment of patients with IgA nephropathy. In: Kremer J, ed. *Medicinal fatty acids in inflammation*. Basel: Birkhauser Verlag, 1998: 125–140.

146. Wigmore SJ, Ross JA, Falconer JS, et al. The effect of polyunsaturated fatty acids on the progress of cachexia in patients with pancreatic cancer. *Nutrition* 1996; 12: S27–30.

147. Bertoux FC, Guerin C, Bertharx P, Burgard G, Alamartine E. One-year randomized controlled trial with omega-3 fatty acid-rich fish oil in clinical renal transplant. *Transplant Proc* 1992; 24: 2578–82.

148. van der Heide HJJ, Bilo HJG, Donker JM, Wilmink JM, Tegzess AM. Effect of dietary fish oil on renal function and rejection in cyclosporine-treated recipients of renal transplants. *N Engl J Med* 1993; 329: 769–73.

149. Maachi K, Berthoux P, Burgard G, Alamartine E, Berthoux F. Results of a 1-year randomized controlled trial with omega-3 fatty acid fish oil in renal transplantation under triple immunosuppressive therapy. *Transplant Proc* 1995; 27: 846–9.

150. Bennett WM, Carpenter CB, Shapiro ME, et al. Delayed omega-3 fatty acid supplements in renal transplantation. *Transplantation* 1995; 59: 352–6.

151. Chang HR, Dulloo AG, Vladoianu IR, et al. Fish oil decreases natural resistance of mice to infection with *Salmonella typhimurium. Metabolism* 1992; 41: 1–2.
152. Mayatepek E, Paul K, Leichsenring M, et al. Influence of dietary (n-3) polyunsaturated fatty acids on leukotriene B4 and prostaglandin E$_2$ synthesis and the time course of experimental tuberculosis in guinea pigs. *Infection* 1994; 22: 106–12.
153. Fritsche KL, Shahbazian LM, Feng C, Berg JN. Dietary fish oil reduces survival and impairs bacterial clearance in C3H/Hen mice challenged with *Listeria monocytogenes. Clin Sci* 1997; 92: 95–101.
154. Clouva-Molyvdas P, Peck MD, Alexander JW. Short-term dietary lipid manipulation does not affect survival in two models of murine sepsis. *JPEN* 1992; 16: 343–7.
155. Rubin RH, Wilkinson RA, Xu L, Robinson DR. Dietary marine lipid does not alter susceptibility of (NZB NZW)F1 mice to pathogenic microorganisms. *Prostaglandins* 1989; 38: 251–62.
156. Venuta A, Spano C, Laudizi L, Bettelli F, Beverelli A, Turchetto. Essential fatty acids: the effects of dietary supplementation among children with recurrent respiratory infections. *J Int Med Res* 1996; 24: 325–30.
157. Black PN, Sharp S. Dietary fat and asthma. Is there a connection? *Eur Respir J* 1997; 10: 6–12.

DISCUSSION

Dr. Haschke: The anti-inflammatory properties of n-3 fatty acids could also be used in therapeutic interventions in enteral nutrition. Are you aware of any use in Crohn's disease, for example, and do you know the outcome?

Dr. Calder: Much literature exists on the use of fish oil in Crohn's disease, ulcerative colitis, and other chronic inflammatory diseases. Many of these studies show changes in biochemical and immunologic variables. Some of them show clinical improvements, although not all. Perhaps the best study is one by Beluzzi (1), where he used a special enterically coated preparation of fish oil and showed very marked maintenance of patients in remission compared with a placebo group, where the patients relapsed.

Dr. Haschke: Is it possible that fish oil might act locally within the gut?

Dr. Calder: I am sure it does. I am sure it acts locally on the gut immune system, on epithelial cells, and on a variety of other cells.

Dr. Haschke: If fish oil is given to premature infants with their very immature immune systems, what could happen if they have a bacterial infection? Many of them do have such infections.

Dr. Calder: This is an important question, but I do not feel confident to answer it because very little information is available on the subject apart from experiments done in animal models, mainly in mature animals. These show a variety of effects, depending on the model and the pathogen. When one gives oils rich in very unsaturated fatty acids, it is important to ensure that the antioxidant protective mechanisms are maintained. In the scenario you are talking about, where there could be diminished reserves or insufficient reserves of antioxidant protectants, it might be very dangerous to give fish oil.

Dr. Meydani: We have shown in humans that a marked decrease in T-cell–mediated immune function occurs following consumption of fish oil (2,3). I think this is important, because these effects are seen particularly in older people who are also more likely to have impaired immunity. We have done studies showing that some of the effect is related to antioxidant status. This could be very important in the case of premature infants. Currently, much interest is expressed in the use of long chain polyunsaturated fatty acids in infant formulas for brain function and so on, but I think we need to be cautious that this use has no adverse effects on immune function.

Dr. Marini: There is a big difference between Europe and the United States in relation to the clinical use of fish oil derivatives in preterm babies. We feel that formulas for preterm babies should contain DHA because such babies are not able to synthesize DHA in sufficient quantity. I think it is also very important to maintain the balance between arachidonic acid and DHA intake in these babies. A recent study by Carlson in St. Louis showed that the addition of DHA plus arachidonic acid to a formula reduced the incidence of necrotizing enterocolitis significantly in the treated group versus a placebo group (4). This may be the answer to Dr. Haschke's question about the local effect of DHA in the intestine.

I have a naive question. At the turn of the 20th Century, people were talking about cholesterol as a defensive factor, as cholesterol is an integral part of the membrane of phospholipids. Now people think that we should lower our cholesterol intake to protect against atherosclerosis. However, during the first years of life maybe a low level of cholesterol could in some way predispose to infection.

Dr. Klish: I feel a need to respond to Dr. Marini's comment about the width of the Atlantic ocean! I think most investigators in the United States are probably not concerned about the addition of these polyunsaturated fatty acids to preterm formulas, as you commented, although the issue with regard to term formula is still unsettled.

Dr. Marini: I am glad that the United States has changed its opinion about supplementation of preterm formula.

Dr. Klish: Let me clarify that. There are no recommendations yet.

Dr. Kotchabhakdi: I would like to raise a few points. No doubt malnutrition and deficiencies of particular nutritional components, including micronutrients, can affect the immune system directly. We are also all aware that the immune system is closely involved with the brain, and that nutrition, whether it be protein, energy, or lipids, also directly affects structure and functional development of the brain, particularly in children. To what extent do you think this effect is caused directly by immune function and how much of it is indirect, via brain immune control? The reason for my question is that in our experience when children suffering from early malnutrition are given nutritional supplements alone, this does not bring about a very rapid improvement, but when food is given together with sensory stimulation the improvement is much more rapid. The use of sensory stimulation in preterm and low birthweight infants appears to improve both the ability to thrive and immune response in these infants.

The second interesting point you brought up was in relation to homeostasis, and how the baby tries to adapt to nutritional deficiency, and how nutrients could be redistributed to the various compartments where their effects are most needed. I remember reading in Myron Winnick's classical text that the brain is relatively spared even in severe malnutrition, but how does it compare with the immune system?

Dr. Calder: In relation to the immune system versus the brain, I think this takes us back to the intimate association between the endocrine system and the immune system. I am sure that situations of stress versus calm can play a role in changing the sensitivity of the immune system to nutritional interventions. For example, it may not be possible for a nutrient to be effective against a very large concentration of a particular stress hormone, whereas if that concentration decreased, it might be possible for the nutrient to exert its effect. I cannot answer specifically on how much these factors are caused by direct or indirect effects, although I think that many of the effects of dietary manipulations can be mimicked in cell culture systems.

Dr. Farthing: I think we accept that some of the studies on inflammatory bowel disease have been beneficial, but fish oil has not found a place in the routine management of these diseases, I think mainly because the effect is not important enough to be clinically useful. Can you tell us what has been done in other inflammatory disorders such as asthma, eczema, and hay fever; and secondly, does feeding fish oil modify the host response to developing a fever?

Dr. Calder: In relation to other inflammatory disorders, much literature is found on rheumatoid arthritis, with results similar to those in inflammatory bowel disease: all the expected biochemical changes, some immunologic changes, and some demonstration of clinical benefit, which include reduced use of other drugs (5). You asked about allergies and asthma. One study that I would draw to your attention to was published in the *American Journal of Clinical Nutrition* in 1997 (6), which involved a very nice fish oil intervention in atopic asthmatics. The authors found some individuals who responded with dramatic clinical improvement, and others whose condition worsened. They were unable to explain the difference between responders and nonresponders, but the responders had markedly increased urinary 5-series leukotriene production, indicating very marked incorporation of EPA and reduced arachidonic acid-derived mediator production. The nonresponders had much less 5-series leukotriene in the urine than the responders. So, some patients can and some cannot respond to this intervention, but the basis of this is not known.

In relation to fever, animal studies quite clearly show that fish oil does modify the fever response. If you feed fish oil and then give the animal a challenge that is normally associated with fever induction, fever is not induced (7). Studies in humans by Rothwell, involving a fish oil intervention, then looked at the induction of fever following injection with a tetanus toxoid vaccine, and showed a reduced fever response (8).

Dr. Meydani: There was also an animal study in guinea pigs looking at anaphylactic response, where they showed worsening of the symptoms with fish oil (9).

Dr. Socha: In relation to the discussion on the treatment of inflammatory bowel diseases in comparison with the use of fish oil supplements in infants, I would like to draw your attention to some differences. First there was a difference in dosage: we use quite high doses of fish oil for the treatment of inflammatory bowel disease, and the effect, therefore, would be very different from supplementation in infants. The other difference is in relation to the type of fatty acid: EPA is the main fatty acid used in the treatment of inflammatory bowel disease, and DHA for supplementing infants.

Dr. Calder: That is a very important point. It seems now from both animal work and human studies that DHA does not have particularly dramatic effects on the immune system, although we know it has important effects on brain development. In contrast, EPA, which as you say is not included in infant formulas, seems to be the immunologically active fatty acid in fish oil. So perhaps functional separation exists there that can be taken advantage of in the preparation of products for different settings.

Dr. Suskind: I think it has been well recognized that children who are severely malnourished have essential fatty deficiency, but the impact of that deficiency on the immune function has not been explored and deserves to be looked at more fully. It could explain some of the rapid reversal in cellular immunity that occurs with refeeding. Have you come across any studies in children dealing with this relationship?

Dr. Calder: Not in humans.

Dr. Tantibhedhayangkul: All mammalian milk contains very large amounts of fat. From the immunologic standpoint, it appears that this is not a good thing. But why would Nature do this if it is not beneficial to the infant?

Dr. Calder: This perhaps raises an important point about differences between adults and infants. The studies I described were carried out in adult volunteers, and they quite clearly showed this effect of high fat feeding. However, it may be that the effect is not exerted earlier in life. This may reflect the composition of human milk, which contains fatty acids at specific positions on the triglyceride molecule. The positional isomerism of the fatty acids and triglycerides may have an important role in maintaining host defenses.

Dr. Woodward: I am wondering how confident it is possible to be that the immunologic effects seen of feeding fish oil versus other types of oil are, in fact, attributable to the EPA or DHA in the fish oil, given the nature of fish oil as a product?

Dr. Calder: If you had asked this question a couple of years ago, I would say that you could not be 100% confident, because what you are alluding to as fish oil contains a variety of other components—vitamin E at different levels from other oils and other fat soluble vitamins at levels that are different from other oils. But I think now, we have very tightly controlled feeding studies on rats fed EPA or DHA with normalization of the other fatty acids and vitamin E, as well as the other vitamins in the diet. So I am reasonably confident that the immunologic effect of fish oil is mainly caused by EPA.

Dr. Woodward: Has that kind of work been done with methyl esters of fatty acids?

Dr. Calder: I think Hamazaki in Japan has done some work with ethyl esters of EPA and DHA and triglycerides of EPA and DHA.

Dr. Griffin: Are there any epidemiologic data looking at different ethnic groups with different dietary fatty acid ingestion? For example, Eskimos compared to Mediterraneans?

Dr. Calder: Epidemiologic observations have been made from the point of view of the incidence of particular disorders that involve a dysfunctional immune response. No associations between fatty acid composition of the diet or serum or cells and immune cell function were found in different ethnic groups. But certainly, the basis of the interest in fish oils and inflammation was the observation that Eskimos have a very low incidence of chronic inflammatory disease, and this was attributed to the change in eicosanoid balance.

Dr. Marini: I would like to comment on the Eskimo diet. On this diet, an increase in serious infectious disease has been shown—not disease in general but the infectious diseases such as sepsis. I do not know whether this is because of the fatty acids or because of other factors in the diet. Another effect of this kind of fish diet is reduced platelet activation. This is probably the reason why Eskimos have less coronary artery disease. DHA is also a very powerful agent against ventricular fibrillation. A study recently presented by the Gruppo Italiano per lo Studio della Sopravvivenza nell'Infarto Miocardio (GISSI)-Prevenzione at the American College of Cardiology (New Orleans, LA, USA March 7–10, 1999), showed that supplementing patients with fish oil after the myocardial infarction can reduce the incidence of ventricular fibrillation by 25%.

Dr. Calder: Fish oil, by virtue of the fatty acids it contains, has a variety of effects that might be responsible for protection against cardiovascular disease. You mentioned at least two of these: platelet aggregation and ventricular fibrillation; a blood lipid lowering effect is also seen. You also mentioned the increase in infectious disease in Eskimos. Tuberculosis in Eskimos is a particular problem, and in one of the animal models I showed, fish oil feeding was associated with increased susceptibility to tuberculosis.

Dr. Meydani: Another observation in Eskimos is that the incidence of diarrheal diseases in children is said to be increased. This might also be related to the effects of the fatty acids in fish oil on immune function.

Dr. Gershwin: I may be the only one here who has lived in Alaska. I should tell you that one of the major staples in the diet of Eskimos, unfortunately, is alcohol, and that plays a significant role in their tuberculosis. I should also say the incidence of rheumatoid arthritis in Eskimos is no different from any other population. Finally, rheumatologists say that feeding fish oils in animal models of systemic lupus erythematosus is effective, but it is only effective if given before the animals get sick. Once the animals have developed lupus, fish oils are relatively ineffective.

Dr. Calder: I think that is a very important point. Maybe using this as a strategy for intervention once the disease has developed is too late, but perhaps these interventions can play a role in the prevention of disease.

REFERENCES

1. Belluzzi A, Brignola C, Campieri M, Pera A, et al. Effect of an enteric-coated fish-oil preparation on relapses in Crohn's disease. *N Engl J Med* 1996; 334: 1557–60.
2. Meydani SN, Endres S, Woods MM, et al. Oral (n-3 fatty acid) supplementation suppresses cytokine production and lymphocyte proliferation: comparison between younger and older women. *J Nutr* 1991; 121: 547–55.
3. Meydani SN, Lichtenstein AH, Cornwall S, et al. Immunological effects of national cholesterol education panel step-2 diets with and without fish-derived n-3 fatty acid enrichment. *J Clin Invest* 1993; 92: 105–13.
4. Carlson SE, Montalto MB, Ponder DL, et al. Lower incidence of necrotizing enterocolitis in infants fed a preterm formula with egg phospholipides. *Pediatr Res* 1998; 44: 491–8.
5. Geusens PP. n-3 fatty acids in the treatment of rheumatoid arthritis. In: Kremer JM, ed. *Medicinal fatty acids in inflammation.* Basel: Birkhauser Verlag, 1998: 111–23.
6. Broughton KS, Johnson CS, Pace BK, et al. Reduced asthma symptoms with n-3 fatty acid ingestion are related to 5-series leukotriene production. *Am J Clin Nutr* 1997; 65: 1011–7.
7. Pomposelli J, Mascioli EA, Bistrian BR, Flores SM. Attenuation of the febrile response in guinea pigs by fish oil enriched diets. *JPEN* 1989; 13: 136–40.
8. Cooper AL, Gibbons L, Horan MA, et al. Effect of dietary fish oil supplementation of fever and cytokine production in human volunteers. *Clin Nutr* 1993; 12: 321–8.
9. Lee TH, Austen KF, Leitch AG. The effects of a fish-oil enriched diet on pulmonary mechanics during anaphylaxis. *Am Rev Respir Dis* 1985; 132: 1204–9.

Nutrition, Immunity, and Infection in Infants and Children, edited by Robert M. Suskind and Kraisid Tontisirin. Nestlé Nutrition Workshop Series, Pediatric Program, Vol. 45. Nestec Ltd., Vevey/Lippincott Williams & Wilkins, Philadelphia ©2001.

Stress, Nutrition, and the Immune Response

Jeffrey S. Kennedy

Department of Cancer Immunology and AIDS, Dana Farber Cancer Institute, Boston, Massachusetts, USA

This chapter highlights the effects of stress on host immunity to disease and reviews the new insights gained over the past few years on the potential therapeutic role of nutrition in altering stress-related disease processes. Recent data suggest that stress may have an effect on both innate and adaptive (specific) immune defenses (1,2). Furthermore, the relation between malnutrition and immune defense indicates a role for nutrition, as many cellular functions are dependent on adequate host nutrition. It is generally accepted that every nutritional deficiency has an effect on the immune system. This has led to the belief that nutritional supplementation can prevent or reduce the impact of disease by augmenting immunity.

The effects of stress and nutrition on innate immune responses has been reviewed elsewhere (3,4). This chapter will focus on the effects of stress on adaptive (specific) immunity. Recent studies demonstrating the effects of stress on immune function have provided important new insights into how individuals vary in their response to different stress loads (allosteric loads). This information is providing a means by which individuals can reduce their risk of stress-associated disease. Interventions such as exercise, nutrition, behavioral modification, or combinations of these may eventually be shown to improve health and prevent disease.

The relation between nutrition and health is especially apparent in the setting of malnutrition. Deficiency of most macro- and micronutrients affects the immune response. This interaction between nutrition and the immune response is bidirectional, with nutrition affecting immune cell response to pathogens, and infectious agents producing detrimental effects on host nutritional status (Fig. 1). There is, however, difficulty in defining optimal nutritional intake when the aim is to augment immune function or prevent disease. Although most investigators agree that suboptimal nutrition increases susceptibility to infectious diseases, we have less understanding of the impact of nutrition in preventing disease. Maintaining the competency of the im-

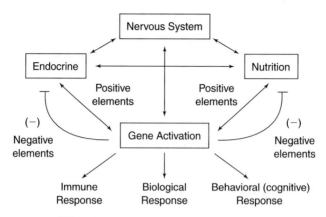

FIG. 1. Neuroendocrine-immune interactions.

mune system during times of stress may serve to decrease the variety of pathogen-related diseases, from infections to cancers and autoimmune diseases.

A landmark review by Scrimshaw *et al.* (5) underscores the effects of malnutrition on the immune response. In the 30 years since this work, numerous reviews have been written on the effects of protein-energy malnutrition on the immune response (6–8). Nutritional deficiencies can affect delayed-type hypersensitivity (DTH), antibody response to pathogens or vaccines, mucosal (immune) integrity, and lymphocyte cytolytic activity against invading pathogens. Generalized malnutrition is a spectrum of deficiencies that can result not only from starvation but also from surgical or medical illness and perhaps strenuous physical or emotional stress. The ensuing acquired immune dysfunction increases host susceptibility to respiratory, intestinal, and systemic infections and assuredly leads to increased morbidity and mortality that is not invariably reversed by nutritional repletion. The interrelation between nutritional status and illness raises questions regarding the role of neuroendocrine responses on the immune system. The influence of the disease process on appetite, intestinal absorption, and end organ utilization must also be considered when attempting to use nutrition as a method of treatment.

Intact adaptive (specific) immunity is essential for host survival. Protein-energy malnutrition suppresses resistance to infections typically encountered in populations in developing countries (9–11). This increased susceptibility to infection appears to be secondary to alterations in T-cell function (12,13). Recovery of immune function following deficiency can be accomplished with nutritional interventions, but it is often delayed when compared with nutritional recovery (14,15). What remains to be determined is whether nutritional supplementation of well-nourished individuals can ameliorate or prevent disease. Clearly, demonstrating a role for nutritional supplements in preventing disease will require studies that delineate, at the molecular level, the mechanisms by which nutrition alters immune cell function and immunity to disease.

IMMUNE FUNCTION: THE ADAPTIVE IMMUNE RESPONSE

The immune system orchestrates the defense against harmful foreign invaders while attempting to spare autologous cells and tissues from injury. First, a protein structure had to be developed, such as an antibody or receptor, which would initiate specific destruction of foreign material. Second, the response to an overwhelming invading force had to be rapid, yet ensure the survival of the host while eliciting for future encounters a memory of the pathogen. Finally, a system would have to evolve that ensured complete destruction of the invading organism, yet protected autologous cells and organs from collateral destruction—a mechanism to distinguish self from nonself.

The human host has developed three distinct but overlapping systems to engage its immune response against pathogens:

1. Antibodies, produced by B lymphocytes and plasma cells, to recognize foreign molecules, called antigens
2. Immune cells specific in recognizing and reacting with antigens on either autologous or foreign cells, called T cells
3. Cytokines and acute phase proteins, designed to maintain immune cell responses and mediate site-directed response to invasion of the host

The specific (or adaptive) immune response is the general term delineating the response of the immune system toward specific antigens. This process involves receptors on T cells that are restricted to recognizing peptide antigens on the surface of cells only when associated with the major histocompatibility complex (MHC), a process referred to as *presentation*. Recognition of protein antigens requires the involvement of antigen-specific helper T cells. This process is fundamental to the initiation of the adaptive (specific) immune response.

The basic elements of the adaptive immune system are cells that process and present antigens. This results in the development of humoral or cytolytic effector responses. Macrophages, and dendritic and Langerhans' cells, although not immunologically specific, are capable of phagocytosis and of processing and presenting antigens to T cells. These cells are important in the secretion of inflammatory cytokines such as interleukins (IL)-1, 2, 6, 10, 12 and tumor necrosis factor-α (TNF-α). These cytokine mediators are important in the induction of fever and innate immune defense molecules such as complement, acute phase proteins, and bactericidal enzymes. Macrophages are, therefore, critical to the initiation of specific immune responses by presenting antigen to T cells and eliciting innate defense mechanisms.

Lymphocytes are immunologically specific cells subdivided into two classes: B and T lymphocytes. B lymphocytes synthesize immunoglobulins and express surface immunoglobulin receptors that recognize soluble intact antigens. T lymphocytes consist of regulatory helper and suppressor cells, and effector T cells, such as cytolytic T cells (CTL) that search and destroy cells bearing specific antigen. The unique specificity of T cells lies in the T-cell receptor which recognizes foreign peptide antigens in association with autologous MHC molecules. The major classes of T cells, as

TABLE 1. *Low-molecular-weight mediators of the acute phase response*

Compound	Effect
Prostaglandins	Vasodilatation
Thromboxane A_2	Vasoconstriction
Leukotriene B_4	Chemotaxis, initiates phagocytosis
Leukotrienes C_4, D_4, E_4	Contraction of smooth muscle
Bradykinin	Mediates activation of pain nerve fibers
Histamine	Chemotaxis, allergic response
Serotonin	
Platelet activating factor	

marked by their surface receptors, location, and effector responses are depicted in Table 1.

The specific immune response can be broken down into two broad types: humoral and cellular immunity. The humoral immune response has been described in detail elsewhere (16). Cellular immunity is essential for survival. Genetic or acquired defects in T-cell function result in increased susceptibility to numerous infections, often to otherwise nonpathogenic organisms (Table 2). Organisms such as *Mycobacterium tuberculosis* (or *M. leprae*), *Listeria*, *Leishmania*, and *Bartonella* have the capacity to replicate within the macrophage. Individuals with impaired cellular im-

TABLE 2. *Markers and distribution of human T and NK cells*

Name	Molecular weight (kd)	Function	Ligand
CD3	γ 25–28 δ 21 ϵ 20 ζ 16 π 21	Signal transduction in T-cell gene activation	Unknown
CD4	60	Coreceptor with the TCR complex for MHC antigen recognition	MHC class II
CD8	α 34 β 34	Maturation and positive selection of MHC class I restricted T cells	MHC class I
CD28	44	Costimulatory molecule signaling independent of TCR	CD86, CD80
TCR	α/β 45/40	$\alpha\beta$: T-cell antigen-specific receptor for MHC-peptide complexes on APC	$\alpha\beta$-MHC-peptide
		$\delta\gamma$: antimicrobial and cytolytic activity	$\gamma\delta$-single molecule, ligand
CD16 (FcγRIIIa)	50–65	Associates with TCRγ and FcϵRI, NK cells, and activated monocytes	IgG immune complexes
CD56 (NCAM)	175–185	Cytotoxicity to NCAM	Unknown
NKB1	70	Inhibits cytotoxicity	HLA-Bw4 alleles
NK1.1	80/38	Murine marker, human equivalent unknown but presumed present activation of cytotoxicity	Unknown

TCR, T-cell antigen receptor; MHC, major histocompatibility complex; APC, antigen-presenting cell; NK, natural killer; NCAM, natural cell adhesion molecule.

munity, as seen in malnutrition, often display accelerated and more lethal consequences when infected by these organisms (17–19).

The clinical integrity of cellular immunity continues to be assessed by the ability of individuals to develop inflammatory skin reactions to recall antigens. The first such test developed involved the ability of individuals previously exposed to *M. tuberculosis* to develop inflammatory skin wheals on re-exposure to intradermally applied tubercle bacillus-derived protein. This test is characterized by local induration, rubor, and swelling, and in rare cases, necrosis, 24 to 48 hours after administration. This subacute reaction, known as the *delayed-type hypersensitivity reaction*, has been subsequently developed for a variety of common bacterial and fungal antigens.

Immunopathologically, the reaction is characterized by perivascular infiltrates of mononuclear cells, is immunologically specific, and is transferred passively by T cells (but only to recipients with matched MHC) but not by plasma. The response is directly linked to macrophage production of IL-2, IL-6, IL-12, and γ-interferon (IFN-γ) by antigen-specific cells. Inhibition of the cytokine response can result in abrogation of the DTH response and is typically seen in disease, malnutrition, and during stress (20,21).

Delayed type hypersensitivity reactions are usually triggered by antigen-mediated stimulation of Th1 effector subset of CD4$^+$ helper T cells (22). These cells produce the cytokines IL-2, IFN-γ, and TNF-α. In a DTH reaction, an antigen stimulates the secretion of these cytokines from Th1 cells that have developed in response to previous exposure to that antigen. The effector response of various cells and cytokines involved in the development of the DTH reaction is depicted in Figure 2. IL-2 promotes expansions of antigen-specific T-cell clones, whereas the other principal cytokines of DTH, IFN-γ and IL-12, initiate an amplification of the response. Other cytokines, which are produced by the Th2 subset of CD4$^+$ helper T cells, function to regulate the DTH reaction. Interleukin-10, an inhibitor of macrophage activation, and IL-4, an antagonist of IFN-γ action, are the principal inhibitory cytokines designed to prevent unchecked tissue injury in DTH reactions.

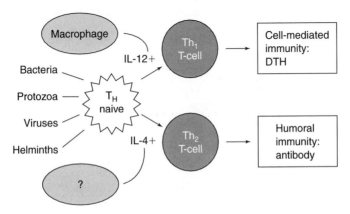

FIG. 2. Cytokine-driven, T-helper cell differentiation.

The immune response to protein antigens is influenced by the differential effect of various antigens on the types of T cells that are induced. Naive CD4$^+$ T cells can be induced to differentiate into either or both effector subsets known as Th1 or Th2 cells. These cell populations produce specific mixtures of cytokines that can be used clinically to mark the type of effector response. The exact mechanisms by which naive T cells differentiate into these effector populations are not completely understood, but the types of cytokine produced locally during antigen exposure appear to be major determinants of differentiation. The pattern of cytokine production as well as signals generated through the T-cell receptor complex may be influenced by disease states (23).

Signals generated through T-cell receptor complex are not sufficient for full activation of T cells. Additional antigen nonspecific co-stimulatory signals through receptors such as CD28 and CTLA-4 are necessary for augmenting IL-2 production and the proliferation and differentiation of effector cell function. Throughout this decade considerable progress has been made in understanding the mechanisms of signal transduction by the T-cell receptor. Various events initiated by T-cell receptor signaling may be important in modulating immune function by hormones, neural input, stress reactions, and nutrition.

Tyrosine phosphorylation is a crucial part of the T-cell signal transduction pathway (Fig. 3). Multiple protein tyrosine-containing motifs, located in the chains of the T-cell receptor complex, are involved in T-cell activation. Two families of protein tyrosine kinases utilize these tyrosine motifs as both substrates and sites for binding, followed by complex formation and activation of downstream signaling events. The *src*-kinase LCK or the *syk*-kinase ZAP-70 play important roles in T-cell receptor signaling, as mutation of either kinase aborts T-cell activation (24,25). These kinases associate with the intracellular chains of T-cell receptor complex (ZAP-70 with the ζ chain and LCK with the ε chain of the complex), initiating a series of downstream events that ultimately direct the T cell to enhance proliferation and IL-2 production (Fig. 4).

The crucial question of how stress can alter response of T cell to MHC presented antigens remains to be explored. Clearly, disruption of DTH and vaccine response

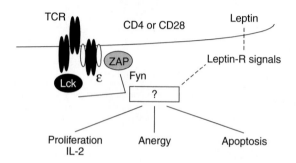

FIG. 3. T-cell signaling and immune response.

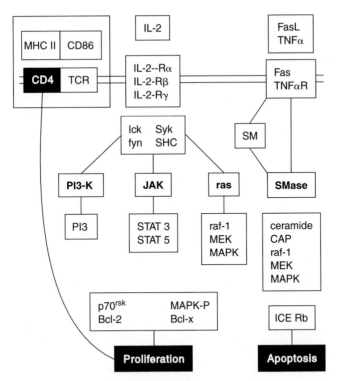

FIG. 4. Signaling components of T-cell activation.

during stress may imply altered T-cell signaling through protein tyrosine kinases. The recent use of altered peptide ligands that engage the same T-cell receptor but induce qualitatively different responses in T cells may help explore the effect of stress on T-cell receptor signaling (26). In addition, antigen-presenting lymphocytes can at times act as antagonists of the T-cell response by altering CD3 phosphorylation through SHP-1 (27). This may be regulated by mitogen and stress-activated protein kinases (MAPK and SAPK) and serine phosphorylation of Lck (28). This altered pattern of ζ-phosphorylation is also associated with a failure to activate ZAP-70 and LCK. These events have been shown to result in loss of IL-2 gene transcription and induction of T-cell anergy in T-cell clones (29). Induction of anergy and lack of lymphocyte proliferation are associated with malnutrition and disease states. It is interesting to speculate about the possible mechanisms underlying this anergic response and the signaling pathways within the T cell and how nutrition may play a role in correcting dysfunctional T-cell responses.

Another area of interest to nutritional immunologists will be the characterization of the process that controls early T-cell development. In both infants and elderly populations, the activation of naive or T-cell progenitors is altered (30). In B cells, a pre–B-cell receptor complex regulates developmental progression and allelic exclusion (16). Recent work has begun to shed more light on the T-cell receptor complex and on the signal transduction pathway and ligand for this receptor (31). Regulation of early T-cell development may be an important area by which nutrition can play a role in disease prevention.

One final area in need of further investigation is the role of T-cell co-stimulatory pathways in the initiation of T-cell responses to pathogens during stress. Much *in vivo* and *in vitro* data have implicated CD28 as a major co-stimulatory receptor on T cells and B7, its ligand, on antigen-presenting cells. The importance of the CD28–B7 interaction in T-cell responses has been confirmed by CD28-deficient mice. T-cell–dependent antibody responses were essentially absent in these mice, as were T-cell responses to some but not all viruses. Subsequent studies have revealed that T-cell proliferation in the presence of antigen-presenting cells was markedly reduced (32). Stress has been shown to affect proliferative response, attenuate IL-2 production, and alter antigen response. Co-stimulatory receptors may also be affected by mediators of the stress response and, therefore, amenable to modulation by nutrition.

CTLA-4 was originally identified as a cDNA expressed in T cells after activation (33). The gene coding for CTLA-4 is highly homologous and is genetically linked to CD28. CTLA-4 binds to B7 with an affinity much higher than CD28, and a soluble form of CTLA-4 has been shown to block T-cell responses *in vivo* and *in vitro*. The function of CTLA-4 remains controversial. Early reports indicated that CTLA-4 might synergize with CD28 to enhance co-stimulation and thereby function to sustain IL-2 production and T-cell proliferation. A more recent report showed that cross linking of CTLA-4 together with T-cell receptor and CD28 resulted in a profound inhibition of IL-2 production and proliferation (34).

Present understanding of the proximal events of signal transduction mediated by CD28 or CTLA-4 is limited. The cytoplasmic domain of CD28 contains a motif, YMNM, that has been shown in other signaling receptor systems to be a site for binding the SH2 domain of phosphoinositide 3-kinase (PI3-kinase). CTLA-4 likewise contains a PI3-kinase domain (YVKM motif) and an association of CTLA-4 with PI3-kinase has been reported (35). PI-3 kinase has recently been shown to be modulated by nutrition (36) and appears to play a role in altered immune function in elderly (37) and aging mouse models (38).

The level of current knowledge regarding the downstream signaling events of CD28 co-stimulation is limited. Augmentation of IL-2 appears to be one important consequence of co-stimulation; however, controversy exists over whether enhanced transcription or mRNA stabilization is the mechanism. At present, it appears that both may play a role. Recent reports of a role for stress-activated protein kinases (SAPK or JNK) in the downstream regulation of induction of IL-2 transcription by T-cell receptor suggest a role of neuroendocrine mediators in modulating T-cell activation during stress.

One intriguing question for the future is whether these biochemical differences can account for the changes in DTH and vaccine response (MHC recognition) seen during stress and malnutrition. Do these changes account for the positive and negative selection in the thymus and can they be reversed by nutrition and other therapeutic approaches?

STRESS, NEUROENDOCRINE RESPONSE, AND IMMUNITY

The relation of stress to immune function has been the subject of much debate and research since the early work of Cannon and Selye. Cannon's summation on the sympathetic nervous system introduced the concept of homeostasis and the intricate balance between the nervous system and health. Selye's notion is that stress is a nonspecific noxious stimulus that elicits an adaptation response encompassing both nervous system elements as well as alterations in the adrenohypophyseal axis (39). The paradox lies in the fact that physiologic systems activated by stress not only protect but may also damage the host. Selye's description of thymolymphatic atrophy in response to stress led to a new understanding of neurohumoral control of the immune response (40).

Stressful experiences, although stimulated by many factors, can best be viewed as acute—in essence *fight or flight*—or chronic, resulting from the cumulative load of day-to-day stress. The latter can be caused by a variety of factors—malnutrition, psychological stress, physical stress, and disease—each influenced by many other factors, as depicted in Figure 5. Genetic factors do not account for all the variability seen in response or sensitivity to stress, as evident from the lack of concordance in identical twin studies (41). Genetic factors also do not explain the differences seen across socioeconomic levels. However, certain factors do appear to have a primary influence on an individual's response to stress. The first relates to how an individual perceives a stressful situation, which is determined not only by genetic factors but also by the person's ability to adjust or habituate to repeated stress and current state of

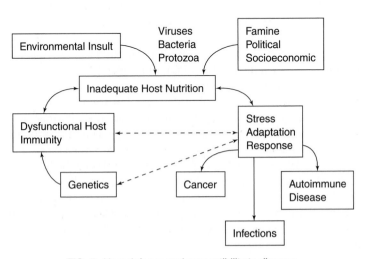

FIG. 5. Host defense and susceptibility to disease.

health; second, and most crucial, is whether the individual perceives a situation as a threat, either psychological or physical (42).

Physiologic and hormonal responses activated by stress can both protect and damage host end organs (43). This paradox confounds our ability to understand the role of stress on disease susceptibility, virulence, and pathophysiologic response. The stress response can be induced by a wide variety of environmental events: cold, sleep deprivation, starvation, and physical injury. The endocrine effects of stress have broad physiologic and metabolic consequences as well as inducing immunologic changes. During acute stress, immune function can be attenuated by the release of glucocorticoids and damage as a result of stress-induced immune activation may be prevented by negative neuroendocrine feedback on immune cells.

The evidence for a relation between stress and disease is compelling. Animal as well as human studies have shown a relation between repeated stress and the development of cancer (44), rheumatoid arthritis (45), and heart disease (46). The available evidence also points to a role of stress in initiating alterations in both specific and nonspecific antigen immunity (47). Numerous studies continue to point toward a role of stress in adversely affecting both arms of adaptive immunity—humoral and cell-mediated (48).

The immune system responds to pathogens by eliciting cellular as well as noncellular immune responses, often referred to as the *acute phase response*. Activation of both the hypothalamic-pituitary axis and the autonomic nervous system during stress has been shown to attenuate the acute phase response and cell-mediated immunity (49). Acute stress results in redistribution of lymphocytes and macrophages throughout the body and margination to certain organ systems such as the skin, lymph nodes, and bone marrow. This margination requires blood vessel endothelial contact, important in *priming* the immune system for the assault against intruders. However, it may also predispose certain individuals toward the development of stress-related disease. As examples, DTH during acute stress is enhanced because of increased trafficking of lymphocytes and monocytes to the site of the acute challenge (50). However, individuals experiencing chronic stress have decreased DTH reactions (51). Individuals afflicted with asthma can exacerbate and enhance the frequency of attacks during periods of emotional stress (52). This latter effect may relate to an increased acute phase response on neutrophil function (53).

These immune-enhancing effects of acute stress last from hours to several days and depend on intact and effective adrenal response. The hypothalamic-adrenal axis functions as a check and balance of the immune response. This allows for heightened surveillance by the immune system and development of immunologic memory to pathogens without self-destructive mechanisms overwhelming the host. It has been suggested that this system, in genetically susceptible individuals, can lead to the development of autoimmune or allergic responses during stress. Chronic or repeated stress has been shown to suppress cellular immunity and lead to inhibited DTH (54), increased severity of viral upper respiratory infections (55), and decreased viral antibody titers (56).

This idea of neuroendocrine control of immune activation has strong support from three models: prolonged physical exertion (exercise-immune model), experimental allergic encephalomyelitis in susceptible strains of rats, and studies in humans and nonhuman primates showing an increased incidence of atherosclerosis and hypertension in situations of chronic high stress (57–59).

Marked individual variation exists in the hypothalamic-pituitary axis response to stress and subsequent effects on systemic immune function (60). The mediator of this systemic response may, in part, be IL-6. The pleiotropic function of IL-6 on immune cells and its involvement in the regulation of endocrine, metabolic, and acute phase response suggests that the role of IL-6 during stress is complex and in need of further study. Recent data from my laboratory suggest a role for IL-6 in the chronic stress response after the usual acute hypothalamic-pituitary axis response of acute stress has subsided. A subset of individuals showed marked changes in T-cell subsets and function, suggesting that extended stress also alters T-cell responses to antigens that could play a role in the development of autoimmune diseases (Table 3).

Integrated homeostatic mechanisms between the nervous and endocrine systems have recently been explained by new information showing that both have important modulating effects on immune function. Regulatory peptides and their receptors, previously thought to be limited to the brain or the immune system, are now known to be expressed in both. This finding helps to explain how stress, particularly the behavioral response to stress, could modify effective immune response to disease.

Toward this end of defining the effect of stress on immune function, research in exercise immunology is guided by the acceptance that strenuous exercise is a model in which to study the effects of stress on the immune system. This model uses exercise as a means of temporarily suppressing the immune system. Disease amelioration and prevention has been the major focus of studies relating exercise and neuroen-

TABLE 3. *Genetic and acquired immunodeficiency and risk of infections*

Disease	Gene defect	Function	Infection risk
SCID	CD3γ	TCR signaling	Intracellular and atypical pathogens
Moderate T-cell immunodeficiency	CD3ε	TCR signaling	Intracellular and atypical infections
X-linked SCID	IL-2Rγ	Lack of circulating T cells	All pathogens
X-linked hyper-IgM	CD40 ligand	Failure of Ig switch	Lethal in first year of life
SCID	Zap-70	TCR signaling	No CD8+ cells; all pathogens
X-linked agamma-globulinemia	Btk	BCR signaling; lack circulating mature B cells	Infections at 5 months with declining maternal antibody; recurrent sinusitis, meningitis, cellulitis
Common variable immunodeficiency	Unknown	B- and T-cell deficits	Autoimmune disease, gastric cancer, sinopulmonary infections

SCID, severe combined immunodeficiency; TCR, T-cell antigen receptor; BCR, B-cell antigen receptor.

docrine or immune function. The role of exercise in cancer prevention, as well as limiting the effects of such diseases as coronary heart disease, osteoporosis, and diabetes, tends to suggest that exercise can have a positive impact on health. In addition, exercise-induced muscle injury represents a model of activating the acute phase response of injury or repair and adds the potential of determining whether nutritional supplements can alter overall immunocompetence and repair mechanisms. Current data are inconclusive to the value of this model in studying the role of nutrition in disease prevention.

Physical exercise has been promoted as a panacea for a host of illnesses (61). However, the complexities and redundancies of the immune system and the unique mechanisms of virulence of specific pathogens confound the role of exercise in altering immune function and human disease processes. Epidemiologic studies point to a reduction in morbidity and mortality from cardiovascular disease, cancer, the human immunodeficiency virus (HIV), osteoporosis, and autoimmune diseases (62–67). Morbidity, and more often mortality, used as outcome measures, make the assumption that they measure the intactness of an integrated host immune defense response. Studies in exercise immunology to date often show abnormalities of lymphocyte subpopulations in peripheral blood or changes in proliferative response to mitogens such as phytohemagglutinin or concavalin A. These assays, although descriptive, lack specificity and fail to define defects in immune function that might be causally linked to disease risk.

Like any other homeostatic system, the immune system is composed of redundant and overlapping mechanisms to ensure adequate response to environmental threats. These overlapping mechanisms are most clearly seen in congenital deficiencies. For example, one of every 500 humans is deficient at synthesizing IgA, which binds pathogens at sites of mucosal defense, yet no increased risk for infectious diseases has been found in these individuals. In contrast, congenital deficiencies of complement can lead to abnormalities in phagocytosis, and in the case of terminal complement deficiency, can lead to increased susceptibility to *Neisseria* infections. This unique quality of the immune response to use several mechanisms in responding to infectious challenges points to a danger in drawing conclusions about the overall resistance to infectious agents based on changes in one isolated mechanism. In addition, defining risk for disease based on immune cell deficiencies requires rigorous analysis of immune function at the cellular and molecular level. This may require future studies to focus, for example, on vaccine antibody response (host), T-cell signaling response (cellular), and MHC genetic polymorphisms (molecular) to adequately define the role of exercise or nutrition in disease risk.

Physical exercise, as with all stressors, can have potential adverse consequences. Severe prolonged exercise and *overtraining syndrome* leads to immunosuppression, resulting in an increased risk of upper respiratory tract infections (68) (Table 3) and immune cell changes consistent with other forms of stress, such as aging and severe psychological stress (69) (Fig. 6). Aging is associated with increased risk of cancer, autoimmune diseases, and infectious diseases. Are the immunologic changes seen with extreme physical stress comparable to the risks of disease inherent in aging?

TABLE 4. *Changes in immune cell populations after a 21-day SFAS training and the risk of upper respiratory tract infection*

	T-cell populations (cells/μl blood)				
	CD4+ (helper)	CD8+ (killer)	IL-4+CD4+ Th2 cells	γIFN+CD4 + Th1 cells	Infection risk over baseline
Day 0 (baseline)	990	545	0.02	83	n.a.
Day 19 (stressed)	780	400	0.35	61	2.3

IL, interleukin; IFN, interferon; n.a., not applicable.

What is the functional impairment of aging that explains this generalized risk of multiple types of illness, and does this impairment exist with prolonged physical stress? Are these processes reversible? Do exercise and nutrition have a role in reducing the risk? By understanding these relations we will be better able to identify at-risk individuals as well as learn how to prevent disease.

The results from animal studies are complicated and the isolated effects of physical stress are difficult to interpret. Models using *swim to exhaustion* may reflect more survival stress than actual mortality observed following infection or diminished resistance to infection. Timing of exercise (rats are nocturnal) can influence the results of studies because sleep deprivation is known to suppress immune function (69). Use of electric shocks to prod the animal to exercise is in itself a proven immunosuppressant. Finally rodents, if given access to their running wheels at night, will typically run several miles a night, which is much more significant exercise than the experimental challenge used during most studies. Additionally, the effect of the exercise on pathogen virulence and susceptibility is less consistent. The swim model of animal exercise has been shown to increase the replication of viruses such as coxsackie A9 (70), B3 (71), and influenza (72), but not bacterial or protozoan infections (72,73). This form of exercise increased mortality secondary to coxsackie B3, influenza, and trypanosomiasis (although perhaps deaths may have been related more to drowning than to the infectious agent). Many of these

	Blood lymphs	Serum Ig	Prolif	IL-2 IL-2R	IL-4 IL-6	CD3
Age > 65	N	N	↓	↓↑	↑↑	↓
Prolonged stress	N	N	↓	↓↑	↑↑	↓

	CD4+	CD8+	CD4CD8+	CD45RA+	CD45RO+
Age > 65	↓	↑	↑	↓	↑
Prolonged stress	↓	↑	↑	↓	↑

FIG. 6. Age- versus stress-related changes in markers of immune function.

studies suffer from the efforts to maximize infection, in that the route of infection (intraperitoneal and intracerebral injection of organisms) may have evaded the typical host immune response and defense mechanisms, leaving the question of whether exercise would have played a role if the normal portals of entry had been used.

Studies conducted in humans emphasize the difficulty in assessing a possible role of exercise in altering immune defense. Two studies (74,75), one of 6 months and the other of 1 year in duration, were used to assess the incidence of upper respiratory infection in young adults active in athletic sports. No correlation was found in either study on risk of upper respiratory infection and exercise activity, although in the former study (74), a negative correlation was found in women. In a study of sedentary obese women, those assigned to a regimen of 15 weeks of supervised walks reported a significantly reduced duration of symptoms when suffering upper respiratory infection. In both studies, a lack of control over the extent and type of pathogen exposure complicates the interpretation of the role played by exercise in reducing upper respiratory infection risk or symptoms. More recently, a large study of 394 subjects given nasal drops containing one of five respiratory viruses versus placebo saline showed that the incidence of infection correlated with measures of psychological stress, but was not related to exercise frequency, intensity, duration, or type (76). This study serves to illustrate that many other factors (*e.g.*, psychological stress) must be controlled for during studies in humans that assess the effects of exercise on immune function.

Acute exercise results in several blood compartment changes in lymphocyte populations. T cells show a decline in both helper ($CD3^+CD4^+CD8^-$) and suppressor ($CD3^+CD4^-CD8^+$) cells as well as declines in B cells ($CD19^+$) and natural killer cells ($CD16^+CD56^+$). Natural killer cell activity has been shown to decline after exercise (77) and it has been hypothesized that this is the cause of the exercise-related risk of upper respiratory tract infection. It has also been shown that antibody production is inhibited and mucosal IgA levels are diminished (77). Whether these cellular changes are associated with altered immune function or risk of disease is not known. Most have only made conjectures from combining the results of several studies.

Several regulatory peptides, first described in immunocompetent cells, are known to have profound effects on both the immune cell and the central nervous system. These include the interleukins and growth factor peptides. Exercise has been shown to induce the acute phase response with the induction of three families of cytokines (IL-1, IL-6, and TNF). Conflicting data are found on the role of IL-1 in the exercise-induced acute phase response. Currently, many studies have reported a lack of IL-1 in the plasma following strenuous exercise (78,79). IL-6, a member of a family of cytokines that triggers gp-130 type receptors (important in the activation of stress kinases), has been shown to be enhanced by strenuous exercise (80). This family of cytokines includes other immunologically important cytokines such as LIF and IL-2, which will be discussed later.

Bruunsgaard *et al.* (80) showed that eccentric exercise (known to induce severe muscle injury) increased plasma IL-6 (fivefold after 2 hours), whereas concentric exercise did not. This study suggests that cytokine production after exercise is connected with activation of the immune response to injury rather than injury itself. In a recent study, it was shown that 21 and 60 days of continuous intense physical training results in a ten to twenty times increase in IL-6, IL-1Ra, and TNFsRp55 (unpublished results). The increase in IL-6 was sustained throughout the duration of the exercise. In addition, these cytokine elevations were not reflective of changes in circulating monocyte or lymphocyte populations, and they were consistent with western blot analysis of lymphocytes that indicated activation of kinases associated with gp130 receptor ligation. The elevation of IL-6 was not associated with significant increases in serum creatine phosphokinase, as seen in eccentric exercise models. It is unlikely, therefore, that muscle injury played a significant role in inducing IL-6 release from immune cells during this training. Other mediators, perhaps in response to stress, may play a more significant role during long-term strenuous exercise.

Immune responses alter neural and endocrine function, although the activity of the latter clearly modifies host immune function. Links are established between neuroendocrine function and response of the immune system to infection and inflammation. The relation between neuroendocrine function and immune responses may explain how emotions, stress, and aging modify individual capacity to fight infection or influence the course of chronic diseases such as cancer and autoimmune disorders. Data from our studies in prolonged stress models show that IL-6 may have a role in the regulation of energy balance. During 60 days of continuous physical and psychological stress, induction of acute phase response and IL-6 was associated with a dramatic decline in plasma leptin levels and diminished T-cell responsiveness following ligation of T-cell receptor (unpublished data). Lymphocytes harvested from these individuals when incubated with leptin showed a return to normal T-cell receptor signaling when compared with controls. A T-cell receptor signaling abnormality seen during stress is consistent with findings from multiple studies indicating that stress alters DTH skin responsiveness and IL-2 production of isolated lymphocytes (81).

Our model used a multistress environment simulating the extreme stress seen during combat, natural disasters, and extended bereavement. This model, involving young men training in US Army Special Operations, enabled us to study the effects of sleep deprivation, mental stress, and intense physical exertion on immune function and risk for infectious diseases. Initial investigations showed that individuals experiencing this stress developed anergic skin DTH at incidences seen in elderly people, people with HIV, and critically ill patients in the hospital (Fig. 7).

Specific immunity is critical to host defense against disease. Medicine today is faced with an array of new technologies geared toward enhancing specific immune response against cancer, autoimmune disease, and pathogens. The role of nutritional supplementation in augmenting host defense mechanisms is only beginning to be explored. The future holds the promise of identifying individuals at risk, which will allow further study of the effects of nutritional interventions on the prevention of disease.

Group	% Anergic
Controls (non-stress)	2%
Children (0.5–2 yrs)	38%
Children (> 2 yrs)	7%
Adults (< 40 yrs)	5–8%
Elderly (> 65 yrs)	15–25%
Continuous Stress	
21 days	25%
60 days	45%
HIV (CD4 = 100–500)	30–60%

FIG. 7. Frequency of anergic skin delayed type hypersensitivity response.

NUTRITION AND STRESS

The study of the effects of dietary nutrients on immune cells and immunity to disease is complicated by the multiple interactions that various types of nutrients have on cellular physiology and metabolism. Dietary proteins, lipids, and complex carbohydrate-based nutrients may act as antigens when absorbed, stimulating mucosal immune responses independent of any innate effects on immune cell function. In addition, the effect of any single nutrient depends not only on its relative concentration in tissues but also on its interaction with other critical nutrients involved in the response measured. For an immunologist, it is, at first glance, difficult to imagine that vitamins or minerals could have effects on immune function except when deficient. However, several nutrients seem to have *pharmacologic value*. In other words, when supplied at levels far in excess of requirements for normal physiologic processes, they exert an effect that appears to alter the relative risk of disease or disease progression. Finally, in many studies of the effects of nutrients on immune function, a nutrient imbalance exists. The duration of this imbalance, as well as factors such as stress, disease, and the age of the host, may influence the measured immune response and cloud the interpretation of the effect of nutrient supplementation.

In 1971, Smythe *et al.* documented the impact of nutrition (protein-energy malnutrition) on cell-mediated immunity (11). This work substantiated a longstanding belief that the cell-mediated immune system bore the brunt of poor nutritional status. This work was supported by later investigations showing that the types of infection seen in malnutrition were consistent with altered cell-mediated immunity (82).

Three specific examples of the interaction of nutrition and the immune cell response serve to illustrate the complexity and difficulties scientists will encounter as they try to elucidate how nutrition can prevent or ameliorate disease. It is widely known that the response to immunization as measured by specific antibodies to an immunogen is often normal in malnutrition, yet cellular immune responses, particularly T-cell function, are impaired. This altered T-cell response correlates with an increased risk of infectious disease morbidity and mortality in malnourished individuals, hospital inpatients, infants, and elderly people. For example, in a child with a recent history of measles, malnutrition increases the risk of death from diarrheal disease (83). This effect appears not to be related to antibody titers against measles virus but rather to be the result of cell-mediated immune suppression induced by the viral infection compounded by malnutrition (84–87).

Measles virus infection can result in near complete suppression of cell-mediated immunity (84). Lymphocytes possess surface molecules called *common differentiation antigens* (CD), which serve as receptors and signal-transducing proteins to initiate the immune system's battle with invading pathogens, as well as to protect the host from cancer and autoimmune diseases. Measles utilizes one such receptor, CD46, a component of the complement system, as a means of binding to lymphocytes and suppressing the immune response. CD46 is upregulated on the surface of lymphocytes during acute inflammation, and the measles virus has adapted to this opportunity, using CD46 as a receptor to enter the cell and evade destruction. Once inside, the virus initiates a series of cytokine effector responses designed to limit host destruction of cells infected with the measles virus.

Normally, the host response to intracellular viruses such as measles involves T-cell production of γ-interferon and IL-2, which elicits a type 1 (Th1) T-cell immune response (88) (Fig. 8). Interestingly, malnutrition also impairs this type of T-cell response (89). The impairment by measles virus of this response is so complete in susceptible hosts (*e.g.*, infants) that other pathogens, in particular enteric bacteria (dysentery), can opportunistically invade a host and cause death.

As a second example, studies by Beck and others (71,90) have extended the concept that nutritional state can alter susceptibility to disease; in this case, virulence and

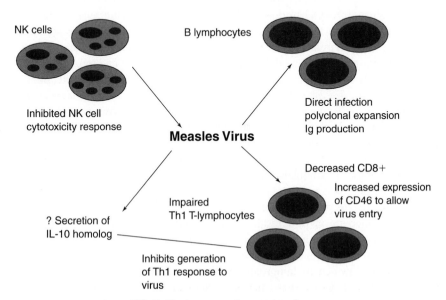

FIG. 8. Host response to measles virus.

pathogenicity of coxsackie B virus for inducing myocarditis during selenium deficiency is increased.

This work serves to illustrate the multidimensional relation between nutrition and immune health. Keshan disease (91) is an endemic cardiomyopathy typically seen in northern China. In endemic areas, individuals have low plasma concentrations of the trace element selenium and repletion of selenium in the diet significantly reduces the prevalence of cardiomyopathy (92). This disease presents an epidemiologic pattern consistent with an infectious agent as a risk factor in endemic selenium deficiency for the development of cardiomyopathy. Initial studies in selenium-deficient mice demonstrated increased heart damage when mice were inoculated with a strain of coxsackie virus (CVB3/20) isolated from individuals with Keshan disease (93). Subsequently, a series of elaborate studies in selenium-deficient mice showed that an animal model with a risk profile similar to that seen in human Keshan disease could be developed (94,95).

Investigators hypothesized that the selenium-deficient environment altered viral genotype, which resulted in increased virulence of the CVB3 virus. In selenium-deficient animals, CVB3 introduced into the animals mutated in six of seven genomic nucleotide positions characteristic of the more virulent strain, CVB3/20. The CVB3/20 virus is the pathogenic strain causing myocarditis (96,97). This hybrid formation occurs *in vivo*, under conditions of selenium deficiency, suggesting that selenium may play a role in altering virulence of a virus (98). The alteration of the viral genome was not unique to selenium, but was also seen under conditions of vitamin E deficiency (99). This later finding suggests, in contradiction to Beck's hypothesis, that altered nutritional status may only be a marker of impaired immune surveillance. Altered immune response may be responsible for the emergence of more pathogenic strains of viruses through natural selection rather than through nutrient deficiency altering viral replication and genetic mutation. Although the exact role of selenium deficiency on CVB3 virulence is unknown, these studies nonetheless point to an important role for nutrition in modulating host immune response and risk of disease.

The role that diet can play in modulating the immune response to infections, as well as in chronic disease states, can be viewed from the role these cytokines play in disease processes. To understand more clearly the role that cytokines, and in particular IL-1, play in disease, one must first understand that the production of cytokines is often only the first step in a cascade of physiologic and cellular responses to inflammation. In septic shock, for instance, the mechanism of action of IL-1 appears to relate to its ability to stimulate the production of small effector molecules such as platelet-activating factor, bradykinins, prostaglandins, and nitric oxide. In rheumatoid arthritis, IL-1 is produced in the synovium of patients, and in animal models intra-articular injection of IL-1 results in the breakdown of cartilage, infiltration of leukocytes, and periarticular bone remodeling. In arteriosclerosis, IL-1 stimulates the proliferation of smooth muscle cells and may play a role in plaque formation by stimulating IL-1 by low density lipoproteins (100). In addition, o-3 fatty acids, known to alter the course of atherosclerosis, have been shown to decrease the production of IL-1 by monocytes in humans fed diets supplemented with *n*-3 fatty acids (101,102). The impact nutrition can have in altering the inflammatory response could influence the morbidity and mortality from many acute and chronic inflammatory diseases. To date, research on the role of nutrition in altering disease or the injury process has been limited. The need for further investigations is quite apparent.

The inflammatory reactions that occur as a part of the host response to infections can occur both before the development of specific immunity and as a component or sequel of the effector phase of specific immune reactions. Inflammation serves a protective function by eliminating infectious agents, and may also cause tissue injury, resulting in local and systemic pathologic abnormalities. As a result, inflammatory reactions that accompany immune responses are often severe and have unique features dependent on the nature of the eliciting antigen and subsequent immune response.

In a recent finding by Lord and others, leptin, a hormone known to regulate body fat stores, was shown to have a profound impact on T-cell immune function. In a mouse model of starvation-induced immunosuppression, leptin administration partially reversed T-cell cytokine, proliferation, and function of the T-helper cell subpopulation (103). In addition, these investigators found that the response to leptin was particularly confined to naive T cells, which may help explain the similar responses seen in human starvation-induced immune suppression. My laboratory has shown a similar response in human subjects experiencing stress coupled with moderate energy deprivation (Kennedy JS, unpublished data; Fig. 9). In this setting, leptin levels correlated with a rise in IL-6 and suppression of T-cell–mediated immune responses. The addition of exogenous leptin to lymphocyte cultures of these individuals reversed the T-cell deficits. Although no leptin was given, the reversal by leptin *ex vivo* suggests that the decreased leptin levels seen during stress may alter T-cell

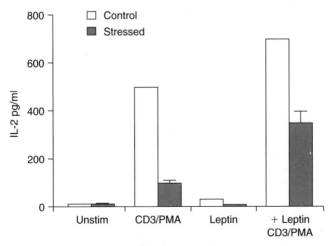

FIG. 9. Effect of leptin on peripheral blood lymphocyte IL-2 production: stressed versus non-stressed humans.

immune function. These advances in understanding the biochemical and molecular mechanisms underlying the effect of malnutrition on immune function will provide the basis in the future with which to make more cogent recommendations regarding supplementation to prevent or treat disease.

The role of nutrition in preventing disease in childhood is becoming well established. A randomized, controlled trial of zinc supplementation in India showed a 21% reduction in the duration of diarrhea (104), improved birthweight following prenatal supplementation, and improved weight gain in infants (105). Vitamin A supplements substantially reduce mortality from severe measles (106), although when supplemented at the time of vaccination they may reduce seroconversion rates in children (107). Recent meta-analysis reviews suggest that the relation between vitamin A supplementation and viral infection (*e.g.*, measles) is more complex (108,109).

The effects of nutrition on disease are reviewed elsewhere in this volume. As research in the field of immunology advances, new and more specific assessments of the impaired immune response during malnutrition will allow investigators to target novel nutritional therapies. I hope the information provided here serves to highlight the new immunologic advances in the area of T-cell signaling, and may influence the development of new approaches to study the effects of stress and malnutrition on T-cell function. I would also like to emphasize the need to develop and fund research projects that incorporate expertise from the fields of immunology, epidemiology, nutrition, and molecular biology. Under rigorous multidisciplinary studies we will learn whether nutrition can have *pharmacologiclike* effects on enhancing immune function and whether these effects can influence disease prevention, susceptibility, morbidity, and mortality.

REFERENCES

1. Wilder R. Neuroendocrine-immune system interactions and autoimmunity. *Annu Rev Immunol* 1995; 13: 307–38.
2. Anisman H, Baines M, Berczi I, et al. Neuroimmune mechanisms in health and disease. *Can Med Assoc J* 1996; 155: 867–74.
3. Khansari D, Murgo A, Faith R. Effects of stress on the immune system. *Immunol Today* 1990; 11(5): 170–5.
4. Irwin M. Stress-induced immune suppression. *Ann NY Acad Sci* 1993; 697: 203–18.
5. Scrimshaw N, Taylor C, Gordon J. *Interactions of nutrition and infection.* Geneva: World Health Organisation, 1968.
6. Redmond H, Shou J, Kelly C, et al. Immunosuppressive mechanisms in protein-calorie malnutrition. *Surgery* 1991; 110: 311–17.
7. Keusch G. Malnutrition, infection and immune function. In: Suskind R, Lewinter-Suskind L, ed. *The malnourished child.* New York: Raven Press, 1990: 37–55.
8. Woodward B. Protein, calories and immune defenses. *Nutr Rev* 1998; 56: S84–92.
9. Chan J, Tran Y, Tanaka K, et al. Effects of protein calorie malnutrition on tuberculosis in mice. *Proc Natl Acad Sci USA* 1996; 93: 14857–61.
10. Mata L. Malnutrition-infection interactions in the tropics. *Am J Trop Med Hyg* 1975; 24: 564–73.
11. Smythe P, Brereton-Stiles G, Grace H, et al. Thymolymphatic deficiency and depression of cell mediated immunity in protein-calorie malnutrition. *Lancet* 1971; ii: 939–43.
12. Woodward B, Miller R. Depression of thymus-dependent immunity in wasting protein-calorie malnutrition does not depend on an altered ratio of helper (CD4$^+$ to suppressor (CD8$^+$) T cells or on a disproportionately large atrophy of the T cell relative to B cell pool. *Am J Clin Nutr* 1991; 53: 1329–35.

13. Chandra R. Numeral and functional deficiency in T helper cells in protein-energy malnutrition. *Clin Exp Immunol* 1983; 51: 126–32.

14. Chevalier P, Sevilla R, Sejas E, Zalles L, Belante G, Parent G. Immune recovery of malnourished children takes longer than nutritional recovery; implications for treatment and discharge. *J Trop Pediatr* 1998; 44: 304–7.

15. Gross R, Newberne P. Role of nutrition in immunologic function. *Physiol Rev* 1980; 60: 188–302.

16. Rudin C, Thompson C. B cell development and maturation. *Semin Oncol* 1998; 25: 435–46.

17. Dye C, Williams B. Malnutrition, age and the risk of parasitic disease: visceral leishmaniasis revisited. *Proc R Soc Lond Biol Sci* 1993; 254: 33–9.

18. Olumese P, Sodeinde O, Ademovo O, Walker O. Protein energy malnutrition and cerebral malaria in Nigerian children. *J Trop Pediatr* 1997; 43: 217–19.

19. Pelletier D, Frongillo E, Schroeder D, Habicht J. The effects of malnutrition on child mortality in developing countries. *Bull World Health Organ* 1995; 73: 443–8.

20. Redmond H, Gallagher H, Shou J, Daly J. Antigen presentation in protein-energy malnutrition. *Cell Immunol* 1995; 163: 80–7.

21. Edelman R. Cell mediated immune response in protein calorie malnutrition—a review. In: Suskind R, ed. *Malnutrition and the immune response*. New York: Raven Press, 1977: 47–75.

22. Tsicopoulos A, Hamid Q, Varney V, et al. Preferential mRNA expression of Th1-type cells (IFNg+,IL-2+) in classical delayed-type (tuberculin) hypersensitivity reactions in human skin. *J Immunol* 1992; 148: 2058–61.

23. Romagnami S. Lymphokine production by human T cells in disease states. *Annu Rev Immunol* 1994; 12: 227–57.

24. Rudd C, Anderson P, Morimoto C, Streuli M, Schlossmann S. Molecular interactions, T cell subsets and role of the CD4/CD8: p56Lck complex in human T cell lymphocytes. *Immunol Rev* 1989; 111: 225–66.

25. Mye D, DiBartolo V, Germain V, Tuosto L, Michel F, Acuto O. Mutation of tyrosine 492/493 in the kinase domain of ZAP-70 affects multiple T cell receptor signaling pathways. *J Biol Chem* 1996; 271: 32644–52.

26. Madrenas A, Wange R, Wang J, Isakov N, Samelson L, Germain R. Zeta phosphorylation without Zap 70 activation induced by TCR antagonists or partial agonists. *Science* 1995; 267: 515–18.

27. Laface D, Couture C, Anderson K, et al. Differential T cell signaling induced by antagonist peptide-MHC complexes and the associated phenotypic response. *J Immunol* 1997; 158: 2057–64.

28. Alberola-Ila J, Forbush K, Seger R, Krebs E, Permutter R. Selective requirement for MAP kinase activation in thymocyte differentiation. *Nature* 1995; 373: 620–3.

29. Li W, Whaley C, Mondino A, Mueller D. Blocked signal transduction to the Erk and JNK protein kinases in anergic CD4$^+$ T cells. *Science* 1996; 271: 1272–6.

30. Whisler R, Newhouse Y, Bagenstose S. Age-related reductions in the activation of mitogen-activated protein kinases p44/ERK1 and p42/ERK2 in human T cells stimulated via ligation of the T cell receptor complex. *Cell Immunol* 1996; 168: 201–10.

31. Imanishi K, Seo K, Kato H, et al. Post-thymic maturation of migrating human thymic single-positive T cells: thymic CD1aCD4$^+$ T cells are more susceptible to anergy induction by toxic shock syndrome toxin-1 than cord blood CD4$^+$ T cells. *J Immunol* 1998; 160: 112–19.

32. Jenkins M. The ups and downs of T cell stimulation. *Immunity* 1994; 1: 443–6.

33. Lord G, Lechler R, George A. A kinetic differentiation model for the action of altered TCR ligands. *Immunol Today* 1999; 20: 33–9.

34. Nishimura Y, Chen Y, Kanai T, Yokomizo H, Matsuoka T, Matsushita S. Modification of human T cell responses by altered peptide ligands: a new approach to antigen-specific modification. *Intern Med* 1998; 37: 804–17.

35. Davis M, Boniface J, Reich Z, et al. Ligand recognition by alpha beta T cell receptors. *Annu Rev Immunol* 1998; 16: 523–44.

36. Dean D, Brozinick J, Cushman S, Cartee C. Calorie restriction increases cell surface GLUT-4 in insulin stimulated skeletal muscle. *Am J Physiol* 1998; 275: E957–64.

37. Kelley K, Meier W, Minshall C, et al. Insulin growth factor-I inhibits apoptosis in hematopoietic progenitor cells. Implications in thymic aging. *Ann NY Acad Sci* 1998; 840: 518–24.

38. Martineau L, Chadan S, Parkhouse W. Age-associated alterations in cardiac and skeletal muscle glucose transporters, insulin and IGF-1 receptors and PI3 Kinase contents in the C57BL/6 mouse. *Mech Ageing Dev* 1999; 106: 217–32.

39. Selye H. A syndrome produced by diverse nocuous agents. *Nature* 1936; 138: 32.

40. Selye H. Thymus and adrenals in the response of the organism to injuries and intoxication. *Br J Exp Pathol* 1936; 17: 238–48.
41. Selye H. Stress and disease. *Science* 1955; 122: 625–31.
42. Ader R, Cohen N. The influence of conditioning on immune responses. In: Ader R, Cohen DL, eds. *Psychoneuroimmunology*, 2nd ed. San Diego: Academic Press, 1996: 611–46.
43. Minowada G, Welch W. Clinical implications of the stress response. *J Clin Invest* 1995; 95: 3–12.
44. Geyer S. Social factors in the development and course of cancer. *Cancer J* 1996; 9: 8–12.
45. Berci I, Barragan F, Chalmers M, Keystone E, Nagy E, Warrington R. Hormones and self tolerance and autoimmunity: a role in the pathogenesis of rheumatoid arthritis? *Autoimmunity* 1993; 16: 45–56.
46. Steptoe A, Fieldman G, Evans O, Perry L. Cardiovascular risk and responsivity to medical stress: the influence of age, gender and risk factors. *J Cardiovasc Risk* 1996; 3: 83–93.
47. Dantzer R, Kelley K. Stress and immunity: an integrated view of relationships between the brain and the immune system. *Life Sci* 1989; 44: 1995.
48. Kort W. The effect of chronic stress on the immune system. *Adv Neuroimmunol* 1994; 4: 1.
49. Chrousos G. The hypothalamic-pituitary-adrenal axis and immune-mediated inflammation. *N Engl J Med* 1995; 332: 1351–62.
50. Dhabhar F, McEwen B. Acute stress enhances while chronic stress suppresses cell mediated immunity in vivo: a potential role for leukocyte trafficking. *Brain Behav Immunol* 1997; 11: 286–306.
51. Dhabhar F. Stress-induced enhancement of cell mediated immunity. *Ann NY Acad Sci* 1998; 840: 359–72.
52. Persoons J, Schornagel K, Breve J, Berkenbach F, Kraal G. Acute stress affects cytokines and nitric oxide production by alveolar macrophages differently. *Am J Respir Crit Care Med* 1995; 152: 619–24.
53. Sternberg E, Chrousos G, Wilder R, Gold P. The stress response and the regulation of inflammatory disease. *Ann Intern Med* 1992; 117: 854–66.
54. Dhabhar F, McEwen B. Enhancing versus suppressive effects of stress hormones on skin immune function. *Proc Natl Acad Sci USA* 1999; 96: 1059–64.
55. Cohen S, Tyrrell D, Smith A. Psychological stress and susceptibility to the common cold. *N Engl J Med* 1991; 325: 606–12.
56. Keller S, Shiflett S, Schliefer S, Bartlett J. Stress, immunity and health. In: Glaser R, Kiecolt-Glaser J, eds. *Handbook of human stress and immunity*. San Diego: Academic Press, 1994: 217–44.
57. Wharborg P. Mental stress and ischemic heart disease: an underestimated connection. *Zur Heart J* 1998; 19 (Suppl. O): O20–3.
58. Mason D, MacPhee I, Antoni F. The role of the neuroendocrine system in determining genetic susceptibility to experimental allergic encephalomyelitis in the rat. *Immunology* 1990; 70: 1–5.
59. Fricchone G, Bilfinger T, Hartman A, Liu Y, Stefano G. Neuroimmunologic implications in coronary artery disease. *Adv Neuroimmunol* 1996; 6: 131–42.
60. Terzolo M. Morning to evening changes of human pituitary and adrenal responses to specific stimuli. *J Endocrinol Invest* 1990; 13: 181–5.
61. Moore M, Park C, Tsuda H. Physical exercise: a pillar for cancer prevention. *Eur J Cancer Prev* 1998; 7: 177–93.
62. Powell K, Caspersen C, Koplan J, Ford E. Physical activity and chronic diseases. *Am J Clin Nutr* 1989; 49: 999–1006.
63. Sothern M, Loftin M, Suskind R, Udall J, Blecker U. The health benefits of physical activity in children and adolescents: implications for chronic disease prevention. *Eur J Pediatr* 1999; 158: 271–4.
64. Brownell K. Diet, exercise and behavioral intervention: the nonpharmacological approach. *Eur J Clin Invest* 1998; 28 (Suppl. 2): 19–22.
65. Dunn A, Marcus B, Kampert J, Garcia M, Kohl H, Blair S. Comparison of lifestyle and structured interventions to increase physical activity and cardiorespiratory fitness: a randomized trial. *JAMA* 1999; 281: 327–34.
66. Bemben D. Exercise interventions for osteoporosis prevention in postmenopausal women. *J Okla State Med Assoc* 1999; 92: 66–70.
67. Loudon C, Corroll V, Butcher J, Rawsthorne P, Bernstein C. The effects of physical exercise on patients with Crohn's disease. *Am J Gastroenterol* 1999; 94: 697–703.
68. Fitzgerald L. Overtraining increases the susceptibility to infection. *Int J Sports Med* 1991; 12 (S5–8).
69. Cannon J. Exercise and resistance to infections. *J Appl Physiol* 1993; 74: 973–81.
70. Tilles J, Preuss T. Mitogenic response of T lymphocytes to exercise training and stress. *J Appl Physiol* 1991; 70: 2535–8.

71. Gatmaitan B, Chason J, Lerner A. Augmentation of the virulence of murine coxsackie B-3 myocardiopathy by exercise. *J Exp Med* 1970; 131: 1121–36.
72. Ilback N-G, Friman G, Beisel W, Johnson A, Berendt R. Modifying effects of exercise on clinical course and biological response of the myocardium in influenza and tularemia in man. *Infect Immun* 1984; 45: 498–504.
73. Elson S, Abelmann W. Effects of muscular activity upon the acute myocarditis of C3H mice with *Trypanosoma cruzi*. *Am Heart J* 1964; 69: 629–36.
74. Schouten W, Verschuur R, Kemper H. Physical activity and upper respiratory tract infections in a normal population of young men and women. The Amsterdam growth and health study. *Int J Sports Med* 1988; 9: 451–5.
75. Osterback L, Qvarnberg Y. A prospective study of respiratory infections in 12 year old children engaged in sports. *Acta Paediatr Scand* 1987; 76: 944–9.
76. Nieman D, Nehlsen-Cannarella S, Markoff P, et al. The effects of moderate exercise training on natural killer cells and acute upper respiratory tract infections. *Int J Sports Med* 1990; 11: 467–73.
77. Pedersen B, Ostrowski K, Rohde T, Bruunsgaard H. Nutrition, exercise and the immune system. *Proc Nutr Soc* 1998; 57: 43–7.
78. Northoff H, Berg A. Immunologic mediators as parameters of the reaction to strenuous exercise. *Int J Sports Med* 1991; 12: S9–15.
79. Cannon J, Meydani S, Fielding R, et al. Acute phase response in exercise. II. Associations between vitamin E, cytokines, and muscle proteolysis. *J Physiol* 1991; 260: R1235–40.
80. Bruunsgaard H, Galbo H, Halkjaer-Kristensen J, Johansen T, MacLean D, Pedersen B. Exercise-induced increase in interleukin-6 is related to muscle damage. *J Physiol* (Lond) 1997; 499: 833–41.
81. Savendahl L, Underwood L. Decreased interleukin-2 production from cultured peripheral blood mononuclear cells in human acute starvation. *J Clin Endocrinol Metab* 1997; 82: 1177–80.
82. Keusch G. Malnutrition and the thymus gland. In: Cunningham-Rundles S, ed. *Nutrient modulation of immune response*. New York: Marcel Decker, 1993: 283–99.
83. Teka T, Faruque A, Fuchs G. Risk factors for deaths in under-age-five children attending a diarrhea treatment center. *Acta Paediatr* 1996; 85: 1070–5.
84. Schlender J, Schnorr J, Spielhoffer P, et al. Interaction of measles virus glycoproteins with the surface of uninfected peripheral blood lymphocytes induces immunosuppression in vitro. *Proc Natl Acad Sci USA* 1996; 93: 13194–9.
85. Nagendra A, Smith C, Wyde P. Evidence that measles virus hemagglutinin initiates modulation of leukocyte function-associated antigen-1 expression. *J Virol* 1995; 69: 4357–63.
86. Kurita M, Yanagi Y, Hara T, Nagasawa S, Matsumoto M, Seya T. Human lymphocytes are more susceptible to measles virus than granulocytes, which is attributable to the phenotypic differences of their membrane cofactor protein (CD46). *Immunol Lett* 1995; 48: 91–5.
87. Addae M, Komada Y, Zhang X, et al. Immunological unresponsiveness and apoptotic cell death of T cells in measles virus infection. *Acta Paediatr Jpn* 1995; 37: 308–14.
88. Ito M, Watanabe M, Kamiya H, Sakurai M. Changes in intracellular cytokine levels in lymphocytes induced by measles virus. *Clin Immunol Immunopathol* 1997; 83: 281–6.
89. Sauerwein R, Mulder J, Mulder L, et al. Inflammatory mediators in children with protein-energy malnutrition. *Am J Clin Nutr* 1997; 65: 1534–9.
90. Beck M. The role of nutrition in viral disease. *Nutr Biochem* 1996; 7: 683–90.
91. Li Y, Wang F, Kang D, Li C. Keshan disease: an endemic cardiomyopathy in China. *Hum Pathol* 1985; 16: 602–9.
92. Group KDR, Sciences CAoM. Observations on the effects of sodium selenite in the prevention of Keshan disease. *Chin J Med* 1979; 92: 471–6.
93. Bai J, Wu S, Ge K, Deng X, Su C. The combined effect of selenium deficiency and viral infection on the myocardium of mice. *Acta Acad Med Sinica* 1980; 2: 31–3.
94. Tracy S, Chapman N, Tu Z. Coxsackievirus B# from an infectious cDNA copy of the genome is cardiovirulent in mice. *Arch Virol* 1993; 122: 399–409.
95. Chapman N, Tu Z, Tracy S, Gauntt C. An infectious cDNA copy of the genome of a non-cardiovirulent coxsackievirus B3 strain—its complete sequence analysis and comparison to the genomes of cardiovirulent coxsackieviruses. *Arch Virol* 1994; 135: 115–30.
96. Beck M, Kolbeck P, Rohr L, Shi Q, Morris V, Levamder O. Increased virulence of a human enterovirus (coxsackie B3) in selenium-deficient mice. *J Infect Dis* 1994; 170: 351–7.

97. Beck M, Kolbeck P, Rohr L, Shi Q, Morris V, Levander O. Amyocarditic coxsackievirus becomes myocarditic in selenium deficient mice. *J Med Virol* 1994; 43: 166–70.
98. Beck M, Shi Q, Morris V, Levander O. Rapid genomic evolution of a non-virulent coxsackievirus B3 in selenium deficient mice results in selection of identical virulent isolates. *Nature Med* 1995; 1: 433–6.
99. Beck M, Kolbeck P, Rohr L, Shi Q, Morris V, Levander O. Vitamin E deficiency intensifies the myocardial injury of coxsackievirus B3 infection in mice. *J Nutr* 1994; 124: 345–58.
100. Endres S, von Schacky C. n-3 Polyunsaturated fatty acids and human cytokine synthesis. *Curr Opin Lipidol* 1996; 41: 203–34.
101. Endres S, Ghorbani R, Kelley V, et al. The effect of dietary supplementation with n-3 polyunsaturated fatty acids on the synthesis of interleukin-1 and tumor necrosis factor by mononuclear cells. *N Engl J Med* 1989; 320: 265–71.
102. Weber P, Leaf A. Cardiovascular effects of omega-3 fatty acids: atherosclerosis risk factor modification by omega 3 fatty acids. *World Rev Nutr Diet* 1991; 66: 218–32.
103. Lord GM, Matarese G, Howard JK, Baker RJ, Bloom SR, Lechler RI. Leptin modulates the T-cell immune response and reverses starvation-induced immunosuppresssion. *Nature* 1998; 394: 897–901.
104. Sazawal S, Black R, Bhan M, Bhandari N, Sinha A, Jalla S. Zinc supplementation in young children with acute diarrhea in India. *N Engl J Med* 1995; 333: 839–44.
105. Ninh N, Thissen J, Collette L, Gerard G, Khoi H, Ketelslegers J. Zinc supplementation increases growth and circulating insulin-like growth factor I (IGF-I) in growth-retarded Vietnamese children. *Am J Clin Nutr* 1996; 63: 514–19.
106. Hussey G, Klein M. A randomized, controlled trial of vitamin A in children with severe measles. *N Engl J Med* 1990; 323: 160–4.
107. Semba R, Munasir Z, Beeler J, et al. Reduced seroconversion to measles in infants given vitamin A with measles vaccination. *Lancet* 1995; 245: 1330–2.
108. Fawzi W, Thomas C, Chalmers T, Herrera M, Mosteller F. Vitamin A supplementation and child mortality. A meta-analysis. *JAMA* 1993; 269: 898–903.
109. Glasziou P, Mackerras D. Vitamin A supplementation in infectious diseases: a meta-analysis. *BMJ* 1993; 306: 366–70.

DISCUSSION

Dr. Griffin: I thought your hepatitis A data were very compelling. I would like to introduce the idea of two other vaccines. The first is an oral vaccine, which would stress the mucosal immune system. I have used, for example, oral cholera vaccine successfully to probe various immune aspects of HIV disease. The other is the possibility of using an intramuscular DNA vaccine. In rodent models, when DNA vaccines are injected into skeletal muscle, the immune response is considerably potentiated when the animal is exercised, and that might be useful in your model because you have these two components of exercise stress and physiologic stress.

Dr. Kennedy: I think those are excellent suggestions. We have become interested in some of the adenoviral vector vaccines as a possible means of looking at the immune response. The difficulty lies in the side effects. We picked hepatitis A because we thought it would have the least side effects of all the vaccines. The subjects we were studying volunteered during a time in their military careers when they were going through a very important course. To do anything that would influence their ability to be successful in that course would have ended our research program!

Dr. Woodward: I firmly believe that in malnutrition at least a shift toward naive-like T cells is real, which has also been observed in elderly subjects (1). I was interested in your leptin results because I believe it is the naive-type cell that responds best to leptin (2). Is that correct?

Dr. Kennedy: Yes, that is correct. We find, as have others, that major shifts occur in memory-naive cell populations. We are not sure what to make of that in terms of either the leptin or the vaccine response, but I agree that the naive cells are probably the ones that are responding most here.

Dr. Woodward: And that is a shift that may occur, not only in the blood, but elsewhere as well. It seems to me that the blood may reflect what is going on elsewhere.

Dr. Kennedy: Yes, but a compelling argument exists that the blood compartment is not where we should be looking, and it may indeed not be reflective of the general immune response. The difficulty with the peripheral blood compartment is getting enough cells. If specific populations of lymphocytes are to be isolated, pints of blood must be drawn, and it becomes a much more difficult approach. Some very interesting ways now use flow cytometry to look at signaling. We have begun to look at calcium signaling and to develop antibodies that will allow us to look at phosphorylation of very specific proteins by flow cytometry after activation. So, I think with flow cytometry we will be able to do some of those studies with fewer cells.

Dr. Farthing: I think you have produced some extremely interesting data, but there is some difficulty in that this was a mixed model: physical stress, psychological stress, and stress from lack of sleep; also, presumably some of these individuals had infections. So, I find it very hard to interpret exactly what was driving what which way in your data. It may be a model that is only relevant to special forces. I presume that they could eat as much as they wanted? Was there any question of limiting their dietary intake?

Dr. Kennedy: There may have been an element of intake limitation in the 60-day model. These individuals had a time limit on their meals and you could see differences between individuals. Some would wolf down 4000 to 5000 calories with a large spoon, but others would be much slower and may not have taken as much as they would have in the mess hall. We think there was probably an appetite suppressing effect. Clear differences appear between individuals in their perception of how hungry they are and what they need.

Dr. Farthing: Those very low leptin levels would be an appropriate response to variation in feed intake.

Dr. Kennedy: The leptin levels were low across the board. After 20 days, occasionally an individual might have a leptin value of 200, but everybody in this group of more than 100 individuals had values of 300 or less, so they all had very significant declines. The standard error bars on those last two time points are very narrow.

Dr. Farthing: During these studies, did you look at the CRH-ACTH-cortisol pathway, because it would seem to be a possible explanation for the depressed appetite?

Dr. Kennedy: We did look at cortisol levels and the blood was drawn at the same time, 5 a.m., at each time point in the studies. We did not find any correlation with simple single point cortisol levels, but we did not do a dexamethasone suppression test, which would be a better way of assessing that axis.

Dr. Gershwin: Did you look at heat shock proteins, or any other stress protein in the model?

Dr. Kennedy: We were very interested in looking at heat shock proteins and these are being analyzed but the data are not available yet. One of our interests is whether or not heat shock proteins are altering the nuclear translocation of phosphorylated transcriptional activators.

Dr. Griffin: Just returning to your point about plasma, or cells in plasma, and reflecting what is going on in the whole immune system, I do not think that is necessarily true. For example, in HIV disease, people have been measuring CD4 kinetics in plasma for a long time, and the finding, of course, is that what is going on in the lymph node is far more important than what is going on in the plasma. A technique is now available for measuring the turnover *in vivo* in humans of any member of the white cell series. This involves the use of 13-carbon glucose, which is metabolized to 13-carbon ribose, enters DNA, and then, providing a cell from plasma can be purified, you can look at its kinetics very easily. With a technique such as that, you could see if the fall in CD4 positive cells was caused by increased removal or decreased production. You could do the same for any of the white cell series that you could sort out and extract DNA from.

Dr. Kennedy: Because of the nature of my research, I am hoping the plasma compartment does mimic the lymph node and spleen compartments! I am not totally convinced that such is the case, but I think that at the moment we are at a point where without some major technical advance it would be difficult to know for certain.

Dr. Keusch: Some of my colleagues have accused me of having a prejudice against animal models, so I would like to try to redeem myself. One very interesting model is the mouse put to exercise on a wheel or a water bath and injected with coxsackie B4 virus. The exercise has a dramatic effect on viral titers of those myotropic strains. So, it might be an interesting model with which to look at the effect of exercise on the immune system and how that might relate to viral proliferation and virus-mediated tissue damage.

Dr. Kennedy: I agree. A paper published about 4 months ago showed exertional rhab-domyolysis in coxsackie B4 virus infection during eccentric exercise (3). The question was raised whether selenium deficiency might alter the inflammatory response and potentiate the virulence factor of coxsackie B4.

Dr. Woodward: It seems to me that a common factor could be oxidant stress. Beck showed the same thing with vitamin E deficiency (4), and more recently with a glutathione peroxidase knock-out mouse (5). It strikes me that the common factor is antioxidants, or at least oxidant stress.

Dr. Kennedy: I agree. I do not think the story is going to be as simple as selenium *per se*, although the selenium may be a key modulating factor.

Dr. Meydani: Data in humans show that eccentric exercise increases oxidative stress, so it could be a common pathway.

Dr. Abu-Zekry: Did you do any studies, or do you know of some studies, relating stress to the development of malignancies or autoimmune diseases?

Dr. Kennedy: That certainly has crossed our minds because of the transformation we see from a TH1 to a TH2 response, and now the alteration in signaling pattern. We are currently interested in the ability of allelic variance to alter the signal transduction pattern, which has a lot to do with autoimmune disease, particularly multiple sclerosis. In a multiple sclerosis model, many of the same signaling pattern abnormalities are seen. Various workers have been focusing on the role of lymphocyte signaling in autoimmune disease states. It is a fairly big leap to suggest that our data show that certain individuals under stress may be more susceptible to autoimmune diseases, but it is an intriguing thought.

Dr. Haschke: Could you comment on whether the changes in immune function that you observed during the period of endurance training in military personnel are comparable to those seen in athletes, for example during endurance training before the Olympic games?

Dr. Kennedy: I am not really sure how it compares with the exercise immunology models that have been done. I would define those studies as models of acute exercise and its effect on immune cells, cytokines, and so on, whereas we deliberately sought a multistress environment. Our primary reason was that we did not want to do all this work and come up with nothing, because we did not stress the subjects enough! We picked our model to ensure that the subjects were as stressed as was ethically possible for a human study. Thus, I am not sure how our model compares with exercise physiology. I would say that if a parallel exists, it is probably best made with what is known as overtraining fatigue of the immune system.

Dr. Haschke: Were the outcome variables that you measured comparable, or similar?

Dr. Kennedy: Some are similar, some are not. The exercise physiology literature is difficult to interpret, because many different studies have indicated different things. I think it is hard to control that environment *per se* and compare one study with another. I think our data are probably more comparable to the aging model in that the changes we see in lymphocyte subpopulations, as well as IL-2, reflect the results obtained by Meydani and others in models of aging.

Dr. Ormisson: I have the same question as Dr. Haschke. Is there any possibility of measuring stress in a very sick baby, say a premature neonate on a respirator surrounded by machines and equipment? What is the stress level under such circumstances?

Dr. Kennedy: I can only speak as an immunologist. It would be a major leap to extrapolate what I have shown to an infant, especially an infant under the age of 2 months, and even more so a premature infant. I think the immune system there reacts in a totally different way to environmental signals, so I am not sure how you would apply our data. However, the assays we did are compatible with work on premature infants in that you do not need a large amount of blood. With well-designed, very specific questions you can be successful with no more than 2 ml of blood.

Dr. Fjeld: I was interested in the disparity between the energy expenditure and the energy intake. I saw Jim Delaney's name mentioned, so I assume you measured energy expenditure by doubly labeled water.

I was wondering whether you looked at the energy density of the weight lost. I did a quick calculation and I see a huge difference in the apparent composition of the weight loss. Did you do that too, and how accurate do you think those data are?

Dr. Kennedy: I think the doubly labeled water data are very accurate. The body composition data are also fairly accurate. We did a subset of individuals by DEXA scan, and the remaining individuals were done by six site caliper.

The caliper body composition data correlated very highly with the DEXA scan data, although our body fat measurements were consistently approximately 1% to 2% higher in the caliper data than in the DEXA data. In all, I think the discrepancy was pretty accurate.

Dr. Fjeld: How did you measure the energy intake?

Dr. Kennedy: We did it mostly by food cards and visual estimation. A period occurs in both these training programs where these individuals go out into the field and it really becomes very, very difficult to do such studies. In those situations, visual estimation was about as accurate as we could get. The recall food survey cards that we had were fairly accurate. They correlated reasonably well with visual estimation, although visual estimation always gave a slightly higher value.

Dr. Suskind: The role of leptin in immunity seems a very important one. It would be interesting to see if leptin levels are a reflection of food intake under conditions of exercise stress.

Dr. Kennedy: I think the leptin levels probably initially reflected the energy deficit and body mass loss. In the first 20 to 30 days, the values were linear and correlated highly in both the 60-day model and the 21-day model. In the 21-day model, we never saw the leptin values plummet. It was only after day 20 or 30 that we see the levels plummet, and then I think there is a dissociation between body fat mass and leptin levels. I believe that is a stress phenomenon, not an energy-deficiency phenomenon.

REFERENCES

1. Lesourd BM. Nutrition and immunity in the elderly: modification of immune responses with nutritional treatment. *Am J Clin Nutr* 1997; 66: 478–84S.
2. Lord GM, Matares G, Howard JK, et al. Leptin modulates the T-cell immune response and reverses starvation-induced immunosuppression. *Nature* 1998; 394: 897–901.
3. Marinella MA. Exertional rhabdomyolysis after recent coxsackie B virus infection. *South Med J* 1998; 91: 1057–9.
4. Beck MA. Increased virulence of coxsackie virus B3 in mice due to vitamin E or selenium deficiency. *J Nutr* 1997; 127: 966–70S.
5. Beck MA, Esworthy RS, Ho Y-S, et al. Glutathione peroxidase protects mice from viral-induced myocarditis. *FASEB J* 1998; 12: 1143–49.

Nutrition, Immunity, and Infection in Infants and Children, edited by Robert M. Suskind and Kraisid Tontisirin. Nestlé Nutrition Workshop Series, Pediatric Program, Vol. 45. Nestec Ltd., Vevey/Lippincott Williams & Wilkins, Philadelphia ©2001.

Iron-Zinc, Immune Responses, and Infection

Ranjit Kumar Chandra

Memorial University of Newfoundland, WHO Centre for Nutritional Immunology, St. John's, Newfoundland, Canada, and Johns Hopkins University School of Hygiene, Baltimore, Maryland, USA

Micronutrients, the immune system and resistance to infection form a veritable trinity. Each one influences the others. Although the influence of diet on risk of infectious disease has been known for centuries, it is only in the last 25 years that the importance of impaired immune responses as an intermediate risk factor has been documented (1,2). It is now established that malnutrition in its broadest definition alters the immune system; the most affected responses include cell-mediated immunity, phagocytes, complement system, mucosal immunity, and the amount and quality of selected antibody responses. The effects of iron and zinc on immunity have been studied extensively.

It is important to recognize the complexity and interdependence of immune responses and the sensitive and functional effects of nutritional intake and status on immunity and susceptibility to infection. This has been reviewed extensively (3–10) and is alluded to in other chapters in this book.

HOST DEFENSES

Host defense mechanisms have been described in depth elsewhere (11,12). For the nonspecialist reader, it may be appropriate to present a simple view of immunity as a protective umbrella (Fig. 1) and as a bridge of life (2) (Fig. 2). The immune responses can be broadly divided into two main tiers: nonspecific and antigen-specific. The nonspecific defenses include the skin and mucous membranes, phagocytic cells, mucus, cilia, complement, lysozyme, interferon, and other humoral factors. These innate processes are naturally present and are not influenced by previous contact with an infectious agent. They act as the first line of protection and retard the establishment of overt infection. Antigen-specific mechanisms include the B-cell system of antibody

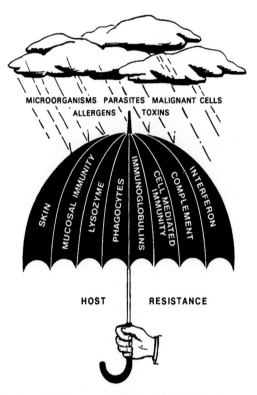

FIG. 1. A simple view of host defenses as a protective umbrella, consisting of physical barriers (skin and mucous membranes), nonspecific mechanisms (complement, interferon, lysozyme, and phagocytes), and antigen-specific processes (antibodies of five immunoglobulin isotypes and cell-mediated immunity). From Chandra RK and ARTS Biomedical Publishers (2); with permission.

production and the T-cell system of cell-mediated immunity. These mechanisms are adaptive and acquired in that they are specific reactions induced by previous exposure to a microorganism or its antigenic determinants. They are effective in checking the spread of infection and eradicating the invading organism. The specific immune responses form the basis of prophylactic immunization against common communicable diseases such as measles, respiratory illness caused by *Haemophilus influenzae*, and systemic disease caused by *Salmonella* organisms. In the body, nonspecific and antigen-specific defenses act in concert.

MICRONUTRIENTS AND IMMUNITY

A few general concepts of the interactions of trace elements, immune responses, and infections disease should be highlighted (13). First, alterations in immune responses occur early in the course of a reduction in micronutrient intake (Fig. 3). Second, the extent of immunologic impairment depends on the type of nutrient involved, its interactions with other essential nutrients, the severity of deficiency, the presence of

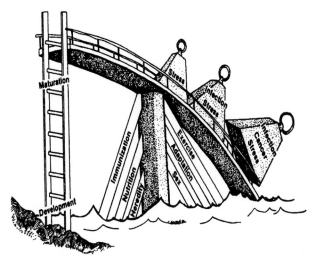

FIG. 2. The immune system is a bridge of life. During fetal and early postnatal life, it undergoes development and maturation. Heredity, sex, adaptation, exercise, immunization, and nutrition are important determinants. Stress, infection, and diseases such as cancer can further impair immunity and end in a fatal outcome. From Chandra RK and ARTS Biomedical Publishers (2); with permission.

concomitant infection, and the age of the subject. Third, immunologic abnormalities predict outcome, particularly the risk of infection and mortality. Fourth, for many micronutrients, excessive intake is associated with impaired immune response. Finally, tests of immunocompetence are useful in titration of physiologic needs and in assessment of safe lower and upper limits of micronutrient intake.

In this chapter, I will present a selective review of the impact of iron status and zinc status on immune responses and susceptibility to infection. The roles played by other

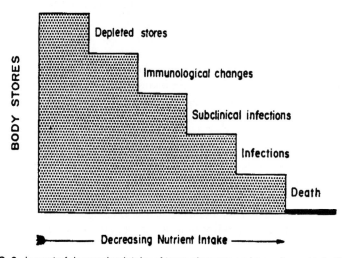

FIG. 3. Impact of decreasing intake of trace elements on immunity and infection.

trace elements (*e.g.*, selenium), vitamins, and fatty acids are discussed in other chapters.

IRON

Iron has been dubbed a *two-edged sword*. On the one hand, the element is required for the *in vitro* growth of most bacteria and fungi, with the exception of lactobacillus. If antibody is added to an iron chelating compound such as lactoferrin, the growth of bacteria such as *Escherichia coli* in the test tube is severely restricted (14). The effect of *excess* iron—that is in amounts that exceed those in normal culture media—has not been well characterized. The extrapolation of these *in vitro* conditions to the *in vivo* situation, particularly in humans, is moot.

Kochan (15) coined the term *iron nutritional immunity* to denote hypoferremia as a common feature of infectious disease and the inhibition of bacterial growth when culture medium is depleted of iron. But clinical data do not support any significant role of iron excess or deficiency as a determinant of the recurrence or severity of infectious disease in humans (16–18).

In this context, it should be emphasized that a similar reduction in serum zinc levels has been noted in infections. Does this imply that reduced zinc availability is a potent host defense? No one seems to suggest that, nor does any objective evidence point to it.

No controversy exists about the deleterious effects of iron deficiency on immune responses; almost all published studies indicate that individuals with iron deficiency show impairment of cell-mediated immunity (delayed cutaneous hypersensitivity responses, T-lymphocyte proliferation response to mitogens and antigens), phagocyte microbicidal function, and mucosal immunity. These findings have been documented in studies reported from many centers. These alterations may well be linked to changes in the activity of scores of iron-dependent enzymes such as myeloperoxidase and ribonucleotide reductase. In addition, physical changes in the mucosal epithelia may also be important. Recently, iron deficiency has been shown to reduce natural killer cell activity and the production of cytokines such as interleukin-2 and interferon-γ (14). A recent study indicates that the presence of iron helped monocytes to suppress the growth of *Mycobacterium tuberculosis* (19). Iron-mediated growth suppression was correlated with selective suppression of tumor necrosis factor-α (TNF-α) release from infected monocytes and iron decreased monocyte sensitivity to exogenously added TNF.

What is apparently controversial is the relation between iron status and risk of infection. This has been reviewed in several publications that purport to present a balanced view of the topic (16–18). The consensus may be stated simply: in humans, iron deficiency is associated with an increased risk of infections and its prevention or treatment may be expected to lower the incidence of common infections. In these circumstances, oral iron administration in conventional doses is safe and effective. In a few selected instances, it is prudent to delay or withhold iron therapy, particularly systemic parenteral therapy; these include very low birthweight infants, young children with severe protein-energy malnutrition and reduced serum transferrin levels, patients with existing bacterial infection, and so on.

Chronic iron overload states such as hemochromatosis with high, almost complete, saturation of transferrin do not result in increased incidence and severity of infection; death is more often caused by cardiac and hepatic failure, hepatoma, and diabetes (20). Nearly 10% of patients do die of infection but then the role of underlying liver disease and diabetes cannot be discounted. In thalassemia, the effective control of iron load may result in serious infection, not when the iron load is at its peak.

Many of the clinical epidemiologic studies on this topic are handicapped by poor study design, inadequate analysis, and biased interpretation of results.

ZINC

The essentiality of zinc for mammals is well documented (17,21,22). In humans, the most dramatic example is the syndrome of acrodermatitis enteropathica in which infants are unable to absorb an adequate quantity of zinc, resulting in a low serum zinc level and the clinical manifestations of zinc deficiency with hair changes, poor growth, diarrhea, rash, and life-threatening infections. Low levels of serum zinc are linked to impaired cell-mediated immunity (23). Before we could diagnose and treat these patients with zinc supplements, they would die in infancy. Today, with appropriate treatment, they can lead an almost normal life. The relation of chronic low zinc intake and poor absorption with growth failure, rash, diarrhea, hypogonadism, and infection was observed in the Middle East. In hospital, in patients on total parenteral nutrition in the 1970s, we also observed many patients with acquired zinc deficiency.

Zinc-dependent enzymes number in the hundreds (21). Many of these are critical for cellular metabolic pathways, including those that mediate the functions of phagocytes and lymphocytes. Zinc regulates the function of superantigens (24). It is not surprising, then, that zinc deficiency results in profound immunodeficiency (25). The salient changes observed are in (*a*) phagocytes—nicotinamide adenine dinucleotide phosphate reduced ingestion of microorganisms, impaired chemotactic migration, decreased activity of reduced oxidase, which is a cofactor for phospholipases A2 and C, instability of cell membranes possibly owing to oxidation of arachidonic acid by iron complexes; (*b*) cell-mediated immunity—reduced lymphocyte proliferation response, decreased CD4:CD8 cell ratio and helper function, impaired natural killer cell function, reduced thymulin activity (Fig. 4); and (*c*) decreased antibody production after challenge with T-cell dependent antigens and alloantigens. The role of zinc in various metabolic and cellular functions is summarized in Figure 5. It should be made clear, however, that further studies are needed to confirm these initial data. A case in point is the importance of zinc in apoptosis.

Several field studies have confirmed the important role of zinc in immunity and risk of infection. For example, young children in underprivileged communities given a zinc supplement (10 mg) daily showed reduced susceptibility to both diarrhea and respiratory infection (26) (Chandra RK, unpublished data, 2000). Boys and the very

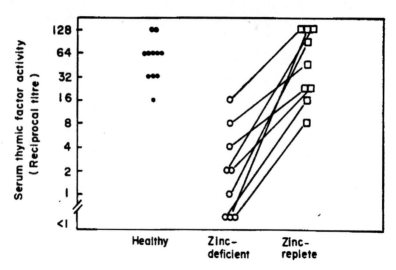

FIG. 4. Serum thymic factor activity in zinc deficiency and effect of zinc treatment.

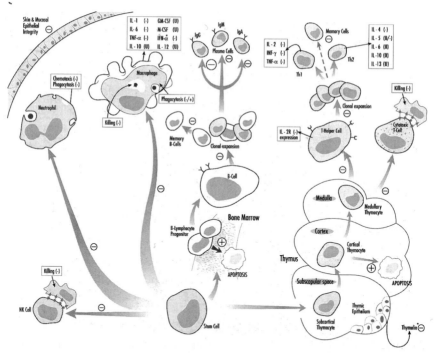

FIG. 5. The effects of zinc on the development and function of certain immunologic cells and cytokines. GM-CSF, granulocyte-macrophage colony-stimulating factor; IG, immunoglobulin; IFN, interferon; IL, interleukin; IL-2R, interleukin-2 receptor; M-CSF, monocyte colony-stimulating factor; NK, natural killer, 0, zinc deficiency has little or no effect on the process or activity; TNF, tumor necrosis factor; U, the effect of zinc deficiency on the particular process or activity is unknown; −, zinc deficiency downregulates or inhibits the process or activity, +, zinc deficiency enhances the process or activity; *, zinc is needed for the structural integrity of the molecule. From the authors Shankar AH and Prasad AS, and the American Society for Clinical Nutrition (21); with permission.

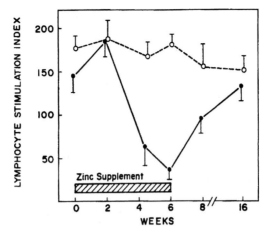

FIG. 6. Lymphocyte stimulation response in healthy adult men given 300 mg zinc supplement daily for 6 weeks (•) compared with results in nonsupplemented controls (○). From the Chandra RK, and the American Medical Association (28); with permission.

young, and those whose initial serum zinc level was low, benefited the most. Whether this benefit is the direct result of zinc or an indirect effect through better availability of other nutrients such as vitamin A needs further study.

In the elderly, zinc is an integral component of the highly effective micronutrient supplement that results in enhanced immunity and reduced incidence of infection (27).

Low birthweight infants show impaired immune responses and an increased incidence of infection. In both preterm and small-for-gestational age infants, zinc supplements (1 mg/kg body weight) enhance immune responses and reduce infection rates (Chandra RK, unpublished data, 2000; in preparation). This topic is reviewed extensively in another part of this book.

Whereas the essentiality of zinc for immunity has been established, it is also true that excessive intake of the element can decrease selected aspects of the immune repertoire (28) (Fig. 6); it may well be that this could enhance risk of infection and other disorders.

In addition, the important interactions between zinc and other trace elements and heavy metals is recognized. For example, zinc supplements abrogate the deleterious immunologic effects of cadmium (29–32).

CONCLUSIONS

Both iron and zinc are essential for the integrity and function of the immune system. For these trace elements, as for nutrition in general, the sane advice is "balance, variety, and moderation."

REFERENCES

1. Chandra RK. Nutrition, immunity and infection: from basic knowledge of dietary manipulation of immune responses to practical application of amelioration of suffering and improving survival. *Proc Natl Acad Sci USA* 1996; 93: 14304–7.
2. Chandra RK. *Nutrition and immunology*. St. John's: ARTS Biomedical Publishers,1992: 7–68.
3. Chandra RK, Newberne PM. *Nutrition, immunity and infection. Mechanisms of interactions*. New York: Plenum, 1977.
4. Suskind R, ed. *Malnutrition and the immune response*. New York: Raven Press, 1977.
5. Keusch GT, Wilson CS, Waksal SD. Nutrition, host defenses, and the lymphoid system. *Archives of Host Defense Mechanisms* 1983; 2: 275–359.
6. Gershwin ME, Beach RS, Hurley LS. *Nutrition and immunity*. New York: Academic Press, 1984.
7. Watson RR, ed. *Nutrition, disease resistance, and immune function*. New York: Marcel Dekker, 1984.
8. Beisel WR. Single nutrients and immunity. *Am J Clin Nutr* 1982; 35: 417–68.
9. Chandra RK. Nutrition and the immune system. *Am J Clin Nutr* 1997; 66: 460–3S.
10. Scrimshaw NS, SanGiovanni JP. Synergism of nutrition, infection, and immunity: an overview. *Am J Clin Nutr* 1997; 66: 464–77S.
11. Chandra RK, ed. *Primary and secondary immunodeficiency disorders*. Edinburgh: Churchill Livingstone, 1983.
12. Roitt IM, Brostoff J. *Immunology*. London: Gower, 1991.
13. Chandra RK. Micronutrients and immune functions. *Ann NY Acad Sci* 1990; 587: 9–16.
14. Chandra RK. 1990 McCollum Award Lecture. Nutrition and immunity: lessons from the past and new insights into the future. *Am J Clin Nutr* 1991; 53: 1087–101.
15. Kochan I. The role of iron in bacterial infections with special consideration of host-tubercle bacillus interaction. *Curr Top Microbiol Immunol* 1973; 60: 1–30.
16. Hershko C, Peto TEA, Weatherall DI. Iron and infection. *BMJ* 1998; 296: 660–4.
17. Puri S, Chandra RK. Trace elements and immune responses. In: Chandra RK, ed. *Trace elements in the nutrition of children*. New York: Raven Press, 1988: 161–7.
18. Walter T, Olivares M, Pizarro F, Muñoz C. Iron, anemia and infection. *Nutr Rev* 1997; 55: 111–24.
19. Byrd TF. Tumor necrosis factor promotes growth of virulent *Mycobacterium tuberculosis* in human monocytes. *J Clin Invest* 1997; 99: 2518–29.
20. Finch SC, Finch CA. Idiopathic hemachromatosis. *Medicine* 1955; 34: 381–430.
21. Shankar AH, Prasad AS. Zinc and immune function: the biological basis of altered resistance to infection. *Am J Clin Nutr* 1998: 68: 447–63S.
22. Bendich A, Chandra RK, eds. *Micronutrients and immune functions*. New York: New York Academy of Sciences, 1990.
23. Chandra RK. Acrodermatitis enteropathica. *Pediatrics* 1980; 66: 789–91.
24. Fraser JD, Urban RG, Strominger JL, Robinson H. Zinc regulates the function of two superantigens. *Proc Natl Acad Sci USA* 1992; 89: 5507–11.
25. Thurnham DI. Micronutrients and immune function: some recent developments. *J Clin Pathol* 1997; 50: 887–91.
26. Sazawal S, Black RE, Bhan MK, et al. Zinc supplementation reduces the incidence of persistent diarrhea and dysentery among low socioeconomic children in India. *J Nutr* 1996; 126: 443–50.
27. Chandra RK. Effect of vitamin and trace-element supplementation on immune responses and infection in elderly people. *Lancet* 1992; 340: 1124–7.
28. Chandra RK. Excessive intake of zinc impairs immune responses. *JAMA* 1984; 252: 1443–6.
29. Chowdhury BA, Fried JK, Chandra RK. Cadmium-induced immunopathology is prevented by zinc administration in mice. *J Nutr* 1987; 117: 1788–94.
30. Hamed A, Chandra RK. Effect of zinc deficiency on cadmium-induced immunopathology. *Immunol Infect Dis* 1992; 2: 35–43.
31. Denduluri S, Chandra RK. Effects of cadmium and zinc and other interactions on immune responses. *Immunol Infect Dis* 1996; 6: 113–19.
32. Denduluri S, Langdon M, Chandra RK. Effect of zinc administration on immune responses in mice. *J Trace Elem Exp Med* 1997; 10: 155–62.

DISCUSSION

Dr. Zoppi: I have a question about iron deficiency and impairment of the immune response. We know that two physiologic conditions exist in the first year of life where the infant has an iron-deficient anemia: physiologic anemia and anemia from cow's milk feeding. Do you think these two conditions can impair the immune response in children in developed countries?

Dr. Chandra: Little information is found on immune responses in the first 3 months of life, when the so-called *physiologic anemia* appears (1). Studies in preterm infants have shown that where there was a more exaggerated reduction in iron level with or without anemia at around 6 or 9 months of age, there was a reduction in immune response (2). Data on the prevalence or incidence of infection are difficult to interpret because of several confounding variables. Nevertheless, there is some suggestion that common infections may be increased in these infants.

Dr. Haschke: In the very low birthweight infant, the view of the US Food and Drug Administration seems to be that uncritical iron supplementation could be dangerous. Those infants with birthweights between 500 g and 1,500 g receive repeated blood transfusions, so they get a lot of iron from that source, and uncritical supplementation with iron-fortified formula is perhaps not the best way to get the iron into the body. One should leave it to the doctor who is treating the baby to decide when and how much iron should be given, in particular in situations where erythropoietin is used as treatment. Would you agree on that?

Dr. Chandra: Yes. With repeated blood transfusions that many very low birthweight babies receive during the first few weeks of life, no need is really seen for additional iron supplementation. Also, iron utilization in the first 3 or 4 months in these babies is very low. The question really is whether an iron-fortified formula should be given from birth so the mother does not have to change formulas around 4 and 6 months, when iron is really needed. It is like giving fluoride supplements in the first 6 months of life, even though they are not needed at that time—you want to condition the mother to start giving them on a regular basis. However, if the mother is intelligent and cooperative and the physician has a good relationship with her, then an iron-fortified formula can and should be started some time after 4 months.

Dr. Marini: Twenty years ago we did a study where we gave 12 mg/d of iron, about 2–3 mg/kg, to one group of low birthweight infants, and another group was given 1 mg/kg. When we looked at these babies at 6 months and 9 months, the babies receiving the higher amount of iron had higher ferritin concentrations and better cardiovascular function, independent of hemoglobin levels (3). This is another example of a nonhematologic effect of iron administration. I remember Oski's study showing that babies with low iron had some impairment of secretion of catecholamines (4). In relation to the risk of infection when giving iron to preterm babies, I think that most intensive care units now give iron because it is necessary to increase the iron intake when giving erythropoietin. Sometimes, in order to achieve an effect and to avoid the need for blood transfusion, we give up to 6 to 8 mg/kg/d of iron to these babies, for about a month. No evidence is seen at all of an increased risk of infection in these babies. So, I think iron is extremely important for preterm babies. The problem of iron toxicity is mainly related to the first week of life, when there may be an increase in free iron in very small preterm babies. This may result in superoxide or free radical damage.

I have a practical question about the clinical value of measuring blood levels of zinc in these babies. When you did your study on zinc supplementation, did you find that zincemia changed in parallel with thymic function, to show that we really need to give zinc to these babies? And is there a relation between zinc and iron, as with calcium and phosphate? Is there an interaction between the two?

Dr. Chandra: I agree with your comments on the nonhematologic effects of iron. So far as your questions are concerned, variations in serum zinc concentration reflect body zinc under conditions of very significant zinc deficiency. The blood pool of zinc is only a very small fraction of total body zinc. Thus, when giving zinc supplements to a zinc-deficient individual, you cannot expect serum zinc to change very dramatically in the short term, even though zinc-dependent functions may change. This is another example where functional changes in enzyme activity and immune responses are more important than measuring levels of serum zinc, which is a notoriously poor indicator of marginal zinc deficiency. So far as the ratio of zinc and iron is concerned, 1:5 or 1:7 would be an optimal ratio that is safe for oral intake.

Dr. Haschke: What about older infants and toddlers, who tend to have a lot of infections and in whom the hemoglobin is on the low side and iron deficiency quite common? In industrialized countries, it has been shown that iron-fortified formulas are safe for infants. Would you say that the same can be said for developing countries? I am not talking about Chile, because in this respect Chile is no longer a developing country, and it has a very low infection rate.

Dr. Chandra: I know of no evidence that iron-fortified formulas would do any harm. Although Chile is different now from many other developing countries, at the time those studies were done, in the urban slums of Santiago (5), the conditions were not very different in terms of sanitation and recovery of fecal pathogenic microorganisms from those in many other developing countries. The consensus of evidence suggests that iron-fortified formulas would do no harm and perhaps could be of benefit to infants, even to toddlers. Of course, other considerations, apart from immunity and infection, are seen. There are the questions of physical activity, temperature regulation, developmental achievement, and many other aspects of body functions impaired by iron deficiency that could be improved by giving an iron-fortified cereal or formula or both. There is also growing concern that the type of iron used in formulas is important. Some types of iron supplement may be more likely to cause oxidative damage than others. Polymaltose, for example, has been shown *in vitro* to be safer than ferrous sulfate or ferrous gluconate. This is a question that has not been looked at adequately so far.

Dr. Coovadia: I have a comment and a question. The comment is in relation to an additional hazard of iron deficiency. This has to do with the rate of vertical transmission of HIV in developing countries. Many risk factors are seen for vertical transmission, but when we looked carefully at our population–they are all Africans and not in the late stages of HIV–we found that one of the more powerful risk factors was anemia in the mother. This raises the prospect of reversal by giving supplements.

My question is related to respiratory infections and micronutrients. On reviewing the literature, I was struck by the variety of definitions of respiratory infection. Some people include the common cold, others talk about *upper respiratory infections*. In the low birthweight baby, what sort of infections are these respiratory infections and how are they diagnosed?

Dr. Chandra: Mostly, these were upper respiratory infections, diagnosed by symptoms such as runny nose, cough lasting 48 or more hours, feeding problems, and pyrexia. In many infants, we had results of ancillary investigations (*e.g.*, total and differential white cell counts, chest radiograph, and C-reactive protein) to support the presence of bacterial infection.

In relation to your comment, I should mention that the type of micronutrient deficiency that is linked to higher or lower transmission rate of HIV from mother to infant seems to vary in different studies. This is a puzzle that I have not been able to solve satisfactorily. In some studies, high vitamin B_{12} levels seem to correlate best with vertical transmission. In others, it is low B_6 level. The same applies to adult patients with HIV in whom nutrient intakes and blood levels correlate with disease progression or CD4 counts. Once again, deficiency of a variety of nutrients has been found to be linked with disease progression. Which of these is the most critical remains to be determined. Perhaps most of these may have some effect, depending on the setting.

Dr. Woodward: With reference to the comments you made about the bactericidal activity of neutrophils in iron deficiency, is there evidence of an influence in the absence of overt infection?

Dr. Chandra: Yes, there is. Even without obvious infection, phagocyte bactericidal capacity is compromised in iron deficiency, which correlates metabolic activity and levels of several of the iron-dependent enzymes (2). Infection causes further impairment of bacterial killing capacity.

Dr. Wasantwisut: I would be interested to hear your comments about malaria infection. Lavender has shown decreased parasite infestation in his selenium-deficient, vitamin E-deficient mice. *Plasmodium burkii* was used as the malaria model. This is in contrast to coxsackie virus, which shows increased virulence in this deficient model. It has also been shown that when malnourished refugees enter camps they have an increase in malaria incidence after they have been fed good food and rehabilitated for some time.

Dr. Chandra: You are right that in those studies by Levander et al., the effects were opposite to what his group later showed for coxsackie virus. The reasons are not clear. I do not think he had an explanation either. The discrepancy might reflect the species of malaria: one species may not be affected by iron status, whereas another might be. Also, in the clinical situation, one must distinguish between the prevalence of parasitemia and the occurrence of symptoms; the two may not go in the same direction. Evidence seems to indicate that symptoms can be exacerbated, whereas parasitemia may not change.

Dr. Keusch: Malaria occupies a very special niche in the host with respect to iron, because it lives in the red cell. In fact, it lives on hemoglobin. It eats the globin portion, uses the amino acids, and spits out the iron. So, there is clearly going to be a very special relationship between malaria and states of iron deficiency or sufficiency. In the context of Dr. Chandra's comment about the species of malaria perhaps being important, it is relevant that iron given to an iron-deficient subject enhances erythropoiesis, and *P. vivax* preferentially lives in young erythrocytes. So, it would be surprising if there was not an increase in the numbers of red cells parasitized and the total number of parasites present in the blood. What is striking is that in very well conducted studies in Papua New Guinea, no effect was seen of iron supplementation in iron-deficient subjects on clinical malaria, as Dr. Chandra pointed out. The only way to interpret that finding, in the face of enhanced parasitemia, is that the iron is also supplementing the immune response and allowing the host to control the enhanced growth of malaria. So it is a very special situation, and the clinical evidence is certainly that iron supplementation in that circumstance does no harm. I think we are ready to close the book on the iron nutrition or immunity hypothesis with respect to dealing with iron deficiency at a population level, and one thing we can do in this conference is to make a very strong statement in that regard.

Secondly, in the context of iron therapy in more acute situations, in protein-energy malnutrition, for example, I do think one has to be careful of loading iron into subjects who are not synthesizing iron transport proteins; under those circumstances, increases in free iron are likely to enhance microbial growth. It is a very special circumstance, but the recommendations are not to use iron in the initial repletion and to wait a week or two. At the point at which transferrin is increasing, it is completely safe to give iron. So, I think it is time to close the chapter on that book.

Dr. Chandra: I wholeheartedly agree. I should also say that once a child with protein-energy malnutrition is put on an appropriate diet, it does not take long—just the matter of a week or 10 days—before transferrin levels begin to rise, so the period during which iron therapy should be withheld is very short [1].

Dr. Coovadia: I was intrigued by your caution over where we should not use iron: severe protein-energy malnutrition, low birthweight babies, and latent infections. How do I translate the last one into practice, and what does it mean?

Dr. Chandra: By that, I mean patients who are, for example, in intensive care units, particularly those with multiple trauma. Some of these may be harboring infections. Even if it is useful to give other forms of nutritional supplementation, including most of the micronutrients, iron should not be given in the first week or 10 days.

Dr. Suskind: Just one comment with regard to the use of iron in protein-energy malnutrition. In several studies that we did in Thailand in the 1970s, we did in fact use iron from the time of admission in children who were severely malnourished, provided that they were on antibiotic coverage for infection. We found that we did not have any problems with aggressively treating the malnourished child with both antibiotics and iron simultaneously. Initially, we used Imferon but then switched to an oral preparation.

Dr. Chandra: There could be a greater concern about the use of iron-dextran, perhaps because of the effect of dextran rather than the iron. Large amounts of dextran may compromise reticuloendothelial function temporarily.

Dr. Klish: One of the issues that is smoldering around iron supplementation in the United States has to do with supplementation of the breast-fed infant, the argument being that iron supplementation saturates lactoferrin, which alters the intestinal milieu, which alters the bacterial mix in the intestinal tract. I am not sure there are any data to support that contention, but do you have any comments about it?

Dr. Chandra: In fact, data are found to the contrary, that iron supplements do not alter microflora (6). So far as the timing of giving iron to breast-fed babies is concerned, supplements are indicated if formula intake is more than 30% of total energy intake. So long as energy intake from formula is less than 30% of the total, supplementary iron is not needed in breast-fed infants up to 6 months of age.

Dr. Valyasevi: In Thailand, there is a high incidence of iron deficiency anemia and at the same time we have a high prevalence of thalassemia. My question is, what are the hazards of iron overload if iron is given as a public health measure in such a population?

Dr. Chandra: Thalassemia is a very special situation where even more caution with respect of iron supplements needs to be exercised, especially for thalassemia major. I do not think it would be a problem with thalassemia minor, where the iron load is minimal at best. I do not know about the prevalence of thalassemia major in Thailand. In certain parts of India, it is of the order of three per 1,000. So you are looking at a very small population and by the time the infants are even 1 year of age, the clinical diagnosis is obvious. A clinician who makes this diagnosis should be cautious about iron intake in such a child, I do not think it should affect national pediatric policy of giving prophylactic iron to prevent iron deficiency. The amount of iron overload is minimal and it takes 10 to 15 years before it becomes significant. Moreover, in the patients of thalassemia who die in the second decade of life or later, the cause of death is liver failure, heart failure, and diabetes, rather than infection.

REFERENCES

1. Vyas D, Chandra RK. Functional implications of iron deficiency. In: Stekel A, ed. *Iron nutrition in infancy and childhood.* New York: Raven Press, 1984: 45–59.
2. Chandra RK. Reduced bactericidal capacity of polymorphs in iron deficiency. *Arch Dis Child* 1973; 48: 864.
3. Clerici Bagozzi D, Gargantini GL, Salice P, et al. Iron haemotological and haemodynamic data in preterm infants up to 6 months of age. *Italian Journal of Pediatrics* 1982; 8: 593(A).
4. Oski FA, Honig A. The effects of therapy on the developmental scores of iron-deficient infants. *J Pediatr* 1978; 92: 21–5.
5. Brunser O, Espinoza J, Araya M, et al. Effect of dietary nucleotide supplementation on diarrhoeal disease in infants. *Acta Paediatr* 1994; 83: 188–91.
6. Chandra RK. Effect of iron supplements on gut microflora of infants. *Nutr Res* 2001 (*in press*).

Nutrition, Immunity, and Infection in Infants and Children, edited by Robert M. Suskind and Kraisid Tontisirin. Nestlé Nutrition Workshop Series, Pediatric Program, Vol. 45. Nestec Ltd., Vevey/Lippincott Williams & Wilkins, Philadelphia ©2001.

The Effect of Vitamin Deficiencies (E and A) and Supplementation on Infection and Immune Response

Simin Nikbin Meydani, *Wafaie W. Fawzi, and Sung Nim Han

*Nutritional Immunology Laboratory, Jean Mayer USDA Human Nutrition Research Center on Aging at Tufts University; and *Department of Nutrition and Epidemiology, Harvard School of Public Health; Boston, Massachusetts, USA*

Nutritional deficiencies contribute to the high incidence of morbidity and mortality from infectious diseases among children in developing countries. Infectious diseases (respiratory and diarrheal) are among the leading causes of death in children around the world. Deficiencies of vitamins E and A have been shown, in animal models and in humans, to impair the immune response and to decrease host resistance to infectious diseases. Furthermore, supplementation with higher than recommended levels of these nutrients in some, but not all cases, was associated with improved immune response and resistance to certain bacterial and viral infections. Several comprehensive reviews have been written on the role of vitamins E and A in the regulation of the immune response. This chapter, therefore, is not intended to be comprehensive; rather, it is a brief summary of past work, with emphasis on recent findings.

VITAMIN A AND IMMUNE RESPONSE

The existence of a relation between vitamin A deficiency and infectious diseases has been known since early in the 20th Century. These earlier studies gained vitamin A the reputation of an *antiinfection* vitamin. As immune function is an important determinant of host resistance to infection, a regulatory role for vitamin A in maintaining the immune response was suggested. Animal and human studies confirmed this speculation, although it is clear that nonimmune-related functions of vitamin A (*e.g.*, maintaining the integrity and differentiation of mucosal epithelial cells and keratinocytes) also contribute to the overall vitamin A-induced resistance to infectious diseases.

Vitamin A Deficiency and the Immune Response

Atrophy of lymphoid organs, including spleen, thymus, and lymph nodes, has been reported in animals deficient in vitamin A (1) (Table 1). However, some of these effects may be caused by loss of appetite and decreased food intake. In addition, changes in spleen cell number are observed in the early stages of vitamin A deficiency and might be a more sensitive indicator of vitamin A deficiency (2). Controversy, however, exists over the effect of vitamin A deficiency on subpopulations of T and B lymphocytes. Some investigators have reported effects of vitamin A deficiency on distribution of T and B lymphocytes and their subpopulations in animal models (1,2), whereas others have reported a selective loss of $CD4^+$ T cells from lymph nodes (3). These latter investigators further demonstrated decreases in the Th2 frequency, resulting in an imbalance in the Th1:Th2 ratio in vitamin A-deficient mice. This was associated with decreased interleukin (IL)-4 and IL-5, and increase in γ-interferon production (4). Further work showed that retinoic acid, through these cytokine changes, has a regulatory role in regulation of B cells and immunoglobulin isotype switching (4,5).

Abnormal T-cell subpopulations were also reported by Semba *et al.* in children with vitamin A deficiency (6). In that study, children with xerophthalmia had a lower $CD4^+$:$CD8^+$ ratio and lower proportions of $CD4^+$ naive T cells and a higher proportion of $CD8^+$ memory cells. Supplementation with vitamin A (60 mg retinol equivalent, RE) for 5 weeks significantly increased the percentage of $CD4^+$ naive cells and the $CD4^+$:$CD8^+$ ratio, and reduced the percentage of $CD8^+$ memory cells compared with the placebo treatment.

Vitamin A deficiency can also affect the function of different cells of the immune system (Table 1). Neutrophils, through their phagocytic function and production of

TABLE 1. *Vitamin A deficiency and immune response*

Variable	Impact of vitamin A or its metabolite
Thymus, spleen, lymph node	Atrophy
Spleen cell number	⇓
T and B cells	⇓ or ⇔
T-cell subpopulation	⇓ or ⇔ in CD4+ T cells
	⇑ CD8+, ⇓ CD4+/CD8+
	Imbalance in Th1/Th2
Cytokines	⇓ IL-4, IL-5, IL-2
	⇓ or ⇑ γ interferon
Natural killer cells	⇓ Cytotoxicity
Neutrophils	⇓ Chemotaxis, adhesion, phagocytosis
	⇓ Oxygen-free radical production
T-cell function	⇓ or ⇑ proliferation
	⇓ or ⇔ DTH
	⇓ or ⇔ T-cell–dependent antibody production
B-cell function	⇓ Antibody production
	⇓ Growth

DTH, delayed type hypersensitivity.

cytotoxic metabolites, are important in providing the first line of defense against infection. Twining *et al.* (7) reported defects in chemotaxis, adhesion, phagocytosis, and the ability to generate reactive oxygen metabolites in neutrophils from vitamin A-deficient rats. Impairment of T- and B-cell function has been reported (2,8). Human leukocytes contain retinol and retinoic acid, as well as other metabolites (9). Retinol has been shown to be necessary as a cofactor in T-cell activation (10,11). Further, retinol through its metabolite, retinol,14-hydroxy-4,14-retroretinol, is reported to be required for B-cell growth (12).

Delayed type hypersensitivity (DTH) skin response, a measure of T-cell–mediated function, was shown to be impaired (2,13) or increased (14) in vitamin A-deficient rats. The difference might be a result of the method of evaluating the DTH. Results from studies evaluating the DTH response in humans have also been inconclusive, as protein-energy malnutrition often coexists with vitamin A deficiency. Furthermore, as can be seen below, vitamin A repletion has not always been successful in restoring DTH in vitamin A-deficient subjects.

Another measure of T-cell function, mitogenic proliferation, has been shown to be reduced when T cells are derived from the spleen, but not from other anatomic locations (1). In general, it appears that when other nutrient deficiencies are controlled, T cells from vitamin A-deficient animals do not show a marked defect in proliferation. In fact, an increase in T-cell proliferation in response to concanavalin A (14) and *Staphylococcus aureus* (15) has been reported. This hyperactivity existed despite lower macrophage phagocytosis and complement activation and a higher incidence of arthritis induced by *S. aureus*. These observations have led Wiedermann *et al.* to propose a proinflammatory role for vitamin A deficiency (15).

Several studies have shown that vitamin A deficiency impairs B-cell function, as indicated by reduced production of both T-cell dependent and independent antibodies (1,2,8). The effect of vitamin A deficiency on antibody production against different antigens has been studied in both experimental animal models and humans. Several investigators have shown impaired primary antibody response to tetanus toxoid in rats (2). The secondary response to this antigen, however, does not seem to be impaired in vitamin A-deficient rats (16). The deficiency in antigen-specific antibody levels exists despite normal to higher serum immunoglobulin levels. Impairment in the production of other T-cell–dependent antibodies, such as sheep red blood cells, keyhole limpet hemocyanin, bovine serum albumin, and *Salmonella pullorum* (13,17,18) has also been reported in rats, mice, and chickens.

In a study by Smith and Hays (13), the primary IgM response was normal, whereas the greatest reduction occurred in the IgG class, particularly IgG1. These investigators attributed the effect of vitamin A to a change in the balance of Th1/Th2 cells and greater production of γinterferon. Others, however, have reported lower γinterferon production in vitamin A-deficient rats (19). The disagreement between these reports could reflect the differences in cell populations used in the two different studies.

The antibody response to T-cell–independent antigens (*e.g.*, *Streptococcus pneumoniae*, type III, or meningococcal polysaccharides) has also been shown to be depressed in vitamin A-deficient rats (20). These defects were corrected following vitamin A repletion. Information related to vitamin A deficiency and antibody production in humans, independent of other nutritional deficiencies, is not available.

Impaired antibody response to viral and parasitic antigens has also been reported in vitamin A deficiency (2). Studies also indicated impaired intestinal IgA production, which is attributed to impairment of gut-associated immune response (21–24).

Vitamin A Supplementation and the Immune Response

As vitamin A deficiency, both in experimental animals and in humans, is associated with an impaired immune response and increased morbidity and mortality from infectious diseases, several investigators have attempted to improve the immune response and, thus, resistance to infection by vitamin A supplementation in vitamin A-deficient subjects. The outcomes of these studies have varied, depending on the vitamin A status of the host, the type of infectious agent, and the immune response evaluated. In general, improvement in immune function and increased resistance to infection is observed if the host was deficient in vitamin A before supplementation.

Several animal experiments have shown that acute, high dose administration of retinoids improves specific and nonspecific immunity, including macrophage phagocytosis, bacterial clearance, cytotoxicity, and complement activation, natural killer (NK) cell activity, antibody production, and *in vitro* measures of T-cell–mediated function (2). Chronic high dose supplementation, however, was shown to decrease antibody production, lymphocyte proliferation, and resistance to infection (25). In that study, diets containing both deficient levels (0 μg/kg) and excess levels (1,000 μg/kg) of vitamin A resulted in higher mortality of chicks from *Escherichia coli* infection compared with adequate vitamin A levels (0.85 μg/kg). Fumarulo *et al.* (26) showed that incubation of human neutrophils with retinoic acid or retinyl acetate (1–100 μM) inhibited in a dose-dependent manner, oxygen-free radical production, chemiluminescence, and degranulation induced by phorbol myristate acetate, *N*-formyl-methionyl-leucyl-phenylalanine, zymosan, or ionophore A23187 in these cells. These studies might explain the apparently increased risk of respiratory infection reported in children supplemented with vitamin A (see below). A study by Gardner and Ross (16) showed that vitamin A supplementation (137.5 or 150 μg RE) given to vitamin A-sufficient nursling rats at the time of tetanus vaccination had no effect on antibody response.

In West Java, Indonesia, Semba *et al.* (27) randomly assigned clinically normal children 3 to 6 years of age or those with mild xerophthalmia to a placebo group or a vitamin A (60,000 μg RE) group for 2 weeks. The children were then vaccinated with intramuscular diphtheria-pertussis-tetanus vaccine, trivalent oral polio vaccine, and trivalent inactivated intranasal influenza vaccine. Children with weight and height less than 80% of median National Center for Health Statistics values were excluded. Serum vitamin A analysis indicated that even some of the clinically normal children had low serum vitamin A levels ($<$ 0.7 μmol/l). Vitamin A-supplemented children in both groups had a greater antibody response to tetanus vaccine. The effect of the other two vaccines was not reported. Three other studies, however, reported no effect of vitamin A supplementation on antibody response to tetanus vaccine (28–30). The lack of the effect in these studies could reflect the use of a single injection of vitamin A at the time of vaccination (28) or the small sample size used (29,30). Rosales and Kjolhede (31) evaluated the effect of vitamin A on antibody response to measles vaccination and on reversing measles-induced suppression of DTH. In Ndola, Zambia, 200 children with acute measles, ranging in age from 5 months to 17 years, were randomly assigned a single dose of placebo or vitamin A (210 μmol retinol or retinyl palmitate and 92 μmol all-rac-α-tocopherol). Antibody titers were evaluated at baseline and 2 weeks after enrollment. DTH was also determined at 1 and 2 weeks after enrollment using Multi-test CMI (Merieux Institute, Miami, FL). Antibody titer increased in both groups and no significant difference was seen between placebo and treatment groups. No difference in DTH response was seen between the two groups, except for a prolongation of DTH unresponsiveness in the treatment group. The results from this study are difficult to interpret or to compare with other studies, as treatment contained tocopherol in addition to retinol, whereas plasma retinol concentrations also increased in both groups.

Semba *et al.* (32) determined the effect on antibody response of 100,000 IU of vitamin A given simultaneously with live measles vaccine in 336 infants aged 6 months in West Java, Indonesia, using a double-blind, placebo-controlled design. More than 50% of the infants had serum retinol levels less than 0.7 μmol/l. The vaccine was standard titer Schwarz measles. A higher percentage of children (33.7%) in the group treated with vitamin A did not seroconvert compared with the placebo group (20.7%). Furthermore, the vitamin A group had a higher percentage of children who did not reach protective serum antibody levels ($>$ 120%). Those treated with vitamin A also developed fewer rashes after immunization. These results indicate that vitamin A supplementation interferes with the establishment of subclinical infection following vaccination and, therefore, reduces host antibody production. A subsequent study by Benn *et al.* (33) showed no adverse effect of vitamin A supplementation on antibody titer against measles vaccine at 6 and 9 months or 9 years of age. Similarly, in a second study in Indonesia by Semba et al., vitamin A supplementation had no effect on seroconversion to measles on any children immunized at age 9 months (34). Thus, recommendations to give vitamin A at the same time as childhood vaccinations need to be further evaluated.

Rahman *et al.* (35) showed that infants given 15 mg of vitamin A when receiving diphtheria, pertussis, and tetanus (DPT) or oral polio vaccine at monthly intervals had a similar DTH response to those treated with the placebo. However, the response was better in well-nourished than in malnourished children. Kramer *et al.* (36) also reported that supplementation with vitamin A (1,500 mg for 6 months) had a modest effect on improving lymphocyte proliferation in response to tetanus and diphtheria. These children had higher serum vitamin A concentrations than those reported in other studies (0.99 μmol/l).

Vitamin A and Infection

In case-control and prospective studies, xerophthalmia and low serum vitamin A concentrations have been associated with increased risk of child mortality and morbidity (37). These observational studies have had limitations, including small sample size and lack of adjustment for confounding variables such as socioeconomic and nutritional status. Here, we focus our discussion on controlled trials examining the efficacy of vitamin A supplements on mortality and morbidity. First, we present community-based trials that examined the effect of supplementation on total mortality. Next, we review hospital-based and community-based studies examining the effect of supplements on measles. Finally, we look at hospital-based and community-based trials that assessed the effect of supplements on the incidence and severity of acute respiratory and diarrheal infections.

Community-Based Mortality Trials

In community-based studies on children aged more than 6 months, the protective effect of vitamin A varied (Table 2). In two studies from the Sudan (38) and Hyderabad, India (39), vitamin A supplements had no effect on total mortality. In other trials, the supplements resulted in a significant reduction in mortality, but the effect ranged from 19% in Ghana (40) to 54% in Tamil Nadu, India (41). Pooling the results from nine studies, vitamin A supplements reduced total mortality by 30% (42). In a study from Tanzania that was completed after the publication of this meta-analysis, a 50% reduction in mortality was noted among children who received vitamin A, with protective effects observed among both human immunodeficiency virus (HIV)-infected and uninfected children (43).

The variability in effect between trials may be explained by various factors (44). The vitamin A status of the study population is important and the supplements are expected to have greater efficacy in geographical areas in which vitamin A deficiency is prevalent. However, the vitamin A status of the children participating in these trials was not measured; consequently, this variable was not examined. The bioavailability of the supplements can also differ among populations: absorption of the lipid

TABLE 2. *Community-based vitamin A and mortality trials in children (>6 months of age)*

Community	Dose	Result	Reference
Tamil Nadu, India	8,333 IU/wk	54% ⇓	Rahmathullah et al., 1990 (41)
Hyderabad, India	200,000 IU/every 6 mo	No effect	Vijayaraghavan et al., 1990 (39)
Sudan	200,000 IU/every 6 mo	No effect	Herrera et al., 1992 (38)
Ghana	200,000 IU/every 4 mo	19% ⇓	Ghana VAST Study Team, 1993 (40)
Meta-analysis		30% ⇓	Fawzi et al., 1993 (42)
Tanzania	200,000 IU (<yearly) or 400,000 IU (>yearly) × (2 at baseline, 2 at 4, 8 mo)	49% ⇓	Fawzi et al., 1999 (43)

TABLE 3. *Community-based vitamin A trials and mortality in children (<6 months old)*

Community	Dose	Result	Reference
Nepal	50,000 IU (<1 mo) 100,000 IU (1–5 mo)	No effect	West et al., 1995, (46)
Meta-analysis		No effect	Vitamin E/Pneumonia Working Group, 1995 (47)
Indonesia	50,000 IU (at birth)	64% ⇓ infant mortality rate	Humphrey et al., 1996 (45)
Multicenter trial in Peru, Ghana, and India	25,000 IU (at 6,10,14, weeks)	No effect	WHO/CHO Study Group, 1998 (48)

soluble supplements is impaired when dietary fat intake is limited. In areas where nutritional deficits are common, deficiency of nutrients essential for the bioavailability of the vitamin (e.g., protein and zinc) can limit the beneficial effects of the supplements. Smaller and more frequent doses of vitamin A appear to protect against mortality more effectively than large periodic doses (42). Thus, small weekly doses in the Tamil Nadu trial, and vitamin A-fortified monosodium glutamate, resulted in a greater reduction in mortality than in trials in which large doses of vitamin A were given every 4 to 6 months. The prevalence of infections at the time of supplementation and the incidence of infections in the period after supplementation are also important factors. Infection at the time of supplementation reduces the absorption of the supplement; a new infection increases the use of vitamin stores and is associated with increased loss of vitamin A, which results in a diminished protective period of the large dose supplement.

A few studies examined the efficacy of vitamin A supplements among children under the age of 6 months (Table 3). In a study from Indonesia, a single dose of vitamin A given to newborns on the day of birth resulted in a significant reduction in the risk of death in infancy (45). In contrast, no effect was observed in a separate trial done in Nepal (46). A meta-analysis examining the effect of the supplements on morbidity and mortality associated with respiratory infections in this age group showed no effect of the supplements (47). Similar findings were noted from a large multicenter trial that was carried out in Peru, Ghana, and India. No differences in mortality or morbidity were observed between children who received placebo or vitamin A at the time of each of the first three doses of DPT or poliomyelitis immunization at 6, 10, and 14 weeks (48).

Hospital- and Community-Based Trials of Vitamin A and Measles

Measles is responsible for nearly 1.5 million deaths every year. Although prevention of measles through immunization is optimal, difficulties in procurement and distribution of the vaccine render millions of children unprotected against the virus.

The efficacy of vitamin A supplements on measles-associated morbidity and mortality has been examined in several hospital-based trials. In a meta-analysis of four

TABLE 4. *Community- and hospital-based trials of vitamin A and morbidity and mortality assoicated with measles*

Community	Dose	Result	Reference
Meta-analysis of community-based studies	Periodic supplement	39% ⇓ in measles-related deaths	Fawzi et al., 1993 (42)
Meta-analysis of four hospital-based studies	Large dose at admission	60% ⇓ in death risk	Fawzi et al., 1993 (42)
Kenya	50,000 IU (<6 mo) 100,000 IU (6–12 mo) 200,000 IU (>12 mo)	No effect on RI/DI	Ogaro et al., 1993 (49)
Zambia	200,000 IU	⇓ Risk of pneumonia	Rosales et al., 1996 (50)

RI, respiratory infection incidence; DI, diarrhea incidence.

studies carried out among children in South Africa, Tanzania, and the United Kingdom, large doses of vitamin A given on admission resulted in a reduction of about 60% in the risk of death overall, and with about 90% reduction among infants (42) (Table 4). In these trials, administration of vitamin A to children who developed pneumonia before or during hospital stays, reduced mortality by nearly 70% compared with control children. The protective effects of the supplements appeared to be greater among infants than older children.

In a later trial from Kenya, vitamin A supplements had no effect on mortality. However, the study had limited power to examine this question (49). Among those with diarrhea on admission to the hospital, vitamin A supplementation resulted in a significantly faster recovery than did the placebo. A trial was carried out among children from Zambia who had measles but whose infection was not severe enough to warrant hospital admission (50). Among children who did not have measles at baseline, there appeared to be a decreased risk of developing pneumonia, but also a decreased risk of recovery from pneumonia among children who had measles at baseline. The sample size of this study was also too small to allow for precise estimation of the associations of interest.

Periodic vitamin A supplements given to apparently healthy children are associated with protective effects against measles. Results pooled from community-based trials with periodic supplementation of vitamin A showed a 39% reduction in measles-related mortality, as well as a decrease in overall mortality (42).

Hospital-Based Studies of Diarrheal and Respiratory Infections

Given the protective effects of vitamin A noted among measles patients, it was natural to examine whether the supplements were similarly beneficial in other serious childhood infections such as pneumonia and diarrhea. In some of the measles trials, vitamin A resulted in a significant reduction in the occurrence and severity of respiratory and diarrheal complications. However, the application of the findings to non-measles infective episodes was not possible.

Four vitamin A efficacy trials were carried out among patients admitted to the hospital with diarrhea (Table 5). In a placebo-controlled study among children from Bangladesh with noncholera watery diarrhea, no differences were found in the duration of illness or the stool output between the two treatment arms (51). Diarrhea was mainly caused by rotavirus and enterotoxigenic *E. coli*. However, in another study from Bangladesh, protective effects of vitamin A supplements were noted among children admitted to the hospital with acute shigellosis (52). A significantly higher proportion of children receiving supplements achieved clinical cure by day 5 of the trial, although no difference was found in bacteriologic cure between the vitamin A and placebo groups. The difference in efficacy between the two studies from Bangladesh could have resulted from differences in the pathogenesis of intestinal infections, reflecting the different etiologic factors. Shigella infection is a serious intestinal disorder associated with mucosal breeches and protein-losing enteropathy, and it is likely to carry an increased risk of complications. Furthermore, in the pathogenesis of shigella, induction of an inflammatory response is important in the passage of the microbe from lateral to basal membrane. The anti-inflammatory role of vitamin A proposed by Wiedermann *et al.* (14) and the well-known role of the vitamin in maintaining endothelial cell integrity might make vitamin A supplementation more effective against this particular infection than against less severe enteric infections.

Vitamin A supplements had no effect on the duration of diarrhea among children in India (53), or malnourished children from the Congo (54), although the cause of diarrhea was not examined in either study. In subgroup analyses in the Indian trial, a significant reduction in the duration of diarrhea was observed among children with severe vitamin A deficiency, as defined by conjunctival impression cytology.

The efficacy of vitamin A supplements on the severity of disease among children admitted to the hospital with pneumonia was examined in several placebo-controlled trials (Table 6). In Guatemala, the supplements had no effect on the length of hospital stay, or on the duration of various signs of respiratory disease, including hypoxia, fever, and rapid respiratory rate (55). In Tanzania, vitamin A-treated and placebo groups were similar in the mean number of days of hospital stay and mean number of days of fever, rapid respiratory rate, and hypoxia (56). In trials from Brazil (57) and Vietnam (58), vitamin A supplements had no effect on the course of pneumonia. In Brazil, an apparently protective effect was seen among a subgroup of children who

TABLE 5. *Vitamin A and diarrheal diseases: hospital-based trials*

Community	Pathogen	Dose/period	Result	Reference
Bangladesh	Rotavirus *Escherichid Coli*	200,000 IU	No effect	Henning et al., 1992 (51)
India	Not known	100,000 IU (<yearly) 200,000 IU (>yearly)	No effect	Dewan et al., 1995 (53)
Congo	Not known	100,000 IU (<yearly) 200,000 IU (>yearly)	No effect	Donnen et al., 1998 (54)
Bangladesh	Shigella	200,000 IU	Protective	Hossain et al., 1998 (52)

TABLE 6. *Vitamin A and respiratory diseases: hospital-based trials*

Community	Dose	Result	Reference
Guatemala	100,000 IU (<yearly) 200,000 IU (>yearly)	No effect	Kjolhede et al., 1995 (55)
United States multicenter	50,000 IU (1–5 mo) 100,000 IU (6–11 mo) 200,000 IU (>12 mo)	No adverse effect	Bresee et al., 1996 (61)
Chile	50,000 IU (1–5 mo) 100,000 IU (6–11 mo) 200,000 IU (>12 mo)	More rapid recovery	Dowell et al., 1996 (62)
United States	100,000 IU	No effect	Quinlan and Hayani, 1996 (60)
Brazil	100,000 IU/d for 2 days (<1 y) 200,000 IU/d for 2 days (1–4 y)	No effect	Nacul et al., 1997 (57)
Vietnam	100,000 IU/d for 2 days (< 1 y) 200,000 IU/d for 2 days (1–4 y)	No effect	Si et al., 1997 (58)
Tanzania	100,000 IU/d for 2 days (<1 y) 200,000 IU/d for 2 days (> 1 y)	No effect	Fawzi et al., 1998 (56)
Peru	150,000 IU/2 d (<yearly) 300,000 IU/2 d (>yearly)	Adverse effect	Stephensen et al., 1998 (59)

had pneumonia severe enough to warrant hospital admission. In Vietnam, the duration of hospital stay was shorter in the vitamin A group among children who were moderately malnourished. In the Tanzania trial, all subjects enrolled were hospital inpatients. No differences in the effect of the supplements were observed among children who had a more severe condition at baseline or among varying categories of age, breast-feeding status, anthropometric status at baseline, or category of dietary vitamin A intake in the 4 months before admission to the hospital. In the same study, no differences were found when the endpoints were examined among a subset with more severe clinical condition at baseline.

Evidence suggests, in some cases, vitamin A supplements can have adverse events when given to children with pneumonia. In a well-designed, placebo-controlled study from Peru, vitamin A supplements resulted in longer duration of clinical signs, including auscultatory evidence of consolidation, a higher prevalence of retractions, and lower oxygen saturation (59) (Table 6). Also, a greater need was seen for supplemental oxygen in the vitamin A group. In the Tanzania study, of the 346 children in the vitamin A group, 13 died in the hospital, in contrast to eight deaths among the 341 children in the placebo group (63% higher mortality in the vitamin A group) (56). This last finding was not statistically significant; however, the study was not designed with statistical power adequate to examine the effect of the supplements on case fatality.

Three trials were carried out to examine specifically the efficacy of vitamin A supplements on children admitted to the hospital with pneumonia caused by the respiratory syncytial virus (RSV). RSV is a paramyxovirus similar to measles, and is also an important cause of bronchiolitis and pneumonia among infants and children. In an American study, children in the supplemented group had longer duration of oxygen treatment and intensive care, although these differences were not statistically significant (60). In a larger, multicenter trial also from the United States, no differences were found in the mean number of days with rapid respiratory rate, nor in the need for supplemental oxygen or intensive care, between the vitamin A and placebo groups (61); however, children who received vitamin A had longer hospital stays than those given a placebo. In contrast, in a third trial done in Santiago, Chile, as a companion to the multicenter trial, vitamin A appeared to result in a more rapid recovery from tachypnea, but this finding was limited to children who had the most significant hypoxemia at baseline ($Po_2 < 12$ kPa; 90 mm Hg) (62). Differences in other environmental factors (e.g., pollution and exposure to other pathogens affecting vitamin A status) might have contributed to differences observed in these two trials.

Community-Based Studies of Diarrheal and Respiratory Infections

Given the protective effects of vitamin A supplements on mortality, it was presumed that the vitamin would have beneficial effects on morbidity. However, in various community trials, vitamin A supplementation had no effect on morbidity despite having a strong protective effect against mortality in the same studies (63) (Table 7). In

TABLE 7. *Vitamin A and diarrheal or respiratory diseases: community-based trials*

Community	Dose	Result	Reference
Tamil Nadu, Southern India	8,333 IU/wk	No effect on DI or RI	Rahmathullah et al., 1991 (66)
Ghana	200,000 IU/every 4 mo	No effect on DI or RI	Ghana VAST Study Team, 1993 (40)
China	100,000 IU A, 40 IU E (2 doses at 3 mo, 9 mo after baseline)	⇓ RI and DI	Lie et al., 1993 (77)
Haiti	200,000 IU/every 4 mo	⇑ RI symptoms	Stansfield et al., 1993 (76)
Brazil	100,000 IU (<12 mo) 200,000 IU (>12 mo)	Significant ⇓ DI; no effect on ALRI	Barreto et al., 1994 (67)
New Delhi, India	200,000 IU	Improvement in DI	Bhandari et al., 1994 (68)
South Africa (HIV+ mothers)	50,000 IU (at 1, 3 mo) 100,000 IU (at 6, 9 mo) 200,000 IU (at 12 mo)	Improvement in DI and RI	Coutsoudis et al., 1995 (69)
India	200,000 IU/every 4 mo	No effect on RI or DI duration	Ramakrishnan et al., 1995 (73)
Indonesia	103,000 IU (<12 mo) 206,000 IU (> 12 mo)	39%⇑ in ALRI 8% ⇑ in ARI	Dibley et al., 1996 (72)
Australia			Pinnock et al., 1988 (75)

DI, diarrhea incidence; RI, respiratory infection incidence; ARI, acute respiratory illness; ALRI, acute lower respiratory illness; HIV, human immunodeficiency virus.

two trials that found an effect on mortality, in Aceh, Indonesia (64,65) and Tamil Nadu, India (41,66), no effect was seen on diarrheal or respiratory infections. In Aceh, morbidity was assessed in the week preceding a 6-month visit, whereas in Tamil Nadu, children were visited on a weekly basis. In these trials, however, mortality was the primary endpoint, and data sufficient to examine fully the effect of the supplements on morbidity were not collected.

Several studies were carried out specifically to examine the effect of the supplements on the incidence and severity of infections. A detailed morbidity profile was assessed on all children using passive and active surveillance of the study populations. In a trial in Ghana in which children were examined on an ongoing weekly basis to determine the rate of morbidity, no significant differences were found between the two treatment arms with respect to the prevalence of diarrheal or respiratory conditions (40). However, children who received vitamin A had fewer visits to clinics and fewer admissions to the hospital. In addition, the supplements resulted in a significant reduction in overall and diarrhea-specific mortality, whereas no effect on respiratory-related deaths was noted. These findings suggest that the protective effect of vitamin A is in reducing the severity rather than the incidence of infections. Among children from Brazil who were visited at home three times a week as part of a vitamin A versus placebo trial, no significant differences were found in the incidence of pneumonia or the frequency of hospital admission between the two groups (67). However, vitamin A resulted in a reduction in the mean daily prevalence as well as in the mean number of episodes of diarrhea, particularly severe episodes, both in this study and in another placebo-controlled study from New Delhi, India (68). In a third trial from South Africa among children born to women infected with HIV, vitamin A supplements resulted in an apparent reduction in the incidence of diarrhea overall, severe diarrhea, and lower respiratory tract infection (69). The protective effects were somewhat stronger among those infected with HIV and presumably more undernourished children than among those children not infected with HIV. However, the statistical power of the study to examine the effect of the supplements on various morbidity endpoints within HIV subgroups was limited. In trials from Brazil (70) and Indonesia (71), children given vitamin A supplement had similar risk and severity of respiratory infection compared with children given a placebo.

Findings from placebo-controlled trials in Indonesia (72) and India (73) suggest that large doses of vitamin A can be harmful when given to well-nourished children. In Indonesia was found a 39% increase in the risk of acute lower respiratory tract infection (ALRI) in the group receiving the vitamin A supplement. This negative effect was limited to children who were not stunted, among whom an 83% increase in ALRI was seen; among stunted children, a 29% reduction in ALRI was observed. Overall, the supplements had no effect on the risk of diarrhea, but vitamin A supplementation resulted in a significantly greater risk of diarrhea among children less than 30 months of age and in a significantly lower risk among older children. However, the effect of the supplements on the risk of pneumonia was not modified by the occurrence of wasting, nor did the effect on diarrhea differ between wasted and stunted children.

Moreover, no differences were seen in the mean duration of ALRI or diarrhea between the vitamin A and placebo arms. In a randomized trial from India, vitamin A supplements did not have a significant effect on either the percentage of time ill or the number of episodes of respiratory infection. Children who received vitamin A had an increased mean duration of diarrheal episodes. Compared with other trials, this population of Indian children had relatively better healthcare, including high coverage of immunization, awareness among mothers about health and nutrition, and routine deworming. These factors may have reduced the chances of finding a protective effect from the supplements.

Results from two trials in Australia and one in Haiti support the hypothesis that vitamin A supplements can increase signs of infection, particularly respiratory signs. In a study of Australian children who received either small doses of vitamin A or a placebo three times a week, children receiving supplement experienced a 12% increase in the mean number of days of cough. However, they also experienced a 9% and a 12% decrease in the number of days with chest and nose or throat symptoms, respectively (74). In a second Australian study of similar design, the group supplemented with vitamin A experienced a 17% increase in the median number of cough days as well as a 9% and a 43% increase in the median number of days with runny nose and sore throat, respectively (75). In a study from Haiti, vitamin A supplementation resulted in a significant increase in the 2-week prevalence of all symptoms of morbidity, including cough, rapid respiration, and diarrhea (76).

In contrast with the above, studies from China (77) and Thailand (78) showed reductions in the incidence of both respiratory infection and diarrhea in children receiving vitamin A supplement compared with control children. An important limitation of both studies was that the control group did not receive a placebo. Therefore, the investigators were not blinded with respect to the treatment arm, raising the possibility of bias by the research staff in ascertaining the outcomes.

Comment

Clear evidence is found of the importance of vitamin A supplementation in cases of measles and malnutrition, including vitamin A deficiency. Vitamin A supplementation may also be beneficial in reducing the severity of disease in some cases of diarrhea. From hospital-based trials among children with pneumonia, no evidence indicates that vitamin A is protective. In some cases, the results suggest a possible increase in risk to patients with pneumonia, as indicated by the increased need for supplemental oxygen in the study from Peru (58) and the apparent increased mortality among Tanzanian children admitted to the hospital with pneumonia (55). In light of these findings, vitamin A supplements should not be given during nonmeasles episodes of pneumonia unless evidence is seen of vitamin A deficiency. The conditions under which vitamin A supplements can be harmful need to be examined further. Given that vitamin A supplementation may reduce diarrheal disease in the period after discharge from the hospital, supplements could be given after recovery from pneumonia and at the time of leaving the hospital.

Large doses of vitamin A provide a potentially quick solution in areas of the world where deficiency is a public health problem. In these communities, vitamin A supplements can reduce total and diarrhea-specific mortality. When periodic dosing is chosen as an intervention strategy, we suggest that these doses be given every 4 months (42). Given the varying degree of protection afforded in different studies, more research is needed on factors that affect the bioavailability of these large doses.

Although periodic large doses of vitamin A are beneficial in the short run, their use as the only approach to the problem of vitamin A deficiency has limitations. Vitamin A deficiency coexists with other nutrient deficits that are not addressed by the supplementation program. In addition, the effectiveness of this approach is limited to the duration of the program, and children who live in distant places and may need the supplement most would be difficult to reach. Furthermore, large dosing programs can put financial and logistic strains on healthcare systems in developing countries. Toxicity caused by ingestion of multiple large doses over a short period of time is a real possibility that needs to be guarded against.

A more sustainable solution to the problem of vitamin A deficiency lies in programs aimed at increasing consumption of vitamin A in the diet. Small, frequent doses (in amounts corresponding to those in the diet) may be more protective against mortality and morbidity than large, periodic doses. Most communities in which vitamin A deficiency is a serious problem have abundant supplies of fruits and vegetables rich in carotenoids with provitamin A activity. Dietary vitamin A intake has been associated with significant reductions in mortality (79), diarrheal and respiratory infection (80), and risks of stunting or wasting (81). Nutrition education programs in these communities should be undertaken in addition to the administration of supplements if the latter strategy is being implemented. In areas of the world where vitamin A foods are not abundant, horticultural approaches should be considered. Vitamin A intervention strategies should be integrated into existing community programs that focus on other health problems rather than implemented as a vertical program. Additional operational research on possible methods of integration is needed.

More studies are needed to determine the mechanism of the effect of vitamin A on morbidity and mortality. Such studies should include both the immune- and nonimmune-related functions of vitamin A, as well as the interaction of vitamin A with the pathogen. Results from these studies would help determine host conditions or infection types for which vitamin A supplementation could be beneficial and those for which it would be harmful.

An important mechanism through which vitamin A exerts both its beneficial and its harmful effects is through modulation of cellular and humoral immunity (see above). Furthermore, vitamin A deficiency can adversely affect the epithelial lining of the gastrointestinal tract (82), leading to decreased secretion of mucus and weakened local barriers to infection. Vitamin A-deficient mice had more severe mucosal changes than normal mice when infected with rotavirus (83), which is a major cause of diarrhea in children.

The positive relationship between vitamin A intake and cough that has been shown in a few studies has three possible explanations (which do not apply to studies that showed other signs of respiratory infection, such as rapid respiration). First, the occurrence of cough may indicate a more competent respiratory epithelium and, hence, these results would suggest that vitamin A intake was protective against respiratory disease. Cough is a defense mechanism by which the body prevents the entry of harmful material into the respiratory system. Although the physiology of cough is not fully understood, it is probably initiated when airway receptors embedded in the tracheobronchial epithelium are stimulated by foreign substances (84). As vitamin A deficiency is associated with keratinization and squamous metaplasia of respiratory epithelium (82), this may adversely affect the cough receptors, leading to the decreased occurrence of cough among children with low levels of vitamin A intake. Alternatively, cough may occur more among vitamin A-deficient subjects, who may be at a higher risk of respiratory infection, in which case the overall association with dietary vitamin A intake indicates that vitamin A is harmful.

VITAMIN E AND THE IMMUNE RESPONSE

Vitamin E is the major chain-breaking antioxidant in membranes. Membrane phospholipids of cells of the immune system have a high content of polyunsaturated fatty acids and are prime targets for free radical reactions. Release of reactive oxygen species by phagocytes on encountering pathogens and rapid lymphocyte proliferation following antigenic stimulation expose the immune cells to high levels of oxidative stress. Thus, it is not surprising that cells of the immune system have a higher vitamin E content than other cells of the body (85).

Both deficiency and supplementation of vitamin E have been shown to affect the immune response and resistance against infection. The influence of vitamin E on immune function has been reported in a variety of species including rodents, chickens, calves, and humans, and has been shown to affect different aspects of immune function including T-cell response, antibody production, NK-cell activity, phagocytic activity, and the production of immunoregulatory molecules. Here, effects of vitamin E deficiency and supplementation on immune functions and their clinical significance will be discussed.

Vitamin E Deficiency and Immune Function

Vitamin E deficiency has been shown to impair both humoral and cell-mediated immune functions in animals and humans.

The effect of vitamin E deficiency on humoral immune response in animals was demonstrated in experiments in which mice fed a diet deficient in vitamin E had fewer plaque-forming cells and a lower hemagglutination titer in response to injection of sheep red blood cells than mice fed a diet adequate in vitamin E (86). Depressed lymphocyte proliferation in response to T-cell mitogen concanavalin A in rats fed a vitamin E-deficient diet indicates that cell-mediated immune response is also impaired in vitamin E deficiency (87,88). Vitamin E deficiency has a significant impact on phagocytic functions. Harris *et al.* (89) reported that chemotactic and ingestive responses of neutrophils were impaired when rats were fed a vitamin E-deficient diet for 2 months. Warschauer *et al.* (90) also showed that vitamin E deficiency augmented the adverse effect of ozone-induced impairments in pulmonary bactericidal capacity following prolonged exposure of rats to low levels of ozone. These effects of vitamin E deficiency might result from increased free radical reactions, oxygen consumption, and hydrogen peroxide release by phagocytosing neutrophils from vitamin E-deficient animals (89).

In humans, primary severe deficiency of vitamin E rarely occurs, whereas secondary deficiency is observed as a consequence of certain diseases such as primary biliary cirrhosis (91), cholestatic liver disease (92), cystic fibrosis (93), and intestinal malabsorption disorders (94). Decreased plasma vitamin E concentrations have been observed in patients with severe viral hepatitis and in children infected with HIV-1 (95,96). In a case report by Kowdley *et al.* (94), *in vivo* and *in vitro* impairment of T-cell function, as well as polyneuropathy, were observed in conjunction with vitamin E deficiency in a woman aged 59 years with progressive systemic sclerosis and malabsorption. Impaired mitogenic responses to concanavalin A and phytohemagglutinin, IL-2 production, and DTH were improved following vitamin E supplementation.

Most premature low birthweight infants have a true deficiency of vitamin E at birth that requires early treatment. Vitamin E deficiency in preterm infants is associated with hemolytic anemia, hyperbilirubinemia, intraventricular hemorrhage, and retinopathy of prematurity (97). Neutrophils from neonates have impaired phagocytic ability, depressed oxidative metabolic responses, and depressed bactericidal activity, as well as a reduced ability to move toward defined chemotactic stimuli, compared with cells from normal adults (98). In healthy children aged 3 years, lower serum vitamin E levels ($<$ 10th centile) were associated with lower lymphocyte proliferation and serum IgM compared with those with higher vitamin E levels ($>$ 90th centile) (99).

Vitamin E Supplementation and the Immune Response

Vitamin E has been shown to have immunostimulatory effects in various species, including humans, when given in quantities exceeding established dietary requirements. Vitamin E supplementation has been shown to affect both humoral- and cell-mediated immune responses.

Dietary supplementation with vitamin E increased lymphocyte proliferation in response to T-cell and B-cell mitogens in mice (100), rats (88), and calves (101). Meydani *et al.* (100) showed that dietary supplementation with 500 ppm vitamin E for 6 weeks increased lymphocyte proliferation and DTH response, and decreased prostaglandin (PG) E_2 production in old mice. In addition, *in vitro* introduction of vitamin E increased the mitogenic response of splenic lymphocytes in mice (102,103). In a coculture study, Beharka *et al.* (103) showed that the *in vitro* addition of vitamin E increased concanavalin A-stimulated cell proliferation when macrophages from old mice were cocultured with purified T cells from either old or young mice, or when macrophages from young mice were cocultured with purified T cells from old mice. IL-2 production was also increased with vitamin E supplementation in cocultures composed of macrophages from old mice and purified T cells from either old or young mice. The immunostimulatory effects of vitamin E supplementation seem to be transferred to the offspring. Chicks hatched from breeders fed diets supplemented with vitamin E had significantly higher tetrahydrofuran-stimulated bursal lymphocyte proliferation and higher concanavalin A and phorbol 12-myristate 13 acetate (PMA) stimulated splenic lymphocyte proliferation compared with control chicks (104). It is suggested that the immunostimulatory effect of vitamin E is mediated by either reduced prostaglandin synthesis (100) or decreased free radical synthesis (105). PGE_2 has been shown to have a direct inhibitory effect on an early stage of T-cell activation, resulting in decreased IL-2 production, decreased IL-2 receptor expression, decreased responsiveness to exogenous IL-2, and decreased proliferation (106).

Vitamin E has been shown to increase antibody production by enhancing humoral immune response or by acting as an adjuvant. Dietary vitamin E supplementation increased the number of plaque-forming cells and hemagglutination titers following immunization with sheep red blood cells and tetanus toxoid in mice (107). Enhancement of humoral immune response to Venezuelan equine encephalomyelitis attenuated live virus vaccine was observed in guinea pigs given intramuscular injections of vitamin E before and after immunization (108). Oral supplementation of vitamin E, begun 2 weeks before vaccination and continued for 3 weeks afterward, did not have an effect on humoral response in this study. Vitamin E supplementation in lambs (20 mg/kg vitamin E diet for 10 weeks) stimulated secondary humoral immune response following parainfluenza 3 virus challenge (109). The adjuvant effect of vitamin E was reported by Francini *et al.* (110). Vitamin E, which partially replaced mineral oil in viral inactivated emulsified vaccines, increased the hemagglutination inhibition titers to the viral antigen (Newcastle disease virus) in chicks.

Several studies have shown that vitamin E supplementation affects immune response in humans. Baehner *et al.* (111) found that administration of 1,600 mg/d of vitamin E for 1 week increased the rate of neutrophil phagocytic activity, but decreased bactericidal activity, which correlated with a reduced level of H_2O_2 release. Vitamin E supplementation has been shown to enhance immune response in the elderly. In a double-blind, placebo-controlled study, Meydani *et al.* (112) found that DTH scores, mitogenic response of peripheral blood mononuclear cells to concanavalin A, and IL-2 production were significantly higher in the elderly subjects (> 60 years of age) supplemented with 800 mg/d vitamin E for 30 days. Decreased PGE_2 production by peripheral blood mononuclear cells and decreased plasma lipid peroxide levels were also observed. In a more recent study, the effect of long-term vitamin E supplementation on *in vivo* indices of immune response in healthy elderly subjects was evaluated (113). After 4 months of vitamin E supplementation at levels of 60, 200, or 800 mg/d, DTH and antibody titer to hepatitis B were significantly increased in the groups supplemented with 200 and 800 mg/d. The largest increase was observed in the 200 mg/d group, which also showed a significant increase in antibody titer to tetanus vaccine. This long-term vitamin E supplementation did not adversely affect the elderly subjects (114). Vitamin E supplementation had no significant effects on plasma concentrations of other nutrients, serum autoantibodies (anti-DNA and antithyroglobulin), liver enzyme function (glutathione peroxidase and superoxide dismutase), or on cytotoxic activity of neutrophils against *Candida albicans*.

Premature infants are under severe oxidative stress as they are faced with an abrupt change to a relatively hyperoxic extrauterine environment and lower levels of antioxidant defenses. In current clinical practice, premature infants usually receive vitamin E in a multivitamin preparation that is added to parenteral formula at a level of 2 to 3 IU/kg body weight (97). Most of the vitamin E supplementation studies on premature infants focus on the outcomes related to retinopathy, bronchopulmonary dysplasia, necrotizing enterocolitis, and sepsis. The effect of vitamin E on the immune function of premature infants is not well documented. The use of vitamin E in premature infants has yielded conflicting results. Pharmacologic levels of α-tocopherol combined with cryotherapy was found to be more effective than cryotherapy alone in decreasing the severity of threshold retinopathy of prematurity in infants weighing less than 1,250 g (115). Although Fish *et al.* (116) reported that necrotizing enterocolitis and sepsis did not occur more frequently in the neonates treated with intramuscular injections of vitamin E, Johnson *et al.* (117) reported an increased incidence of necrotizing enterocolitis and neonatal sepsis associated with vitamin E treatment (oral, intravenous, or intramuscular application). Necrotizing enterocolitis is a condition that results in widespread intestinal necrosis and often leads to perforation of the bowel and peritonitis. The difference in outcomes of the studies by Fish *et al.* (116) and Johnson *et al.* (117) might reflect the difference in target serum vitamin E levels: 0.5 to 3.5 mg/dl in the study by Fish *et al.* and 5.0 mg/dl in the study by Johnson *et al.* In fact, nearly 43% of infants supplemented with vitamin E had serum vitamin E levels greater than 5.0 mg/dl in the study by Johnson *et al.* Sobel *et al.* (118) reported an increased incidence of necrotizing enterocolitis associated with serum levels of vitamin E greater than 3.5 mg/dl, whereas Finer *et al.* (119) reported an increased incidence in association with an oral dose (200 mg) of vitamin E, which may have been related to hyperosmolarity of the preparation. Mino (120) investigated the effect of oral vitamin E supplementation on leukocyte function of premature infants: no effect was seen on zymosan-induced superoxide anion formation by neutrophils following the administration of 40 mg/kg of all-rac-tocopherol nicotinate to the infants for 8 to 14 days. Chirico *et al.* (121) reported improved neutrophil function with intramuscular injections totalling 120 mg/kg vitamin E to healthy premature infants during the first 13 days after birth. Enhanced index and frequency of phagocytosis were observed at 5 days of age. As clinical outcomes of vitamin E treatment in premature infants vary with dose, the route of administration, and the preparation of vitamin E used, administration to premature infants should be done with caution, with dose and route of administration carefully examined.

Vitamin E and Infection

Vitamin E Deficiency and Infection

Beck *et al.* (122) showed that vitamin E deficiency can be detrimental to mice infected with coxsackievirus. Vitamin E deficiency in mice exacerbated the cardiac damage caused by a virulent myocarditic strain of the coxsackievirus and allowed the nonvirulent amyocarditic CVB3/0 strain to become myocarditic. Viral passage experiments showed that the increased virulence of both these viral strains was caused by phenotypic change in the viruses as a result of their replication in a vitamin E-deficient host. It is thought that the nonspecific effect of oxidative stress is responsible for these results as N,N'-diphenyl-p-phenylenediamine, a synthetic antioxidant structurally unrelated to vitamin E, was active in protecting vitamin E-deficient mice against the cardiotoxic effects of the coxsackievirus (123). On the other hand, pro-oxidant dietary conditions (menhaden fish oil-enriched and vitamin E-deficient) produce beneficial effects against lethal *Plasmodium yoelii* infection in mice that lack the ability to produce an acquired antimalarial immune response (124).

Whereas vitamin E deficiency has an effect on the outcome of infection, infection can alter vitamin E status of the host as well, leading to exacerbation. In animals, decreased vitamin E concentration in lung and liver was observed following influenza infection (125). Furthermore, retrovirus infection significantly reduced vitamin E levels in the liver, spleen, and thymus (126). These decreases in vitamin E levels may reflect increased oxidative stress that follows viral infection. In humans, plasma vitamin E concentrations were significantly lower in patients with acute or chronic viral hepatitis with high disease activity (95). Furthermore, significantly lower serum concentrations of α-tocopherol were observed in papillomavirus-positive patients with cervical intraepithelial neoplasia (127). Circulating α-tocopherol values were lower in patients infected with HIV; this decrease corresponded with increased malondialdehyde levels (128). Results from a study by Tang *et al.* (129) suggest that high serum levels of vitamin E can be associated with lower HIV-1 disease progression. Men in the highest quartile of serum vitamin E levels showed a 34% lower risk of progression to the acquired immunodeficiency syndrome compared with those in the lowest quartile.

Vitamin E Supplementation and Infectious Diseases

The immunostimulatory effect of vitamin E supplementation was shown to confer resistance against infection with different pathogens, in different species of animals. Lower mortality from *E. coli* infection in chicks (130), fewer clinical cases of mastitis in cows (131), faster recovery from chlamydia infection in lambs (132), higher survival from *Diplococcus pneumoniae* type I infection in mice (133), higher resistance to *Mycoplasma pulmonis* infection in rats (134), and lower influenza viral titers in mice (135) were observed with vitamin E supplementation. In a study by Hayek *et al.* (135), dietary supplementation with 500 ppm vitamin E significantly reduced lung viral titers in old mice infected with influenza virus. It was suggested that the effect of vitamin E may be caused, in part, by preservation of antioxidant status and NK cell activity. Wang *et al.* (136) also reported that vitamin E supplementation prevented retrovirus-induced suppression of splenocyte proliferation and NK activity and partially restored production of IL-2 and γ-interferon by splenocytes. *In vitro* addition of RRR-α-tocopheryl succinate to splenocytes from avian erythroblastosis virus-infected chickens resulted in normalization of T-cell response to concanavalin A and phytohemagglutinin, which is suppressed in infected animals (137).

Few studies have investigated the direct effect of vitamin E supplementation on the incidence of infectious diseases in humans. Harman and Miller (138) gave supplement (200 or 400 mg/d of vitamin E for 6 months) to 103 patients in a chronic care facility and determined the serum antibody titers to influenza virus vaccine and the number of cases of pulmonary, urinary tract, and other infections. No effect was seen of vitamin E on the serum titers or the incidence of infectious diseases. Unfortunately, because data on subjects' health status, medication use, and other relevant variables were not reported, it is hard to determine the effect of confounding factors. Meydani *et al.* (113) reported a nonsignificant (p = 0.09) 30% lower incidence of self-reported infection in elderly subjects receiving vitamin E supplement compared with a placebo group. Chandra (139) gave a multinutrient supplement formulation to 96 healthy elderly individuals for 12 months. The supplemented group had a greater antibody response to influenza vaccine and less infection-related illness than the placebo group. It is impossible to attribute the effect to a particular nutrient because the intervention included multinutrients. However, vitamin E was the only nutrient provided at greater than 400% of the recommended daily allowance (RDA); other nutrients were provided at 30% to 200% of the RDA. Results from the Alpha-Tocopherol Beta-Carotene Cancer Prevention (ATBC) study showed no effect of 50 mg/d vitamin E supplementation on symptoms of chronic obstructive pulmonary disease (e.g., chronic cough, phlegm, or dyspnea) over a period of 5 to 8 years in male smokers (140).

Vitamin E supplementation has been used to improve the clinical outcomes of several infectious disease states, including viral hepatitis, chronic respiratory tract infection, and sepsis in humans and animals. In a randomized, double-blind, placebo-controlled study by von Herby *et al.* (141), treatment of patients with hepatitis C with 800 IU/d RRR—tocopherol for 12 weeks improved clinical indices indicative of liver damage. Alanine aminotransferase and aspartate aminotransferase levels were lowered after 12 weeks of vitamin E treatment. Andreone *et al.* (142) also reported improved biochemical and virologic outcomes in chronic hepatitis B with 3 months of vitamin E supplementation (600 mg/d). However, Yurdakök and Kanra (143) did not observe beneficial effects of vitamin E therapy (300 mg/d intramuscular injection for 7 days) in children with acute viral hepatitis. These conflicting results may reflect difference in the duration of treatment.

Comment

Vitamin E deficiency, both in animal models and in humans, impairs the immune response and renders the host (animal models) more susceptible to infectious diseases.

Severe primary vitamin E deficiency rarely occurs. However, marginal deficiency is observed in premature infants, in malnourished children, and following viral and bacterial infection. Further studies are needed to determine the role of vitamin E status in the resistance of premature or malnourished infants to infectious disease.

Clinical trials in the aged have shown significant improvement in immune response. This effect in animal models is associated with increased resistance to influenza infection. Such information is not yet available in humans. At least two clinical trials in the United States and Europe are currently addressing this question. Similarities exist between immunologic changes in the elderly and in malnourished children. The success of vitamin E supplementation in improving the immune response in elderly people suggests that vitamin E may produce similar results in malnourished children. Studies are needed to determine the role of vitamin E supplementation in maintaining the host defense of malnourished, low birthweight infants against pathogens.

Research is needed to determine the mechanisms by which vitamins E and A exert their effect, as well as those of supplementation on immune response and infection. Such information will help in developing more effective intervention strategies. In particular, such information is needed to determine the type of infection and host conditions most conducive to effective interventions.

Acknowledgments: This material is based on work supported by the US Department of Agriculture (USDA), under agreement No. 58-1950-9-001. Any opinions, findings, conclusions, or recommendations expressed in this publication are those of the authors and do not necessarily reflect the view of the USDA. This work was also supported by the National Institute of Child Health and Human Development (NICHD R01 32257) and the Fogerty International Center (NIH D43 TW00004). The authors would like to thank Joanne Meegan for preparation of this manuscript.

REFERENCES

1. Nauss K. Influence of vitamin A status on the immune system. In: Bauernfeind C, ed. *Vitamin A deficiency and its control*. New York: Academic Press, 1986: 207–43.
2. Ross A. Vitamin A status: relationship to immunity and the antibody response. *Proc Soc Exp Biol Med* 1992; 200: 303–20.
3. Carman J, Smith S, Hayes C. Characterization of a helper T-lymphocyte defect in vitamin A deficient mice. *J Immunol* 1989; 143: 388–93.
4. Cantorna M, Nashold F, Chun TY, et al. Vitamin A down-regulation in IFN-γ synthesis in cloned mouse Th1 lymphocytes depends on the CD28 costimulatory pathway. *J Immunol* 1996; 156: 2674–9.
5. Tokuyama Y, Tokuyama H. Retinoids as Ig isotype-switching modulators. *Cell Immunol* 1996; 170: 230–4.
6. Semba R, Muhilal, Griffin D, et al. Abnormal T-cell subset proportions in vitamin A-deficient children. *Lancet* 1993; 341: 5–8.
7. Twining S, Schulte D, Wilson P, et al. Vitamin A deficiency alters rat neutrophil function. *J Nutr* 1997; 127: 558–65.
8. Semba R. The role of vitamin A and related retinoids in immune function. *Nutr Rev* 1998; 56: S38–48.
9. Sklan D, Trifon S, Kedar O, et al. Retinoid metabolism in human leucocytes. *Br J Nutr* 1995; 73: 889–95.

10. Garbe A, Buck J, Hammerling U. Retinoids are important cofactors in T cell activation. *J Exp Med* 1992; 176: 109–17.
11. Allende L, Corell A, Madrono A, et al. Retinol (vit A) is a cofactor in CD3-induced human T-lymphocyte activation. *Immunology* 1997; 90: 388–96.
12. Buck J, Myc A, Garbe A, et al. Differences in the action and metabolism between retinol and retinoic acid in B lymphocytes. *J Cell Biol* 1991; 115: 851–9.
13. Smith S, Hayes C. Contrasting impairments in IgM and IgG responses of vitamin A-deficient mice. *Proc Natl Acad Sci USA* 1987; 84: 5878–82.
14. Wiedermann U, Chen X, Enerback L, et al. Vitamin A deficiency increases inflammatory responses. *Scand J Immunol* 1996; 44: 578–84.
15. Wiedermann U, Tarkowski A, Bremell T, et al. Vitamin A deficiency predisposes to *Staphylococcus aureus* infection. *Infect Immun* 1996; 64: 209–14.
16. Gardner E, Ross A. Immunologic memory is established in nursling rats immunized with tetanus toxoid, but is not affected by concurrent supplementation with vitamin A. *Am J Clin Nutr* 1995; 62: 1007–12.
17. Krishnan S, Bhuyan U, Talwar G, et al. Effect of vitamin A and protein-calorie undernourishment on immune responses. *Immunology* 1974; 27: 383–92.
18. Panda B, Combs G. Impaired antibody production in chicks fed diets low in vitamin A, pantothenic acid or riboflavin. *Proc Soc Exp Biol Med* 1963; 113: 530–4.
19. Bowman T, Goonewardene I, Pasatiempo A, et al. Vitamin A deficiency decreases natural killer cell activity and interferon production in rats. *J Nutr* 1990; 120: 1264–73.
20. Pasatiempo A, Bowman T, Taylor C, et al. Vitamin A depletion and repletion: effects on antibody response to the capsular polysaccharide of *Streptococcus pneumoniae*, type III (SSS-III). *Am J Clin Nutr* 1989; 49: 501–10.
21. Chandra R. Reduced secretory antibody response to live attenuated measles and poliovirus vaccines in malnourished children. *Br Med J* 1975; 2: 583–5.
22. Puengtomwatanakul S, Sirisinha S. Impaired biliary secretion of immunoglobin A in vitamin A-deficient rats. *Proc Soc Exp Biol Med* 1986; 182: 437–42.
23. Majumder M, Abdus Sattar A, Mohiduzzaman M. Effect of vitamin A deficiency on guinea pig Peyer's patches. *Nutr Res* 1987; 7: 539–45.
24. Majumder M, Abdus Sattar A. Peyer's patch immune function of vitamin A deficient guinea pigs. *Nutr Rep Int* 1987; 36: 143–50.
25. Friedman A, Meidovsky A, Leitner G, et al. Decreased resistance and immune response to *E. coli* in chicks with low or high intakes of vitamin A. *J Nutr* 1991; 121: 395–400.
26. Fumarulo R, Conese M, Riccardi S, et al. Retinoids inhibit the respiratory burst and degranulation of stimulated human polymorphonuclear leukocytes. *Agents Actions* 1991; 34: 339–44.
27. Semba R, Muhilal, Scott A, et al. Depressed immune response to tetanus in children with vitamin A deficiency. *J Nutr* 1992; 122: 101–7.
28. Brown K, Rajan M, Chakraborty J, et al. Failure of a large dose of vitamin A to enhance the antibody response to tetanus toxoid in children. *Am J Clin Nutr* 1980; 33: 212–17.
29. Kutty P, Mohanram M, Reddy V. Humoral immune response in vitamin A deficient children. *Acta Vitaminol Enzymol* 1981; 3: 231–5.
30. Bhaskaram P, Jyothi S, Rao K, et al. Effects of subclinical vitamin A deficiency and administration of vitamin A as a single large dose on immune function in children. *Nutr Res* 1989; 9: 1017–25.
31. Rosales F, Kjolhede C. A single 210-μmol oral dose of retinol does not enhance the immune response in children with measles. *J Nutr* 1994; 124: 1604–14.
32. Semba R, Munasir Z, Beeler J, et al. Reduced seroconversion to measles in infants given vitamin A with measles vaccination. *Lancet* 1995; 345: 1330–2.
33. Benn C, Aaby P, Bale C, et al. Randomised trial of effect of vitamin A supplementation on antibody response to measles vaccine in Guinea-Bissau, West Africa. *Lancet* 1997; 350: 101.
34. Semba R, Akib A, Beeler J, et al. Effect of vitamin A supplementation on measles vaccination in nine-month-old infants. *Public Health* 1997; 111: 257.
35. Rahman M, Mahalanabis D, Alvarez J, et al. Effect of early vitamin A supplementation on cell-mediated immunity in infants younger than 6 mo. *Am J Clin Nutr* 1997; 65: 144–8.
36. Kramer T, Udomkesmalee E, Dhanamitta S, et al. Lymphocyte responsiveness of children supplemented with vitamin A and zinc. *Am J Clin Nutr* 1993; 58: 566–70.
37. Sommer A, Katz J, Tarwojto I. Increased risk of respiratory disease and diarrhea in children with pre-existing mild vitamin A deficiency. *Am J Clin Nutr* 1984; 40: 1090–5.

38. Herrera M, Nestel P, El Amin A, et al. Vitamin A supplementation and child survival. *Lancet* 1992; 340: 267–71.
39. Vijayaraghavan K, Radhaiah G, Prakasam B, et al. Effect of a massive dose of vitamin A on morbidity and mortality in Indian children. *Lancet* 1990; 336: 1342–5.
40. Ghana VAST Study Team. Vitamin A supplementation in northern Ghana: effects on clinic attendance, hospital admissions, and child mortality. *Lancet* 1993; 342: 7–12.
41. Rahmathullah L, Underwood B, Thulasiraj R, et al. Reduced mortality among children in southern India receiving a small weekly dose of vitamin A. *N Engl J Med* 1990; 323: 929–35.
42. Fawzi W, Chalmers T, Herrera M, et al. Vitamin A supplementation and child mortality: a meta-analysis. *JAMA* 1993; 269: 898–903.
43. Fawzi W, Mbise R, Hertzmark E, et al. A randomized trial of vitamin A supplements in relation to mortality among HIV infected and uninfected children in Tanzania. *Pediatr Infect Dis J* 1999; 18: 127–33.
44. Fawzi W. Environmental factors that impact the efficacy of vitamin A supplements among children. *Environ Nutr Interact* 1997; 1: 299–333.
45. Humphrey J, Agoestina T, Wu L, et al. Impact of neonatal vitamin A supplementation on infant morbidity and mortality. *J Pediatr* 1996; 128: 489–96.
46. West K, Katz J, Shresta S, et al. Mortality of infants <6 mo of age supplemented with vitamin A: a randomized, double-masked trial in Nepal. *Am J Clin Nutr* 1995; 62: 143–8.
47. The Vitamin E and Pneumonia Working Group. Potential interventions for the prevention of childhood pneumonia in developing countries: a meta-analysis of data from field trials to assess the impact of vitamin A supplementation on pneumonia morbidity and mortality. *Bull World Health Organ* 1995; 73: 609–19.
48. WHO/CHD Immunization-Linked Vitamin A Supplementation Study Group. Randomized trial to assess benefits and safety of vitamin A supplementation linked to immunization in early infancy. *Lancet* 1998; 352: 1257–63.
49. Ogaro F, Orinda V, Onyango F, et al. Effect of vitamin A on diarrhoeal and respiratory complications of measles. *Trop Geogr Med* 1993; 45: 283–6.
50. Rosales F, Kjolhede C, Goodman S. Efficacy of a single oral dose of 200,000 IU of oil-soluble vitamin A in measles-associated morbidity. *Am J Epidemiol* 1996; 143: 413–22.
51. Henning B, Stewart K, Zaman K, et al. Lack of therapeutic efficacy of vitamin A for non-cholera, watery diarrhoea in Bangladeshi children. *Eur J Clin Nutr* 1992; 46: 437–43.
52. Hossain S, Biswas R, Kabir I, et al. Single dose vitamin A treatment in acute shigellosis in Bangladeshi children: randomized double blind controlled trial. *BMJ* 1998; 316: 422–6.
53. Dewan V, Patwari A, Jain M, et al. A randomized controlled trial of vitamin A supplementation in acute diarrhea. *Indian Pediatr* 1995; 32: 21–5.
54. Donnen P, Dramaix M, Brasseur D, et al. Randomized placebo-controlled clinical trial of the effect of a single high dose or daily low doses of vitamin A on the morbidity of hospitalized, malnourished children. *Am J Clin Nutr* 1998; 68: 1254–60.
55. Kjolhede C, Chew F, Gadomski A, et al. Clinical trial of vitamin A as adjuvant treatment for lower respiratory tract infections. *J Pediatr* 1995; 126: 807–12.
56. Fawzi W, Mbise R, Fataki M. Vitamin A supplements and severity of pneumonia among children admitted to hospital in Dar es Salaam, Tanzania. *Am J Clin Nutr* 1998; 68: 187–92.
57. Nacul L, Kirkwood B, Arthur P, et al. Randomized, double blind, placebo controlled clinical trial of efficacy of vitamin A treatment in non-measles childhood pneumonia. *BMJ* 1997; 315: 505–10.
58. Si N, Grytter N, Vy N, et al. High dose vitamin A supplementation in the course of pneumonia in Vietnamese children. *Acta Paediatr* 1997; 86: 1052–5.
59. Stephensen C, Franchi L, Hernandez H, et al. Adverse effects of high-dose vitamin A supplements in children hospitalized with pneumonia. *Pediatrics* 1998; 101: e3.
60. Quinlan K, Hayani K. Vitamin A and respiratory syncytial virus infection. *Arch Pediatr Adolesc Med* 1996; 150: 25–30.
61. Bresee J, Fischer M, Dowell S, et al. Vitamin A therapy for children with respiratory syncytial virus infection: a multicenter trial in the US. *Pediatr Infect Dis J* 1996; 15: 777–82.
62. Dowell S, Papic Z, Bresee J, et al. Treatment of respiratory syncytial virus infection with vitamin A: a randomized, placebo-controlled trial in Santiago, Chile. *Pediatr Infect Dis J* 1996; 15: 782–6.
63. Beaton G, Martorell R, L'Abbe K, et al. *Effectiveness of vitamin A supplementation in the control of young child morbidity and mortality in developing countries: summary report.* Toronto: University of Toronto, 1993.

64. Sommer A, Tarwotjo I, Djunaedi E. Impact of vitamin A supplementation on childhood mortality. A randomized controlled community trial. *Lancet* 1986; i: 1169–73.
65. Abdeljaber M, Monto A, Tilden R, et al. The impact of vitamin A supplementation on morbidity: a randomized community intervention trial. *Am J Public Health* 1991; 81: 1654–6.
66. Rahmathullah L, Underwood B, Thulasiraj R, et al. Diarrhea, respiratory infections, and growth are not affected by a weekly low-dose vitamin A supplement: a masked, controlled field trial in children in southern India. *Am J Clin Nutr* 1991; 54: 568–77.
67. Barreto B, Santos L, Assis N, et al. Effect of vitamin A supplementation on diarrhoea and acute lower-respiratory tract in young children in Brazil. *Lancet* 1994; 344: 228–31.
68. Bhandari N, Bhan M, Sazawal S. Impact of massive doses of vitamin A given to preschool children with acute diarrhoea on subsequent respiratory and diarrhoeal morbidity. *BMJ* 1994; 309: 1404–7.
69. Coutsoudis A, Bobat R, Coovadia H, et al. Effect of vitamin A supplementation on the morbidity of children born to HIV-infected women. *Am J Public Health* 1995; 85: 1076–81.
70. Nacul L, Arthur P, Kirkwood B, et al. The impact of vitamin A supplementation given during a pneumonia episode on the subsequent morbidity of children. *Trop Med Int Health* 1998; 3: 661–6.
71. Kartasasmita C, Rosmayudi O, Deville W, et al. Plasma retinol level, vitamin A supplementation and acute respiratory infections in children of 1–5 y in a developing country. *Tuber Lung Dis* 1995; 76: 563–569.
72. Dibley M, Sadjimin T, Kholhede C, et al. A supplementation fails to reduce the incidence of acute respiratory illness and diarrhea in preschool-age Indonesian children. *J Nutr* 1996; 126: 434–42.
73. Ramakrishnan U, Latham M, Abel R, Frongillo E. Vitamin A supplementation and morbidity among preschool children in south India. *Am J Clin Nutr* 1995; 61: 1295–303.
74. Pinnock C, Douglas R, Badcock N. Vitamin A status in children who are prone to respiratory tract infections. *Aust Paediatr* 1986; 22: 95–9.
75. Pinnock C, Douglas R, Martin A, et al. Vitamin A status in children with a history of respiratory syncytial virus infection in infancy. *Aust Paediatr* 1988; 24: 286–9.
76. Stansfield S, Pierre-Louis M, Lerebours G, et al. Vitamin A supplementation and increased prevalence of childhood diarrhea and acute respiratory infections. *Lancet* 1993; 342: 578–82.
77. Lie C, Ying C, En-Lin W, et al. Impact of large-dose vitamin A supplementation on childhood diarrhea, respiratory disease, and growth. *Eur J Clin Nutr* 1993; 47: 88–96.
78. Bloem M, Wedel M, Egger R, et al. Mild vitamin A deficiency and risk of respiratory diseases and diarrhea in preschool and school children in northeastern Thailand. *Am J Epidemiol* 1990; 131: 332–9.
79. Fawzi W, Herrera M, Willett W, et al. Dietary vitamin A intake and the risk of mortality among children. *Am J Clin Nutr* 1994; 59: 401–8.
80. Fawzi W, Herrera M, Willett W, et al. A prospective study of dietary vitamin A and the incidence of diarrhea and respiratory infections among Sudanese children. *J Nutr* 1995; 125: 1211–21.
81. Fawzi W, Herrera M, Willett W, et al. Dietary vitamin A intake in relation to child growth. *Epidemiology* 1997; 8: 402–7.
82. Wolbach S, Howe P. Tissue changes following deprivation of fat-soluble A vitamin. *J Exp Med* 1925; 42: 753–77.
83. Ahmed F, Jones D, Jackson A. The interaction of vitamin A deficiency and rotavirus infection in the mouse. *Br J Nutr* 1990; 63: 363–73.
84. Braga P, Alegra L. *Cough*. New York: Raven Press, 1989.
85. Hatman LJ, Kayden HJ. A high-performance liquid chromatographic method for the determination of tocopherol in plasma and cellular elements of the blood. *J Lipid Res* 1979; 20: 639–45.
86. Tengerdy R, Heinzerling R, Brown G, et al. Enhancement of the humoral response by vitamin E. *Int Arch Allergy Immunol* 1973; 44: 221–32.
87. Eskew ML, Scholz RW, Reddy CC, et al. Effect of vitamin E and selenium deficiencies on rat immune function. *Immunology* 1985; 54: 173–80.
88. Bendich A, Gabriel E, Machlin L. Dietary vitamin E requirements for optimum immune response in rats. *J Nutr* 1986; 116: 675–81.
89. Harris R, Boxer L, Baehner R. Consequences of vitamin E deficiency on the phagocytic and oxidative functions of the rat polymorhponuclear leukocyte. *Blood* 1980; 55: 338–43.
90. Warschauer D, Goldstein E, Hoeprich P, et al. Effect of vitamin E and ozone on the pulmonary antibacterial defense system. *J Lab Clin Med* 1974; 83: 228–40.

91. Munoz S, Heubi J, Balistreri W, et al. Vitamin E deficiency in primary biliary cirrhosis: gastrointestinal malabsorption, frequency and relationship to other lipid-soluble vitamins. *Hepatology* 1989; 9: 525–31.

92. Sokol R, Balistreri W, Hoofnagle J, et al. Vitamin E deficiency in adults with chronic liver disease. *Am J Clin Nutr* 1985; 41: 66–72.

93. Sitrin M, Lieberman F, Jensen W, et al. Vitamin E deficiency and neurologic disease in adults with cystic fibrosis. *Ann Intern Med* 1987; 107: 51–4.

94. Kowdley K, Meydani S, Cornwall S, et al. Vitamin E deficiency and impaired cellular immunity related to intestinal fat malabsorption. *Gastroenterology* 1992; 102: 2139–42.

95. von Herby A, Stahl W, Niederau C, et al. Diminished plasma levels of vitamin E in patients with severe viral hepatitis. *Free Radic Res* 1996; 25: 461–6.

96. Periquet B, Jammes N, Lambert W, et al. Micronutrient levels in HIV-1 infected children. *AIDS* 1995; 9: 887–93.

97. Stone W. Oxidative stress and antioxidants in premature infants. In: Papas AM, ed. *Antioxidant status, diet, nutrition, and health.* Boca Raton: CRC Press, 1998: 277–97.

98. Miller M. Phagocytic function in the neonate: selected aspects. *Pediatrics* 1979; 64: 5709–12.

99. Vobecky J, Vobecky J, Shapcott D, et al. Nutritional influences on humoral and cell-mediated immunity in healthy infants. *J Am Coll Nutr* 1984; 3: 265.

100. Meydani SN, Meydani M, Verdon CP, Shapiro AC, Blumberg JB, Hayes KC. Vitamin E supplementation suppresses prostaglandin E_2 synthesis and enhances the immune response of aged mice. *Mech Ageing Dev* 1986; 34: 191–201.

101. Reddy P, Morrill J, Minocha H, et al. Vitamin E is immunostimulatory in calves. *J Dairy Sci* 1987; 70: 993–9.

102. Corwin L, Shloss J. Influence of vitamin E on the mitogenic response of murine lymphoid cell. *J Nutr* 1980; 110: 916–23.

103. Beharka AA, Wu D, Han S-N, et al. Macrophage prostaglandin production contributes to the age-associated decrease in T cell function which is reversed by the dietary antioxidant vitamin E. *Mech Ageing Dev* 1997; 94: 157–65.

104. Haq A, Bailey C, Chinnah A. Effect of β-carotene, canthaxanthin, lutein, and vitamin E on neonatal immunity of chicks when supplemented in the broiler breeder diets. *Poult Sci* 1996; 75: 1092–7.

105. Corwin LM, Shloss J. Role of antioxidants on the stimulation the mitogen response. *J Nutr* 1980; 110: 2497–505.

106. Vercammen C, Ceuppens J. Prostaglandin E_2 inhibits T-cell proliferation after crosslinking of the CD3-Ti complex by directly affecting T cells at an early step of the activation process. *Cell Immunol* 1987; 104: 24–36.

107. Nockels C. Protective Effects of supplemental vitamin E against infection. *FASEB J* 1979; 38: 2134–8.

108. Barber T, Nockels C, Jochim M. Vitamin E enhancement of Venezuelan equine encephalomyelitis antibody response in guinea pigs. *Am J Vet Res* 1977; 38: 731–4.

109. Reffett J, Spears J, Brown J. Effect of dietary selenium and vitamin E on the primary and secondary immune response in lambs challenged with parainfluenza virus. *J Anim Sci* 1988; 66: 1520–8.

110. Francini A, Canti M, Manfreda G, Bertuzzi S. Vitamin E as adjuvant in emulsified vaccine for chicks. *Poult Sci* 1991; 70: 1709–15.

111. Baehner RL, Boxer LA, Allen JM, et al. Autooxidation as a basis for altered function by polymorphonuclear leukocytes. *Blood* 1977; 50: 327–35.

112. Meydani SN, Barklund MP, Liu S, et al. Vitamin E supplementation enhances cell-mediated immunity in healthy elderly subjects. *Am J Clin Nutr* 1990; 52: 557–63.

113. Meydani SN, Meydani M, Blumberg JB, et al. Vitamin E supplementation enhances in vivo immune response in healthy elderly subjects: a randomized controlled trial. *JAMA* 1997; 277: 1380–6.

114. Meydani S, Meydani M, Blumberg J, et al. Assessment of the safety of supplementation with different amounts of vitamin E in healthy older adults. *Am J Clin Nutr* 1998; 68: 311–18.

115. Johnson L, Quinn G, Abbasi S, et al. Severe retinopathy of prematurity in infants with birth weights less than 1250 grams: incidence and outcome of treatment with pharmacologic serum levels of vitamin E in addition to cryotherapy from 1985 to 1991. *J Pediatr* 1995; 127: 632–9.

116. Fish W, Cohen M, Franzek D, Williams J, Lemons J. Effect of intramuscular vitamin E on mortality and intracranial hemorrhage in neonates of 1000 grams or less. *Pediatrics* 1990; 85: 578–84.

117. Johnson L, Bowen F, Abbasi S, et al. Relationship of prolonged pharmacologic serum levels of vitamin E to incidence of sepsis and necrotizing enterocolitis in infants with birth weight 1,500 grams or less. *Pediatrics* 1985; 75: 619–37.

118. Sobel S, Gueriguian J, Troendle G. Vitamin E in retrolental fibroplasia. *N Engl J Med* 1982; 306: 867.
119. Finer N, Peters K, Hayek Z, et al. Vitamin E and necrotizing enterocolitis. *Pediatrics* 1984; 73: 387–93.
120. Mino M. Clinical uses and abuses of vitamin E in children. *Proc Soc Exp Biol Med* 1992; 200: 266–70.
121. Chirico G, Marconi M, Colombo A, et al. Deficiency of neutrophil phagocytosis in premature infants: effect of vitamin E supplementation. *Acta Paediatr Scand* 1983; 72: 521–4.
122. Beck M, Kolbeck P, Rohr L, et al. Vitamin E deficiency intensifies the myocardial injury of coxsackievirus B3 infection in mice. *J Nutr* 1994; 124: 345–58.
123. Beck M, Levander O. Dietary oxidative stress and the potentiation of viral infection. *Annu Rev Nutr* 1998; 18: 93–116.
124. Taylor D, Levander O, Krishna V, et al. Vitamin E-deficient diets enriched with fish oil suppress lethal *Plasmodium yoelii* infections in athymic and scid/bg mice. *Infect Immun* 1997; 65: 197–202.
125. Hennet T, Peterhans E, Stocker R. Alterations in antioxidant defenses in lung and liver of mice infected with influenza A virus. *J Gen Virol* 1992; 73: 39–46.
126. Wang Y, Liang B, Watson R. Suppression of tissue levels of vitamin A, E, zinc, and copper in murine AIDS. *Nutr Res* 1994; 14: 1031–41.
127. Kwasniewska A, Tukendorf A, Semczuk M. Content of α-tocopherol in blood serum of human papillomavirus-infected women with cervical dysplasias. *Nutr Cancer* 1997; 28: 248–51.
128. Malvy D-M, Richard M-J, Arnaud J, et al. Relationship of plasma malondialdehyde, vitamin E and antioxidant micronutrients to human immunodeficiency virus-1 seropositivity. *Clin Chim Acta* 1994; 224: 89–94.
129. Tang A, Graham N, Semba R, et al. Association between serum vitamin A and E levels and HIV-1 disease progression. *AIDS* 1997; 11: 613–20.
130. Likoff R, Guptill D, Lawrence L, et al. Vitamin E and aspirin depress prostaglandins in protection of chickens against *Escherichia coli* infection. *Am J Clin Nutr* 1981; 34: 245–51.
131. Smith K, Harrison J, Hancock D, et al. Effect of vitamin E and selenium supplementation on incidence of clinical mastitis and duration of clinical symptoms. *J Dairy Sci* 1984; 67: 1293–300.
132. Stephens LC, NcChesney AE, Nockels CF. Improved recovery of vitamin-E treated lambs that have been experimental infected with intratracheal chlamydia. *Br Vet J* 1979; 135: 291–3.
133. Heinzerling RH, Tengerdy RP, Wick LL, et al. Vitamin E protects mice against *Diplococcus pneumonia* type I infection. *Infect Immun* 1974; 10: 1292–5.
134. Tvedten H, Whitehair C, Langham R. Influence of vitamins A and E on gnotobiotic and conventionally maintained rats exposed to *Mycoplasma pulmonis*. *J Am Vet Med Assoc* 1973; 163: 605–12.
135. Hayek MG, Taylor SF, Bender BS, et al. Vitamin E supplementation decreases lung virus titers in mice infected with influenza. *J Infect Dis* 1997; 176: 273–6.
136. Wang Y, Hwang DS, Licing B, et al. Nutritional status and immune responses in mice with murine AIDS are normalized by vitamin E supplementation. *J Nutr* 1994; 124: 2024–32.
137. Kline K, Sanders B. RRR-α-Tocopheryl succinate enhances T cell mitogen-induced proliferation and reduces suppressor activity in spleen cells derived from AEV-infected chickens. *Nutr Cancer* 1991; 15: 73–85.
138. Harman D, Miller RW. Effect of vitamin E on the immune response to influenza virus vaccine and the incidence of infectious disease in man. *Age* 1986; 9: 21–3.
139. Chandra RK. Effect of vitamin and trace-element supplementation on immune responses and infectious disease in elderly subjects. *Lancet* 1992; 340: 1124–7.
140. Rautalahti M, Virtamo J, Haukka J. The effect of alpha-tocopherol and beta-carotene supplementation on COPD symptoms. *Am J Respir Crit Care Med* 1997; 156: 1447–52.
141. von Herby A, Stahl W, Niederau C, et al. Vitamin E improves the aminotransferase status of patients suffering from viral hepatitis C: a randomized, double-blind, placebo-controlled study. *Free Radic Res* 1997; 27: 599–605.
142. Andreone P, Gramonzi A, Bernardi M. Vitamin E for chronic hepatitis B. Ann *Ann Intern Med* 1998; 128: 156–7.
143. Yurdakök M, Kanra G. Vitamin E in the treatment of viral hepatitis. *Turkish J Pediatr* 1985; 27: 209–12.

DISCUSSION

Dr. Cochran: It has been mentioned many times during this conference that it is uncommon clinically to see isolated nutrient deficiencies. This morning both you and Dr. Chandra have shown not only that nutrient deficiency adversely affects the immune system, but also that excess nutrients can have adverse effects too. I would like your opinion, in a case where an individual is deficient in both iron and vitamin E and only a therapeutic dose of iron is given without supplementing vitamin E, whether that will adversely affect the immune system?

Dr. Meydani: My guess would be yes. If there is vitamin E deficiency, reversing that will be beneficial. However, this has not been well studied.

Dr. Chandra: I think that, with the sole exceptions of iodine, iron, and vitamin A deficiencies, we often deal with multiple nutrient deficiencies as a result of a reduced dietary intake. This applies to all age groups in the elderly. Therefore, for arguments that I have made elsewhere (1–3), I do believe very strongly that supplements of a single nutrient, be it a trace element or a vitamin, sometimes cause more problem than benefit. You never know what other nutrients may become conditionally deficient if you give large amounts of a single nutrient. So, I would be very cautious, particularly in people who are already immunocompromised, of giving very large amounts of one nutrient that may induce problems of absorption, interaction, and requirements of another nutrient.

Dr. Meydani: I do not totally agree with Dr. Chandra's statement because I believe we need to know what particular deficiencies exist, or what nutrients are a problem for specific situations, and deal with these. I think the idea of supplementing the whole range of nutrients for every situation will not really help us in understanding how we need to deal with each situation. So, I think we need to understand better what are the particular nutrient problems that exist in different situations and deal with them directly.

Dr. Zoppi: In a study published in 1982 in the *Journal of Pediatric Gastroenterology and Nutrition* (4), we studied infants fed from birth with soy milk. We showed that T-cell immunity was impaired in those children. We think that could have resulted from a deficiency of vitamin A or zinc because of the presence of phytates. I would like your opinion on that.

Dr. Meydani: I do not believe it has been shown that feeding soy-based formulas or soy protein to animal models causes vitamin A or zinc deficiency.

Dr. Chandra: Earlier soya-based formulas did have problems with zinc absorption, but with the additional amounts of zinc that are currently being used, that is no longer a problem.

Dr. Novelli: The National Institutes of Health is about to start a large vaccination program on elderly patients, giving varicella vaccine to prevent herpes zoster. I might have missed it in your talk, but does vitamin E supplementation in elderly patients prevent zoster or decrease its incidence?

Dr. Meydani: We have not looked at that. Currently, we are doing a large study with 600 nursing home residents, looking at the effect of vitamin E supplementation on infectious disease. Our emphasis is on respiratory infections but we certainly will be looking at other types of infection as well.

Dr. Woodward: With regard to the community-based vitamin A supplementation studies showing decreased childhood mortality, my impression has been that the programs are successful in populations in which protein-energy malnutrition manifests primarily as a stunting disease. Is that true?

Dr. Meydani: My understanding is that the effect was independent of protein-energy malnutrition; in other words, it was also effective in children who were not severely malnourished or who had stunting.

Dr. Kennedy: I think you have a unique opportunity to study a population that is at risk for T-cell immune defects. My comments are more from an immunologist's point of view. We have begun to use our large T-cell model as a mechanism with which to screen micronutrients. Based on your work and that of Dr. Chandra and others, we picked three nutrients: vitamin E, zinc, and vitamin D_3. We have used different stimulants. We looked at the interleukin 2 gene and asked what specifically was going to activate IL-2 gene transcription in humans. We focused on T-cell antigen receptor ligation and whether or not co-stimulatory molecules such as a CD28 or possibly inhibitory molecules such as CTLA4 would be influenced by supplementation with these molecules. Looking at CD3 and CD28 stimulation, we found that vitamin E actually suppressed IL-2 and did not increase it, but when we applied stimulation, such as with phytohemagglutinin (PHA), there was an increase in comparison with controls. Thus, the IL-2 response generated by vitamin E plus PHA was augmented compared with control plus PHA. We found IL-2 levels consistent with yours, from 100 to 200 pg/ml per culture. When we looked at anti-CD3 cross-linking and anti-CD3 with co-stimulation with CD28, we found that vitamin E was actually inhibitory compared with control; we had IL-2 levels of about 900 pg/ml per culture, but when we added vitamin E, we got about 300 to 400 pg/ml. We hypothesized that vitamin E may be actually affecting the response by activating PI3 kinase. Therefore, we started looking at CTLA4 interactions, as PI3 kinase is clearly involved with CTLA4, maybe as a shut-off mechanism. When we used cross-linking with CTL4 along with anti-CD3, we found that vitamin E was probably having its effect by activating PI3 kinase, because we found an even more pronounced inhibition of IL-2. Do you think that in this situation vitamin E may be playing a role in augmenting immune response by attenuating some of these reactions?

Dr. Meydani: Certainly. I did not have time to go into the mechanism-related work that we have done. It is interesting that you see suppression in your large T-cell model. I wonder if that is something specific to the particular cell, because we have done studies with purified T cells from mice looking at anti-CD3 and anti-CD28 and certainly in that situation we see an enhancement similar to what we see with PHA. In purified T cells from both young and old animals, there was an enhancement with vitamin E, so I am curious to the reason for the difference. Like you, we hypothesized that vitamin E, as well as inhibiting prostaglandin formation by macrophages which is one way of enhancing T-cell function, has some direct effect on the T cells by affecting signal transduction or perhaps by affecting nuclear transcription factors. In some other cell lines, in fibroblasts for example, vitamin E has been shown to affect AP1 activation.

Dr. Kennedy: I agree. Our cell lines do not express CTLA4 to any large extent, so we need to transfect them and get them to express CTLA4. They have already been exposed to a plasmid *pathogen*, so there may be some influences there. We have only begun to look at gene transcription. My next question: In your isolated cells do you see activation of transcriptional regulators?

Dr. Meydani: We have not got that far. So far, we have just demonstrated an effect occurs on purified T cells. That is the next step.

Dr. Kennedy: Have you stimulated your cells with things like anti-CD3?

Dr. Meydani: Yes, that is what we have done. We used anti-CD3 and then anti-CD3 in combination with anti-CD28, which is where we actually see an increase in proliferation. That is interesting, because in other transformed cell lines vitamin E does inhibit proliferation. If you look at fibroblasts, for example, it inhibits proliferation. I think it has to do with the type of cell. When we test purified T cells using the same stimuli, we see enhancement.

Dr. Coovadia: I want to comment on your reference to a study on the return of delayed hypersensitivity and vitamin A in measles (5–6). The point I want to make is that when you choose the wrong test and do it at the wrong time you will get the wrong result. There is no question in my mind that vitamin A is useful in measles. So the question is, what tests do you do? That study tested delayed hypersensitivity, but delayed hypersensitivity correlates very poorly with outcome in measles. Furthermore, the test was done at 2 weeks, and it takes about 6 weeks for the immune response and its various manifestations to return to normal after measles.

Dr. Meydani: I totally agree. Thank you for pointing that out.

Dr. Keusch: In some of the vitamin A studies that showed no effect of supplementation, I wonder if that was because there was no effect of vitamin A, or because vitamin E had a significant effect and was used as the control.

Dr. Meydani: I was surprised at those results. It seems that in the vitamin A field nobody is aware of what vitamin E does to immune function! I was disturbed to see it being used as a placebo; although the levels were low, they were certainly high enough to have an effect. That is an excellent point and needs to be pursued.

REFERENCES

1. Chandra RK. Nutrition, immunity and infection: from basic knowledge of dietary manipulation of immune responses to practical application of amelioration suffering and improving survival. *Proc Natl Acad Sci USA* 1996; 93: 14304–7.
2. Denduluri S, Chandra RK. Effects of cadmium and zinc and other interactions on immune responses. *Immuno Infect Dis* 1996; 6: 113–9.
3. Chandra RK. Nutrition and the immune system. *Am J Clin Nutr* 1997; 66: 460–3S.
4. Zoppi G, Gerosa F, Pezzini A, et al. Immunocompetence and dietary protein intake in early infancy. *J Pediatr Gastroenterol Nutr* 1982; 1: 175–82.
5. Coovadia HM, Wesley A, Brain P, et al. Immunoparesis and outcome in measles. *Lancet* 1977; 1: 619–21.
6. Coovadia HM, Wesley A, Brain P. Immunological events in acute measles influencing outcome. *Arch Dis Child* 1978; 53: 861–7.

Nutrition, Immunity, and Infection in Infants and Children, edited by Robert M. Suskind and Kraisid Tontisirin. Nestlé Nutrition Workshop Series, Pediatric Program, Vol. 45. Nestec Ltd., Vevey/Lippincott Williams & Wilkins, Philadelphia ©2001.

Eating Disorders (Obesity, Anorexia Nervosa, Bulimia Nervosa), Immunity, and Infection

A. Marcos, A. Montero, S. López-Varela, and *G. Morandé

*Instituto de Nutrición y Bromatología, Facultad de Farmacia, Ciudad Universitaria, Madrid, Spain; and *Servicio de Psiquiatría Infantil, Hospital del Niño Jesús, Madrid, Spain*

IN PURSUIT OF A DESIRABLE WEIGHT

Obesity, anorexia nervosa, and bulimia nervosa are significant public health concerns affecting a large section of the population; they are even considered to be epidemics. These disorders have a common problem—the failure to maintain a desirable weight. Treatment focused on making obese people thin is clearly not working and might even cause more harm than good (1). Many obese people give up attempting to lose weight because most of them fail in their efforts to achieve and maintain their desired weight (2). At the other extreme, overemphasis on thinness is contributing to an increasing incidence of anorexia nervosa and bulimia nervosa (3), which can present greater risks than obesity. The desired weight goal of patients with anorexia nervosa and bulimia is very far from the ideal body weight, and the medical complications of these conditions can ultimately be very serious.

OBESITY

Obesity, defined as an excess of body fat relative to lean body mass, is the consequence of a chronic imbalance between energy intake and energy expenditure; evidence also indicates that obese people have an increased tendency to deposit dietary fat as body fat (4). A high intake of fat may be important in both the cause and the maintenance of obesity; in fact, obese individuals have a preference for eating fatty foods and they consume a higher proportion of fat in their diets than normal weight individuals (5). Despite this well-defined cause of obesity, it is not yet clearly established whether the main abnormality responsible for the increase in body fatness is a chronic excess intake of energy, a defect in energy expenditure, or perhaps a combination of both (6).

Obesity can be classified in a clinically useful way according to the body mass index (BMI) (7): grade 0, BMI 20 to 24.9 (normal weight); grade I, BMI 25 to 29.9; grade II, BMI 30 to 40; grade III, BMI more than 40.

The BMI range of 20 to 24.9, classified as normal, coincides well with the normal mortality ratio derived from the Metropolitan Life Insurance tables (8). The mortality ratio begins to increase at BMI levels above 25, at which point health professionals should be concerned. Although the increase in mortality in grade I is not great, it is of importance because it is transitional to grades II and III, which create more serious health risks for the individual (5).

ANOREXIA NERVOSA

Anorexia nervosa is a syndrome that includes three particular features: a marked fear of fatness, a disturbed perception of body size (body image), and an obsessive desire to lose increasing amounts of weight (9). Other symptoms and characteristics of this disorder are shown in Table 1. Anorexia as such is not usually associated with the syndrome of anorexia nervosa, and appetite in this condition remains normal or is even increased until late in the course of the illness (10).

BULIMIA NERVOSA

As in anorexia nervosa, patients with bulimia pursue thinness. However, in bulimia the distinguishing feature is binge eating, which is the rapid consumption of a large quantity of food in a short period of time, usually less than 2 hours, invariably followed by purging. Table 1 summarizes the main features of patients with bulimia nervosa according to the fourth edition of the *Diagnostic and Statistical Manual of Mental Disorders* (DSM-IV) (11).

Anorexia nervosa and bulimia nervosa are psychiatric illnesses characterized by abnormal eating patterns. People with these disorders respond in a different way from normal individuals to the macronutrient content of food (fat, carbohydrate, and protein). These abnormal responses seem to reflect the development of particular attitudes toward the macronutrient profiles of foods (12).

INTERACTIONS BETWEEN NUTRITION, IMMUNITY, AND INFECTION

The complexity of the interactions between nutrition, immunity, and infection is well recognized (13). Nutrients are known to play an important role in the appropriate maintenance of the immune mechanisms involved in host defense systems (14).

Epidemiologic data also suggest that the incidence and severity of infectious illness are higher in obese than in nonobese individuals (15). The mechanisms respon-

TABLE 1. *DSM-IV diagnostic criteria for anorexia nervosa and bulimia nervosa*

Anorexia nervosa	Bulimia nervosa
A. Refusal to maintain body weight over a minimally normal weight for age and height (*e.g.,* weight loss leading to maintenance of body weight 15% below that expected), or failure to make expected weight gain during period of growth, leading to body weight below 15% of that expected. B. Intense fear of gaining weight or becoming fat, even though underweight. C. Disturbance in the way in which one's body weight or shape is experienced, undue influence of body shape and weight on self-evaluation, or denial of the seriousness of current low body weight. D. In postmenarchal females, amenorrhea (i.e., the absence of at least three consecutive menstrual cycles). (A woman is considered to have amenorrhea if her periods occur only following hormone, *e.g.,* estrogen administration.) Restricting type: During the episode of anorexia nervosa, the person does not regularly engage in binge eating or purging behavior (i.e., self-induced vomiting or the misuse of laxatives or diuretics). Binge eating/purging type: During the episode of anorexia nervosa, the person regularly engages in binge eating or purging behavior (*i.e.,* self-induced vomiting or the misuse of laxatives or diuretics).	A. Recurrent episodes of binge eating. An episode of binge eating is characterized by both of the following: 1. Eating in a discrete period of time (*e.g.,* within any 2-hour period), an amount of food that is definitely larger than most people would eat in a similar period of time in similar circumstances; and, 2. A sense of lack of control over eating during the episode (*e.g.,* a feeling that one cannot stop eating or control what or how much one is eating). B. Recurrent inappropriate compensatory behavior to prevent weight gain, such as self-induced vomiting; misuse of laxatives, diuretics, or other medications; fasting; or excessive exercise. C. The binge eating and inappropriate compensatory behaviors both occur, on average, at least twice a week for 3 months. D. Self-evaluation is unduly influenced by body shape and weight. E. The disturbance does not occur exclusively doing episodes of anorexia nervosa. Purging type: The person regularly engages in self-induced vomiting or the misuse of laxatives or diuretics. Nonpurging type: The person uses other inappropriate compensatory behaviours (e.g., fasting or excessive exercise), but does not regularly engage in self-induced vomiting or the misuse of laxatives or diuretics.

DSM-IV, Diagnostic and Statistical Manual of Mental Disorders, 4th ed.

sible for the increased risk of infection and altered immunity among obese persons are unknown but they may be linked to the effects of hyperglycemia, hyperinsulinemia, and hyperlipidemia on the glucose uptake and function of certain immune cells (16). Obesity can promote the development of diabetes, which can also alter the immune state (17).

It is also necessary, however, to take into account the fact that weight reducing diets are the most common treatment for obesity and, therefore, most obese persons are subjected to energy restricted diets. The effects of such restricted diets on immunocompetence have not been widely reported, which is the reason why the effects of weight reduction on immunity are still disputed (18). Some investigators have speculated that a decrease in nutrient intake during weight loss might explain subsequent

TABLE 2. *Body mass indices (in kg/m²) frequently used to define desirable and obese weights in adults*

Source	Recommended*		Overweight or obese†	
	Males	Females	Males	Females
Metropolitan Life 1959‡	22.0	21.5	26.4	25.8
Metropolitan Life 1983‡	22.7	22.4	27.2	26.9
NHANES I§	24.5	23.0	—	—
NHANES II§	24.3	23.2	27.8	27.3
NHANES III§	24.9	24.1	—	—
Guidelines for Americans‖				
<35	19–25	19–25	—	—
>35	21–27	21–27	—	—
US Army¶	—	—		
17–20	—	—	25.8	22.8
21–27	—	—	26.4	23.5
28–39	—	—	27.1	24.1
>40	—	—	27.5	24.9

* Midpoint of desirable range for Metropolitan Life Insurance height and weight tables in 1959 and 1983; 50th percentile for NHANES (National Health and Nutrition Examination Survey) I, II, and III, phase 1; and healthy weights in the dietary guidelines for Americans.

† One hundred twenty percent of midpoint for Metropolitan Life Insurance tables in 1959 and 1983, 85th percentile for NHANES II, and discharge weights for obesity by the US Army, provided certain fat percentages are not met.

‡ Metropolitan Life Insurance, 1959;1983.

§ Kuczmarski *et al.* (1994), *JAMA* 272:205–11.

‖ Linsted *et al.* (1991), *Int J Obes Relat Metab Disord* 15:397–06; US Department of Health and Human Services, (1989)

¶ BMIs Friedl *et al.* (1989), *Army Res Inst Environ Med.*

changes in immune function (15). Diets for weight reduction should optimally provide adequate amounts of all necessary nutrients except energy. It is very difficult, however, to maintain an adequate intake of micronutrients with energy intakes below 1,000 kcal/d unless supplements are provided (15).

Weight reduction, if adequate, has been reported to restore immunity in obese persons, although other effects secondary to the diet itself, or to stress during a very low energy diet, cannot be excluded (16).

Obese individuals have underlying impairment of lymphocyte responsiveness, although this can be reversed with adequate weight reduction. In those who are obese, this impairment, in conjunction with the risks incurred by a restricted diet (19), can cause further deterioration in immune function and ultimately produce manifestations of disease (20).

By contrast, many reports have suggested that anorexic patients, even though severely malnourished, remain relatively free of infectious disease (21) and show an unexpectedly high resistance to malignancy (22), at least until they enter the advanced stages of debilitation (23).

On the basis of various clinical observations, an association between refeeding and infection (24) has been suggested, in that starvation may suppress and refeeding may activate certain infections. The fact that the usual anorectic diet is deficient in carbohydrate and energy while being relatively sufficient in protein and fat (25) could explain the apparently low likelihood of infection, with only a moderate deficiency of copper, zinc, and iron-binding proteins, and, rarely, vitamin deficiency (26). These conditions, therefore, are different from primary protein-energy malnutrition, although affected individuals have been classed as being "relatively protein-calorie malnourished" (27).

Studies of immune function of patients suffering from eating disorders have shown them to have multiple impairments similar to those occurring in simple malnutrition (27,28). Thus, although some of the immune impairments found in anorexia nervosa are similar to those observed in primary malnutrition, they are less common and less severe, and immune function seems to be better preserved than would be expected, considering the highly undernourished state of these individuals (29). The difference between simple starvation and anorexia nervosa may reflect the individual variability in the micronutrient and macronutrient intake in the latter (22).

CHANGES IN THE IMMUNE SYSTEM

Nutrient excesses and deficits affect immune responses both directly and indirectly through their effects on metabolism (17). It is also important to take into account that both obesity (30) and anorexia nervosa or bulimia (29) are associated with increased plasma cortisol. Epidemiological, clinical, and experimental evidence now indicate that obesity, weight reduction treatment for obesity, and anorexia nervosa and bulimia are all associated with impairment of immune function, although this has received relatively little attention. The results, however, are controversial (15,31,32).

Obesity and dieting are associated with altered intake and metabolism of nutrients that are known to affect immune responses (6,14,15). Although B- and T-lymphocyte counts, polymorphonuclear (neutrophil) phagocytosis, and serum immunoglobulins and complement components have been found to be normal in obese adolescents, impaired delayed type hypersensitivity (DTH) testing responses, mitogen-stimulated proliferation, and bactericidal capacity of neutrophil phagocytosis have been reported in more than 30% of these individuals (14). The impaired immune function in obesity could be a result of micronutrient deficiencies, even when relatively mild (17). A high prevalence of vitamin deficiency, especially of the antioxidant vitamins, has been found in obese women (33). However, immune responses can be enhanced in obese children on supplementation (34).

With respect to anorexia nervosa and bulimia, little information is presently available on alterations to the immune system, and the results obtained so far suggest a large between-patient variability in the effects of these disorders on immune response (32).

These observations imply that the protocol used for restricting energy intake or refeeding, depending on the pathology, can affect many variables. This shows the importance of investigating the interactions between metabolic, biochemical, and immunologic factors with respect to diet, weight loss or gain, and, most importantly, nutritional status (35).

In addition, nutritional and neuroendocrine status are among the factors likely to be involved in modulation of immune responses, both in obesity, as a result of dieting and weight reduction during obesity treatment (15), and in patients with anorexia nervosa because of their abnormal eating behavior (22).

IMMUNOCOMPETENT CELLS

Immunocompetent cell populations are well known to be affected by nutritional status, and either an excess or a deficient dietary intake, as in dieting to lose weight or refeeding to gain weight, can affect their number and function.

Obesity has been related to higher blood cell counts of total leukocytes, neutrophils, lymphocytes, and monocytes; these have been identified as independent risk factors for cardiovascular disease and cancer (36). Thus, decreases in numbers of these cells with weight loss could be interpreted as being consistent with lowered risk status. In fact, a decrease in total leukocyte, neutrophil, lymphocyte, and monocyte counts has been found in obese subjects during dietary treatment or following weight loss, although this is relatively modest. However, these altered white blood cell values are not outside the normal range (18,36), and no changes have been found in the leukocyte pattern of obese subjects after the ninth week on a very low energy diet or by the end of the program (37).

Studies of immune function in anorexia nervosa and bulimia nervosa, on the other hand, have provided additional information on the immunologic consequences of long-term dietary energy deficits and large weight losses in humans. Although it is currently accepted that hematologic values in patients suffering from these syndromes are within the normal range, studies on immunohematologic variables suggest an aberrant immunologic status (32). Thus, low values have been found in anorexia nervosa, and a tendency is seen to leukopenia together with a relative lymphocytosis in both anorexia nervosa (27) and bulimia, especially when the diagnosis is delayed (> 3.5 years) (28). However, when the diagnosis of bulimia nervosa is early (< 1.5 years), neither an alteration in the neutrophil or monocyte counts nor a relative lymphocytosis occurs. Nevertheless, lymphocyte counts are lower than in controls, which is a sign that malnutrition is occurring in the bulimia patients (38). It is important, therefore, to diagnose such patients early to lessen the likelihood of their becoming seriously malnourished and to avoid prolonged damage to their immunocompetent cells (32).

IMPLICATION OF LYMPHOCYTE SUBSETS IN THE DETECTION OF SUBCLINICAL SITUATIONS OF MALNUTRITION

The percentage of T-helper (CD4) cells has been shown to decrease in obese dieters at weeks 4 and 6 of dieting (370 kcal/d), with no change in the number of T suppressor (CD8) cells; this outcome results in a fall in the CD4:CD8 ratio. On refeeding, however, the percentage of T-helper cells and the CD4:CD8 ratio return to baseline values (18). Nevertheless, normal CD4$^+$ counts have been reported in obese subjects after 6 months of dieting (800 kcal/d for 3 months followed by 3 months of food rein-troduction). Although the numbers and percentage of CD8 lymphocytes in obese di-eters do not differ significantly from the values in controls, significant decreases oc-cur during and after dieting, reaching levels below controls at the end of the study period (39). One of the lymphocyte subsets that is most affected by dieting is the nat-ural killer (NK) cells, which do not return to prerestriction levels after refeeding on an adequate dietary energy intake (40).

In contrast to other types of starvation characterized by low $CD4^+$ counts (14), however, some investigators have found normal $CD4^+$ counts in patients with anorexia nervosa and suggest that this could explain the lack of increased infection risk in affected individuals (39).

Cytofluorometric studies of immune function do not show a significant impair-ment of the immune system in adolescents admitted to the hospital for anorexia ner-vosa (29). On the other hand, significant reductions in the numbers of T lymphocytes and CD4, CD8, and CD57 cells have been found in comparison with controls (41,42). Some of these differences could be explained by the characteristics of the populations chosen for study, reflecting variations in age and the duration of illness. It is very im-portant to take into account not only the degree of malnutrition in the patient but also the evolution of the illness, the time after diagnosis, and whether the patient has re-ceived adequate treatment (32).

In early studies, no modifications in CD4 cells were observed in outpatients suf-fering from anorexia nervosa who had received inadequate treatment at the onset of the illness. However, the CD8 subset was increased, leading to a lower CD4:CD8 ratio (27), which is considered to be an index of malnutrition (43). On the other hand, in a 1 year follow-up study of patients diagnosed early, admitted to the hos-pital, and submitted to both psychiatric and nutritional therapy from the onset of the illness, the CD4:CD8 ratio remained unmodified in comparison with controls, even though the numbers of CD2, CD3, CD4, CD8, and CD57 cells were lower than in the control group. However, an increase in CD2, CD3, and CD4 subsets was ob-served after the period of hospital admission (which lasted ~1 month), although curiously this was less when the patients had been living at home for a month (41) (Fig. 1).

Naive cells have been shown to be particularly sensitive to malnutrition (42). Thus, a reduction in naive $CD4^+CD45RA^+$ cells and an increase in cytotoxic $CD8^+$ cells have been reported in patients with anorexia nervosa (age range 14 to 18 years) by Allende et al. (44). According to these investigators, although the $CD4^+$ subset is al-tered in malnourished patients with anorexia nervosa (BMI < 17.5), the percentage of $CD4^+$ cells increases after refeeding when the patients tested have a BMI greater than 17.5; the increase particularly involves naive $CD4^+CD45RA^+$ cells, with no significant change in the memory $(CD^+CD45RO^+)$ cells. Obviously the $CD45RA^+:CD45RO^+$ ratio reached its lowest value in the group with a BMI of less than 17.5. The CD4:CD8 ratio was also particularly reduced in the patients with the lowest BMI (< 17.5), although higher values were restored when BMI increased to more than 17.5, becoming similar to controls.

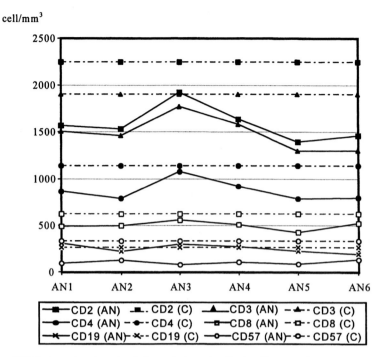

FIG. 1. Lymphocyte subsets in controls and patients with anorexia nervosa.

As mentioned, it is important to specify the age range of the patients tested. Thus, in patients with anorexia nervosa (aged between 14 and 42 years), with a great variation in duration of illness (from 1 to 21 years), the most affected cells were memory $CD4^+$ and $CD8^+$ ($CD45RO^+RA^-$) cells, which increased after refeeding. This finding could be related to the perceived lack of common viral infections in underweight anorexic patients, and their return with weight recovery (45). In our research group, we consider the development of a febrile illness during hospital treatment of anorexia to be a sign of improvement and a reason for congratulating the patient (32).

With regard to bulimia, CD2 and CD4 counts have been shown to be reduced by 39% and 56%, respectively, compared with control in patients with illnesses lasting 3.5 years or more and with a normal BMI (28). This might reflect a deterioration in cell-mediated immunity (43). However, CD8 levels have been found to be unaltered, so the CD4:CD8 ratio reaches values below 57% of those in the controls. If the disease evolves over a shorter time course (<1.5 years), the CD4:CD8 ratio appears to be within the normal range, although the lymphocyte subsets show lower values than in controls (41). Vomiting has also been shown to affect lymphocyte subsets (38) (Fig. 2).

As well as the T-lymphocyte subset count findings cited above, it is important to take into account thymocyte function in these eating disorders, which will depend on weight fluctuation, diet restriction, and malnutrition status.

Unstimulated and mitogen-stimulated proliferation of lymphocytes decreases significantly in obese dieters after being on a 6-week, all protein, very low energy diet (370 kcal/d), and except for the response to one mitogen combination, this returns to baseline on refeeding (18). A decrease in the intracellular incorporation of [³H]-thymidine on stimulation of T lymphocytes with either phytohemagglutinin or concanavalin A (Con A) has been found in obese subjects compared with nonobese controls, with an increase in T-lymphocyte response to both these mitogens after weight reduction (16). Similarly, a significantly lower phytohemagglutinin-stimulated proliferative response has been reported in obese than in nonobese children and adolescents (34). However, exercise may enhance the impaired immune system in obese persons, and it has been reported that exercise reverses the impaired mitogen-stimulated lymphocyte proliferation and NK-cell activity in obese Zucker rats (46).

Delayed type hypersensitivity test responses to six antigens in obese dieters were not affected by the diet, although a trend was seen toward an increase in the size of the cutaneous response (18). However, in a study carried out in middle-aged obese women before and 2 months after a weight loss of 21 kg achieved over a 6 month period, reduced cutaneous responses were found after the weight loss. The change in DTH response may be directly related to changes in BMI (the more weight lost, the greater the decrease in average induration size). This outcome suggests that large

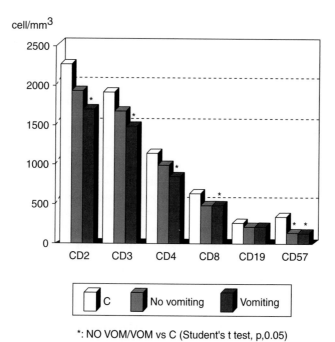

*: NO VOM/VOM vs C (Student's t test, p,0.05)

FIG. 2. Lymphocyte subsets in controls and patients with bulimia with and without vomiting.

weight losses in obese persons result in a decrease in the functional capacity of the cell-mediated immune system (15). An impairment of the cutaneous DTH responses has been found by other investigators (36). Nevertheless, according to Chandra and Kutty (34), all the obese patients tested in their study showed a DTH response to at least one antigen.

When the DTH response to seven recall antigens was determined in overweight women after energy restriction, following a high fat or a low fat diet, no changes were found (40). According to the authors of that paper, the reason was likely to be that the women were all healthy, which is the reason why it is important to stress that prolonged or drastic energy restriction should obviously be supervised by physicians.

Similar hemagglutination inhibition titers against different viral antigens (and in the tuberculin test) have been found in patients with anorexia nervosa in comparison with a control group (47). A normal reactive skin test response has been reported in anorexic patients where *Candida albicans* was one of the five antigens used (48). Likewise, cellular immune function (evaluated by means of an anergy panel including candida, streptokinase/streptodornase, and mumps antigens) has been shown to be preserved in patients suffering from anorexia nervosa until weight loss is far advanced (23). However, reduced cutaneous reactions against other antigens have been reported (21). Our group (49) observed reduced responses to a delayed hypersensitivity skin test in patients with anorexia nervosa and bulimia compared with a control population (839 women aged from 16 to 25 years): it seemed that the most severe impairment of the cellular immunity occurred in patients with bulimia; however, this could be a reflection of the longer period of illness in the bulimia patients (3.75 years) in comparison with the anorexia nervosa patients (1.77 years).

Cell-mediated immunologic reaction to stimulation, as expressed by T-lymphocyte proliferative response to the phytohemagglutinin stimulus, seems to be well preserved in anorexic patients, as an unmodified T-lymphocyte proliferative response is seen to this stimulus, both under basal conditions and after the acute administration of corticotropin-releasing hormone in comparison with a control group (22). This is in contrast with the blunted responses observed in simple starvation (43) and might be one of the factors explaining the resistance to infection and malignancy observed in patients with anorexia nervosa (22).

The basis of these contradictory results could be qualitative nutritional differences reflecting different degrees of malnutrition. Patients with anorexia nervosa, although severely malnourished, usually have a relatively well-preserved protein intake (22), and it is well known that in primary malnutrition the blunted proliferative response to mitogens is related more to protein deficiency than to a globally reduced energy intake (18).

CYTOKINE REGULATION AND THE IMMUNE RESPONSE

Cytokines are modulated by nutrients and their participation is essential in triggering certain mechanisms involved in the infection process (50). Interesting data suggest that expression of at least one cytokine, tumor necrosis factor (TNF), is affected by adiposity. Thus, increased expression of TNF mRNA in adipocytes from fat biopsies has been found in obese subjects, possibly related to the degree of adiposity. Interestingly, the levels of TNF mRNA fall consistently with a reduction in body weight (51). It is important to stress that obese subjects do not comprise a homogeneous group and significant differences can be found, depending on the degree of adiposity, the distribution of body fat (which is affected by sex), and the origin of the obesity (17).

The Interrelationship Between Leptin and Cytokines in Obesity

Leptin, the protein encoded by the ob gene, is known to regulate appetite and energy expenditure. Obese (ob/ob) mice fail to produce leptin and show hyperphagia, decreased energy expenditure, and obesity. When such mice are treated with recombinant leptin, their food intake decreases and they lose weight (31).

An interrelation is also seen between cytokines and leptin levels. Thus, exogenous leptin has been reported to stimulate phagocytic function and activate macrophages to produce proinflammatory cytokines, such as TNF-α, interleukin (IL)-6, and IL-12 in ob/ob mice (31). This implies a novel function for leptin as an upregulating factor in inflammatory immune responses.

In addition, ob/ob mice are known to show increased sensitivity to endotoxin-induced liver injury and lethality, suggesting a potential link between leptin deficiency and the dysregulated expression of endotoxin inducible cytokines (52).

In a recent hypothesis of body weight control and the regulation of metabolism, it has been established that adipocytes secrete leptin, a molecule that has a secondary cytokine structure correlating with the amount of fat tissue. In addition, adipocytes express TNF-α locally, which also reduces lipoprotein lipase activity in white adipocytes. Moreover, increased leptin levels downregulate appetite and increase sympathetic activity and thermogenesis in the hypothalamus. Diet-induced weight loss reduces adipose TNF-α expression and serum leptin levels (53).

Cytokine Changes in Anorexia Nervosa

Lymphocytes of anorectic patients have been shown to display major functional defects related to cytokines (54). Thus, an impairment of lymphocyte production of interferon has been reported during protein starvation (55). However, no substantial differences in the 2'-5' oligoisoadenylate synthetase activity or interferon system activation have been reported in anorexia nervosa patients in comparison with healthy controls on a regular diet (56).

It is important to stress that infection-induced malnutrition, the most common form of cytokine-induced malnutrition, results from the actions of proinflammatory cytokines (TNF, IL-1, IL-6), which are capable of activating the hypothalamic-pituitary-adrenal axis (57). These cytokines are known to be capable of initiating an acute phase reaction that is stereotyped, including loss of appetite (35), fever, cellular hypermetabolism, and multiple endocrine and enzyme responses (58) (Fig. 3). How-

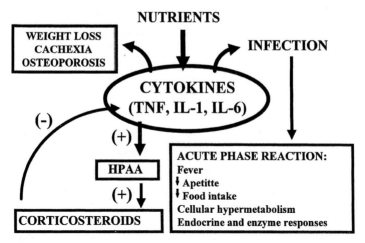

FIG. 3. Interrelations among cytokines, nutrients, and infection.

ever, we are reporting specific types of malnutrition here, and patients with anorexia nervosa and bulimia do not show the same stereotyped reaction observed in infection-induced malnutrition.

Synthesis of TNF has been found to be inhibited in anorexia nervosa (56). The lack of detectable levels of TNF-α in the serum of anorexic patients could be a result of the short plasma half-life of this cytokine (54). Others have reported raised TNF-α levels when lean body mass is depleted (59), and then normalizes after weight gain (35,56).

The production of IL-1 has been shown to be impaired in protein-energy malnutrition (60); however, synthesis of IL-1, whether spontaneous or after lipopolysaccharide stimulation, has not been found to differ significantly between patients with anorexia nervosa and a control group (61). The clinical significance of such *in vitro* laboratory observations is unclear, as patients with anorexia nervosa tend to be free of infectious disease, at least until they enter the advanced stage of debilitation (41).

Transforming growth factor-β (TGF-β) is an anti-inflammatory cytokine that can act as a brake on the immune system and suppress immune responses (10) by inhibiting proinflammatory cytokine-induced immunologic or inflammatory processes. As a persistent state of hypercortisolism is found in anorexia nervosa (29) and as glucocorticoids may trigger TGF-β production and release (62), the undetectable serum levels of TNF-α found in some studies (54) may be explained by the actions of TGF-β. This could be the reason why immunosuppression is one of the characteristics of patients with eating disorders.

Raised serum IL-6 concentrations have been found in patients with anorexia nervosa, which may partially be attributable to the increased TGF-β levels (54). IL-6 has been detected in high concentrations in the serum of some tumor-bearing animals with cancer-associated cachexia (63). Interrelations exist between IL-6 and other cytokines: not only is IL-6 capable of modulating IL-1 (64), but the release of IL-6 is also modulated by a variety of stimuli, including cytokines such as IL-1 (65), TNF-α, and TGF-β (66). In addition, IL-6 has been shown to play a major role in the pathogenesis of postmenopausal osteoporosis (66). Thus, a raised IL-6 concentration could contribute to osteoporosis in anorexia nervosa (54).

Phytohemagglutinin-stimulated peripheral blood mononuclear cells from patients with anorexia nervosa show a lower capacity to produce IL-2 than cells obtained from healthy subjects. However, an enhanced stimulatory effect of the patients' serum has been shown on the secretion of IL-2 by blood mononuclear cells from healthy controls (61). This supports the hypothesis that the patients' plasma not only contains inhibitors of immune function but also sufficient nutrients to sustain a normal lymphocyte transformation response (22). This is the reason why the presence of a stimulation factor in the serum of patients with anorexia nervosa has been suggested, which could compensate for the reduced capacity of their own peripheral blood mononuclear cells to produce IL-2. Such a mechanism provides a relatively normal immune response and could explain why patients with anorexia nervosa are not susceptible to infections despite reduced cytokine production by their peripheral blood mononuclear cells (61).

CONCLUSIONS

Because of the controversial results in published reports, research in this field should be focused on groups of patients who are as homogeneous as possible. Thus, any studies in this area should be undertaken only after careful selection of patients on the basis of their age at the time of study and at the onset of the disorder; their psychological and physiologic characteristics; and the duration of the appropriate treatment and the illness. Furthermore, as there are different types of anorexia nervosa and bulimia, different degrees of obesity, and different applications of very low energy diets, the frequency and length of weight fluctuations must be taken into account because of their important role in prognosis, disease evolution, and cure.

In this chapter, we have tried to update research related to immunocompetent cells and cytokines involved in infectious processes. Although the literature consulted has been vast, assessment of correlations between the immune system and other systems in the organism, such as the central nervous system and the endocrine system, would be of great interest in exploring the mechanisms involved (Fig. 4). This information could be important in determining appropriate therapy and avoiding lengthy treatments that may even interfere with the possibility of early recovery from these eating disorders. Professionals involved in the field should take into account the fact that anorexia nervosa and bulimia, and very often obesity, are psychological disorders that result in adverse somatic consequences, causing chaos throughout the organism. Thus, both psychotherapy and pharmacotherapy should be used appropriately according to what is known about the psychological characteristics of these disorders but also about the disturbances in function related particularly to their neuroendocrine and immunologic effects.

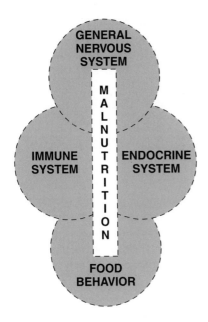

FIG. 4. Interactions among the central nervous, endocrine, and immune systems in situations of malnutrition.

REFERENCES

1. Abernathy RP, Black DR. Healthy body weights: an alternative perspective. *Am J Clin Nutr* 1996; 63: 448–51S.
2. Wooley SC, Garner DM. Obesity treatment: the high cost of false hope. *J Am Diet Assoc* 1991; 91: 1248–51.
3. Brownell KD. Dieting and the search for the perfect body: where physiology and culture collide. *Behav Ther* 1991; 22: 1–12.
4. Thomas CD, Peters JC, Reed GW, Abumrad NA, Sun M, Hill JO. Nutrient balance and energy expenditure during "ad libitum" feeding of high-fat and high carbohydrate diets in humans. *Am J Clin Nutr* 1992; 55: 934–42.
5. Pi-Sunyer FX. Obesity. In: Shils ME, Olson JA, Shike M, eds. *Modern nutrition in health and disease*. Philadelphia: Lea and Febiger, 1994: 984–1006.
6. Saris WHM. Physical inactivity and metabolic factors as predictors of weight gain. *Nutr Rev* 1996; 54: 110–15S.
7. Garrow JS. *Treat obesity seriously*. Edinburgh: Churchill Livingstone, 1981: 3.
8. Metropolitan Life Insurance Company. Metropolitan height and weight tables. *Stat Bull Metrop Insur Co* 1983; 64: 2–9.
9. American Psychiatric Association. *Diagnostic and statistical manual of mental disorders*, 3rd ed. Washington DC: American Psychiatric Association Press, 1987.
10. Comerci GD. Medical complications of anorexia nervosa and bulimia nervosa. *Med Clin North Am* 1990; 74: 1293–310.
11. American Psychiatric Association. *Diagnostic and statistical manual of mental disorders*, 4th ed. Washington DC: American Psychiatric Association Press, 1994.
12. Drewnowski A, Pierce B, Halmi KA. Fat aversion in eating disorders. *Appetite* 1988; 10: 119–31.
13. Scrimshaw NS, SanGiovanni JP. Synergism of nutrition, infection, and immunity: an overview. *Am J Clin Nutr* 1997; 66: 464–77S.
14. Chandra RK. Nutrition and the immune system: an introduction. *Am J Clin Nutr* 1997; 66: 460–3S.
15. Stallone DD. The influence of obesity and its treatment on the immune system. *Nutr Rev* 1994; 52: 37–50.
16. Tanaka S, Inoue S, Isoda F, et al. Impaired Immunity in obesity: suppressed but reversible lymphocyte responsiveness. *Int J Obes Relat Metab Disord* 1993; 17: 631–6.

17. Keith ME, Jeejeebhoy KN. Immunonutrition. *Baillieres Clin Endocrinol Metab* 1997; 11: 709–38.
18. Field CJ, Gougeon R, Marliss Eb. Changes in circulating leukocytes and mitogen response during very-low-energy all-protein reducing diets. *Am J Clin Nutr* 1991; 54: 123–9.
19. Corman LC. Effects of specific nutrients on the immune response. Selected clinical applications. *Med Clin North Am* 1985; 69: 759–91.
20. Gross RL, Newborne PM. Role of nutrition in immunological function. *Physiol Rev* 1980; 60: 188–302.
21. Golla AG, Larson LA, Anderson CF, et al. An immunological assessment of patients with anorexia nervosa. *Am J Clin Nutr* 1981; 34: 2756–62.
22. Brambilla F, Ferrari E, Brunetta M, et al. Immunoendocrine aspects of anorexia nervosa. *Psychiatr Res* 1996; 62: 97–104.
23. Wade S, Bleiberg F, Mossé A, et al. Thymulin (Zn-facteur thymique sérique) activity in anorexia nervosa patients. *Am J Clin Nutr* 1985; 42: 275–80.
24. Hart BL. Behavioral adaptations to pathogens and parasites: five strategies. *Neurosci Biobehav Rev* 1990; 14: 273–94.
25. Crisp AH, Stonehill E. Relation between aspects of nutritional disturbances and menstrual activity in primary anorexia nervosa. *BMJ* 1971; iii: 149–51.
26. Casper RC, Kirschner B, Sanstead HH, et al. An evaluation of trace metal, vitamins and taste function in anorexia nervosa. *Am J Clin Nutr* 1980; 33: 1801–8.
27. Marcos A, Varela P, Santacruz I, et al. Nutritional status and immunocompetence in eating disorders. A comparative study. *Eur J Clin Nutr* 1993; 47: 787–93.
28. Marcos A, Varela P, Santacruz I, et al. Evaluation of immunocompetence and nutritional status in patients with bulimia nervosa. *Am J Clin Nutr* 1993; 57: 65–9.
29. Silber TJ, Chan M. Immunologic cytofluorometric studies in adolescents with anorexia nervosa. *Int J Eat Dis* 1996; 19: 415–18.
30. Vettor R, Macor C, Novo F, et al. Corticosteroid receptors in mononuclear leukocytes of obese subjects. *J Endocrinol* 1998; 156: 187–94.
31. Loffreda S, Yang SQ, Lin HZ, et al. Leptin regulates proinflammatory immune responses. *FASEB J* 1998; 12: 57–65.
32. Marcos A. The immune system in eating disorders: an overview. *Nutrition* 1997; 13: 853–62.
33. Moor de Burgos A, Wartanowicz M, Ziemlanski. Blood vitamin and lipid levels in overweight and obese women. *Eur J Clin Nutr* 1992; 46: 803–8.
34. Chandra RK, Kutty KM. Immunocompetence in obesity. *Acta Paediatr Scand* 1980; 69: 25–30.
35. Vaisman N, Hahn T, Dayan Y, et al. The effect of different nutritional states on cell-mediated cytotoxicity. *Immunol Lett* 1990; 24: 37–41.
36. Nieman DC, Nehlsen-Cannarella SL, Henson DA, et al. Immune response to obesity and moderate weight loss. *Int J Obes Relat Metab Disord* 1996; 29: 353–60.
37. Pekkarinen T, Mustajoki. Use of very low-calorie diet in preoperative weight loss: efficacy and safety. *Obes Res* 1997; 5: 595–602.
38. Marcos A, Varela P, Toro O, et al. Evaluation of nutritional status by immunological assessment in bulimia nervosa. Influence of BMI and vomiting episodes. *Am J Clin Nutr* 1997; 66: 491–7S.
39. Fink S, Eckert E, Mitchell J, et al. T-lymphocyte subsets in patients with abnormal body weight: longitudinal studies in anorexia nervosa and obesity. *Int J Eat Dis* 1996; 20: 295–305.
40. Kelley DS, Daudu PA, Branch LB, et al. Energy restriction decreases number of circulating natural killer cells and serum level of immunoglobulins in overweight women. *Eur J Clin Nutr* 1994; 48: 9–18.
41. Marcos A, Varela P, Toro O, et al. Interactions between nutrition and immunity in anorexia nervosa. A one year follow-up. *Am J Clin Nutr* 1997; 66: 485–90S.
42. do Carmo I, Palma-Carlos ML, Melo A, et al. Characterization of leukocytes, lymphocytes and lymphocyte subsets in eating disorders. *Allergy Immunol* 1997; 29: 261–8.
43. Chandra RK. Immunocompetence is a sensitive and functional barometer of nutritional status. *Acta Pediatr Scand* 1991; 374: 129–32S.
44. Allende LM, Corell A, Manzanares J, et al. Immunodeficiency associated with anorexia nervosa is secondary and improves after refeeding. *Immunology* 1998; 94: 543–51.
45. Mustafa A, Ward A, Treasure J, et al. T lymphocyte subpopulations in anorexia nervosa and refeeding. *Clin Immunol Immunopathol* 1997; 82: 282–9.
46. Moriguchi S, Kato M, Sakai K, et al. Exercise training restores the decreased cellular immune functions in obese Zucker rats. *J Appl Physiol* 1998; 84: 311–17.
47. Armstrong-Esther CA, Lacey JH, Bryant TN, et al. An investigation of the immune response of patients suffering from anorexia nervosa. *Postgrad Med J* 1978; 54: 395–9.

48. Pertschuk MJ, Crosby LO, Barot L, Mullen JL. Immunocompetency in anorexia nervosa. *Am J Clin Nutr* 1982; 35: 963–72.
49. Muñoz-Velez A, Santacruz I, Varela P, et al. Inmunoglobulinas séricas en anorexia nerviosa. *Nutr Clin* 1989; 9: 37–40.
50. Grimble RF. Malnutrition and the immune response. 2. Impact of nutrients on cytokine biology in infection. *Trans R Soc Trop Med Hyg* 1994; 88: 615–19.
51. Kern PA, Saghizadeh M, Ong JM, et al. The expression of tumor necrosis factor in human adipose tissue. *J Clin Invest* 1995; 95: 2111–19.
52. Yang SQ, Lin HZ, Lane MD, et al. Obesity increases sensitivity to endotoxin liver injury: implications for the pathogenesis of steatohepatitis. *Proc Natl Acad Sci USA* 1997; 94: 2557–62.
53. Halle M, Berg A, Northoff H, et al. Importance of TNF-alpha and leptin in obesity and insulin resistance: a hypothesis on the impact of physical exercise. *Exerc Immunol Rev* 1998; 4: 77–94.
54. Pomeroy C, Eckert E, Hu S, et al. Role of interleukin-6 and transforming growth factor-β in anorexia nervosa. *Biol Psychiatry* 1994; 36: 836–9.
55. Mengheri E, Nobili F, Crocchioni G, et al. Protein starvation impairs the ability of activated lymphocytes to produce interferon-γ. *J Interferon Res* 1992; 12: 17–21.
56. Schattner A, Steinbock M, Tepper R, Schonfeld A, Vaisman N, Hahn T. Tumor necrosis factor production and cell-mediated immunity in anorexia nervosa. *Clin Exp Immunol* 1990; 79: 62–6.
57. Swain MG, Maric M. Tumor necrosis factor-alpha stimulates adrenal glucocorticoid secretion in cholestatic rats. *Am J Physiol* 1996; 270: 987–91.
58. Beisel WR. Herman Award Lecture, 1995. Infection-induced malnutrition—from cholera to cytokines. *Am J Clin Nutr* 1995; 62: 813–19.
59. Holden RJ, Pakula IS. The role of tumor necrosis factor alpha in the pathogenesis of anorexia and bulimia nervosa, cancer cachexia and obesity. *Med Hypotheses* 1996; 47: 423–38.
60. Muñoz C, Arévalo M, López M, et al. Impaired interleukin-1 and tumor necrosis factor production in protein-calorie malnutrition. *Nutr Res* 1994; 14: 347–53.
61. Bessler H, Karp L, Notti I, et al. Cytokine production in anorexia nervosa. *Clin Neuropharmacol* 1993; 16: 237–43.
62. Ayanlor-Batuman O, Ferrero AP, Diaz A, et al. Regulation of transforming growth factor 1 gene expression by glucocorticoids in normal human T lymphocytes. *J Clin Invest* 1991; 88: 1574–80.
63. Billingsley KG, Fraker DL, Strassmann G, et al. Macrophage-derived tumor necrosis factor and tumor-derived of leukemia inhibitory factor and interleukin-6: possible cellular mechanisms of cancer cachexia. *Ann Surg Oncol* 1996; 3: 29–35.
64. Zhou D, Shanks N, Riechman SE, et al. Interleukin 6 modulates interleukin-1 and stress-induced activation of the hypothalamic-pituitary-adrenal axis in male rats. *Neuroendocrinology* 1996; 63: 227–36.
65. Romero LI, Kakucska I, Lechan RM, et al. Interleukin-6 (IL-6) is secreted from the brain after intracerebroventricular injection of IL-1 beta in rats. *Am J Physiol* 1996; 270: R518–24.
66. Girasole G, Jilka RL, Passeri G, et al. 17 Beta-estradiol inhibits interleukin-6 production by bone marrow-derived stromal cells and osteoblasts in vitro: a potential mechanism for the antiosteoporotic effect of estrogens. *J Clin Invest* 1992; 89: 883–91.

DISCUSSION

Dr. Zoppi: It is important to stress that anorectic infants and children also have high levels of cholesterol in the blood. Dr. Suskind reported these results in his book on infant nutrition. It is possible to have such a lipid pattern in anorexia nervosa as well. The reason is that if the dietary energy intake is low, the percentage of fat may be relatively high compared with the calories ingested.

Dr. Marcos: Rather than the percentage of fat being relatively high, it is the percentage of protein which is high. In fact, patients with anorexia nervosa eat almost no fat but still have high levels of cholesterol. I think their metabolism is completely altered.

Dr. Chandra: One of the possible explanations for high cholesterol in these patients is the reduction in lipoprotein synthesis and also the mobilization of fat from the liver, and reduction in lipoprotein lipase activity. All these factors could be responsible for the higher cholesterol levels.

Dr. Suskind: You mentioned the difference between the anorectic and the marasmic child in terms of the factors that may play a role in their maintaining their immune response. You pointed out a very important point relating to the intake of vitamins and minerals helping to maintain the immune system, which otherwise would be compromised by starvation. I was wondering if you might elucidate that a little bit further.

Dr. Marcos: Differences are seen between the situation of a child with protein-energy malnutrition (PEM) and the adolescent suffering from anorexia nervosa. The most important thing to take into account is that the children with PEM do not have the opportunity to eat enough, because they cannot. In anorexia nervosa, the patients can eat whatever they want, but they do not want to eat; they only want to lose weight. That is why I believe you have to take into account the role played by neurotransmitters, as these have to be involved in all these mechanisms. Cytokines must be involved in the food behavior too, because in the end all of these factors are interlinked.

Dr. Suskind: Could that information be valuable in terms of the treatment of anorexia, as far as the cytokines or leptin are concerned? Have leptin levels and TNF-α been measured in anorexia and bulimia? And if they have, do you happen to know what the values are?

Dr. Marcos: Leptin levels have been measured in anorexia nervosa (1), and the results are the opposite to obesity (2)—TNF-α has been shown to be higher in anorexia nervosa than in control subjects (3). In one study, TNF-α was similar to the control group (4), but if measured *in vitro* the production is much higher than in controls.

Dr. Marini: I was impressed by the figures that Dr. Suskind gave yesterday concerning the number of babies who become obese after being malnourished—maybe as many as 20%. I think this may be related to the genetic constitution of these subjects. I believe they are more efficient at conserving energy: their membrane sodium-dependent adenosine triphosphatase works better than in other individuals, so they can save energy. Thus, when they resume a normal diet, they become obese. It is just a genetic selection of these cases.

Another point is about leptin. When you look to the intrauterine growth retarded babies (and this fits very well with Barker's theories), these babies have very high levels of leptin, despite the fact that they are very thin. Maybe this high level of leptin causes downregulation of receptors, so that later on they develop obesity (5). We have recently evaluated the outcome in babies born from diabetic mothers kept under very tight metabolic control (6). These women had very low glucose blood levels, which was maintained very carefully to avoid the usual fetal complications. The newborn infants appeared to be perfectly normal, with no macrosomia at all. When we followed-up these subjects, some of whom are now 30 years of age, we found an extremely high rate of obesity (~55%). This is very high compared with other series of babies born from diabetic mothers managed conventionally (7), where the incidence of obesity is usually around 20%. Thus, it appears that if the supply of glucose to the fetus is reduced too much during fetal life, a risk may be incurred of developing obesity in later life. A possible explanation, involving the IGF-system has recently been suggested (8).

Dr. Wasantwisut: You said that the eating disorders group remained mainly free of infection. I wonder whether this is because that group is more likely to come from the well-to-do end of society and so has reduced exposure to infection. Most eating disorders occur in the well-to-do communities.

Dr. Marcos: Regarding the lack of infection in anorexia nervosa patients, the ones we studied were admitted to the hospital, usually for between 1 and 3 months, so they had the opportunity to become infected because they were in a hospital environment. Another finding was that, although some of the patients had suffered from allergies before the onset of anorexia nervosa, when the anorexia began their allergies disappeared. It is as though anorexia was a cure for allergy. We believe the reason why they were not infected is that there was a modulation of the immune system. We have recently measured T-helper 1 and T-helper 2 cells and found a decrease in T-helper 1 but no decrease in memory T cells. We think that may be the reason why the patients in the study did not get infected. Related to the high socioeconomic levels, today, at least in Spain, anorexia nervosa patients come from all levels of society. However, some years ago, the professionals involved in this field thought that they came mainly from high socioeconomic levels as they were the only people who could afford private psychiatric treatment.

Dr. Woodward: With regard to the lesser impact on immune competence of anorexia nervosa in the adolescent than in the marasmic infant or child, it seems to me that this is more likely to be related to different stages of immune system development at which the nutritional stress is imposed rather than to micronutrient intake differences, which I know are often suggested as a cause. I have no precise idea why imposing such a stress earlier in the development of the immune system might make the situation worse, but intuitively that makes sense. Could you comment on that?

Dr. Marcos: As these people eat fruit and vegetables their intake of micronutrients could be at a reasonable level. However, as their intakes are extremely low, not more than about 500 kcal/d at most, their micronutrient intakes are also correspondingly very low. That is why I think that other factors must be involved in the apparent resistance to infection.

Dr. Woodward: It seems to me that a critical difference in the response to a somewhat similar nutritional stress at a different stage in development is the important factor here; that is, the infant responds with a much more profound depression of immune function than the adolescent. So, it strikes me that rather than trying to explain that difference in terms of nutritional intake, we need to understand it in terms of the individual's stage of development.

Dr. Tontisirin: What are the major causes of death in patients with anorexia nervosa and bulimia? If it is infection, that suggests a similar response to infants and young children with malnutrition.

Dr. Marcos: The mortality is caused by suicide and sudden death from heart failure. These patients do not usually die of infections; in fact, they have to be really cachectic to get a fatal infection. That is why this condition is so different from other types of malnutrition in developing countries.

Dr. Farthing: Are there any similar groups that have been studied with regard to their immune function, such as prisoners on hunger strike? They would comprise a similar group to anorexics: they would be adults and probably come from a similar cultural background.

Dr. Marcos: I believe they have been studied but I am not aware of any data about alterations in the immune system in such populations.

Dr. Farthing: Could I just ask you a question then about the mechanisms of anorexia nervosa. Some years ago, a study suggested that cholecystokinin (CCK) was increased, both basal levels and in response to food, in these individuals. I wonder today whether you think CCK is an important mediator of the continuing anorexia, because it is an important satiety peptide?

Dr. Marcos: We measured this too, and it was really high but I cannot explain why.

Dr. Suskind: As a pediatrician, and not knowing very much about anorexia, it is hard to believe that such a vast difference exists between a marasmic child and an anorectic adult or teenager. I just wonder if this is primarily because we have not studied anorexia in enough depth in relation to the immune system, gut flora, and so on. Maybe sudden death in these patients could be caused by endotoxic shock from septicemia, with no fever but usually an elevated white count. We have studied the malnourished child in depth over the years, but have we studied the malnourished anorectic adult in sufficient depth?

Dr. Marcos: It is true that not many studies have been done in this field, and even fewer on the immune system. But I think that there are great differences between the two situations: a malnourished child is malnourished from around the time of birth, whereas the anorexia nervosa patient usually develops the condition at around 11 or 15 years of age. So, during their first 10 years at least they are well nourished. Then they lose approximately 10 to 15 kg in a very few months. The mechanisms involved in the adaptation of the organism to that new situation must be different from the situation in the malnourished child. Besides not finding any cases of fever, we found low white blood counts showing even a tendency to leukopenia.

Dr. Chandra: Although it is true that patients, mostly girls, with anorexia have fewer infections, once they get infections they can be devastating. Many report patients dying, not only of heart failure, or so-called heart failure (for which not much objective evidence is seen), but also of severe terminal infection. I would agree with Dr. Suskind that if an autopsy is done on these patients, endotoxin levels and other evidence of possible infections should be measured and documented. A small additional nutritional point is that zinc has been measured in patients with anorexia nervosa and found to be somewhat low, and many centers use zinc supplements in an attempt to improve taste and appetite. No controlled trials have been done, but the clinical impression is that it might be helpful.

I know of at least two other situations wherein voluntary starvation has been associated with impaired immune response. These are people who for religious or other reasons stop eating for periods of from 7 to 15 days; and secondly, in patients with rheumatoid arthritis, where it has been recommended that periodic starvation might help the clinical symptoms. Indeed, studies have shown that after about 6 to 7 days of almost total starvation, a reduction in the immune response occurs, which may have beneficial effects on symptoms. Cell-mediated immunity and complement levels fall in these patients.

I would support Dr. Woodward's suggestion that perhaps the age at which starvation occurs may be critical. Many of the patients we were talking about yesterday have had malnutrition from birth or soon after, when the immune system is developing, and that could be quite different from a mature individual with well-established immune responses.

Dr. Marcos: I agree with Dr. Chandra; however, when we measured zinc levels they were very high in the serum, three to four times as high as in controls and the zinc-dependent enzymes were low, so the whole metabolism is very altered. More research should be carried out to elucidate which mechanisms are involved.

Dr. Keusch: I was trying to recall the studies by Cerami and his group when they rediscovered TNF and called it cachectin (9). When TNF, or cachectin, was administered to mice on a daily basis, a reduction in food intake and loss of weight occurred, which continued for several days. However, the effect then dissipated, and I think the weight began to increase again, which suggested that a counter-regulatory cytokine network of interactions might have occurred to counteract the initial effect of TNF on food intake and weight loss. In relation to the question that Dr. Farthing was raising about CCK as being a possible factor in the sustained anorexia in those patients, tachyphylaxis of the cytokine-induced appetite suppression and weight loss might require the added effect of, for example, CCK to reverse it.

Dr. Kennedy: Just a comment on immunology and the cytokines: I agree with Dr. Keusch and some of his comments, but a recent paper reported on Bosnian concentration camp survivors. They found that the immunologic changes were very similar to marasmus, and different from anorexia, so I would not be surprised to find that the infection rates in patients with anorexia were different. Probably what we are dealing with here is a very interesting model of neuroendocrine influences on immune function and the ability to manipulate cytokines by neuroendocrine inputs.

Dr. Marcos: I agree with you. Elite gymnasts comprise another group that is similar in a way to patients with anorexia nervosa. Their physical exercise is on a very high level, 48 hours a week, that is 8 hours a day including Saturdays. Their behavior is very similar to that of anorexics and their food intake is very low. But for some reason these people get many more infections than anorexics. So it is not only the starvation—it is more than that.

Dr. Suskind: One thing that you mentioned with regard to the anorexics that may explain this difference is the fact that they take supplements. Perhaps what you are seeing is the impact of severe malnutrition on the immune system being mitigated by the vitamin and mineral supplements they are taking, so they do not have the same changes in their immune system as, for instance, a severely malnourished adult or child would have. In relationship to obesity, I agree with you that it is important to make certain that any child or adult who is on a weight reduction program is on one that is safe in terms of maintaining lean body mass as well as immune function. I do not think we look at that seriously enough, but the fact is that if you put a child or an adult on a very low energy diet–500 or 600 kcal, high protein, low fat, low carbohydrate–it is also critical that these patients have vitamin and mineral supplements. I think that those of us who are working in the area of adult and childhood obesity should be looking at what happens to the immune system. We have been looking at lean body mass and how it is maintained on these low energy diets, but we have not looked at the immune system.

Dr. Marcos: We carried out a trial of supplements on our anorexic patients, and the most important result was that they gained more lean body mass than patients without supplements. The delayed hypersensitivity skin test was improved as well, but nothing else. We think that they probably needed more supplements than we gave, so we are going to start another trial giving more.

REFERENCES

1. Grinspoon S, Gulick T, Askari H, et al. Serum leptin levels in women with anorexia nervosa. *J Clin Endocrinol Metab* 1996; 81: 3861–3.
2. Geldszus R, Mayr B, Horn R, et al. Serum leptin and weight reduction in female obesity. *Eur J Endocrinol* 1996; 135: 659–62.
3. Schattner A, Steinbock M, Tepper R, et al. Tumour necrosis factor production and cell-mediated immunity in anorexia nervosa. *Clin Exp Immunol* 1990; 79: 62–6.
4. Brambilla F, Bellodi L, Brunetta M, et al. Plasma concentrations of interleukin-1β, interleukin-6 and tumor necrosis factor-α in anorexia and bulimia nervosa. *Psychoendocrinology* 1998; 23: 439–47.
5. Shekhawat PS, Garland JS, Shivpuri C, et al. Neonatal cord blood leptin: its relationship to birth weight, body mass index, maternal diabetes and steroids. *Pediatr Res* 1998; 43: 338–43.
6. Marini A, Cattaneo F. Control of diabetes in pregnancy and metabolic alterations in the neonate. *Acta Paediatr* 1998; 87: 711–16.
7. Whitaker RC, Pepe MS, Seidel KD. Gestational diabetes and the risk of offspring obesity. *Paediatrics* 1998; 101: E9.
8. Cianfarani S, Germani D, Branca F. Low birthweight and adult insulin resistance: the "catch-up growth" hypothesis. *Arch Dis Child Fetal Neonatal Ed* 1999; 81: F71–73.
9. Cerami A, Ikeda Y, Le Trang N, et al. Weight loss associated with an endotoxin-induced mediator from peritoneal macrophages: the role of cachetin (tumor necrosis factor). *Immunol Lett* 1985; 11: 173–7.

Nutrition, Immunity, and Infection in Infants and Children, edited by Robert M. Suskind and Kraisid Tontisirin. Nestlé Nutrition Workshop Series, Pediatric Program, Vol. 45. Nestec Ltd., Vevey/Lippincott Williams & Wilkins, Philadelphia ©2001.

Allergy and Infection

Ricardo U. Sorensen and Mary Catherine Porch

Louisiana State University Medical Center, New Orleans, Louisiana, USA

It is well established that some infections and parasitic diseases predispose patients to allergic sensitization and trigger allergic reactions, whereas allergic inflammation predisposes them to skin and mucosal infections. Our understanding of the relationship between allergy and infection is currently undergoing a change. Several studies have provided evidence for a worldwide increase in allergic diseases over the last decades (1). Although environmental factors (*e.g.*, such as air pollution, cigarette smoke exposure, and increased indoor allergen exposure) have probably all contributed to this change, a decrease in childhood infections has also been suggested as a possible cause of the rise of allergic diseases in children (2). In this chapter, we discuss our present understanding of the immunologic aspects of the relationship between infections and allergy, and explore ways in which this knowledge might be used to decrease both.

ALLERGY AS A PREDISPOSING FACTOR FOR INFECTIONS

Allergic diseases lead to infections whenever allergic inflammation contributes to barrier breakdown or decreased function in bacterial clearance mechanisms. Allergic rhinitis, for example, is a well-known cause of secondary infectious sinusitis, as well as otitis media. Inflammation with increased secretion and decreased ciliary beating reduces the normal elimination of bacteria from sites of colonization (nasopharynx) and promotes their entry into normally sterile sites (*e.g.*, sinus cavities and the middle ear). Decreased secretory IgA in some allergic patients plays an additional role.

In atopic dermatitis, skin inflammation leads to a breakdown of the natural barrier preventing infection. Staphylococcal skin infections are a common cause of exacerbation and complications in atopic dermatitis. Furthermore, through the induction of antistaphylococcal IgE antibodies, an additional allergic reaction may occur or compound the chronic allergic reactions to foods and inhalant allergens known to cause atopic dermatitis (3).

INFECTIONS AS PREDISPOSING FACTORS FOR ALLERGY

Viral, bacterial, fungal, and parasitic infections can all trigger the production of IgE and, in some instances, of allergic reactions. In areas where parasitic infections have become rare, viruses are the main infectious agents associated with allergic diseases. The association between viral infections of the respiratory tract and asthma has been well established in several studies in children and adults (4–7). The different mechanisms whereby infections can increase IgE production and lead to subsequent allergic diseases can be illustrated by examining the effect of various viral infections on these two aspects of the allergic response.

Several viruses induce an IgE response to their antigens, the presence of which then produces symptoms attributable to allergic inflammation in addition to the direct viral cytopathic effect. In the first 2 years of life, the infectious agents most commonly isolated from the airways of wheezing infants have been (in descending order): respiratory syncytial virus (RSV), parainfluenza viruses, adenoviruses, rhinoviruses, and *Mycoplasma pneumoniae* (8). Welliver *et al.* demonstrated the presence of IgE bound to exfoliated nasopharyngeal cells in 70% to 80% of infants infected with RSV. Cell-bound IgE persisted in 73% to 80% of patients who developed wheezing, but in only 27% of patients with respiratory infections or pneumonia alone (9). Similarly, wheezing infants have a higher titer of RSV-specific IgE in the nasal secretions than nonwheezing infants (10). Finally, infants with RSV infection who had the highest nasal IgE response developed recurrent episodes of wheezing at up to 48 months of age compared with IgE nonresponders (11).

Although in the aforementioned examples the development of antiviral IgE antibodies relates to the pathogenesis and symptoms of respiratory disease caused by viral infections, IgE not related to recognizable symptoms of allergy can also be produced in response to viral infections. For instance, IgE concentrations are increased in A, B, and delta hepatitis without a known pathogenic effect (12).

A single virus can induce different types of IgE responses. A typical example is the human immunodeficiency virus (HIV), which induces the production of specific IgE antibodies that can be used for diagnostic purposes (13). In addition, HIV produces raised circulating IgE concentrations not correlated with allergen-specific IgE antibodies (14) or with manifestations of allergic diseases (15). Some patients infected with HIV develop a syndrome resembling the hyper-IgE syndrome: a primary immunodeficiency with eosinophilia, very high IgE concentrations, and recurrent skin and deep-seated infections (16).

In contrast to the aforementioned viral infections, children with Epstein–Barr virus infections in the first years of life tend to have lower total IgE concentrations (17).

INFECTIONS AND VACCINES PROTECTING AGAINST ALLERGY

Although infections have commonly been associated with an increased incidence of allergic diseases (6,7), recently several instances of a protective effect have also been described. For example, increasing numbers of siblings in a family have been observed to have a slight protective effect against eczema, hay fever, and asthma (18). However, this protection against atopic disease by larger sibships could not be explained by a history of common childhood infections such as rubella, varicella, mumps, or pertussis. Only a history of measles after the age of 3 years showed a weak protective effect against asthma. A role for measles infections protecting against allergy was also suggested by a study in Guinea-Bissau, where young adults who had had measles were significantly less likely to have immediate skin test reactivity to house mites (19).

Similarly, Shirakawa *et al.* reported a negative association between tuberculin responses and atopic disorders in Japan (20), concluding that a decline in the incidence of tuberculosis could be a factor in the increased prevalence and severity of atopic diseases there. As the tuberculin reactivity detected in this study was more likely to have been caused by bacille Calmette–Guérin (BCG) immunization than by active tuberculosis, a possible protective effect of BCG immunization was subsequently postulated and investigated in a cohort of 1,314 newborns followed over 5 years (21). Total and specific IgE were determined at 12, 24, 36, and 60 months of age. Life-time prevalence of allergic diseases was lower in the BCG-vaccinated group, with differences decreasing over time and no longer present at 60 months of age. Obstructive bronchitis, atopic dermatitis, and food allergy were not significantly lower in the BCG group. Intraindividual time courses for total and specific IgE did not differ at any point. The lack of a pronounced protective effect of BCG against atopic disease or IgE sensitization can be attributed to genetic differences in the induction and persistence of tuberculin reactivity (22,23). These differences should be taken into account in further studies of the possible effect of BCG immunization on IgE responses.

IMMUNOGLOBULIN E PRODUCTION AND TH1-TH2 BALANCE

The host components needed for an immediate-type allergic reaction are IgE antibodies directed at specific epitopes on the allergen, and mast cells capable of releasing mediators responsible for the allergic reaction. The response is initiated when an allergen penetrates a mucosal surface and initiates the production of IgE. The allergen is taken up by antigen-presenting cells (APCs) and presented to T-helper cells in the context of histocompatibility antigens on the surface of the APCs. T-helper cells regulate IgE production by two signals: the production of cytokines (interleukin (IL)-4 and IL-13), and the cognate T–B cell interactions through complementary surface molecules such as CD40-CD154 (formerly CD40 ligand) (Fig. 1).

Two types of mature T-helper cells, Th1 and Th2, both derive from naive Th0 cells. For all antigens, including allergens, the predominant T-helper cell subtype present at the mucosal surface helps to determine whether the immune response will be mediated by IgE and antibody or by a cell. The Th1 subset produces IL-2 and γ-interferon, promoting delayed type hypersensitivity and protection against intracellular pathogens (24). The Th2 subset produces IL-4 and IL-5 which, with the help of CD40L, shift the immune response to IgG and or IgE antibody production (Fig. 1) (25).

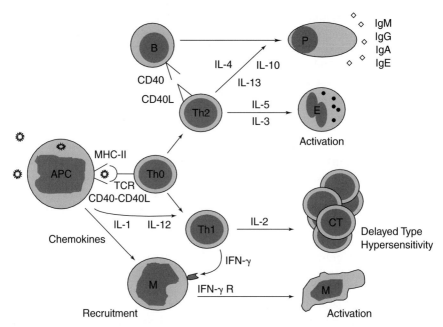

FIG. 1. Regulation of antibody-mediated immunity and delayed type hypersensitivity by Th1 and Th2 cells. APC, antigen presenting cell; Th0, naive T-helper cells; Th1 and Th2, type 1 and 2 T-helper cells; IFN-γ, γ interferon; M, monocytes or macrophages; B, B lymphocytes. See text for explanation.

Interleukin-4 is responsible for the isotype switch in B cells allowing IgE production (26), IL-3 and IL-4 are responsible for mast cell growth, and IL-5 is responsible for eosinophil differentiation (27). Th2 cells also produce IL-10, which is responsible for inhibition of Th1 cell cytokine production (28). Because γ-interferon, which is produced by Th1 cells, inhibits the proliferation of Th2 clones, a reciprocal relationship exists between IL-4 and γ-interferon levels in the regulation of IgE production.

Although currently much emphasis is placed on the development and regulation of these two types of T helper cells and their cytokines, it is important to remember that in reality these cells are just one component of a much more complex network of cells and cytokines activated by infections, vaccines, or exposure to allergens.

ONTOGENY OF IMMUNOGLOBULIN E PRODUCTION

Immunoglobulin E production and allergic reactions can occur at any age. IgE does not cross the placenta but is produced by the fetal liver by 11 weeks and in the lung by 21 weeks (29). Raised newborn IgE levels, reflecting *in utero* sensitization, have been used as a marker for an increased risk of developing allergy in infancy and childhood (30). The development of IgE in infancy and early childhood is driven by exposure to various allergens (Fig. 2).

The first allergens encountered in an individual's life are food allergens (31). *In utero* sensitization to food allergens from the mother can be inferred from observations of neonates who developed reactions within the first 72 hours of life when fed cow's milk (32). Infants can next become sensitized to food proteins in breast milk or infant formulas, followed by solid food allergens. Cow's milk, soy formula, wheat, peanut proteins (often present as an additive in other foods), and egg are the most important allergens in early infancy. Allergy to cow's milk proteins is estimated to develop in 2% to 7% of all infants receiving cow's milk in the first year of life (33), increasing to as high as 74% in infants at risk for atopy (34).

Viral antigens are the next sensitizing agents to which infants are exposed (4). Because viral infections also induce protective IgG antibodies, individual viruses usually do not recur and viral allergens decrease in importance after the first 3 years of life.

Indoor inhaled antigens (aero allergens) and then outdoor aero allergens are next in the sequence of sensitization. Indoor allergens include mites, cockroaches, cat and dog dander, and molds. The relative importance of these allergens varies from region to region, as well as from household to household. Outdoor allergens, including outdoor mold, grass, weed, and tree allergens, show a seasonal pattern and a defined geographic distribution.

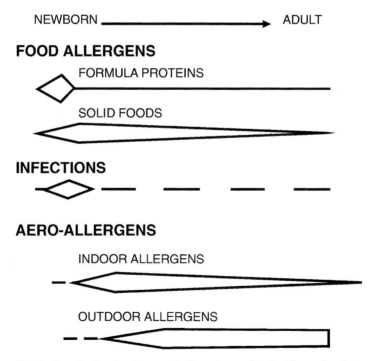

FIG. 2. Sensitization to allergens at different ages. See text for explanation.

Allergic diseases caused by sensitization to the allergens discussed also tend to follow a well-defined sequence: food allergy and atopic dermatitis in infancy, followed by allergic rhinitis and asthma later in life. This would suggest that early sensitization to food allergens may in itself become a risk factor for subsequent sensitization to environmental allergens responsible for respiratory diseases.

An important question not answered by the observations discussed above is why some individuals become allergic and others do not, and why an initial allergic sensitization may be an added risk factor for sensitization to other, unrelated allergens. As some exposure to the main allergens listed is unavoidable for all individuals, a genetic predisposition for the development of allergy in only some individuals has been postulated. Several studies of parents and their offspring support some genetic regulation of the process of sensitization (35). Studies of identical twins found a 60% concordance in the development of allergic symptoms. However, this also means that in 40% of twin pairs, other factors lead to the development of allergy in one but not the other twin (35a). Current evidence suggests an important role for Th1/Th2 balance in defining which infant will become allergic and which will be protected.

ONTOGENY OF TH1/TH2 CELLS

It appears that, during pregnancy, fetal survival depends on a shift of the maternal Th1/Th2 balance to a Th2 pattern of cytokine production. If this does not occur and there is a predominance of Th1 cytokines, unexplained recurrent abortion may result (36). Newborns also have a predominance of Th2 cells, with decreased production of the Th1-produced γ-interferon (37). Maturation of the immune system during infancy can be understood as a gradual change of the fetal and newborn immune response from a predominant TH1 to a predominant TH2 response (38). This development is probably driven by infections and vaccines, whereas exposure to allergens may have a negative effect, delaying or preventing the shift to a Th1 predominance (39) (Fig. 3).

For each immune response to an antigen, the development of either Th1 or Th2 from TH0 cells is influenced by IL-12 secreted by APCs and by interferon (Fig. 1) (40). The triggering of an antigen receptor in the presence of IL-12 and interferon will lead to the development of Th1 cells, whereas naive Th0 cells triggered in the presence of IL-4 will become Th2 cells, which can promote IgE production. It is interesting to note, however, that not all patients with high IgE concentrations have a typical Th2 response. Patients with the hyper-IgE syndrome, caused by either HIV infection or the presence of a primary immunodeficiency syndrome, have increased IgE concentrations despite deficient $CD4^+$ cells that include a Th2 cell population (16,41).

MODIFYING THE ALLERGIC RESPONSE

Allergen immunotherapy, traditionally performed to decrease the IgE response in favor of IgG and cellular immune responses, is now also understood as a way to change

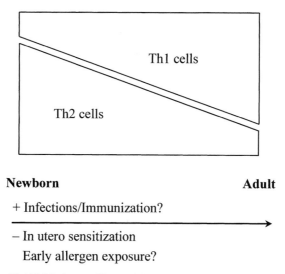

FIG. 3. Shift in the Th1/Th2 balance with age. Infections and immunizations accelerate the shift to a Th1 predominance, whereas *in utero* sensitization and early allergen exposure maintain a Th2 predominance.

the Th1/Th2 balance. Immunotherapy has been shown to increase the production of Th1 cytokines and decrease that of Th2 cytokines (42). Thus, although some allergens induce a Th2 response, allergen immunotherapy modifies the immune response in the opposite direction.

Unfortunately, immunotherapy is not available for some of the most prevalent or severe forms of allergy (*e.g.*, severe asthma and food-induced anaphylaxis). Food is an important cause of severe acute hypersensitivity reactions, including fatal anaphylaxis (43). Severe reactions to foods can occur at all ages, from infants receiving cow's milk or casein or whey hydrolysate formulas to children, adolescents, and adults (44,45). Although some reactions caused by milk formula proteins in infants may decrease in intensity with age, the risk of severe reactions to other foods remains present for long periods of time, even in the absence of exposure (46).

The early onset and high prevalence and severity of allergic reactions in infancy and childhood has led to an intense search for strategies to prevent sensitization to food proteins and inhalant allergens. General measures to decrease allergen exposure include promotion of breast-feeding in infancy and of a healthy environment. Specific measures of prevention should be suggested for individuals at risk, particularly newborns and infants, based on the identification of risk for the development of allergy.

PREDICTION OF ALLERGY RISK

A study of allergic rhinitis, asthma, and atopic dermatitis in parents and children in 6,665 families in southern Germany revealed an increased risk for rhinitis, asthma, or atopic dermatitis in a child if one parent was affected by the same allergic disease (47). An influence of parental sensitization on the Th1/Th2 balance of infants was suggested by the observation that parental skin test reactivity inversely correlated with γ-interferon production of their infants at 6 months of age (48).

The risk for developing any form of allergy can usually be predicted based on family history. Summarizing the results of 12 studies, Zeiger estimated the incidence of allergic disorders at 70% where both parents have a history of allergy, 50% with one parent involved, and 12% with no parental history (35).

However, difficulties are seen with using parental history as a predictor. Among 130 infants enrolled in a study of the prevention of sensitization in New Orleans, 39% had only one parent available for evaluation (49). Furthermore, some parents may have underreported symptoms, despite the use of a detailed questionnaire that included inquiries about symptoms of allergic rhinitis, asthma, atopic dermatitis, and food and drug allergies. In all, 190 parents answered the questionnaire and underwent skin prick testing to common inhaled and food allergens. Of 143 parents with a positive history, 93 (65%) had a positive skin prick test, whereas 19 of 47 parents with a negative history had a positive skin prick test (40%). Interestingly, fathers were five times more likely to report a negative history for allergy and have a positive skin prick test than mothers. The predictive value of the presence of parental allergic sensitization, defined by a positive history and a positive skin prick test, for the development of symptoms of food allergy by 12 months of age was evaluated in 62 children in the same study. Of 25 children with two allergic parents, three (12%) had symptoms of food allergy, whereas among the remaining 37, who had only one allergic parent, seven (19%) had symptoms of food allergy. Thus, in this study little distinction was found between children with one and those with two allergic parents. These findings suggest that more reliable determinants of risk are needed.

PREVENTING THE DEVELOPMENT OF FOOD ALLERGY IN INFANCY

The high incidence of allergy to cow's milk has led to the development of extensively hydrolyzed casein and partially hydrolyzed whey formulas. Avoiding exposure to cow's milk in infants at risk decreases allergic sensitization to cow's milk proteins (50). In addition to preventing specific sensitization to milk protein, allergen avoidance may also prevent the development of a Th2 predominance that leads to a sensitization to other allergens. This secondary protective effect against all forms of allergy by early dietary intervention is suggested by the work of Chandra showing decreased food and respiratory allergies in breast-fed infants and infants fed a partial whey hydrolysate compared with infants receiving conventional cow's milk formula (51).

We recently concluded a comparison of breast-feeding and partially and extensively hydrolyzed infant formulas that showed these formulas do decrease allergic sensitization in infants at risk (49). However, in all feeding groups, we identified infants who, by 12 months of age, had developed raised IgE concentrations or IgE an-

TABLE 1. *Correlation between symptoms, laboratory findings, and skin testing at 12 months of age in children at risk for allergy*

	Feeding groups					
	Breast-fed		Partially hydrolyzed whey		Extensively hydrolyzed casein	
	Symptomatic (n = 5)	Asymptomatic (n = 12)	Symptomatic (n = 13)	Asymptomatic (n = 25)	Symptomatic (n = 6)	Asymptomatic (n = 13)
IgE ≥ 16.3 IU/ml	1 (20%)	0	3 (43%)	4 (25%)	1 (20%)	1 (8%)
RAST to milk >3% binding	0	0	0	1 (7%)	1 (25%)	0
Positive SPT to food and aeroallergens	1 (20%)	3 (25%)	6 (13%)	2 (8%)	2 (33%)	0

RAST, radioallergosorbent test; SPT, skin prick test.

tibodies to cow's milk or aeroallergens (Table 1). We also found evidence of allergic sensitization in all feeding groups, despite the presence or absence of respiratory, gastrointestinal, or dermatologic symptoms suggestive of allergy. Symptomatic infants had higher percentages of sensitization in the hydrolyzed milk feeding groups, but some asymptomatic infants receiving the partially hydrolyzed whey also had evidence of sensitization.

Two conclusions can be drawn from these observations: none of the three feeding groups was completely free of sensitization, and evidence of sensitization could be detected even in some infants who showed no clinical evidence of allergy. The evidence of sensitization in some infants receiving hydrolyzed formulas from birth indicates that additional strategies for allergy prevention must be developed. This brings us back to the issue of infections and immunizations.

PROJECTIONS: PREVENTION OF ALLERGY AND INFECTIOUS DISEASES IN THE GENERAL POPULATION

The evidence reviewed in this chapter shows a close relationship between infections and allergic disease. Although generally one seems to lead to the other, the possible synergistic effect of allergy prevention and the prevention of infectious diseases must also be explored. The increase in allergic sensitization has been linked repeatedly to the decrease in infectious diseases that may shift the Th1/Th2 balance to a Th2 predominance. As preventive dietary manipulations and environmental protection alone are either ineffective or impossible to achieve, it is reasonable to combine our efforts to prevent infectious diseases with those designed to decrease allergic diseases. In other words, major breakthroughs in the prevention of allergic sensitization and disease may be linked to effective prevention of infectious diseases.

The traditional method of modifying the immune response is to use immunizations against infectious diseases and immunotherapy against allergies. The effectiveness of immunization is measured by its ability to decrease the incidence of infections and to elicit protective immunity. The effect of immunization on the function of immune cells and on the Th1/Th2 balance is just beginning to be understood (52).

Many issues must be considered before general recommendations can be made. For instance, recent experimental work by Power showed that the dose of mycobacteria determined the resulting Th1/Th2 balance: low doses lead to a predominant Th1 pattern, whereas higher doses induced both Th1 and Th2 cells independently of the route of administration (53). It is likely that similar differences may be seen with different vaccines in humans.

We have reviewed epidemiologic evidence that measles vaccine, as well as BCG, may decrease the incidence of allergic sensitization, and that BCG and pneumococcal polysaccharide vaccines have measurable effects on monocyte activation and Th1/Th2 cytokine patterns. Each of these two T-helper cell subsets may play a beneficial or a detrimental role in human disease. Th1 responses are essential for the control of major infectious diseases caused by intracellular pathogens, including HIV and tuberculosis, but they are also implicated in immunologic diseases such as rheumatoid arthritis, multiple sclerosis, and diabetes (54,55), where a predominance of Th2 responses may have a protective effect. Th2 responses are involved in the development of IgG antibodies that confer long-term protection against many infections caused by extracellular pathogens, yet they have been implicated in the excess production of IgE and, therefore, of atopy and allergic diseases. A critical challenge for modern immunology is to understand the fine regulation of these differences so that they can be used to our advantage in new prevention and treatment strategies.

Childhood immunizations, where antigens are delivered in known doses at known ages and stimulation can be routinely repeated several times, would be a far better modulator of the immune balance of an individual than infections. The varying severity, age, and treatment of infections probably explain the variable results reported by investigators trying to determine a protective effect of natural infections with various agents against atopic disease.

ACKNOWLEDGMENT

We acknowledge and thank Patricia A. Giangrosso for her editorial assistance.

REFERENCES

1. Woolcock AI, Peat JK, Trevillion LM. Is the increase in asthma prevalence linked to increase in allergen load? *Allergy* 1995; 50: 935–40.
2. Shaheen SO. Changing patterns of childhood infection and the rise in allergic disease. *Clin Exp Allergy* 1995; 25: 1034–7.
3. Moore C, Ehlayel MS, Junprasert J, et al. Topical sodium cromoglycate in the treatment of moderate-to-severe atopic dermatitis. *Ann Allergy Asthma Immunol* 1998; 81: 452–8.
4. Duff AL, Pomerantz ES, Gelber LE, et al. Risk factors for acute wheezing in infants and children: viruses, passive smoke, and IgE antibodies to inhalant allergens. *Pediatrics* 1993; 92: 535–40.
5. Martinez FD. Viral infections and the development of asthma. *Am J Respir Crit Care Med* 1995; 151: 1644–8.
6. Folkerts G, Busse WW, Nijkamp FP, et al. Viral infections and airway hyperresponsiveness. *Am J Respir Crit Care Med* 1998; 157: 1708–20.

7. Atmar RI, Guy E, Guntupalli KK, et al. Respiratory tract viral infections in inner-city asthmatic adults. *Arch Intern Med* 1998; 158: 2453–9.

8. Henderson FW, Collier AM, Sanyal MA, et al. A longitudinal study of respiratory viruses and bacteria in the etiology of acute otitis media with effusion. *N Engl J Med* 1982; 306: 1377–83.

9. Welliver RC, Kaul TN, Ogra PL. The appearance of cell-bound IgE in respiratory tract epithelium after respiratory syncytial virus infection. *N Engl J Med* 1980; 303: 1198–202.

10. Welliver RC, Wong DT, Sun M. The development of respiratory syncytial virus specific IgE and the release of histamine in nasopharyngeal secretions after infection. *N Engl J Med* 1981; 305: 841–6.

11. Welliver RC, Sun M, Rijnaldo D. Predictive value of respiratory syncytial virus specific IgE responses for recurrent wheezing following bronchiolitis. *J Pediatr* 1986; 109: 776–80.

12. Gutierrez D, Guardia P, Delgado J, et al. Increased serum IgE in acute type A, B and delta hepatitis. *J Investig Allergol Clin Immunol* 1997; 7: 119–121.

13. Miguez-Burbano MJ, Hutto C, Shor-Posner G, et al. IgE-based assay for early detection of HIV-1 infection in infants. *Lancet* 1997; 350: 782–3.

14. Goetz DW, Webb EL, Whisman BA, et al. Aeroallergen-specific IgE changes in individuals with rapid human immunodeficiency virus disease progression. *Ann Allergy Asthma Immunol* 1997; 78: 301–6.

15. Babcot BK, Paul ME, Navarro M, et al. Objective measures of allergic diseases in children with human immunodeficiency virus infection. *J Allergy Clin Immunol* 1997; 100: 707–11.

16. Paganelli R, Scala E, Mezzaroma I, et al. Immunologic aspects of hypergammaglobulinemia E-like syndrome in patients with AIDS. *J Allergy Clin Immunol* 1995; 95: 995–1003.

17. Alessandri CM, Rosengard PG, Di Caro A, et al. Correlation between Epstein Barr virus antibodies, serum IgE and atopic disease. *Pediatr Allergy Immunol* 1997; 8: 91–6.

18. Bodner C, Godden D, Seaton A. Family size, childhood infections and atopic diseases. *Thorax* 1998; 53: 28–32.

19. Shaheen SO, Aaby P, Hall AJ, et al. Measles and atopy in Guinea-Bissau. *Lancet* 1996; 347: 1792–6.

20. Shirakawa T, Enomoto T, Shimazu T, et al. The inverse association between tuberculin responses and atopic disorders. *Science* 1997; 275: 77–9.

21. Gruber C, Kulig M, Guggenmoos-Holzmann I. Total IgE, specific sensitization, and atopic disease in BCG-vaccinated and non-vaccinated children. *Allergy & Clinical Immunology International* 1997; (Suppl 4: 97).

22. Sepulveda RL, Heiba IM, King A, et al. Evaluation of tuberculin reactivity in BCG-immunized siblings. *Am J Respir Crit Care Med* 1994; 149: 620–4.

23. Sepulveda RL, Heiba IM, Navarrete C, et al. Tuberculin reactivity after newborn BCG immunization in mono- and dizygotic twin pairs. *Tuber Lung Dis* 1994; 75: 138–43.

24. Constant SL, Bottomly K. Induction of TH1 and TH2 CD4$^+$ T cell responses: alternative approaches. *Annu Rev Immunol* 1997; 15: 297–322.

25. Paul WE, Seder RA. Lymphocyte responses and cytokines. *Cell* 1994; 76: 541–51.

26. DelPrete G, Maggi E, Parronchi P. IL-4 is an essential co-factor for the IgE synthesis induced in vitro by human T cell clones and their supernatants. *J Immunol* 1988; 140: 4193–8.

27. Clutterbuck EJ, Hirst EM, Sanderson CJ. Human interleukin-5 (IL-5) regulates the production of eosinophils in human bone marrow cultures: comparison and interaction with IL-1, IL-3, IL-6, and GMCSF. *Blood* 1989; 73: 1504–12.

28. Moore KW, Vieira P, Fiorentino DF, et al. Homology of cytokine synthesis inhibitory factor (IL-10) to the Epstein-Barr virus gene BCRFI. *Science* 1990; 248: 1230–4.

29. Miller DL, Hirvonen T, Gitlin D. Synthesis of IgE by the human conceptus. *J Allergy Clin Immunol* 1973; 52: 182–8.

30. Kjellman NI, Croner S. Cord blood IgE determination for allergy prediction—a follow-up to seven years of age in 1,651 children. *Ann Allergy* 1984; 53: 167–71.

31. Sorensen RU, Moore C. Immunology in the pediatrician's office. *Pediatr Clin North Am* 1994; 41: 691–714.

32. Firer MA, Hosking CS, Hill DJ. Effect of antigen load on development of milk antibodies in infants allergic to milk. *BMJ* 1981; 283: 693–6.

33. Schrander JJP, van den Bogart JPH, Forget PP, et al. Cow's milk intolerance in infants under 1 year of age: a prospective epidemiological study. *Eur J Pediatr* 1993; 152: 640–4.

34. Halken S, Host A, Hansen LG, et al. Effect of an allergy prevention programme on incidence of atopic symptoms in infancy. A prospective study of 159 "high risk" infants. *Allergy* 1992; 47: 545–53.

35. Zeiger RS. Development and prevention of allergic disease in childhood. In: Middleton EJ, Reed CE, Ellis EF, Adkinson NF, Yunginger JW, Busse WW, eds. *Allergy. Principles and practice*, 4th ed. St Louis: CV Mosby, 1993: 1137–71.

35a. Edfors-Bubs ML. Allergy in 7000 twin pairs. *Acta Allergol* 1971; 26: 249–85.

36. Picini MP, Romagnani S. Regulation of fetal allograft survival by a hormone-controlled Th1- and Th2- type cytokines. *Immunol Res* 1996; 15: 141–50.
37. Wilson CB, Westall J, Johnston LL, et al. Decreased production of interferon-gamma by human neonatal cells. *J Clin Invest* 1986; 77: 860–7.
38. Bona C, Bot A. Neonatal immunoresponsiveness. *The Immunologist* 1997; 5: 5–9.
39. Romagnani S. The TH1/TH2 paradigm. *Immunol Today* 1997; 18: 263–6.
40. Rogge L, Sinigaglia F. Regulation of IL-12 receptor expression in developing T helper cell subsets. *The Immunologist* 1998; 6: 142–5.
41. Rodríguez MF, Patiño PJ, Montoya F, et al. García de OD. Interleukin 4 (IL-4) and interferon-γ (IFN-γ) secretion by antigen and mitogen stimulated mononuclear cells in the hyper-IgE syndrome: no TH-2 cytokine pattern. *Ann Allergy Asthma Immunol* (in press).
42. Bellinghausen I, Metz G, Enk AH, et al. Insect venom immunotherapy induces interleukin-10 production and a Th2 to Th1 shift, and changes surface marker expression in venom-allergic subjects. *Eur J Immunol* 1997; 27: 1131–9.
43. Yocum MW, Khan DA. Assessment of patients who have experienced anaphylaxis: a three year survey. *Mayo Clin Proc* 1994; 69: 16–23.
44. Yunginger JW, Sweeney KG, Sturner WQ, et al. Fatal food-induced anaphylaxis. *JAMA* 1988; 260: 1450–2.
45. Sampson HA, Mendelsohn IM, Rosen JP. Fatal and near-fatal anahylactic reactions to food in children and adolescents. *N Engl J Med* 1992; 327: 380–4.
46. Bock SS. The natural history of food sensitivity. *J Allergy Clin Immunol* 1982; 69: 173–7.
47. Dold S, Wjst M, von Mutius E, et al. Genetic risk for asthma, allergic rhinitis, and atopic dermatitis. *Arch Dis Child* 1992; 67: 1018–22.
48. Martinez FD, Stern DA, Wright AL, Holberg CJ, Taussig LM, Halonen M. Association of interleukin-2 and interferon-γ production by blood mononuclear cells in infancy with parental allergy skin tests and with subsequent development of atopy. *J Allergy Clin Immunol* 1995; 96: 652–60.
49. Porch MC, Shahane AD, Leiva LE, et al. Influence of breast milk, soy or two hydrolyzed formulas on the development of allergic manifestations in infants at risk. *Nutr Res* 1998; 18: 1413–24.
50. Halken S, Jacobsen HP, Host A, et al. The effect of hypo-allergenic formulas in infants at risk of allergic disease. *Eur J Clin Nutr* 1995; 49: S77–83.
51. Chandra RK. Five-year follow-up of high risk infants with family history of allergy who were exclusively breast-fed or fed partial whey hydrolysate, soy, and conventional cow's milk formulas. *J Pediatr Gastroenterol Nutr* 1997; 24: 380–8.
52. Sorensen RU, Butler B, Ortigas A, et al. Upregulation of CD40 ligand and IL-4 mRNA expression, but not of IL-12 and IFN-γ mRNA after immunization with the 23-valent pneumococcal vaccine in children with recurrent respiratory infections. *Pneumococcal vaccines for the world*. Washington, DC, 1998.
53. Power CA, Wei G, Bretscher PA. Mycobacterial dose defines the Th1/Th2 nature of the immune response independently of whether immunization is administered by an intravenous, subcutaneous, or intradermal route [Abstract]. *Infect Immun* 1998; 66: 5743–50.
54. Nicholson LB, Carrizosa AM, Kuchroo VK. Pathogenic versus protective repertoires in autoimmune disease—tuning the balance. *The Immunologist* 1998; 6: 151–7.
55. Bach J-F. Immune dysregulation in organ-specific autoimmune diseases: the case of type I diabetes. *The Immunologist* 1998; 6: 158–60.

DISCUSSION

Dr. Meydani: Could you comment on the observation that in the elderly is seen a decline in TH1 response and an increase in TH2 response, yet the incidence of allergies goes down with aging. Secondly, do you see the same changes in cytokines if an oral vaccine is given?

Dr. Sorensen: You probably realize that I really do not believe in this TH1, TH2 paradigm. There may be some truth in it: these two types of cells indeed exist. But what we have not differentiated clearly is when a TH2 cell promotes IgE or when it promotes IgG. That is an essential question that we have to answer, and the literature does not help us. The key to this is probably other cytokines that are produced concomitantly and which, if present, can push the response toward IgG as opposed to IgE. In the elderly is seen another very interesting issue—a shift from IgG1 to IgG2 responses. In relation to pneumococcal antibodies, a very sharp increase occurs in the total concentration of antibodies against the various serotypes around adolescence. Adults have very high concentrations of antibodies. However, in the elderly they are not functional. In part, this is explained by a shift from the IgG1 type to the IgG2 type. This is a very fertile area of investigation, particularly as many countries have now introduced routine pneumococcal immunization in the elderly.

Regarding cytokines, obviously what we know about cytokines in vaccines refers only to the pneumococcal polysaccharide vaccine and the pneumococcal conjugated vaccine, and we are about to learn more about BCG. But what about all the rest? Somebody needs to do all those studies. We have had no chance to do them, in part because of the sad situation in the United States, where it is very hard to do any follow-up studies. That is the reason why we do so many studies in Latin America, where follow-up is so much easier.

Dr. Gershwin: Can you share your thoughts on the use of the whooping cough vaccine in children with an atopic family history?

Dr. Sorensen: I do not have any data nor do I recall any reports about whooping cough vaccine and family histories of allergy. Could you elaborate on why this is an issue? Maybe you know things that I do not know!

Dr. Gershwin: The reason I asked is that one of the best ways to elicit an IgE response in an animal is to use pertussis as the adjuvant; however, concern is seen about pertussis and the subsequent development of asthma and atopy in humans. Some pediatricians do not recommend pertussis vaccine in children who already have asthma. I have a related question about respiratory syncytial virus vaccine because of concerns that it may lead to a higher incidence of asthma.

Dr. Sorensen: With respect to whooping cough, I do not know the data on allergy, but I do know that in England a campaign was waged against pertussis vaccine in the 1980s, when a few very vocal doctors begun to stir up public opinion against it. This resulted in many people refusing the vaccine for their children, with disastrous results the following year, when there were multiple hospital admissions with whooping cough. So I think you have to select what you prefer: whooping cough or a very slight likelihood of asthma.

Dr. Gershwin: I do not disagree with the cost-benefit analysis. If I understand the numbers correctly, however, about 9% of individuals in the United States have asthma, mortality is going up in every country in the world, and I know there is concern about pertussis. I think that is why the new pertussis vaccine is going to be offered soon. Can you give us an update on the status of the respiratory syncytial virus vaccine in the United States?

Dr. Sorensen: The early RSV vaccine was a disaster; the vaccine was based on killed virus, which actually modified the immune system in such a way that it made the disease worse. Currently, the trend is to use hyperimmune gamma globulin and monoclonal antibodies. I do not know where the development of new vaccines is at this point. I think everybody got very scared with the experience in the 1970s with the killed virus vaccine.

Dr. Gershwin: You are absolutely correct: children who received the vaccine and subsequently developed RSV had a significant mortality rate. A new RSV vaccine is being field tested right now, but I do not know how things stand now. It is a recombinant vaccine. Perhaps we will hear about it in the future.

Dr. Sorensen: About 40 vaccines are in the pipeline. The next issue will be how many vaccines we can really give to our children.

Dr. Griffin: With regard to the United Kingdom and the whooping cough vaccine you alluded to, the problem was not one of allergy, it was one of encephalopathy. When it was looked at epidemiologically, it was found not to be a problem at all. It was the antivaccine campaigners who were whipping up antivaccine feeling. The vaccine was not in fact withdrawn, it was maintained, but there was a great fall in uptake because parents were alarmed. We still use whole cell vaccine.

Dr. Novelli: Among general practitioners in the late 1970s was a feeling that a history of allergy was a contraindication to pertussis vaccination. I think that probably was a throwback to the time when smallpox vaccination was in use, and that vaccine was contraindicated for children with eczema or a history of eczema. This then became one of the mythical contraindications to pertussis vaccination, and a lot of general practitioners and even consultant pediatricians really did not think that pertussis should be given to patients with a history of allergy. That has all changed now, obviously.

Dr. Sorensen: Thank you for that. One of the advantages of performing studies in different countries is that you can do comparative analyses. It is fascinating to me that in New Orleans, we have patients who have no antibodies at all to pneumococcal polysaccharides before immunization, at all ages. In Brazil and in Chile, that simply does not happen. I think one of the differences, and something we have not mentioned yet, may be the overuse of antibiotics, which I suspect may have quite an important effect.

Dr. Haschke: I have a question bringing us back to nutrition. You indicated that you do not believe in the TH1/TH2 story. But are there any recent reports on the change in TH2 to TH1 environment in infants at high risk of allergy who are breast-fed versus those who receive formula? Is there any influence of antigen exposure and if so, are there any data on the effects of hydrolysates?

Dr. Sorensen: No, I am not aware of any. Let me correct you on one point: I do think there is some truth in the TH1/TH2 paradigm, but it is not as simple as currently represented. The studies you mention need very much to be done. I am glad that you asked your question, because I do not think we should abandon the idea of introducing diets early on that may be hypoallergenic or nonallergenic. We need to consider them along with other host factors, and those should be fascinating studies to do.

Dr. Marini: Together with Dr. Chandra, we have had almost 15 years' experience in preventing allergy in very high risk atopic babies with a hypoallergenic formula (1,2). I think that your last suggestion of treating all the population to prevent allergic disease would be a real magic bullet, if it worked. I think that in attempting to prevent allergic disease you have to take care of two aspects: the nutritional aspect and the environmental aspect. It is difficult to achieve good results if first, you do not provide a suitable diet in the early years, with a substantial delay in introducing solid foods (which is extremely important for avoiding allergic disease) followed by the selective introduction of solids in the first few years; and second, if you do not limit exposure to environmental allergens. This makes for a very cumbersome program, and only mothers with a very high familial risk are likely to be motivated enough to follow such a program. One important point is the role of infection. In our program, we avoid daycare centers for the first 2 years of life, because we thought that attendance at such centers increases the risk of infection. In our control group, which was not on a preventive program, we showed that going to the daycare center was a significant factor in the development of allergy on multivariate analysis. I think this is probably because those babies had greater exposure to RSV in their early years (3).

I would like to ask you about your statement that the most important thing was to switch from IgE to IgG production. What do you think about the Spanish data (4) on the use of nucleotides to enhance the production of IgG β-lactoglobulin in preterm babies. Do you think this could be a protective factor?

Dr. Sorensen: I cannot answer your question about nucleotides as I have not seen the paper or considered the issue. In relation to infection, in the United States if we were to suggest that the solution to allergy was to avoid daycare centers, that would be a real problem; for families where both parents are working, daycare centers are essential. A researcher named Martinez has been following 1,200 children in Tucson from birth onward and has published many papers on what promotes and what decreases allergy (5). He even proposes that babies be taken to households where there is another baby with an infection, so the baby will acquire this infection, thus preventing the development of allergy! I think the truth may be along the lines you mentioned: avoid RSV, which is a known promoter of IgE production, and maybe use vaccines that will promote, if not a TH1 response, then at least the kind of TH2 response that will not lead to allergy.

Dr. Klish: The idea of exposing children to disease to decrease the prevalence of allergy is an area I have been thinking about a lot lately in relation to breast-fed children having a decrease in hypersensitivity or allergy. The reason for this could be that breast milk is perhaps the dirtiest thing that a child can drink—in the sense that is full of antigen from mother. In some way, that milk is inducing tolerance rather than intolerance, and we may be focusing our attention in completely the wrong direction when we try to eliminate exposure to antigens, when perhaps we should be increasing the exposure to antigens.

Dr. Sorensen: Thank you for bringing up the issue of oral tolerance, which I think we need to pay more attention to. It is a fascinating idea. Perhaps going for more and more elemental formulas is exactly the wrong way to go, because they may not induce the tolerance we need. I would love to propose a big study that could include all these factors, but it is a very difficult thing to do.

Dr. Griffin: With regard to adjuventicity, one of the five components in the acellular vaccine, which I believe it is pertactin, is a very strong adjuvant, as is the beta subunit of cholera toxin, and concern exists that if these vaccines are given intranasally their adjuventicity may cause sensitization to allergens in the atmosphere and give rise to atopy. That is theoretic, but it is certainly possible.

I entirely agree with your comment about TH1 and TH2. It is a useful concept that cells may produce different forms of cytokines, but when you consider that our immune response to an infection or an antigen consists of a host of responses at the mucosal surface as well as trafficking, and when you are looking at cells only from blood and saying this is a TH1 response, this is totally naive when all the other components are ignored.

My final point is about BCG, and your data showing the increase in TNF production in subjects given it. That is explicable quite simply by an interaction between macrophages and T cells. If you have primed T cells interacting with a macrophage, you get a massive release of TNF. I am sure your experiments contain some contaminating T cells.

Dr. Sorensen: You are quite right. When we were doing those experiments 10 years ago, we had no idea what we would find; we were after something else. But the fact is that these changes can be detected many months after the actual immunization. So my point is that immunizations have a long-lasting effect on certain aspects of the immune system.

Dr. Eigenmann: Studies have shown that if you immunize neonatal mice with diphtheria and tetanus vaccine they have a TH2-like response; if you immunize them later, however, they have more of a TH1-like response. My question is about DNA vaccine. People are talking about this more and more, not only for prevention but also for treatment. Do you have a comment on that?

Dr. Sorensen: Not really. It is a fascinating area, but I still have not figured out exactly what these vaccines will do to us.

Dr. Eigenmann: They are a long way from using them in humans, but studies are underway in mice to treat food allergy with DNA vaccines, using adjuvants such as CPG which induce a TH1-type response (6). Maybe in a couple years we will know more about that.

Dr. Embree: Maybe I can contribute with some information from the infectious disease/HIV world. TH1/TH2 has been very well discussed and one thing that came out was the dose of antigen received, with a high dose in theory producing a TH2 response and a low dose a TH1 response. This was such a good theory that it brought the HIV immunization program to a halt and promoted the use of DNA low-dose vaccines. However, the early results of these have shown that low-dose HIV vaccine gives rise not only to cell-mediated immunity but also to IgA immunity, which does not make sense according to the proposed paradigm. So in terms of your talk, it is the dose of antigens that children get at a young age that determines whether they produce IgE, so we should be ensuring that when children get infected, they get infected with a lot of antigen rather than just a little!

Dr. Sorensen: Thank you for that comment. Following our work with pneumococcal vaccines, proposals are now before the National Institutes of Health to investigate the use of pneumococcal vaccines in attempting to prevent the development of diabetes, which is supposed to be a TH1 reaction. So, things are getting rather interesting. We are facing a new world as infections decrease and allergy and autoimmunity become important issues.

Dr. Chandra: Although the paradigm of TH1/TH2 remains controversial and much more detail needs to be filled in, individuals who are atopic or who develop allergic disease later do show a higher production of IL-4 and decreased synthesis of γ-interferon; for example, children who have higher production of IL-4 and relatively less γ-interferon in the first months of life often develop atopic eczema or recurrent wheezing. Several studies now confirm this. May I ask a question about the elderly? You mentioned that they appear to have a switch of immunoglobulin subclass isotype from G1 to G2. If that is true, they should be better protected against the polysaccharide antigen than the other way around.

Dr. Sorensen: This is not really suggested by opsonophagocytosis studies that we have done in collaboration with the Centers for Disease Control. Elderly patients with high concentrations of IgG antibodies measured by enzyme-linked immunosorbent assay have almost no opsonophagocytic activity, which probably reflects a combination of the subclass component and the avidity of the antibodies. Regarding your comments about γ-interferon and IL-4, I agree, but our results show that we are inducing a tremendous IL-4 response and that the patients in general get better. It is an interesting problem.

Dr. Suskind: We briefly discussed the issue of the malnourished child with hyper-IgE and eosinophilia, which we have noticed for the past 30 years but which remains unexplained. Could the switch from TH1 to TH2 explain the eosinophilia and hyper-IgE? And should we be looking at these children later on in life to see if they have a greater prevalence of allergy?

Dr. Sorensen: That is what this conference is all about: our bringing different ideas together and seeing what can be done to learn from each other.

REFERENCES

1. Marini A, Agosti M, Motta G, et al. Effects of a dietary and environmental prevention programme on the incidence of allergic symptoms in high atopic risk infants: three years' follow-up. *Acta Paediatr Suppl* 1996; 414: 1–21.
2. Chandra RK. Five-year follow-up of high-risk infants with family history of allergy who were exclusively breast-fed or fed partial whey hydrolysate, soy and conventional cow's milk formulas. *J Pediatr Gastroenterol Nutr* 1997; 24: 380–8.

3. Strannegard O, Cello J, Bjarnason R, et al. Association between pronounced IgA response in RSV bronchiolitis and development of allergic sensitization. *Pediatr Allergy Immunol* 1997; 8: 1–6.
4. Martinez-Augustin O, Boza JJ, Del Pino JI, et al. Dietary nucleotides might influence the humoral immune response against cow's milk proteins in preterm neonates. *Biol Neonate* 1997; 71: 215–23.
5. Dodge R, Martinez FD, Cline MG, et al. Early childhood respiratory symptoms and the subsequent diagnosis of asthma. *J Allergy Clin Immunol* 1996; 98: 48–54.
6. Li X, Huang CK, Schofield BH, et al. Strain-dependent induction of allergic sensitization caused by peanut allergen DNA immunization in mice. *J Immunol* 1999; 162: 3045–52.

Nutrition, Immunity, and Infection in Infants and Children, edited by Robert M. Suskind and Kraisid Tontisirin. Nestlé Nutrition Workshop Series, Pediatric Program, Vol. 45. Nestec Ltd., Vevey/Lippincott Williams & Wilkins, Philadelphia ©2001.

The Metabolic Effects of Infection on Nutritional Status

Carla R. Fjeld

Fjeld and Associates, Bethesda, Maryland, USA

WHY FOCUS ON AMINO ACIDS AND FUNCTIONAL PROTEINS?

Stunted growth in many children from developing countries is caused by the synergistic effects of infection or inflammation and malnutrition. As has been shown many times over, children's growth can be impeded through the effects of infection on intake, metabolism, and partitioning of nutrients. The impact of infectious disease on nutritional status is so profound that infections are thought to be responsible for as much of the malnutrition in children in developing countries as the lack of suitable food (1–4). Moreover, the cumulative effects on nutritional status of chronic or multiple infections without full recovery in between probably outweigh those of single acute episodes (1).

Most of our current understanding of the synergy between infection and malnutrition was derived from studies done in patients with severe infection. However, differences in the pathogenicity of the infectious agent or the immunocompetence of the host determine whether an infectious challenge results in clinical disease. Observations made in studies of animals, and others, although fewer, in children, suggest that even those challenges that do not result in clinical disease have potentially negative effects on nutritional status and, thus, give rise to the hypothesis that chronic subclinical or *unapparent* infections can also compromise nutritional status, net anabolism, and growth (5).

Severe infections trigger a host of responses which, in turn, alter nutrient intake, most major metabolic pathways, and the relations between many clinical and functional assessments of nutritional status and dietary intake. The metabolic effects of infection are mediated through cytokine activation and the ensuing amplification of host defense mechanisms. These factors favor the partitioning and redistribution of dietary and endogenous nutrients away from the maintenance of host nutritional status (6), body composition, and growth and toward support of the immune response and the increase in the hepatic synthesis of some proteins (positive acute phase reactants) and involve most major metabolic pathways. It is now more than 20 years since Beisel developed a generalized model to portray the relationship between the sequential phases of an acute infection and the major metabolic events just listed (7).

Are these metabolic events also altered during immune stimulation that is not manifested as a clinical infection? Evidence suggesting that they may be is to be found in the fact that alterations in body composition and nitrogen balance are initiated during the incubation (presymptomatic) phase, and that catabolic losses persist even when clinical signs of infection have abated and child's appetite has been restored (1,8,9). Studies in elderly persons, even those without clinically detectable infection or inflammation, have also shown that chronic immune stimulation contributes to a deterioration in lean body mass, a process referred to as *sarcopenia* in the elderly (10). Such observations provide further support for the hypothesis that chronic immune stimulation caused by subclinical infection is a significant environmental cause of reduced lean body cell mass in undernourished, or inappropriately nourished, populations.

Further evidence of the metabolic effects of subclinical infection comes from studies of micronutrient nutrition. Micronutrient deficiencies that persist despite micronutrient supplementation and which are accompanied by low levels of circulating nutrient transport proteins in children with raised C-reactive protein but no clinical signs of infection, suggest that low levels of transport proteins (*e.g.* albumin or transferrin) lead to micronutrient diversion and sequestration in less accessible body pools (6,11), and that these alterations occur as a secondary effect of infection.

GOAL OF THE REVIEW

There are three general modes of action by which infection inhibits growth:

- Reduced exogenous supply of substrates through anorexia and malabsorption
- Nutrient–endocrine interaction: decreased production of insulinlike growth factor 1 (IGF-1) caused by increased interleukin (IL)-6 production
- Resetting metabolic priorities and competition for substrates: increased demand for amino acid substrates for acute phase protein synthesis leading to catabolic losses, inhibition of anabolic processes, and diversion of amino acid substrates for nutrient transport

The main purposes of this chapter is to discuss the nutrient-endocrine and substrate competition mechanisms, as food intake will be discussed in other chapters in this book. Within this framework, I will attempt to put into perspective the alterations in metabolic priorities that involve the redistribution of dietary and endogenous amino acids from growth and maintenance of body composition toward support of the immune response, including synthesis of the acute phase proteins, and to speculate how amino acid metabolism can negatively affect nutrient status, even in subclinical infection. Although infection alters the major metabolic pathways involving most nutrients, focus is mainly on amino acids because of the multitude of nutritional roles that they play; for example, as substrates for both the positive nutrient transport and export or transport proteins (referred to here as negative acute phase proteins), and in anabolism and growth. Moreover, stable isotope methods are available for tracing specific amino acids and specific proteins that have had only limited application in children in developing countries but which would be highly useful in conducting the studies needed to increase our understanding of the relationship between infection, amino acid metabolism, micronutrient status, and growth, and also to improve our capacity to intervene.

MECHANISMS OF EFFECTS OF CYTOKINES ON MAINTENANCE OF BODY CELL MASS AND GROWTH

Chronic inflammation or recurrent infection can lead, within hours, to increased production of IL-6 and other cytokines (12), which have both systemically and locally produced effects. The cytokines that have the most documented effects on metabolism and nutrition are tumor necrosis factor (TNF), IL-1, and IL-6, partly because they were discovered earlier than the other cytokines. The acute phase response is associated with species-specific increases and decreases in the rates of secretory protein synthesis and is controlled at least in part at the transcriptional level. It involves upregulation in the synthesis and mobilization of substrates for the positive acute phase proteins (*e.g.*, C-reactive protein, serum amyloid A, α_1-acid glycoprotein, haptoglobin, fibrinogen) and decreased plasma concentrations of transport proteins (*e.g.*, albumin, transferrin, and retinol binding protein) (13). The metabolic effects are both direct, mediated by binding of cytokines to cell receptors in the responding tissue, and indirect, elicited by stimulation of the release of cytokines, glucocorticoids, and prostaglandins, and decreased production of IGF-1.

WHAT ELEMENTS OF EXPERIMENTAL DESIGN ARE RATE-LIMITING IN DETERMINING THE NUTRITIONAL EFFECTS OF CYTOKINES?

Before discussing the evidence for the various mechanisms by which infection or inflammation affect growth, I will comment on the difficulties in determining the effects of cytokines.

1. Cytokine concentrations in the plasma do not represent their rates of synthesis or predict their effects. This is because cytokines are synthesized both locally and systemically but with different time courses; they are present in very low concentrations in blood, turn over very rapidly, and their modes of action are affected by various inhibitory mechanisms. Therefore, the impact on nutritional outcomes from circulating cytokine levels is hard to establish.

2. Stimuli for the production of early response cytokines (e.g., IL-1 and TNF) are varied and include the bacterial lipopolysaccharide of gram-negative organisms, peptidoglycan of gram-positive organisms, antigen-antibody complexes, and viral interactions with host cells. Within this complex set of stimuli, some cytokines act to induce other cytokines and some act together to cause stereotypical host responses, which are well described in an excellent review of the interactions between nutrition and infection by Keusch (14).

3. Cytokines directly and indirectly mediate a wide range of host responses which, in turn, affect or confound their nutritional significance.

4. Most of the human studies of the effects of infection on nutritional status were done during severe infections. Thus, studies in animal models involving both febrile and afebrile responses, in which any of the cytokines, crude or recombinant, were infused at either high or low dose, provide some understanding of the mechanisms whereby infection perturbs growth and body mass, but do not speak directly to the issue of chronic, and particularly chronic subclinical, infection. The latter is especially relevant, given that subclinical infection is widespread among young children in developing countries. For example, 35% (6) to 50% (15) of the children in field studies in Guatemala and Ghana, respectively, were found to have subclinical infections. Furthermore, their poor nutritional status seemed to result from metabolic alterations or rearrangements during those infections more than from inadequate intake of micronutrients.

5. Because subclinical infections are not easily detectable but may, in fact, be chronic, a fourth methodologic issue is that much of the evidence that subclinical infection is a cause of malnutrition is anecdotal. Thus, another complication of the study of the nutritional effects of cytokines is that malnutrition may blunt the acute phase response, so it is less vigorous in undernourished than in well-nourished individuals. This point is addressed in other chapters in this book.

6. How nutritional status and the nutritional outcomes are defined and measured are further challenges to clarifying the relationship between infection and nutritional status.

CYTOKINE-INDUCED REARRANGEMENTS IN AMINO ACID METABOLISM

Nutrient–Endocrine Interactions

The next step is to try to pinpoint the mechanisms of cytokine actions on growth. An endocrine–nutrient growth inhibitory role of IL-6 was discussed by De Benedetti *et al.* (16), who studied children with systemic juvenile rheumatoid arthritis, a chronic inflammatory disorder characterized by raised circulating levels of IL-6. In patients with this disease, IL-6 is known to be markedly increased. In the first part of that particular study, De Benedetti *et al.* worked with colonies of transgenic mice carrying a neurospecific enolase promoter that drives the expression of IL-6 cDNA, leading to overexpression of IL-6. The control group was a colony of wild-type mice. The primary measurements made were of IGF-1, IL-6, TNF, food intake, and weight gain. Food intake (g/g body weight) did not differ between the two mouse types. Nevertheless, the wild-type mice gained significantly ($p < 0.05$) more body weight between days 0 and 21 and between days 29 and 35 of the 35-day study, suggesting a growth inhibitory effect in the IL-6 transgenic mice, despite the fact that feed intake per gram of body weight did not differ between the two groups.

The next experiment was to inject a monoclonal antibody (15-A7) to neutralize the IL-6 receptor and enable further study of the mechanism of the growth suppression in the mice. The 30% to 50% reduction in body weight that the transgenic mice showed without the antibody was partially reversed by the antibody. The attribution of the effect specifically to IL-6 was strengthened by the reproduction of the effects in the wild-type mice treated with IL-6. The hypothesis that the decreased growth rate reflected a behavioral disorder leading to a decrease in food intake was ruled out by the observation of equal food intake and conversion per gram of body weight. The hypothesis that the overexpression of IL-6 had an effect on the function of the pituitary was ruled out by the observation that the distribution of the cells that produce growth hormone and thyroid-stimulating hormone, and the circulating concentrations of the two hormones, were the same in the transgenic as in the wild-type littermates.

In further studies on children with systemic juvenile rheumatoid arthritis, De Benedetti *et al.* reported a consistently negative correlation between serum IL-6 and plasma IGF-1 Z-scores ($p = 0.004$). Together, these findings strongly suggest that the IL-6–mediated decrease in IGF-1 production is a major mechanism whereby chronic inflammation limits growth.

Resetting Metabolic Priorities and Competition for Substrates

The conclusions drawn from the types of endocrine-nutrient studies just discussed do not explain the profound catabolic responses that occur with severe infections (1), of which the classical indices are increased urinary nitrogen excretion, depletion of muscle protein, nutrient wastage, and peripheral wasting (4). The description and understanding of infection-induced muscle wasting has evolved over at least the last 100 years. In 1910, a German case was cited in which the nitrogen equivalent of 2.5 kg of muscle was lost in 8 days of fever (17). By the end of the 19th Century, the nitrogen equivalent of muscle lost during a febrile episode had already been calculated, and Voit had made the observation (in dogs) that carbohydrate can reduce protein catabolic degradation during induced septic fever (18).

Reorganization of amino acid metabolism occurs to support the hepatic synthesis of acute phase proteins and the synthesis and secretion of factors involved in host defense (12). As hypothesized by Powanda and Beisel in 1982 (19), these host defense mechanisms are dependent on the ability of the host tissue or cells to provide amino acid and other substrates in sufficient quantity for the formation of the positive acute phase proteins, and deficiencies of amino acids can depress the synthesis of the proteins that contribute to host defense.

Such deficiencies can occur through reduced influx of protein and energy substrates; through anorexia or malabsorption, or both; through increased metabolic rates from hyperthermia or fever; or by the transcriptional activation and inhibition of hepatic genes involved in the synthesis of the positive and negative acute phase proteins (14). Some of the nutritional significance of limitations on the influx of nutrients, through anorexia and malabsorption, is discussed by others in this volume. However, the fact that catabolic and oxidative losses of endogenous nitrogen exceed those resulting from fasting alone and persist even when patients become afebrile and asymptomatic, resume an adequate dietary intake, and are no longer malabsorbing, speaks to the importance of the other two main types of mechanism listed at the beginning of this review, which may lead to the depletion of body nitrogen and amino acid substrates.

Scrimshaw *et al.* hypothesized in 1957 (20) and again in a classic monograph (21) that "the internal diversion of nutrients for the synthesis of compounds involved in the response to infection contributes importantly to the depletion of body stores." The fact that the cytokine network modulates protein synthesis and breakdown enzymes and that it inhibits the regulatory actions of anabolic hormones on protein synthesis (22) suggests a basis for the competition for amino acid and other substrates, particularly under the stress of dietary insufficiency.

In 1976, Bostian *et al.* reported the changes in serum concentrations of certain proteins during typhoid fever infection, and speculated that meeting the demand for increased hepatic output of positive acute phase proteins altered protein balance (23). Other early evidence indicated that the acceleration of the synthesis of acute phase proteins altered protein balance by altering the demand for specific amino acids.

Experiments based on infusion of crude, and later recombinant, cytokines have shown induction by cytokines of muscle proteolysis in both animals and humans. Some of those have been done using skeletal muscle isolated from either animals or humans, with or without the addition of inhibitors or stress hormones; others have been done *in vivo* in animals and humans, again with or without other stress hormones. Some have used bolus or continuous high doses of cytokines to simulate sepsis, whereas others have used bolus or continuous lower levels of the cytokines and hormones. However, very few have looked at the combined effects of marginal malnutrition and chronic immunostimulation, such as may occur among children living in crowded, unhygienic environments, so some initial information can be gleaned from studies on the metabolic effects of sepsis.

CYTOKINE-MEDIATED SYNTHESIS AND BREAKDOWN OF PROTEIN

One of the earliest studies on the metabolic effects of sepsis was published by Clowes *et al.* (24), who conducted a series of experiments to elucidate the relations between muscle protein synthesis and breakdown in sepsis. The first step was to determine how the rates of protein synthesis and degradation in muscle tissue from septic patients differ from the rates in metabolically normal people. To do this, they obtained specimens of the rectus abdominus muscles from septic and nonseptic surgical patients. For comparison of the human with an animal model they also obtained rat muscle tissue: they first starved the rats for 3 days, then induced peritonitis by cecal ligation, after which the rats were killed and the soleus muscle of each hind leg extracted; one group of control animals was studied to assess the effect of 3-day starvation alone. Protein breakdown was measured *in vitro* in both human and rat muscle from the rate of tyrosine appearance in the incubating medium (to which no measurable contribution from free intracellular tyrosine was seen). Protein synthesis was measured from the intracellular incorporation of UL-^{14}C-tyrosine in the human and rat studies. Rates of *in vitro* protein breakdown were compared with *in vivo* rates by measuring tyrosine release from leg muscles obtained from both the septic and aseptic humans. Finally, to understand the proteolysis-inducing influence of factors in the plasma itself, plasma from patients with or without sepsis was added to the incubating medium, which contained either muscle tissue from aseptic patients or aseptic rats. The investigators concluded that sepsis induced a 212% increase in the rate of protein breakdown and a modest increase in protein synthesis in human muscles. In rats, a modest acceleration in synthesis was accompanied by a 190% increase in the rate of degradation. The rats that were only starved but not infected showed an increase in degradation of 24%, so that the calculated rate of protein degradation that could be attributed to infection alone was approximately 164% of the control value. Incubation of normal human muscle with plasma from septic patients caused a small increase in synthesis and a 192% increase in protein degradation, a finding that contributed to the isolation and identification of cachectin, as TNF was first called.

At least in sepsis, TNF has been found to stimulate muscle protein catabolism and the net release of amino acids from peripheral muscle (7,14,25–31) and may involve the release of adrenocorticotropin and cortisol (32,33) to stimulate muscle catabolism. In experiments designed to disaggregate the effects of these activators, Raina and Jeejeebhoy (33) gave 100 g TNF/kg/d to rats and compared the effects on measures of protein metabolism between those rats and rats infused with TNF and corticosterone, the most abundant circulating steroid in rats. Carcass weight was used as an index of change in lean body mass and, thus, of catabolic effects. By this index, lean body mass, as a percentage of body weight, was significantly reduced by TNF. The fact that urinary nitrogen output was not increased but that an increase in total protein content of the liver was observed suggests that amino acid substrates were redirected from peripheral muscle for acute phase protein synthesis in the liver by TNF alone, as well as by TNF plus corticosterone.

Blocking the effect of TNF in rats by giving TNF antiserum reduced mortality from 25% to 5%, had no effect on muscle protein synthesis, but reduced rates of total protein breakdown and myofibrilar protein breakdown, as shown by increases in the rates of release of tyrosine and 3-methylhistidine, respectively (34).

LESSONS FROM THE BIRDS

Building on the knowledge that microbial challenges, which rarely result in clinical disease produce significant immune responses in poultry, and on the long established practice of giving antibiotics as feed supplements to poultry in insanitary environments, Klasing *et al.* (35–38) conducted a series of studies in poultry to explain the mechanisms and nutritional significance of subclinical infection on metabolism, specifically on the growth inhibition of the subclinical infections. For example, they found that asymptomatic chickens reared in typical unsanitary environments and fed antibiotics grew significantly better ($p < 0.05$) than nonantibiotic-treated chickens (38). In other words, antibiotics appeared to reverse the growth inhibition caused by immunologic stress. Importantly, the antibiotic treatment also resulted in greater weight gain per gram feed consumed than in the nontreated controls (i.e., it improved the efficiency of feed conversion: $p < 0.05$) (38). The overall conclusions from these and other studies done by Klasing's team are that decreased growth, decreased feed efficiency (gram gain per gram feed), and changes in nutrient requirements all result from subclinical, asymptomatic immune stimulation. If the immune system has an especially high demand for nutrients, then animal nutritionists must consider immunity when setting dietary requirements and predicting or evaluating the efficiencies of feed conversion. Are similar paradigms relevant to understanding the net efficiencies of anabolism in children living in unhygienic environments?

SUBSTRATE COMPETITION DURING INFECTION IN CHILDREN

Referring back to the hypothesis that the growth inhibition of IL-6 is a secondary effect of its causing decreased concentrations of IGF-1 (16), Reeds *et al.* emphasized that the diversion of nitrogen from somatic protein to the synthesis of the acute phase proteins would result in nitrogen conservation and, thus, would not explain the increases seen in urinary nitrogen and protein oxidation, and the net losses of nitrogen from the body during infection (39). To look further into the mechanism whereby nitrogen is irreversibly lost from the body, we compared the gross amino acid composition of the major acute phase proteins synthesized by humans with those of mixed muscle (39). Four of the six acute phase proteins (C-reactive protein, amyloid A, haptoglobin, and α_1-antitrypsin) contain high contents of phenylalanine, three of them (α_1-acid glycoprotein, haptoglobin, and amyloid A) contain high amounts of tyrosine, and five of them (C-reactive protein, fibrinogen, α_1-acid glycoprotein, haptoglobin, and amyloid A) are rich in tryptophan.

By contrast, mixed muscle protein has a relatively low content of phenylalanine, tyrosine, and tryptophan, whereas it is rich in the branched chain amino acids. Thus, if the major source of amino acids used in the synthesis of acute phase proteins is from endogenous sources (mainly muscle), then during the catabolic response the demands for the aromatics and tryptophan together would require the mobilization of substantially more muscle protein than would be gained as acute phase protein (Fig. 1).

Based on data published by Colley *et al.* (40) and Kushner (41), Reeds *et al.* (39) estimated the amino acid requirements for synthesis of a typical mix of acute phase proteins. Acute phase proteins synthesized under conditions of infection increased by 850 mg protein per kilogram body weight per day. On the basis of those results and

FIG. 1. Amino acid equivalencies of proteins synthesized in the acute phase and muscle protein catabolized to provide amino acid substrate. From Reeds PJ, Fjeld CR, Jahoor F (39).

the amino acid composition of the acute phase proteins, we calculated the quantity of each amino acid that would have been incorporated into the acute phase protein mixture. We then calculated the quantity of muscle protein that would have to be catabolized to supply a sufficient amount of each amino acid to support acute phase protein synthesis. The figure of 850 mg was actually a conservative estimate, given Waterlow's estimate of a peak synthetic rate of 1.2 g acute phase proteins per kilogram body weight per day (13). In any case, by our calculations, the quantity of phenylalanine in 850 mg of the mixture of acute phase proteins represents the quantity of phenylalanine contained in 1,980 mg of muscle protein. Assuming that the phenylalanine is used completely in acute phase protein synthesis, we then calculated the difference between the quantity of each amino acid in 1,980 mg muscle protein and that in 850 mg acute phase protein. Including the needs for the aromatic amino acids, which by these calculations are the limiting amino acids when skeletal muscle provides the amino acid substrates for acute phase proteins, results in a surfeit of the branched chain amino acids because they are so much more abundant in muscle than in the acute phase proteins. This excess has to be catabolized, as it cannot be recycled into body protein because phenylalanine becomes limiting to further synthesis. The total of the nitrogen contained in this excess is 130 mg/kg body weight, which, according to Reeds et al.(39), is close to a typical daily loss of body nitrogen following uncomplicated trauma.

One of the conclusions from our study was that 2 g of muscle protein must be broken down to support the synthesis of 1 g of the mixture of positive acute phase proteins; therefore, a significant proportion of the net loss of body nitrogen results from the excessive demands for aromatic amino acids (phenylalanine, tyrosine), the limiting amino acids for synthesis of acute phase proteins when amino acids contained in muscle provide the substrate. Theoretically, these *surplus* amino acids would be deaminated and the carbon skeletons lost through oxidation. According to this analysis, the source of the protein oxidized and the nitrogen lost is the muscle amino acids that remain after the relatively greater demands for phenylalanine for synthesis of acute phase proteins have been satisfied, or the available phenylalanine runs out.

ISOTOPIC STUDIES OF AMINO ACID OXIDATION DURING INFECTION

In October of 1992, the International Atomic Energy Agency in Vienna released a Request for Proposals for studies relating infection to protein metabolism in marginally nourished children from developing countries. Proposals were reviewed and a coordinated research program was founded. Initially, the program involved researchers from seven developing and four industrialized countries. However, it became clear that a set of assumptions, measurements, and study design elements was common (or could be common) to each study. By an iterative process, those elements were forged into a *generic protocol* for studying the effects of subclinical infection on protein oxidation in marginally nourished, free-living children.

The team was composed of researchers from the Center for Studies of Sensory Impairment, Aging and Metabolism in Guatemala City, Guatemala; the International Centre for Diarrhoeal Disease Research, Bangladesh in Dhaka, Bangladesh; St. John's Hospital, Bangalore, India; the Tropical Metabolism Research Unit in Kingston, Jamaica; the Instituto de Investigación Nutricionál in Lima, Peru; the Queen Elizabeth Central Hospital, Balantyre, Malawi; the Children's Nutrition Research Center, Houston, Texas, USA; Washington University School of Medicine, St. Louis, Missouri, USA; Johns Hopkins University, Baltimore, Maryland, USA; and the International Atomic Energy Agency, Vienna, Austria. The expert advice of F. Jahoor, P. Reeds, D. Halliday, and G. Keusch contributed substantially to the development of that protocol, which was published and used as the foundation for subsequent studies in most of the developing country research sites (42).

The generic protocol and, thus, each of our studies tried to achieve several things:

1. Standardize the infectious challenge and the markers thereof
2. Standardize the characterization of nutritional status
3. Preclude the substitution of exogenous protein for amino acids that, under home feeding conditions, might have been provided from exogenous supplies
4. Develop and validate a study design that could be implemented in children and would require no blood (i.e., only urine and breath)
5. Study the metabolic effects of infection at an approximately uniform point in the course of the infection or challenge

One of the main achievements of the Coordinated Research Program was to unite developing country scientists in their mutual interest in the effects of chronic immune challenges or infection on growth, a pre-eminent concern in most developing country settings. This Program also resulted in several publications (43–46) and substantial experience in the uses of stable isotopic research methods in nutrition research in developing country settings, where typically access to these kinds of methods may be limited.

The central hypothesis of each of the studies was that obtaining sufficient quantities of the aromatic amino acids for synthesis of the acute phase proteins, using skeletal muscle as the sources of the amino acid substrates, would result in a relative surfeit of the branched chain amino acids, which would be oxidized after the amino acids that limited synthesis were exhausted. If true, this could explain some of the increases in amino acid oxidation that occur along with the negative nitrogen balance that is observed during infection. Our interest in the issue of nitrogen wasting was based in no small part on the hypothesis put forward by Scrimshaw in 1959 (17) and elaborated further by Solomons *et al.* (5): the occurrence of *unapparent* infections in children (i.e., no clinically apparent infection but a raised erythrocyte sedimentation rate and white cell count) is responsible for the diversion of nutrients from anabolic pathways and, thus, explains some of the growth faltering and malnutrition among children in developing countries. Thus, we were interested in the following:

1. Finding out whether a subclinical infection would result in increased oxidative losses of leucine, a branched chain amino acid present in relatively greater abundance in skeletal muscle than in acute phase proteins—as had been observed during *in vivo* infusions of crude IL-1 which resulted in increased excretion of N-methylhistidine, hydroxyproline, and creatinine (47) and increased leucine oxidation (48);
2. The dietary modification of the oxidative losses, if indeed they were shown to occur;
3. The practicalities and accuracies of orally administered stable isotope tracers given non-invasively for these kinds of studies.

To simulate a subclinical infection, we used a diphtheria, tetanus, and pertussis (DTP) vaccine. The particular field work discussed below was carried out in Bangalore, India, by a team that combined researchers at St. John's Medical College in Bangalore, India and at the Children's Nutrition Research Center at the Baylor College of Medicine in Houston, Texas, USA. The research program's interest was in evaluating the putative effects of subclinical infections on amino acid substrate partitioning, and particularly in developing practical alternatives to the intravenous tracer infusion methods to evaluate amino acid kinetics in children. The group, thus, had been working to elaborate the theoretic basis and practical application of a minimally invasive protocol (42,46).

Tracer studies of leucine metabolism were conducted using carbon-13 as a tracer of leucine and bicarbonate. A protocol in which isotopes were given orally to the children was run in parallel with a more conventional protocol for the intravenous administration of the isotopes in adults (46). The children were undernourished (weight for age Z-score, -2.3) and the adults had an average body mass index of 16.3 kg/m^2. Tracer protocols and breath collections performed during the fed state enabled the measurement of the rate of leucine oxidation and the rates of protein synthesis and breakdown. During the 6-hour studies, subjects were given small, frequent feeds of wheat starch biscuits (protein-free) at 30-minute intervals; breath, blood (adults only), and urine samples were collected according to the respective protocols. Our results showed significant increases in the rate of protein breakdown ($p < 0.05$) and a significant (17%) increase in the rate of leucine oxidation in the children following vaccination with DTP ($p < 0.01$). In adults, the DTP vaccination had no significant effect on whole body protein synthesis, but did cause a significant acceleration in the rates of protein breakdown, leucine flux, and leucine oxidation (21% increase; $p < 0.01$). The main conclusion from the study was that minor infections increase the irreversible oxidative loss of leucine, the amino acid that becomes available in disproportionately large amounts when muscle is catabolized to provide amino acid substrates. Thus, the process of redirecting amino acid metabolism appears to contribute to the irreversible loss of nitrogen and nitrogen wasting. This study was purposely controlled to preclude confounding effects of the dietary amino acid intake on the rate of leucine oxidation.

EFFECTS OF TUMOR NECROSIS FACTOR IN DOGS

Leucine released from the body protein mass must either be reutilized for *de novo* protein synthesis or be irreversibly lost to oxidation. Sakurai *et al.* (49) infused ^{13}C-leucine and ^{14}HCO$_3$ into conscious dogs along with recombinant tumor necrosis factor (rTNF) (bolus 2.5 μmol/kg plus a continuous infusion of 62.5 ng/kg/min), collected expired air through tracheostomy tubes, and took blood samples in which they measured isotopic enrichments and cytokine concentrations to study the effects of TNF on amino acid kinetics. Their observation of a 49% increase in the rate of leucine oxidation, which was significantly greater than the loss to nonoxidative disposal (*i.e.*, synthesis), along with a significant increase in the rate of urea production ($p < 0.05$ at each time point), suggested that net losses of leucine occurred from the body protein pool and that the leucine was irreversibly lost to oxidation. This finding supports the hypothesis that during infection or immune challenge, the body draws on the protein pool as a source of amino acids, reutilizes the amino acid substrates needed to mount the acute phase response, and oxidizes the surfeit that arises when muscle is catabolized to synthesize acute phase proteins.

NEGATIVE ACUTE PHASE PROTEINS

As stated, the negative acute phase proteins are the export or transport proteins, the synthetic rates of which decrease during infection (thus *negative acute phase*) through hepatic transcriptional inhibition of genes that code for these proteins (14). In this context, how might a chronic immune challenge or chronic infection or inflammation affect micronutrient status? To my knowledge, we do not know what effect leukocytes have in this relation; if cytokines are involved, however, then some effects are potentially attributable to infection. Cytokines inhibit the synthesis and release of transport proteins such as serum albumin, transthyretin, retinol-binding protein, and transferrin, among others. Those with reduced synthetic rates during the acute phase are referred to as *negative acute phase proteins*, such as transferrin and albumin. The reduction in the circulating levels of transport proteins results in decelerations in nutrient transport and in the redistribution of nutrients and, thus, is another mechanism whereby infection affects nutritional status.

Serum albumin concentration has been one of the tools relied on in the clinical evaluation of undernourished children in developing countries. It is thought to reflect both protein status and recent infection. One nutritionally relevant effect of TNF is a reduction in serum albumin, which can occur by two mechanisms. First, TNF decreases albumin gene transcription and steady state albumin mRNA levels (50) and, thus, reduces hepatic albumin synthesis (51). Second, the increased vascular permeability that cytokines induce leads to leaking of albumin into interstitial spaces and to loss of albumin through the gastrointestinal tract (52).

The acute phase is associated with low concentrations of plasma retinol; reduced concentrations of retinol-transport proteins, retinol-binding protein, and transthyretin; and a reduced abundance of retinol-binding protein mRNA in the liver (53). Thus, the reduced hepatic synthesis of retinol-binding protein and secretion of the retinol-to-retinol binding protein complex is a mechanism by which hyporetinolemia occurs in infection and explains the unreliability of plasma retinol concentration alone as an indicator of vitamin A status during or following an acute phase response. The mechanism whereby synthesis of acute phase proteins supersedes synthesis of transport proteins is, I believe, unknown. Recently, Mitra *et al.* (54) observed that serum retinol concentrations abruptly rebounded in patients during early convalescence from infection without administration of vitamin A, suggesting that hyporetinolemia is induced by the cytokine-mediated response to infection rather than being directly related to the hepatic retinol stores. In an accompanying review of the work by Mitra et al., Beisel (55) raised the question of whether the transient reduction in serum retinol during infections is a secondary consequence of cytokine-induced inhibition of retinol-binding protein and transthyretin production, or whether it should be classified, along with the effects on iron and copper, as an apparently purposeful cytokine-induced component of the acute phase reaction. The extent to which the competition for amino acid substrates under conditions of infection and an inadequate dietary intake blunts the synthesis of the nutrient transport proteins involved in vitamin A nutrition is an issue that can be explored using the isotopic methods for tracing amino acid metabolism.

Putting the research results into the challenging context of marginally nourished children living in crowded, unhygienic condition, Ruz *et al.* (6) postulated that some of the growth faltering in children results from the immunostimulation that occurs secondary to chronic exposure to insanitary environmental conditions, and the hypothesis has come to be known as *Noel's dirty chicken hypothesis*. At issue is the extent to which the crowded unhygienic living conditions foster *unapparent* or occult infections in children and thereby explain part of the syndrome of malnutrition in children. Some fundamental experimental evidence for this hypothesis came from studies by Klasing *et al.* on the effects of antibiotic treatment on growth in chickens (35–38), showing that chickens grew more poorly when reared in unsanitary conditions than when reared under the same conditions but were given antibiotics.

The main goal of this review has been to provide further evidence for the afore-mentioned hypothesis by reviewing evidence for the redistribution of amino acid substrates during infection, effects that could have particular relevance to anabolism under the pressure of chronic dietary deficiency. Evidence has been provided to support the hypothesis that the diversion of anabolic substrates from the peripheral skeletal muscle to support acute phase protein synthesis increases the oxidative disposal of indispensable amino acids. Furthermore, it was shown that growth inhibition by nonpathogenic microbes is reversed in asymptomatic poultry by antibiotic treatment. An *insanitary environment* may trigger a sufficient acute phase response to effect a redistribution of amino acids from nutrient transport and growth to maintenance of an acute phase response, where the duration of the *phase* may be most of early childhood. For many children in developing countries, and for some adults in developed countries (*e.g.*, elderly people and those in hospital) the concurrence of malnutrition and infection is a reality. Despite this, little is known about the chronic effects of cytokines on either the positive or the negative acute phase proteins in subclinical or *unapparent* infections. Growth faltering in asymptomatic children may result from either or both of the following factors: a diversion of anabolic substrates, and a cytokine effect on IGF-1, with a secondary effect on the growth hormone receptor. Oxidative disposal of exogenous amino acids, which cannot be used in the synthesis of acute phase proteins, partially explains the negative nitrogen balance in infection, including subclinical infection.

DIRECTIONS FOR FUTURE RESEARCH

Future research should take heed of the hypothesis made 40 years ago (20) that "the internal diversion of nutrients for the synthesis of compounds involved in the response to infection contributes importantly to the depletion of body stores." We need to learn more about the conditions under which, and to what extent, subclinical infections can cause a reorientation of amino acid metabolism such that growth or micronutrient status are altered. This research would need to be done in the field, where the children are living, and would benefit from the use of stable isotope tracers of amino acid metabolism such as have been used for decades but not applied extensively in developing countries. Less invasive methods, which are based on the oxidation of the limiting amino acid and breath collections or oral infusions and breath collections, may make these studies more practical for developing country settings.

Specific Goals or Questions for Future Research

1. A method to detect subclinical chronic infection in children, preferably based on urinary rather than plasma measures, is needed.
2. Characterization of the magnitude and mechanisms of growth inhibition in marginally nourished children (general or pathogen-specific) particularly in terms of:
   - Decreasing synthesis of visceral proteins, especially IGF-1 (the nutrient-endocrine axis)

- Catabolism of structural proteins, enzymes, or nutrient transport proteins to provide amino acid substrates under conditions when exogenous intake cannot satisfy the priority need to make the acute phase proteins (competition for substrates mechanism)

3. Reversal of the growth inhibitory effects of chronic infection in children by giving cytokine antibodies and determining the effect on the variables listed above
4. Reversal or blunting of the growth inhibitory effects listed above
5. Testing the hypothesis that the drive to provide sufficient substrates for the synthesis of acute phase proteins competes for substrates, energy, or in related ways compromises the synthesis of nutrient transport proteins and, thus, contributes to micronutrient malnutrition and possibly growth faltering. (Jahoor's group at the Children's Nutrition Research Center in Houston, Texas, working with researchers at the TMRU in Kingston Jamaica, has recently published a series of papers [56–60] that provide fundamental conceptual and methodologic insights into the experimental model needed to test this hypothesis, particularly with regard to modeling nutrient transport protein kinetics.)

ACKNOWLEDGMENTS

Comments and suggestions on drafts of this manuscript provided by Drs. William Beisel, Jerry Keusch, Kirk Klasing, Noel Solomons, and Bob Suskind are greatly appreciated.

REFERENCES

1. Scrimshaw NS. Effect of infection on nutrient requirements. *JPEN* 1991; 15: 589–600.
2. Mata LJ, Kromal RA, Urrutia JJ, et al. Effect of infection on food intake and the nutritional state: perspectives as viewed from the village. *Am J Clin Nutr* 1977; 30: 1215–27.
3. Martorell R, Ho TJ. Malnutrition, morbidity and mortality. In: Mosley H, Chen L, eds. Child survival: strategies for research. *Population Development Review* 1984; 10 (Suppl.): 49–68.
4. Waterlow JC. Protein turnover with special reference to man. *Q J Exp Physiol* 1984; 69: 409–38.
5. Solomons NW, Mazariegos M, Brown KH, Klasing KC. The underprivileged developing country child: environmental contamination and growth failure revisited. *Nutr Rev* 1993; 51: 1–6.
6. Ruz M, Solomons NW, Mejia LA, Chew F. Alteration of circulating micronutrients with overt and occult infections in anaemic Guatemalan preschool children. *Int J Food Sci Nutr* 1995; 46: 257–65.
7. Beisel WR. Magnitude of the host nutritional responses to infection. *Am J Clin Nutr* 1977; 30: 1236–47.
8. Beisel WR. Herman Award Lecture, 1995: Infection-induced malnutrition—from cholera to cytokines. *Am J Clin Nutr* 1995; 62: 813–19.
9. Beisel WR, Sawyer WD, Ryll ED, Crozier D. Metabolic effects of intracellular infections in man. *Ann Intern Med* 1967; 67: 744–79.
10. Roubenoff R. Inflammatory and hormonal mediators of cachexia. *J Nutr* 1997; 127:1014–16S.
11. Beisel WR. Metabolic and nutritional consequences of infection. In: Draper HH, ed. *Advances in nutritional research.* New York: Plenum Publishing, 1972; 1:125–143.
12. Klasing KC. Nutritional aspects of leukocytic cytokines. *J Nutr* 1988; 118: 1436–46.
13. Waterlow JC. *Protein-energy malnutrition.* London: Edward Arnold, 1992.
14. Keusch GT. Infection: nutritional interactions. In: Sadler MJ, Strain JJ, Caballero B, eds. *Encyclopedia of human nutrition.* New York: Academic Press, 1998.
15. Filteau SM, Morris SS, Abbott RA, et al. Influence of morbidity on serum retinol of children in a community-based study in northern Ghana. *Am J Clin Nutr* 1993; 58: 192–7.

16. De Benedetti F, Alonzi T, Moretta A, et al. Interkeukin 6 causes growth impairment in transgenic mice through a decrease in insulin-like growth factor-I. *J Clin Invest* 1997; 99: 643–50.
17. Scrimshaw NS, Taylor CE, Gordon JE. Interactions of nutrition and infection. *Am J Med Sci* 1959; 237: 367–403.
18. Beisel WR. Impact of infection on nutritional status: definition of the problem and objectives of the Workshop. *Am J Clin Nutr* 1977; 30: 1206–10.
19. Powanda MC, Beisel WR. Hypothesis: leukocyte endogenous mediator/endogenous pyrogen lymphocyte-activating factor modulates the development of nonspecific and specific immunity and affects nutritional status. *Am J Clin Nutr* 1982; 35: 762–8.
20. Scrimshaw NS, Behar M, Viteri F, Arroyave G, Tehada C. Epidemiology and prevention of severe protein malnutrition (kwashiorkor) in Central America. *Am J Public Health* 1957; 47: 53–67.
21. Scrimshaw NS, Taylor CE, Gordon JE. *Interactions of nutrition and infection.* Geneva: World Health Organisation, 1968.
22. Cooney RN, Kimball SR, Vary TC. Regulation of skeletal muscle protein turnover during sepsis: mechanisms and mediators. *Shock* 1997; 7: 1–16.
23. Bostian KA, Blackburn BS, Wannemacher RW, McGann VG, Beisel WR, DuPont HL. Sequential changes in the concentration of specific serum proteins during typhoid fever infection in man. *J Lab Clin Med* 1976; 87: 577–585.
24. Clowes GHA, George BC, Villee CA, Saravis CA. Muscle proteolysis induced by a circulating peptide in patients with sepsis or trauma. *N Engl J Med* 1983; 308: 545–52.
25. Warren RS, Starnes HF, Gabrilove JL, et al. The acute metabolic effects of tumor necrosis factor administration. *Arch Surg* 1987; 122: 1396–400.
26. Zamir O, Hasselgren PO, Kunkel SL, et al. Evidence that tumor necrosis factor participates in the regulation of muscle proteolysis during sepsis. *Arch Surg* 1992; 127: 170–4.
27. Espat NJ, Copeland EM, Moldawer LL. Tumor necrosis factor and cachexia: a current perspective. *Surg Oncol* 1994; 3: 255–62.
28. Chang HR, Bistrian B. The role of cytokines in the catabolic consequences of infection and injury. *JPEN* 1998; 22: 156–66.
29. Ling PR, Schwartz JH, Jeevandandam M, et al. Metabolic changes in rats during a continuous infusion of recombinant interleukin 1. *Am J Physiol* 1996; 270: E305–12.
30. Ling PR, Schwartz JH, Bistrian BR. Mechanisms of host wasting induced by administration of cytokines in rats. *Am J Physiol* 1997; 272: E333–9.
31. Darling G, Fraker DL, Jensen JC, et al. Cachectic effects of recombinant human tumor necrosis factor in rats. *Cancer Res* 1990; 50: 4008–13.
32. Milenkkovic L, Rettori V, Snyder GD, Beutler B, McCann SM. Cachectin alters anterior pituitary hormone release by a direct action in vitro. *Proc Natl Acad Sci USA* 1987; 86: 2418–22.
33. Raina N. Jeeheebhoy KN. Changes in body composition and dietary intake induced by tumor necrosis factor alpha and corticosterone—individually and in combination. *Am J Clin Nutr* 1998; 68: 1284–90.
34. Zamir O, Hasselgren PO, Kunkel SL, et al. Evidence that tumor necrosis factor participates in the regulation of muscle proteolysis during sepsis. *Arch Surg* 1992; 127: 170–4.
35. Klasing KC, Austic RE. Changes in protein degradation in chickens due to an inflammatory challenge. *Proc Soc Exp Biol Med* 1984; 176: 292–6.
36. Klasing KC, Laurin DE, Peng RK, Fry DM. Immunologically mediated growth depression in chicks: influence of feed intake, corticosterone and interleukin-1. *J Nutr* 1987; 117: 1629–723.
37. Klasing KC, Barnes DM. Decreased amino acid requirements of growing chicks due to immunologic stress. *J Nutr* 1988; 118: 1158–64.
38. Roura E, Homedes J, Klasing KC. Prevention of immunologic stress contributes to the growth-permitting ability of dietary antibiotics in chicks. *J Nutr* 1992; 122: 2383–90.
39. Reeds PJ, Fjeld CR, Jahoor F. Do the differences between the amino acid compositions of acute-phase and muscle proteins have a bearing on nitrogen loss in traumatic states? *J Nutr* 1994; 124: 906–10.
40. Colley CM, Fleck A, Goode AW, Muller BR, Myers MA. Early time course of acute-phase protein response in man. *J Clin Pathol* 1983; 36: 203–7.
41. Kushner I. The phenomenon of the acute phase response. *Ann NY Acad Sci* 1982; 389: 39–48.
42. Fjeld CR, ed. Application of stable isotope tracer methods to studies of amino acid, protein, and energy metabolism in malnourished populations of developing countries. Report of the First Research Coordination Meeting. Vienna: International Atomic Energy Agency, 1994.

43. Manary MJ, Brewster DR, Broadhead RL, Crowley JR, Fjeld CR, Yarasheski KE. Protein metabolism in children with edematous malnutrition and acute lower respiratory infection. *Am J Clin Nutr* 1997; 65: 1005–10.
44. Manary MJ, Brewster DR, Broadhead RL, et al. Whole-body protein kinetics in children with kwashiorkor and infection: a comparison of egg white and milk as dietary sources of protein. *Am J Clin Nutr* 1997; 66: 643–8.
45. Manary MJ, Broadhead Rl, Yarasheski KE. Whole-body protein kinetics in marasmus and kwashiorkor during acute infection. *Am J Clin Nutr* 1998; 67: 1205–9.
46. Kurpad AV, Jahoor F, Borgonha S, et al. A minimally invasive tracer protocol is effective for assessing the response of leucine kinetics and oxidation to vaccination in chronically energy-deficient adult males and children. *Am J Clin Nutr* 1999; 129: 1537–44.
47. Yang RS, Moldawer LL, Sakamoto A, et al. Leukocyte endogenous mediator alters protein dynamics in rats. *Metabolism* 1983; 32: 654–60.
48. Sobrado J, Moldawer LL, Bistrian BR, Dinarello CA, Blackburn GL. Effect of ibuprofen on fever and metabolic changes induced by continuous infusion of leukocytic pyrogen (interleukin 1) or endotoxin. *Infect Immun* 1983; 42: 997–1005.
49. Sakurai, Y, Zhang XJ, Wolfe RR. Effect of tumor necrosis factor on substrate and amino acid kinetics in conscious dogs. *Am J Physiol* 1994; 266: E936–45.
50. Brenner DA, Buck M, Freitelberg SP, Chojkier M. Tumor necrosis factor-alpha inhibits albumin gene expression in a murine model of cachexia. *J Clin Invest* 1990; 85: 248–55.
51. Rothwell NJ, Grimble RF. Metabolic and nutritional effects of TNF. In: Beutler B, ed. *Tumor necrosis factor*. New York: Raven Press, 1992.
52. Henning B, Hinckel R, Goldblum SE, et al. Tumor necrosis factor mediated hypoalbuminemia in rabbits. *J Nutr* 1988; 118: 1586–90.
53. Rosales FJ, Ritter SJ, Zolfaghari R, Smith JE, Ross AC. Effects of acute inflammation on plasma retinol, retinol-binding protein, and its mRNA in the liver and kidneys of vitamin A-sufficient rats. *J Lipid Res* 1996; 37: 962–71.
54. Mitra AK, Alvarez JO, Wahed MA, Fuchs CJ, Stephensen CB. Predictors of serum retinol in children with shigellosis. *Am J Clin Nutr* 1998; 68: 1088–94.
55. Beisel WR. Infection-induced depression of serum retinol—a component of the acute phase response or a consequence? *Am J Clin Nutr* 1998; 68: 993–4.
56. Morlese JF, Forrester T, Jahoor F. Acute-phase protein response to infection in severe malnutrition. *Am J Physiol* 1998; 275: E112–17.
57. Morlese JF, Forrester T, Del Rosario M, Frazer M, Jahoor F. Repletion of the plasma pool of nutrient transport proteins occurs at different rates during the nutritional rehabilitation of severely malnourished children. *J Nutr* 1998; 128: 214–19.
58. Morlese JF, Forrester T, Del Rosario M, Frazer M, Jahoor F. Transferrin kinetics are altered in children with severe protein-energy malnutrition. *J Nutr* 1997; 127: 1469–74.
59. Morlese JF, Forrester T, Dadaloo A, Del Rosario M, Frazer M, Jahoor F. Albumin kinetics in edematous and nonedematous protein-energy malnourished children. *Am J Clin Nutr* 1996; 64: 952–9.
60. Jahoor F, Sivakumar B, Del Rosario M, Frazer EM. Isolation of acute-phase proteins from plasma for determination of fractional synthesis rates by a stable isotope tracer technique. *Anal Biochem* 1996; 236: 95–100.

DISCUSSION

Dr. Keusch: I wanted to make a comment about the dirty chicken, and the concept that antibiotics exert their growth-promoting action by an antibacterial effect. That may not be the case. Studies were carried out in the 1950s and 1960s using the dregs from tetracycline production, which have no antimicrobial activity but were fed to domestic animals for testing growth promotion. They were found to have a growth-promoting effect that was similar to the fractions that had antibiotic activity. Human experiments were also carried out by Scrimshaw in Guatemala, using a β-lactam and a protein synthesis inhibitor (tetracycline, I think). What they observed in children, which depended somewhat on the antibiotic, was some initial growth promotion and then a failure to show any effect as the experiment continued, which is unlike what you see in animal husbandry (1). So, even though a growth-promoting effect of antibiotics may be seen in humans, it is not sustained, and we would have to try to explain that on the basis of alterations in the flora, which makes it a lot more complicated than you were implying.

This brings me to question the hypothesis about latent infection, and extrapolating from your experiment with DTP to asymptomatic infections. After all, DTP immunization is not asymptomatic; it causes an inflammatory response, typically with fever, whereas the situation that you are talking about with latent infection would be asymptomatic. Whether or not an activation of the acute phase response occurs that is sufficient to cause a sustained effect remains to be proved, I think. Your experiment does not address that, although it is very provocative in terms of mild inflammatory stimuli. But to give you the benefit of the doubt, under conditions of limiting diet, small changes might be important over the long run.

Dr. Griffin: Following on from that, we studied a vaccination model in the same way as you did in adults, using the Burroughs-Wellcome monovalent typhoid vaccine, which induces a beautiful acute phase response over about 36 to 48 hours. We applied stable isotope technology with ^{15}N guanidino-labeled nitrogen in arginine to see if nitric oxide is part of this acute phase response. In the 12 humans we looked at, no increased conversion to 15N nitric oxide was seen in this 48-hour period. So, we can rule out nitric oxide in vaccine-induced acute phase responses as a potential for therapy.

Dr. Meydani: Can you predict whether you would see the same effect or a different effect if you were to do the same experiments in well-nourished children or adults?

Dr. Fjeld: I think the point is that if the dietary intake is not adequate to support that diversion, then the endogenous source becomes the source of substrates. So, it is a low dietary quality situation that we are most interested in, but the metabolic effect should still hold in the well-nourished individual if dietary intake is short circuited during that time.

Dr. Zoppi: You said at the beginning of your presentation that there is an impairment in growth hormone efficiency and secretion. Do you have any experience in the administration of growth hormone to infants who are infected in order to improve nutritional status and growth?

Dr. Fjeld: Reports have been made of children in developing countries where growth hormone concentrations have been measured and found to be normal. Normal growth hormone concentrations were also found in juvenile rheumatoid arthritis. It seems that the expression of the receptor on the hepatocyte is reduced by the changes in IL-6 and IGF-1 (2). I do not have any experience with the administration of growth hormone to infected children, although I do have some in relation to children with short stature. It can enhance growth in the short term, but the effect is generally not sustained in the long term.

Dr. Klish: In your DTP immunization studies, I would assume that you could affect your leucine kinetics by the nutritional status of the individual at the time the kinetics were done. You mentioned the children were on an equilibration diet, but it was only for 2 days. I would be curious to know what the equilibration diet was. Did you maintain the children in catabolism or convert them to anabolism?

As a comment, everybody who has discussed growth faltering in relation to infection has used Mata's weight data. I have a slide in my collection of his height data, which I think tells more about the impact of negative nitrogen balance in infected children. Every time one of these children became infected, they would stop growing in height. After recovery, they would begin to grow again, but would not quite catch up to normal before they became infected again. As a result, you can see persistent height faltering over the 3- to 4-year period they were studied.

Dr. Fjeld: The people in Bangalore who did the study have excellent dietitians who measured the customary dietary intake. They then concocted a diet for the equilibration phase that would keep the subjects in energy balance but that would give them all a similar background abundance of ^{13}C, which varies in the different foodstuffs in the diet. Thus, the diet was tailored to meet their energy needs, but gave a consistent amount of $^{13}CO_2$ as background.

Dr. Klish: Were 2 days enough to do that?

Dr. Fjeld: I hope so.

Dr. Gershwin: I like the thesis and I do not think we should be overly concerned about re-exploration of studies that were done in the 1950s and 1960s. But for the data to be reconciled, we are going to have to consider the nature of the flora and what the specific organisms are, because obviously there are going to be differences.

Dr. Marini: Do you feel that the reaction of the body to acute infection is independent of the agent—gram-positive or gram-negative bacteria, fungi, and so on—or does it depend on the agent to some extent? In neonates, differences are seen according to the agent causing the sepsis.

Dr. Fjeld: My intuition tells me that the responses have to differ markedly, but that is certainly not in my area of expertise.

Dr. Marini: I asked the question because in the baby with gram-negative sepsis is found hyperglycemia and hyperinsulinemia, in other words insulin resistance. When we manage these babies with total parenteral nutrition, they do better when we add medium chain triglycerides.

Dr. Griffin: In your balance experiments with muscle protein and acute phase proteins, did you take into account the negative synthesis of albumin during the acute phase response, which would be contributing to the amino acid pool for the acute phase proteins?

Dr. Fjeld: No, we looked at overall muscle composition and overall acute phase protein composition. Those are described in our 1994 paper in the *Journal of Nutrition* (3).

Dr. Griffin: During the acute phase response albumin synthesis falls considerably.

Dr. Fjeld: That is right, the nutrient transport proteins in general fall precipitously. An extension of this hypothesis is that a driving force may exist: if the host is trying to synthesize the acute phase proteins, that may be a factor in reducing the synthesis rate of the nutrient transport proteins.

Dr. Griffin: That is transcriptionally controlled. The lack of amino acids going into those pools will contribute to your acute phase pool as well.

Dr. Fjeld: But the idea that phenylalanine and other amino acids of that group are limiting would still hold true.

Dr. Suskind: Some years ago, when we first started looking at the endocrine changes in malnutrition, we found that these children had very high growth hormone levels and very low IGF-1 levels. We began looking at recovery of IGF-1 during renutrition and it seemed to follow the other visceral proteins. So it appeared that IGF-1 was a very sensitive visceral protein for assessing recovery from malnutrition and also from infection, which was obviously a major factor in the low IGF-1 levels. I was wondering whether you might comment on the relative roles of infection and growth. Perhaps what is happening is that the increase in production of cytokines is traded against the production of visceral proteins and that one of those visceral proteins is IGF-1; when the infectious insult is over, this can return to normal to allow a normal endocrine profile and, hence, normal growth to be re-established.

The second point I would like you to comment on is the question of whether it could be the products of muscle catabolism that promote the loss of zinc, water-soluble vitamins, vitamin A, and other nutrients. I wonder if you might comment on that to try to put the whole picture together in terms of the catabolic response.

Dr. Fjeld: I think your explanation about the downregulation of the IGF-1 as a visceral protein is a lovely idea; it certainly fits with this whole hypothesis. With regard to your second point, I have not made a quantitative assessment, but one can appreciate the concept that when skeletal muscle is catabolized, not only is there a loss of nitrogen but also of the other constitutive elements of lean body mass, including potassium and the micronutrients. Also, there is downregulation of the rate of synthesis of the nutrient transport proteins such as retinol-binding protein and transferrin, and that is partly why we see, for instance, more vitamin A loss from the body during times of infection.

Dr. Wasantwisut: I would like to hear your comments on the implications in terms of protein quality for a population at high risk of infection. In the past, only the absolute amount of protein in the diet has been considered and this is usually derived mainly from plant protein in developing countries. You imply that it may be important to have animal protein.

Dr. Fjeld: I think that is the key question. We do not have enough data yet; however, as I see it, this brings into question some of our fundamental concepts about protein requirements, given that metabolic demands may be placed on protein that determine what levels of individual amino acids are best suited to the individual under particular conditions. Most data on amino acid requirements are based on nitrogen balance studies, which are less sensitive to flux of single amino acids than the tracer studies that can now be carried out internationally. The International Dietary Energy Consultancy Group met a few years ago in London and examined the question of whether protein requirements needed to be reconsidered in infected children. It was considered that the data were too sparse to support such a re-evaluation. However, this notion can now be explored with newer tracer methodology that allows us to follow the flux of individual amino acids under defined conditions.

Dr. Coovadia: I would like to comment on an issue that was raised earlier: although it is important to look at the host, it may be very important to look at the agent too. Your elegant methods may help to unravel some important clinical problems. I want to illustrate this by experiences that go back over many years. Not all infections are associated with weight loss, and the rate of weight loss is quite different in different infections. Anyone who has seen a child with measles knows how rapid the weight loss can be, but in a child with chronic gastrointestinal tuberculosis weight is lost by a much more gradual attrition. And you have to see a case of the acquired immunodeficiency syndrome to know what real marasmus is. So, different agents produce different patterns. Even more interesting is the fact that some infections are not associated with malnutrition at all, and the impact of the disease on nutritional state is minimal. One example is streptococcal infection causing nephritis. This starts with a streptococcal sore throat, but it then causes an immune reaction in the kidney with resulting glomerulonephritis. This nearly always occurs in well-nourished children and the weight loss during the disease is minimal. The other condition is meningitis. In our setting, where malnutrition is prevalent, meningitis is rarely associated with severe malnutrition. So the point I am making is that your methods could be used to elucidate the impact of different agents on nutrition.

Dr. Farthing: I think we would all agree that the mobilization of amino acids from muscle during the acute phases is vital in terms of the initial host defense, but I sometimes wonder whether the body responds excessively. For example, I wonder whether a 50 times increase in C-reactive protein is really necessary. Dr. Keusch brought to our attention the fact that a very important part of the interaction between organism and host is host generated, and that a lot of diseases, for instance in the intestine, are actually generated by the host immune system. Good examples are shigellosis and enterohemorrhagic *Escherichia coli*, where most of the damage is produced by host immune cells. So, do we really need this magnitude of acute phase response or is the body overreacting to a stimulus? My question is, do you think that there would ever be a time when one might consider modulating the acute phase response to limit the amount of somatic damage? Are there any clever ways whereby we might at least modulate it? Particularly, as we know that nutritional restoration in the acute phase of the illness is never going to entirely restore the negative nitrogen balance and somatic mass?

Dr. Fjeld: I could think about blunting the nutritional effect of the acute phase response, but I do not think I can comment on whether it is an exaggerated response relative to the biological need.

Dr. Farthing: But I think it is an interesting research question.

Dr. Woodward: It seems to me that we can let the body give us the answer, or at least initiate an answer. By which I mean that we can now say the body for some reason places a high metabolic priority on maintaining acute phase protein concentrations in the blood, regardless of metabolic status; this is done even in the marasmic child, although interestingly by a different mechanism from what is accepted for you and me (4). We seem to increase synthesis, whereas the marasmic child accomplishes the same endpoint by decreasing catabolism. We need to find out the reason for this high priority, but in the meanwhile I would suggest that as acute phase proteins are maintained at a high level even under extreme circumstances, there must be an important protective reason. Of course, antioxidant defense is among them.

Dr. Griffin: If you look at animal models of infection and you remove some of the cytokine effect, for example by blocking TNF in salmonella models in rodents, the immune response is almost completely ablated and mortality increases greatly. In *Listeria* models, you see the same effect if you block TNF or IL-6. In humans, in the intensive care situation, given high dose methyl prednisolone, mortality from secondary infections is greatly increased, and that treatment is now contraindicated, of course, in the ICU setting. If we start to manipulate the acute phase response, we must be very careful not to remove crucial elements of the response. I do not think we are in a position yet to know what they are. Tuberculosis is a prime example. TNF is crucial in the formation of granulomas and the sequestration of that organism; if you ablate that response, you get much more profound metabolic change and death in animal models. So, I would advise caution.

Dr. Meydani: I can offer two examples from our own work where a nutritional manipulation was effective in reducing some of the effects associated with the acute phase response. One example is a study looking at IL-1 induced weight loss in an animal model, where we used fish oil to reduce the production of prostaglandin E_2, and, therefore, obviate the weight loss that you normally see (5,6). In that case, the effect of limiting the acute phase response was beneficial. Also, in our vitamin E studies in influenza infection, we were able to reduce the weight loss associated with influenza without really affecting several other mechanisms, for example TNF production or IL-6 production or some of the inflammatory mediators that probably will be needed for defense against the infection. So, I think the key question is how to manipulate the response without, as Dr. Griffin said, affecting crucial functions. In that regard nutritional manipulation might be somewhat different from using antibodies against specific cytokines, where you would totally reduce or inactivate the function of the cytokine.

Dr. Roberton: Do you have any specific suggestions for the immune outcome in your immunization model? The purpose of the protein catabolism and of nutritional restitution, it is hoped, is to mount a more efficient inflammatory response. The acute phase response has a lot of nonspecific elements to it that create an immediate inflammatory response, but also some longer term components. Do you have any suggestions how you might measure the efficiency of the immune response in your immunization model as a long-term effect resulting from the transient nutritional supplementation? What are the outcome indicators that would be useful?

Dr. Fjeld: One of the indicators we would be interested in is turnover—how much futile cycling of amino acids there is. We would want to get the most synthesis out of the least amount of breakdown. We may be also interested in the rate at which nutrient transport proteins are synthesized, and the relative compromise between the positive acute phase proteins and the decrement in nutrient transport proteins. For instance, we know that children who are asymptomatic in the field but who have a raised leukocyte count also have disturbances in micronutrient nutrition. We think these are caused, at least partially, by the unavailability of transport proteins, so the lack of those transport proteins seems to be compromising the child's micronutrient status, with all its attendant consequences. So, we want to look at the balance between the synthesis of the acute phase proteins and the maintenance of adequate nutrient transport proteins, for instance. And both of those things could be looked at using a tracer methodology.

Dr. Suskind: If we were to provide the limiting amino acids for the acute phase reaction, such as phenylalanine, tyrosine, and tryptophan, during the infectious state, do you think the loss of nitrogen would be mitigated, thereby providing us an approach to treatment in the acutely infected patient?

Dr. Fjeld: It is tempting to say yes, but I am sure many other nutrient and dietary factors need to be considered along with that. It would not simply be a matter of including those amino acids.

REFERENCES

1. Guzman MA, Scrimshaw NS, Bruch HA, et al. Nutrition and infection field study in Guatamalan villages, 1959–64. Physical growth and development of preschool children. *Arch Environ Health* 1968; 17: 107–18.
2. Chikanza IC. Neuroendocrine immune features of pediatric inflammatory rheumatic diseases. *Ann NY Acad Sci* 1999; 22: 71–80.
3. Reeds PJ, Fjeld C, Jahoor F. Do the differences between the amino acid compositions of acute-phase and muscle proteins have a bearing on nitrogen loss in traumatic states? *J Nutr* 1994; 124: 906–10.
4. Morelese JF, Forrester T, Jahoor F. Acute-phase response to infection in severe malnutrition. *Am J Physiol* 1998; 275: E112–7.
5. Hellerstein M, Meydani SN, Meydani M, et al. Interleuken-1-induced anorexia in rats: influence of prostaglandins. *J Clin Invest* 1989; 84: 228–235.
6. Han SN, Wu D, Ha WK, et al. Vitamin (E) supplementation increases splenocyte IL-2 and interferon-γ production of old mice infected with influenza virus. *FASEB J* 1998; 12: A819.

Nutrition, Immunity, and Infection in Infants and Children, edited by Robert M. Suskind and Kraisid Tontisirin. Nestlé Nutrition Workshop Series, Pediatric Program, Vol. 45. Nestec Ltd., Vevey/Lippincott Williams & Wilkins, Philadelphia ©2001.

Anorexia and Cytokines in the Acute Phase Response to Infection

Michael J.G. Farthing and Anne B. Ballinger

Digestive Diseases Research Centre, St. Bartholomew's and The Royal London School of Medicine and Dentistry, London, UK

The cardinal clinical features of systemic infection are fever, anorexia, myalgia, and lethargy sometimes leading to sleep. During the acute phase of infection, these symptoms are judged to have a net benefit for the host, as the adaptive value of fever is thought to enhance immune responses and stabilize cell membranes; anorexia supervenes at a time when it may be more difficult for the host to obtain food; and myalgia and somnolence reduce mobility, thus limiting the body's demands for energy during the acute phase response. Anorexia, reduced food intake, and loss of body weight usually reverse rapidly in self-limited infections (*e.g.*, influenza), but when infection persists, reduced food intake is probably the major contributor to energy deficits, which in infants and young children can lead to retarded growth and development. Thus, understanding the mechanisms of anorexia and reduced food intake during infection could have important therapeutic implications in the future, as the possibility of modulating the unwanted effects of mediators of the acute phase response becomes an increasing reality.

INFECTION AND ANOREXIA

Irrefutable evidence indicates that most systemic and many single organ infections produce anorexia and reduced food intake (1–4). Mata *et al.* clearly demonstrated the relationship between infection and growth faltering: respiratory and gastrointestinal (GI) infections, bacterial meningitis, pertussis, and viral infections such as rubella and varicella all interrupted linear growth and produced weight loss which, on the basis of dietary studies, was attributed predominantly to reduced food intake during the infection (1). Martorell *et al.*, also working in Guatemala, performed a 4-year longitudinal study in 477 children (2). During this period, home visits were made to assess the incidence of illness, and related this to food intake in the cohort by assessing

24-hour dietary recall. When children were ill, daily energy intake diminished on average by about 25%. Hoyle *et al.* measured 24-hour food and breast milk intake in 41 Bangladeshi children aged 6 to 35 months (3). Fifteen children had standard hospital care; the mothers of a second group of 15 children received dietary education in which the importance of feeding during illness was heavily endorsed; and a third group of 11 healthy control children were recruited through their mothers who were attending family planning clinics. Children with diarrhea had energy intakes that were 42% less than healthy controls, and dietary education failed to have any impact on energy intake. This indicates that anorexia is the major determinant of reduced energy intake, not food withholding, which had been thought to be a factor in the past when mothers were advised to stop feeding during acute diarrheal illness. The intake of breast milk, however, did not change significantly in ill children, indicating that this is a useful route to provide energy during diarrheal disease and should be continued during the illness at all costs. Food intake has been shown to be reduced in Nigerian children with intestinal parasites and in *Ascaris lumbricoides* infection; dietary intake of protein and energy was inversely related to the severity of the infection.

Food intake has also been shown to be reduced in a variety of animal models of infection including *Ascaris suum* infection in the pig, *Nippostrongylus brasiliensis* in the rat, and *Toxoplasma gondii* (5) and influenza virus infection (6) in mice.

The weight loss commonly associated with the human immunodeficiency virus (HIV) infection appears, at least in the United Kingdom, to be entirely caused by reduced energy intake secondary to anorexia (7). The situation may be more complex in the poorer countries of the world such as Africa, where opportunistic infections are more difficult to treat and nutrient losses from the GI tract and increased energy expenditure may be contributory factors (8). Nevertheless, HIV infection remains a highly relevant clinical example of the effect of a systemic virus infection on appetite and food intake (9).

The mechanisms by which infectious diseases modulate appetite and food intake will be discussed in more detail below. However, it is evident from the data reviewed so far that anorexia occurs both in systemic infections such as those caused by viruses (influenza, rubella, varicella, malaria, and HIV) and also in localized infections such as those limited to a specific organ (pneumonia, meningitis, gastroenteritis). Infections of the GI tract can have special additional effects on food intake, as ingestion of food may exacerbate abdominal pain and diarrhea, and delayed gastric emptying and ileus associated with infection, produce sensations of abdominal bloating and early satiety. Vomiting is common during the early phase of many GI infections, which is a major disincentive to the sufferer to take food or fluids by mouth. Thus, these observations indicate that infections can modulate appetite through their systemic effects and also through local effects in the gastrointestinal tract.

APPETITE CONTROL IN HEALTH

Appropriate feeding behavior is vital for survival. Feeding is essential, not only for the provision of essential macro- and micronutrients but for its fundamental role in maintaining overall energy homeostasis. Body energy stores in the form of adipose tissue are maintained over long periods of time by variations in feeding behavior that are dependent on fluctuations in energy requirements.

Central Mechanisms

Following a period of food deprivation, central feeding pathways in the hypothalamus are activated, partly in response to low circulating levels of insulin and leptin (Fig. 1). The most well-characterized signaling pathway within the hypothalamus is the arcuate nucleus–paraventricular nucleus, neuropeptide Y (ARC–PVN NPY) pathway (10,11). Axons project from NPY containing cell bodies in the arcuate nucleus to the paraventricular nucleus which is an important central site for the integration of energy homeostasis. NPY receptors (Y1 and Y5) are plentiful in the paraventricular nucleus, and central administration of NPY increases feeding behavior. Repeated administration of NPY can produce obesity. The ARC–PVN projection is stimulated by conditions of energy deficit and weight loss, notably fasting. These conditions increase NPY mRNA levels in the ARC, raise NPY levels in the paraventricular nucleus, and enhance NPY release in the paraventricular nucleus. The activity of the ARC–PVN projection only returns to normal when overeating has restored body weight to control values. NPY is considered to drive hunger and hyperphagia in these energy-deficient states. The increase in hypothalamic NPY mRNA

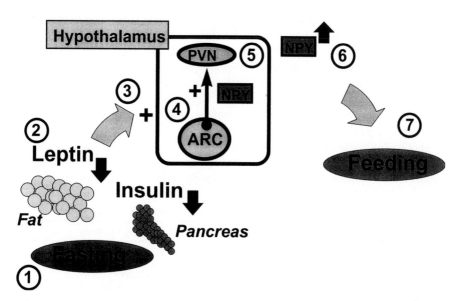

FIG. 1. The neuroendocrine response to fasting. An early response to fasting (1) is a decrease in circulating levels of insulin and leptin, and the anorectic hormone secreted by adipocytes (2). In response to these changes (3), the arcuate nucleus (ARC) increases synthesis and release of neuropeptide Y (NPY) (4), which is released into the paraventricular nucleus (PVN) (5). This increase in NPY (6) induces hunger and feeding behavior (7). Other mediators are almost certainly involved, although the insulin–leptin NPY pathway is the best characterized to date.

that occurs with fasting can be attenuated by administration of insulin and leptin. Although the ARC–PVN NPY pathway is the most extensively studied, other signaling molecules have been implicated in increasing feeding behavior following fasting. Deletion of the NPY gene in mice does not appear to affect food intake or body weight. Thus, it would appear that other systems are able to compensate and maintain feeding behavior in the absence of NPY. Signaling molecules of particular interest include other hypothalamic neuropeptides such as melanin-concentrating hormone (12) and the recently described orexins A and B (Table 1).

As soon as energy homeostasis has been restored, it is essential that feeding should terminate. Several signaling molecules have been implicated, including corticotrophin-releasing hormone, which is synthesized in paraventricular nucleus neurons; the melanocortins, particularly α-melanocyte–stimulating hormone (α-MSH); and serotonin (5-hydroxytryptamine, 5-HT) (Table 1). Leptin is also thought to act by activation of the melanocortin and corticotrophin-releasing hormone pathways. Serotonergic neurons project from the median raphé to the paraventricular nucleus and, when activated, inhibit the release of NPY from the nucleus. A new satiety peptide, cocaine and amphetamine regulated transcript (CART), has recently been described and is thought to be closely associated with leptin and NPY pathways (13).

Peripheral Mechanisms

Cholecystokinin (CCK) is thought to be an important satiety regulator (14,15). On feeding, CCK is released both in the central nervous system (CNS) and from the gastrointestinal tract. Administration of CCK reduces meal size but chronic administration does not alter body weight. Experimental animals can compensate by taking an increased number of smaller meals. CCK-A knockout mice gain weight. It is considered that CCK has its major effect through vagal afferent pathways rather than through direct effects in the CNS, as distal vagotomy abolishes the satiety effect. Other proposed satiety peptides include bombesin, somatostatin, and glucagonlike peptide-1 (Table 1).

Another long-established putative mechanism for postprandial satiety is gastric distension. Distension receptors are present within the gastric wall and evidence indicates that larger, more bulky meals induce satiety earlier than those of smaller bulk

TABLE 1. *Central nervous system modulators of food intake*

Feeding promoters	Feeding inhibitors
Neuropeptide Y	Cholecystokinin
Galanin	Corticotrophin-releasing hormone
Melanin-concentrating hormone	α-Melanocytes stimulating hormone
Orexin A and B	Cocaine and amphetamine regulated transcript
Peptide YY	Insulin
Norepinephrine	Glucagon-like peptide-1
β-Endorphin	Serotonin
Dynorphin	Bombesin
Gonadotrophin-releasing horomone	Calcitonin gene-related peptide

but of the same energy value. However, it is unlikely that this phenomenon is mediated directly by the vagus because vagotomy does not abolish the satiety effect, indicating the involvement of a humoral mechanism. Bombesin appears to be the most likely candidate as its effects are preserved following complete denervation of the stomach.

Thus, feeding behavior and energy homeostasis rely on a variety of inhibitory and stimulatory signals from the periphery which are integrated within the hypothalamus. Understanding these mechanisms will ultimately lead to the development of agents directed at key sites within these pathways to reduce feeding behavior in the obese and to reverse anorexia in those with disease. Current evidence from studies in humans and experimental animal models indicates that the proinflammatory cytokines tumor necrosis factor-α (TNF-α), interleukin (IL)-1, IL-6, and possibly IL-8 are likely to be the most important mediators of anorexia in infectious diseases, cancer, and chronic inflammatory disorders.

CYTOKINES AND INFECTIOUS DISEASES

Most clinically significant infectious diseases produce an immune or inflammatory response in the host. In some, this may be exquisitely localized (*e.g.*, a minor skin infection), whereas in others evidence may point to extensive systemic immune activation (16,17). Cytokines are produced by a variety of immunocytes and other inflammatory cells and by other cell types (*e.g.*, epithelial cells) not generally regarded as playing an active role in the immune response. Cytokines coordinate the immune and inflammatory response, having a variety of roles that can be broadly classified as proinflammatory and anti-inflammatory. The chemokines, an important class of cytokines of which now more than 40 have been described, play a major role in the pathogenesis of infective and inflammatory disease because of their ability to act as leukocyte chemoattractants (18–20). Depending on the chemokine, a wide range of chemoattractant activities can be directed toward eosinophils, basophils, monocytes, resting and activated T cells, dendritic cells, neutrophils, and natural killer cells. Perhaps one of the most interesting recent discoveries is that a variety of microorganisms can induce chemokine synthesis and release by nonimmune cells, thereby initiating a local inflammatory response before classic antigen-mediated immune pathways have been activated (21–23). It is likely that this forms part of an early innate, nonimmune host defense response, although the consequence of this inflammatory response may have deleterious effects for the host.

Various proinflammatory cytokines have been identified as being important in infectious diseases because of both their central role in the acute phase response, including the production of acute phase proteins, and their potentially damaging nutritional consequences (24). IL-1, IL-6, and other cytokines have been detected in the cerebrospinal fluid of patients with the acquired immunodeficiency syndrome (AIDS), indicating that these cytokines are either generated within the CNS or are able to gain access to it during infection and in other states that produce systemic immune activation (10).

Tumor Necrosis Factor-α

TNF-α, identified as having antitumor activity in 1975, was subsequently shown to be the humoral mediator of cachexia in *Trypanosoma brucei* infection in cattle and experimental animals (16). TNF is produced predominantly by macrophages and monocytes that have been activated, for example, by bacterial lipopolysaccharide (25). TNF-α has been implicated as a key endogenous mediator of endotoxic shock associated with serious gram-negative infections. TNF-α is an important inflammatory mediator in many infectious diseases including cerebral malaria and HIV infection. We have shown evidence of major systemic immune activation in patients with AIDS in Zambia, with extremely high plasma levels of neopterin and soluble TNF receptor (sTNF-R55). sTNF-R55 concentrations correlated negatively with measures of nutritional status such as body mass index (8). The concentrations of sTNF-R55 were significantly higher than local HIV-negative control subjects with tuberculosis, indicating the magnitude of the immune activation in HIV infection. TNF-α, the prototype proinflammatory cytokine, is particularly important because of its ability to promote the synthesis and secretion of other proinflammatory cytokines including IL-1, IL-6, granulocyte-macrophage colony-stimulating factor, and a variety of chemokines, including IL-8 (16,25).

Interleukin 1

Previously known as endogenous pyrogen, IL-1 is another important proinflammatory cytokine produced during most infective febrile illnesses. In addition to fever, IL-1 induces thermogenesis, hypophagia, and cachexia (26,27) and has various neuroendocrine effects that are mediated through corticotrophin-releasing factor and result in the release of adrenocorticotrophic hormone from the pituitary gland.

Interleukin 6

The proinflammatory cytokine IL-6 is increased in infections associated with marked tissue inflammation, particularly invasive infections of the GI tract, such as shigellosis. IL-6 is the major stimulus to the production of acute phase proteins (28), although an interaction with IL-1 or TNF-α is required for the induction of C-reactive protein and serum amyloid A. In addition, IL-6 produced in the brain stem is required for the production of fever, and IL-6 has also been implicated in the central modulation of feeding behavior.

Interleukin 8

Intraventricular administration of the chemokine IL-8 has also been shown to induce anorexia in rats, although its effect was less potent than IL-β but similar to TNF-α (27). The most profound suppression of feeding behavior was achieved by a combination of IL-1β, TNF-α, and IL-8.

Proinflammatory cytokines also have effects in the liver that may be relevant to the growth inhibitory effects of some chronic infections. IL-1β and TNF-α produce decreased responsiveness to growth hormone, with reduced plasma concentrations of insulinlike growth factor 1 (IGF-1), at least in part, because of a decrease in the expression of growth hormone receptors on hepatocytes. IL-6 may have a similar role as transgenic mice that overexpress this cytokine have reduced plasma concentrations of IGF-1 and are growth retarded (29).

Thus, the increased production of proinflammatory cytokines during acute and chronic infection may not only modulate their well-recognized clinical manifestations (*e.g.*, fever and septic shock), but also directly influence appetite and feeding behavior. In addition, proinflammatory cytokines may retard growth in young children, an effect that is independent of that on food intake.

MECHANISMS BY WHICH CYTOKINES PRODUCE ANOREXIA

Administration of TNF-α, IL-1, IL-6, and IL-8 induce hypophagia and weight loss in experimental animals. Implantation of tissue culture cell lines into mice that overexpress TNF-α or IL-6 also produces anorexia and weight loss in them. Important questions remain, however, as to the precise mechanisms by which these proinflammatory cytokines influence feeding behavior. Identification of the central signaling pathways involved in feeding behavior requires the use of experimental models of infection or inflammation. For a model to be informative, it is important in the first place that the experimental intervention resembles, at least in part, a human infection or systemic immune activation; second, that it will identify which cytokine or cytokines are responsible for anorexia and decrease in body weight; and third, that it is appropriate for assessing the central hypothalamic neural pathways involved in feeding behavior. Various models have been developed that activate components of the infection or inflammation anorectic pathways.

Systemic Immune Activation Models

Administration of low-dose lipopolysaccharide to rats increases circulating levels of proinflammatory cytokines (including IL-1, IL-6, and TNF-α) and inhibits feeding behavior (27). In addition, lipopolysaccharide increases IL-1β mRNA in the CNS, indicating that lipopolysaccharide not only promotes cytokine production in the periphery but also has direct effects in the CNS (30). Pretreatment of mice with an IL-1 receptor antagonist (rA) prevents the IL-1β–induced reduction in feeding behavior in mice.

Specific Cytokine Models

An alternative experimental approach is to administer individual proinflammatory cytokines, either centrally or peripherally (27), or to create a cytokine generator system such as implanting a tissue culture cell line that overexpresses an individual cytokine (31) or producing a cytokine overexpressing transgenic animal (29). Using these approaches, evidence shows that TNF-α, IL-1β, IL-6, and IL-8 inhibit feeding behavior. Although the mechanisms have not been fully elucidated in this experimental system, it has been shown that IL-1β causes release of serotonin which would inhibit feeding behavior. IL-1β and other cytokines (IL-2, IL-6, IL-12 and TNF-α) promote release of corticotrophin-releasing hormone in the paraventricular nucleus, which inhibits ARC NPY gene expression, resulting in decreased ARC NPY and anorexia (10).

Models of Infection and Inflammation

Various models have been used to mimic human infection or inflammatory disorders. Administration of an influenza virus to mice inhibits feeding behavior and produces loss of body weight, which can be partially reversed by administration of IL-1ra, given either by repeated subcutaneous injection or by continuous subcutaneous infusion by osmotic minipumps (6). These observations suggest that IL-1β is a major mediator of hypophagia during experimental influenza virus infection, although it is unlikely that it accounts completely for the alteration in feeding behavior.

A model of bowel inflammation using trinitrobenzensulphonic acid (TNBS) in ethanol has been used to study feeding behavior and the central pathways involved in appetite control. TNBS colitis produces an early and profound reduction in food intake and loss of body weight, which gradually recovers over a 7-day period. It is assumed, therefore, that this represents an acute phase response to intestinal inflammation (32). We have shown that the reduction in food intake is accompanied by inappropriately low concentrations of 5-HT in the paraventricular nucleus and increased 5-HT release (33). This increased hypothalamic 5-HT neuronal activity would suppress the drive to eat and produce hypophagia. In pair-fed animals (i.e., healthy but food restricted to match the food intake of colitic animals), a marked increase was seen in paraventricular nucleus 5-HT concentration and an appropriate reduction in 5-HT release, which would tend to promote feeding behavior in response to energy restriction.

We have also studied the role of NPY in the central mediation of anorexia in TNBS colitis (34). NPY release from the paraventricular nucleus was appropriately increased in both pair-fed rats and rats with colitis, indicating that anorexia cannot be explained simply by impaired synthesis and release of NPY. However, Million *et al.*, using the same model, have shown that hypothalamic ARC NPY mRNA expression is reduced in rats with colitis, in contrast to the previous study (35). This same group, however, did show that central administration of NPY in rats with colitis failed to stimulate feeding behavior, which suggests that, in the presence of inflammation, the hypothalamus is partially refractory to the effects of NPY (36).

Increasing evidence indicates that the proinflammatory cytokines, particularly IL-1β, produce anorexia, at least in part through the ARC-PVN NPY pathway (Fig. 2). IL-1 suppresses neuronal activity in hypothalamic nuclei and, when administered centrally, antagonizes the promotional effects of NPY on feeding. Chronic central administration of IL-1 increases TNF-α mRNA in the hypothalamus, suggesting the

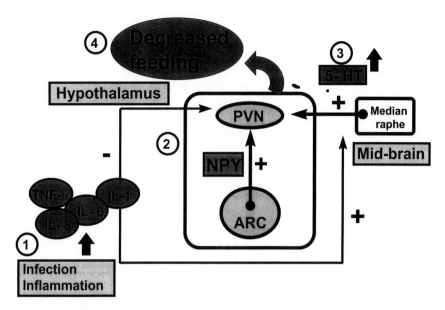

FIG. 2. Central effects of proinflammatory cytokines on feeding behavior. Several proinflammatory cytokines (IL-1β, IL-6, TNF-α and possibly IL-8) (1) have been shown to inhibit feeding behavior, either in response to direct intraventricular injection in the central nervous system, as a result of peripheral generation following administration of bacterial lipopolysaccharide (LPS), or in experimental models of infection or inflammation. Evidence suggests that IL-1β acts directly on the ARC-PVN NPY pathway to inhibit the effect of NPY (2), thereby preventing the compensatory changes in feeding behavior that would restore energy deficit. Evidence also indicates that IL-β can stimulate 5-hydroxytryptamine activity in the PVN (3), which would also have an inhibitory effect on feeding behavior (4). Similar modes of action may also be relevant for the other proinflammatory cytokines.

potential for a local anorectic cytokine network. Evidence also shows that autoregulatory positive and negative feedback involves other cytokines.

The anorectic peptide leptin, which is thought to act through the ARC-PVN NPY pathway (11), has also been investigated as a possible mediator of anorexia in infective and inflammatory states. However, we failed to find inappropriately high leptin concentrations in plasma in patients with chronic inflammatory bowel disease or in severely wasted patients with AIDS (37). Nevertheless, plasma leptin is increased in the early phase of TNBS colitis in the rat and may be implicated in anorexia in this model (38). Plasma leptin concentrations rapidly return to normal even before the colitis and anorexia has resolved, indicating that autoregulatory mechanisms are promptly activated.

CYTOKINES, ANOREXIA, AND GROWTH RETARDATION

The relationship between infection, undernutrition, and growth retardation in infants and young children is well established. A continuing question, however, is whether growth retardation relates solely to anorexia and reduced food intake or whether an independent effect of infection or inflammation has an impact on growth and development (39). We have used the TNBS model of colitis to induce growth retardation in young rats and have shown that the reduction in linear growth in rats with colitis is greater than in pair-fed controls. These findings indicate that inflammation and reduced food intake have independent effects on linear growth (40). Rats with colitis had inappropriately low plasma growth hormone concentrations and markedly reduced plasma concentrations of IGF-1 compared with pair-fed animals. Linear growth in rats with colitis could be partially reversed by administration of recombinant human IGF-1 and by supplemental feeding (41). IL-6 has been implicated as a mediator of growth failure in transgenic mice overexpressing IL-6, with the supposition that IL-6 directly inhibits IGF-1 production in the liver (29). Figure 3 summarizes possible mechanisms by which proinflammatory cytokines generated during infection and inflammation might impair growth and development. Further studies are

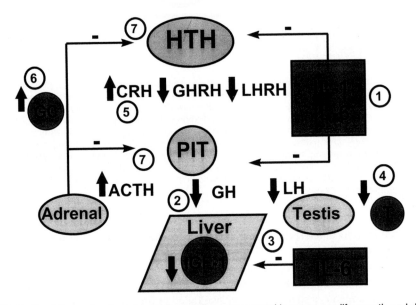

FIG. 3. Possible mechanisms by which proinflammatory cytokines can modify growth and development. IL-1 and IL-6 have been shown to act directly on the hypothalamus and pituitary to inhibit synthesis and release of growth hormone-releasing hormone (GHRH) and luteinizing hormone-releasing hormone (LHRH), with resulting decreased circulating levels of growth hormone (GH) and luteinizing hormone (LH) (1). The reduced circulating levels of GH may be partly responsible for the decreased synthesis and release of insulinlike growth factor-1 (IGF-1) (2), but evidence also suggests that IL-6 directly reduces IGF-1 synthesis in the liver (3). The latter may be the most important site of action for this proinflammatory cytokine and where it has its major impact on the pathogenesis of growth retardation. The reduced LH will decrease testosterone and dihydrotestosterone synthesis and release by the testes (4). Hypogonadism is a common feature of chronic infective and inflammatory conditions. In addition, IL-1 and IL-6 will increase synthesis of corticotrophin-releasing hormone (CRH) (5), which will activate the hypothalamic-pituitary-adrenal axis, increasing the circulating concentrations of glucocorticoids (6), which will then activate a negative feedback pathway on the hypothalamus and pituitary to decrease GH and LH synthesis (7).

required to determine whether this is an important mechanism in infection and inflammatory disorders.

FUTURE RESEARCH

Further work is required to delineate the alterations in central and peripheral control mechanisms during infection, to determine whether these differ according to the type of infection, and to explore ways of modifying central and peripheral anorectic pathways that would have beneficial effects on food intake without compromising the host's ability to respond to the infection.

REFERENCES

1. Mata LJ, Urrutia JJ, Albertazzi C, Pellecer O, Arellano E. Influence of recurrent infections on nutrition and growth of children in Guatemala. *Am J Clin Nutr* 1972; 25: 1267–75.
2. Martorell R, Yarborough C, Yarborough S, Klein RE. The impact of ordinary illnesses on the dietary intakes of malnourished children. *Am J Clin Nutr* 1980; 33: 345–80.
3. Hoyle B, Yunus M, Chen LC. Breast-feeding and food intake among children with acute diarrheal disease. *Am J Clin Nutr* 1980; 33: 2365–71.
4. Brown KH, Black RE, Robertson AD, Becker S. Effects of season and illness on the dietary intake of weanlings during longitudinal studies in rural Bangladesh. *Am J Clin Nutr* 1985; 41: 343–55.
5. Arsenijevic D, Girardier L, Seydoux J, et al. Metabolic-cytokine responses to a second immunological challenge with LPS in mice with *T. gondii* infection. *Am J Physiol* 1998; 274: E439–45.
6. Conn CA, McClellan JL, Maassab HF, Smitka CW, Majde JA, Kluger MJ. Cytokines and the acute phase response to influenza virus in mice. *Am J Physiol* 1995; 268: R78–84.
7. Macallan DC, Noble C, Baldwin C, et al. Energy expenditure and wasting in HIV infection. *N Engl J Med* 1995; 333: 83–8.
8. Kelly P, Summerbell C, Ngwenya B, et al. Systemic immune activation as a potential determinant of wasting in Zambians with HIV-related diarrhoea. *Q J Med* 1996; 89: 831–7.
9. Keusch GT, Farthing MJG. Nutritional aspects of AIDS. *Annu Rev Nutr* 1990; 10: 475–501.
10. Schwartz MW, Dallman MF, Woods SC. Hypothalamic response to starvation: implications for the study of wasting disorders. *Am J Physiol* 1995; R949–57.
11. Woods SC, Seeley RJ, Porte D, Schwartz MW. Signals that regulate food intake and energy homeostasis. *Science* 1998; 280: 1378.
12. Qu D, Ludwig DS Gammeltoft S, et al. A role for melanin-concentrating hormone in the central regulation of feeding behaviour. *Nature* 1996; 380: 243–7.
13. Kristensen P, Judge ME, Thim L, et al. Hypothalamic CART is a new anorectic peptide regulated by leptin. *Nature* 1998; 393: 72–6.
14. Morley JE. Appetite regulation by gut peptides. *Annu Rev Nutr* 1990; 10: 383–95.
15. Ballinger A, McLoughlin L, Medbak S, Clark M. Cholecystokinin is a satiety hormone in humans at physiological post-prandial plasma concentrations. *Clin Sci* 1995; 89: 375–81.
16. Tracey JK, Cerami A. Tumor necrosis factor in the malnutrition (cachexia) of infection and cancer. *Am J Trop Med Hyg* 1992; 47: 2–7.
17. Grunfeld C, Feingold KR. Metabolic disturbances and wasting in the acquired immunodeficiency syndrome. *N Engl J Med* 1992; 327: 329–37.
18. Adams DH, Lloyd AR. Chemokines: leucocyte recruitment and activation cytokines. *Lancet* 1997; 349: 490–5.
19. Friedland JS. Chemokines and human infection. *Clin Sci* 1995; 88: 393–400.
20. Luster AD. Chemokines—chemotactic cytokines that mediate inflammation. *N Engl J Med* 1998; 338: 436–45.
21. Eckmann L, Jung HC, Schurer-Maly C, Panja A, Morzycha-Wroblewska E, Kagnoff MF. Differential cytokine expression by human intestinal epithelial cell lines: regulated expression of interleukin 8. *Gastroenterology* 1993; 105: 1689–97.

22. Eckmann L, Kagnoff MF, Fierer J. Epithelial cells secrete the chemokine interleukin-8 in response to bacterial entry. *Infect Immun* 1993; 61: 4569–74.
23. Yang S-K, Eckmann L, Panja P, Kagnoff MF. Differential and regulated expression of C-X-C, C-C and C-chemokines by human colon epithelial cells. *Gastroenterology* 1997; 113: 1214–23.
24. Bendtzen K. Interleukin-1, interleukin-6 and tumour necrosis factor in infection, inflammation and immunity. *Immunol Lett* 1988; 19: 183–91.
25. Bazzoni F, Beutler B. The tumor necrosis factor ligand and receptor families. *N Engl J Med* 1996; 334: 1717–25.
26. Dinarello CA, Wolff SM. The role of interleukin-1 in disease. *N Engl J Med* 1993; 328: 106–13.
27. Sonti G, Ilyin SE, Plata-Salaman CR. Anorexia induced by cytokine interactions at pathophysiological concentrations. *Am J Physiol* 1996; 270: R1394–402.
28. Gabay C, Kushner I. Acute-phase proteins and other systemic responses to inflammation. *N Engl J Med* 1999; 340: 448–54.
29. De Benedetti F, Alonzi T, Moretta A, et al. Interleukin-6 causes growth impairment in transgenic mice through a decrease in insulin-like growth factor-1. *J Clin Invest* 1997; 99: 643–50.
30. Gayle D, Ilyin SE, Flynn MC, Plata-Salaman CR. Lipopolysaccharide following acute fasting: characterization of brain cytokine and neuropeptide systems mRNAs. *Brain Res* 1998; 795: 77–86.
31. Plata-Salaman CR, Ilyin SE, Gayle D. Brain cytokine mRNAs in anorectic rats bearing prostate adenocarcinoma tumor cells. *Am J Physiol* 1998; 275: R566–73.
32. McHugh KJ, Collins SM, Weingarten HP. Central interleukin-1 receptors contribute to suppression of feeding after acute colitis in the rat. *Am J Physiol* 1994; 266: R1659–63.
33. El-Haj T, Ballinger AB, Perrett D, Williams G, Farthing MJG. Increased activity of hypothalamic 5-HT neuronal activity in a model of colitis-associated anorexia. *Gastroenterology* 1999; 116: A712.
34. Ballinger AB, El-Haj T, Corder R, Williams G, Farthing MJG. The role of hypothalamic neuropeptide Y in anorexia associated with experimental colitis. *Gastroenterology* 1999; 116: A590.
35. Million M, Kresse A, Saperas E, Tache Y. Body weight loss induced by chronic colonic inflammation in rats: role of hypothalamic neuropeptide Y (NPY) [Abstract]. *Gastroenterology* 1997; 112: A894.
36. Million M, Kresse A, Tache Y. Acute colitis inhibits central neuropeptide Y (NPY)-induced increase in food intake and body weight without affecting the hypothalamic NPY and mRNA expression in rats [Abstract]. *Gastroenterology* 1998; 114: A1595.
37. Ballinger AB, Kelly P, Hallyburton E, Besser R, Farthing MJG. Plasma leptin in chronic inflammatory bowel disease and HIV: implications for the pathogenesis of anorexia and weight loss. *Clin Sci* 1998; 94: 479–83.
38. Barbier M, Cherbut C, Aube AC, Blottiere HM, Galmiche JP. Elevated plasma leptin concentrations in early states of experimental intestinal inflammation in rats. *Gut* 1998; 43: 783–90.
39. Koniaris SG, Fisher SE, Rubin CT, Chawla A. Experimental colitis impairs linear bone growth independent of nutritional factors. *J Pediatr Gastroenterol Nutr* 1997; 25: 137–41.
40. Ballinger AB, Azooz O, Farthing MJG. Mechanisms of linear growth failure associated with intestinal inflammation [Abstract]. *Gastroenterology* 1998; 114: A1126.
41. Azooz O, Farthing MJG, Ballinger AB. IGF-1 deficiency but not IGF-1 resistance in a model of colitis associated with linear growth retardation. *Gastroenterology* 1999; 116: A538.

DISCUSSION

Dr. Zoppi: I would like to make a clinical comment. We have experience in treating very young children with severe infection with total parenteral nutrition (TPN) and total enteral nutrition. We have seen that if we treat such children with TPN during acute or chronic infection, clinical status improves, and we can prevent the anorexia and the loss of appetite. Do you have any comment on that?

Dr. Farthing: Your experience is common to many, and many reports have been published reports of the positive effect of nutritional supplementation in both acute and chronic situations. The model that we use for chronic inflammation is Crohn's disease, because I see a lot of children and adolescents with this condition, and the evidence is that nutritional supplementation alone without control of inflammation does not fully restore growth. My clinical staff are well aware of growth problems and we routinely measure the children's heights and weights. Yet, when we audited our results that were purely centered around nutritional supplementation, we still did not achieve optimal growth in many. So I believe, as this model suggests, that nutrition is only half the story.

Dr. Keusch: With respect to the last comments in your summary on potential mechanisms to modulate the effects of proinflammatory cytokines, I think we have some human data that are consistent with your hypothesis. These are data that we published from studies of individuals with HIV in central Africa (1). We looked at a group of women who had been enrolled in a perinatal transmission study approximately 5 years before. We were able to reconfirm that they were in fact HIV infected, so they had been infected for at least 5 years. They had remained asymptomatic over this period and had done well clinically. A moderate reduction was seen in CD-4 and a moderate effect on body composition, so the question was, why had they done well? We looked at their cytokine levels in plasma and found they had sky high levels of IL-1 and TNF, as high as you ever see in severe meningitis or in experimental conditions (e.g., after the injection of proinflammatory stimuli), yet these individuals were afebrile, eating reasonably well, and had maintained their weight. Next, we looked at the anti-inflammatory cytokine molecules such as IL-1 receptor antagonist and the TNF P55 soluble receptor, and these were off into the stratosphere! The molar excess of the inhibitory cytokines was approximately what you would have to add *in vitro* to block the effects of IL-1 or TNF. So, clearly in these individuals, the balance of anticytokines and proinflammatory cytokines was sufficient to mitigate the effect of these very high levels of the proinflammatory cytokines. We have no idea why these women were able to do that, and it may relate to genetic polymorphism or to stimuli that we do not yet understand, but it supports your view that blocking the biological activity of the inflammatory cytokines *in vivo* can have the effects you described.

Dr. Farthing: Thank you. Our own work in African patients shows that the degree of systemic immune activation in HIV, with or without infection, is absolutely enormous. Markers such as the soluble TNF receptors are an order of magnitude higher than in tuberculosis, for instance. These are highly immune-activated individuals. I think your observations of the downregulation by the body are very interesting. Although we need to proceed with caution, I believe the potential exists for therapeutic intervention in individuals who are unable to generate those anti-inflammatory responses themselves.

Dr. Keusch: I should add that in a group of women with clinical AIDS and wasting, that molar ratio of very high antagonist to agonist did not exist. So, clearly, a clinical correlation existed between levels of anti-inflammatory and proinflammatory cytokines to clinical manifestations.

Dr. Wakelin: Could I ask you to extrapolate a little from what you said about the central effects of proinflammatory cytokines to what might happen in the pregnant woman who is suffering from chronic inflammation, in terms of the growth of the fetus?

Dr. Farthing: I believe there is evidence that shows that the fetus is smaller and fails to grow in women with chronic inflammatory disease, malignant disease, or chronic infections. It would be surprising if this was not the case. I am sure some people here have had more direct experience than I have.

Dr. Marini: I would say that the growth of the fetus is related mainly to the oxygen supply through the placenta. If not enough oxygen is delivered, it is very bad for the fetus if you increase the amount of nutrient supply. None of the trials I have done trying to increase amino acid levels in the mother to improve the growth of the fetus have been successful, because we were unable to increase the oxygen supply to the fetus.

I have a comment about 5-hydroxytryptamine and reduction of appetite. In the mid-1980s, it was suggested that babies could be made quieter by giving a formula with increased tryptophan and reduced valine, because increasing the level of tryptophan increases the level of 5-HT in the brain!

Dr. Farthing: You have touched on a highly controversial area. Studies suggest that you can drive 5-HT levels by dietary tryptophan and, indeed, tryptophan was used as an antidepressant for awhile. It was on sale in the United Kingdom as Optimax and it appeared to work. However, I find it a very difficult concept. The idea that a dietary nutrient can drive brain levels directly seems counter-intuitive to me. It would make the brain very vulnerable. To have a very large tryptophan meal one day and suddenly find your brain levels of 5-HT shooting up does not sound reasonable biologically. We have looked at this again, and we do not agree with the tryptophan/5-HT hypothesis.

Dr. Marini: But is there no rationale in providing chocolate in survival rations because the tryptophan it contains diminishes appetite?

Dr. Farthing: I think it is the caffeine that would diminish the appetite.

Dr. Kennedy: The studies in patients with HIV are interesting. One other mechanism that may be relevant with regard to fever and CNS interactions is that probably IL-1 and TNF in the circulation are not inducing fever directly or centrally; they probably interact with the endothelial cell, and then it is IL-6 centrally that induces the fever. This raises an interesting question because when you are dealing with leptin and energy expenditure, and the response to leptin in the immune system, you are dealing with GP130 receptors. A great deal of research has been done in recent months looking at whether or not in the DV mouse, which has leptin receptor insensitivity, there are effects on IL-6 receptor. Nobody has been able to show yet that, despite the abnormality in leptin receptor response or signaling, a signaling problem exists in IL-6. So my question to you: Have you looked at DV mice in terms of their colitis response and whether or not they showed similar type changes?

Dr. Farthing: Not yet, but it is a very good suggestion. I will take it back with me.

Dr. Meydani: I have two questions. First, you said that infection caused nutritional deficiencies. I wonder if you really meant that, or is it that there is redistribution of nutrients, or perhaps limited availability for certain functions? Second, have you or anyone else used cyclic oxygenase inhibitors to look at growth in the colitis model? Because in the case of colitis, for example, Cox-2 expression is certainly increased.

Dr. Farthing: I meant that infection interferes with nutritional status through intake, but also through redistribution internally. Second, no, we have not looked at Cox inhibitors. The difficulty with these is that they often precipitate inflammation. It was hoped that one could use Cox-2 inhibitors, but they have been very disappointing. I do not think, in this model, it would be a very helpful intervention.

Dr. Suskind: Given your findings with respect to the impact of cytokines on appetite regulators and inflammation, would you like to comment on the relevance of this to anorexia nervosa, which is another model that might clarify the changes in neuropeptide Y and 5-HT? In individuals who are obese and who are put on very low energy diets, a degree of anorexia occurs which is thought to be mediated by ketone bodies. Could you comment on that in relation to the control of appetite? Is there a role for ketone bodies in appetite regulation?

Dr. Farthing: The anorexia question is a difficult one, because it is hard to study the brain of people with eating disorders. I think ways will be found to do this in the future. Certainly, functional magnetic resonance imaging is now possible, and one of the ways in which we are now moving forward is to do studies in humans using noninvasive functional tests in the brain.

I speculate that changes will be found, but from yesterday's discussions it seems that these may be primarily psychologically driven, with failure to compensate appropriately. Once a major cortical input exists, you may completely change the way in which the hypothalamus responds.

Your second question about ketones and obesity is an interesting one. I am not aware of any recent studies looking at the effect of ketones on appetite. Maybe this should be looked at again.

Dr. Haschke: Products used in the treatment of obesity that have high protein, high carbohydrate, and very low fat content are now regulated even by the European Union. How do these work? Is there evidence that they influence satiety peptides?

Dr. Farthing: Very little has been done to study this. We assume that energy deprivation alone eventually resets the obesity regulator. What it actually does in the hypothalamus in humans is uncertain, but one would imagine that it affects both sides of the drive: the neuropeptide Y axis is suppressed by low levels of insulin and leptin and, ideally, the hypothalamus is retrained. However, we know how difficult that is because once people come off these diets, history tells us that most of them regain weight. Similarly, if you use a drug like fenfluramine, which alters the 5-HT pathway and maybe causes release of 5-HT and suppression of appetite, again the effect is short lived. So a real question exists about reprogramming the hypothalamus that has learned to respond to stimuli inappropriately.

Dr. Wakelin: TNBS is a very dramatic way of inducing colitis, and you described very rapid changes as results of exposing the gut to that trauma. From your experience with more chronic forms of colitic inflammation, would you expect to see the same changes?

Dr. Farthing: We are indeed studying an acute model. Ways exist to extend the model—by multiple dosing, for example, which will create an illness that lasts for about 10 days. It would certainly be as interesting to do these experiments, as it would be to translate this model into a more clinically relevant infection.

Dr. Calder: Branched chain amino acids compete with free tryptophan taken to the brain. I wonder, therefore, if some role is seen for the apparently wasteful oxidation of branched chain amino acids that Dr. Fjeld mentioned in regulating tryptophan metabolism in the brain in inflammation and infection?

Dr. Farthing: That is an interesting suggestion. I do not know of any work in that area, but it would certainly be an interesting experiment to do. We could look directly at what is going on in the central pathways.

Dr. Calder: About 10 years ago, Blomstrand et al. (2) did some studies feeding branched chain amino acids to rats and looking at 5-HT and 5-HIAA in different brain regions. She showed significant differences, which reflected the administration of the branched chain amino acids and also the exercise regimen that the animals had been on.

Dr. Farthing: I think it is true to say, however, that the effects have been disappointing in terms of the systemic response in muscle.

REFERENCES

1. Thea DM, Porat R, Nagimbi K, et al. Plasma cytokines, cytokine antagonists and disease progression in African women infected with HIV-1. *Ann Intern Med* 1996; 124: 757–62.
2. Blomstrand E, Perrett D, Parry-Billings M, et al. Effect of sustained exercise on plasma amino acid concentrations and on 5-hydroxtryptamine metabolism in six different brain regions in the rat. *Acta Physiol Scand* 1989; 136: 473–81.

Nutrition, Immunity, and Infection in Infants and Children, edited by Robert M. Suskind and Kraisid Tontisirin. Nestlé Nutrition Workshop Series, Pediatric Program, Vol. 45. Nestec Ltd., Vevey/Lippincott Williams & Wilkins, Philadelphia ©2001.

Relations Between Gastrointestinal Infections and Childhood Malnutrition

Kenneth H. Brown

Program in International Nutrition and Department of Nutrition, University of California, Davis, California, USA

More than 90% of the world's children live in low income countries, where infectious diseases are the predominant cause of the increased rates of childhood mortality and morbidity that are typical of these settings (1). With regard to gastrointestinal infections (GI) in particular, the World Health Organization estimates that nearly one billion episodes of diarrhea occur annually among children aged less than 5 years in the developing world, resulting in more than three million deaths (2). These illnesses are more likely to occur in children with pre-existing nutritional deficits and the episodes to be of longer duration, of greater severity, and to result in death in malnourished children. Moreover, the illnesses themselves contribute further to malnutrition in affected children (Fig. 1). This article reviews some of the relations between GI infection and children's nutrition from both of these perspectives, relying primarily on the results of clinical research and community-based epidemiologic studies. Other chapters focus on the immunologic mechanisms involved, so these will not be re-examined here.

EFFECTS OF GASTROINTESTINAL INFECTIONS ON HOST NUTRITION

There is general scientific consensus that gastrointestinal infections affect the host's nutritional status adversely, although the magnitude of this effect can vary considerably, depending on the cause, severity, and anatomic site of the infection, as well as on the underlying health and nutritional status of the host and the treatment provided during and after illness. Moreover, because the nutritional consequences of illness can be assessed in various ways, such as measurement of physical growth (anthropometry), nutrient balance, or biochemical indicators of micronutrient status, the ap-

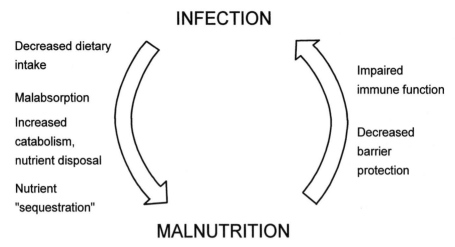

FIG. 1. Relationship between gastrointestinal infections and malnutrition.

parent nutritional impact can vary according to the type of nutritional outcome selected. For example, changes in body weight often become evident fairly rapidly following the onset of an episode of acute diarrhea, but may no longer be identifiable several weeks or months after the episode (3,4). By contrast, differences in linear growth induced by diarrhea may be detectable only as the cumulative effect of multiple days of illness monitored over longer periods of time (5).

For these reasons, it is extremely difficult to quantify the overall impact of GI infections on children's nutritional status. Nevertheless, it is possible to draw general conclusions about the effect of these infections on dietary intake and intestinal absorption, which are probably the major pathways leading to secondary malnutrition. The metabolic consequences of infection, which may also undermine host nutritional status, are described in a separate chapter by Fjeld.

EFFECT OF GASTROINTESTINAL INFECTIONS ON APPETITE AND DIETARY INTAKE

The effect of gastrointestinal infections on dietary intake has been examined both in hospital inpatients (6–8) and in children participating in longitudinal, community-based studies (9–14). Most of these studies detected reduced energy intake during illness, although the results are somewhat variable (15). In general, children who were admitted to the hospital for diarrhea (and who presumably had more severe illness) had greater reductions in energy intake during illness than those evaluated in community-based studies. Even among the field studies, however, considerable variability was seen in the effect of illness on food consumption. For example, two reports from Guatemala, which included only children who were completely weaned from the breast, noted a reduction of about 15% to 20% in energy intake during illness

(9,10). By contrast, breast-fed infants and young children in both Bangladesh and Peru, who received about half their energy intake from breast milk, had substantially smaller decrements in energy intake during illness, presumably because of the protective effect of breast-feeding (11,12). Indeed, when energy intakes from breast milk and other foods were examined separately in the Peru study, only the intakes from milk sources other than the breast declined during illness. Thus, part of the difference in the results of published studies may be explained by the protective effect of breast-feeding in those children who were still nursing at the breast.

Most previous studies have failed to consider the possibility that the effect of illness on energy consumption might be modified by the nature of the diet. Marquis *et al.* (14) explored whether dietary viscosity influenced the amount of energy consumed by Peruvian children during and after illness. They compared intakes by groups of children who received either an amylase-treated, low-viscosity, potato-based diet or an untreated, higher viscosity diet of similar food and nutrient composition during and after diarrhea. Although both groups had lower intakes during illness than following recovery, no apparent benefit was seen of the reduced viscosity diet at any stage of illness. Additional studies are needed to determine whether other dietary factors might influence consumption patterns during illness.

Several investigators have studied the role of disease severity on energy intake. For example, Brown *et al.* (16) examined factors associated with caregivers' reports of poor child appetite during longitudinal observations in Peru. Initial exploration of the relationship between reported anorexia and energy intake on days when dietary intake was observed and measured quantitatively indicated that the caregivers' reports of low child appetite were associated with a 12% to 15% reduction in energy intake, depending on the age of the child. Reported anorexia was most commonly associated with diarrhea and respiratory illness. When the illness syndromes were accompanied by fever, the likelihood of anorexia was considerably greater than when fever was absent. Diarrhea-related anorexia was also more likely to occur when the episode was associated with a greater number of daily bowel movements and during rotavirus infections and episodes of dysentery. In another study of risk factors for poor appetite among young children admitted to hospital for diarrhea, Brown and Perez (17) reported that low serum bicarbonate and raised urine-specific gravity at the time of admission were the two characteristics that independently identified children with low food intakes during the first day of hospital admission. Thus, they concluded that the appropriate therapeutic intervention to reduce diarrhea-related anorexia is to provide adequate rehydration therapy to prevent dehydration and acidosis.

EFFECT OF GASTROINTESTINAL INFECTIONS ON INTESTINAL ABSORPTION

Intestinal absorption is often diminished during diarrhea as a result of (*a*) damage to the enterocyte caused either directly by pathogens and the host immune responses that they induce or through release of microbial toxins; (*b*) aberrations of intestinal motility; and (*c*) increased fecal loss and/or bacterial hydrolysis of bile acids (18,19).

The effects of enteric infections on macronutrient absorption have been reviewed (20,21). Briefly, abnormalities of digestion and mucosal transport of carbohydrates, protein, and fat occur frequently as a result of enteric infections. Maldigestion of carbohydrates is of special importance for several reasons. First, the superficial location of brush border carbohydrases makes them particularly vulnerable to the effects of enteric infections. Moreover, a large proportion of dietary energy is usually provided by sugars and starches, and the amount of individual carbohydrates that are ingested may overwhelm the digestive capacity of remaining brush border hydrolytic enzymes. Even though some of these incompletely digested carbohydrates can be metabolized by colonic bacteria and absorbed by the colon as organic acids, this process is not fully efficient when sizable carbohydrate loads enter the colon (22). The sum of nondigested fecal carbohydrate, unabsorbed organic acids, and the cations associated with both these substances induces further stool water loss and thereby contributes to diarrhea severity. Incomplete absorption of carbohydrates seems to be especially problematic during rotavirus infections (23).

Several studies have also found increased fecal excretion and net negative balances of selected micronutrients during diarrhea. For example, studies by Castillo-Duran *et al.* in Chile (24) described negative balances of zinc and copper during the early stage of acute diarrhea that were directly proportional to the severity of stool losses. Increased loss of B vitamins has also been reported (25).

Recent research has also shown that altered intestinal permeability to test sugars, an indication of intestinal mucosal dysfunction, occurs frequently during diarrhea and persists for a variable period thereafter (26,27). Importantly, studies in west Africa have found a strong association between abnormal intestinal permeability and impairment of children's growth (28). Although the causal direction of this association is uncertain, it is conceivable that GI infections can continue to affect nutritional status adversely through subclinical malabsorption, even after the clinical symptoms subside. Several studies suggest that continued feeding during illness and supplementation with specific nutrients (*e.g.*, zinc) may diminish the frequency and duration of abnormal intestinal mucosal permeability (26,29–31). These observations may have important implications not only for longer term nutritional outcomes as described above (28) but also for the risk of sensitization to dietary proteins and future occurrence of food allergy (26).

COMMUNITY-BASED LONGITUDINAL STUDIES OF THE EFFECT OF DIARRHEA ON NUTRITIONAL STATUS

Several groups of investigators have attempted to quantify the cumulative impact of diarrheal incidence or prevalence on children's weight increments and linear growth (3–5,32–38). Most studies have documented a negative relationship between diarrheal prevalence and physical growth, although the magnitude of this effect varies considerably across studies. As indicated, one explanation for these differences among studies is the duration of the observation period, with deficits in weight gain being more obvious in the short term and reductions in length gain detectable only after longer periods of observation. Because the impact of diarrhea seems to depend on the total number of days of illness (5,38), those studies that considered only incidence and not prevalence of disease were less likely to conclude that diarrhea had a major impact. By the same token, studies that used infrequent surveillance for illness and, therefore, identified fewer episodes and days of illness, generally identified a smaller total impact of diarrhea on growth. It is notable that persistent episodes of diarrhea—those lasting at least 14 days—appear to exert the greatest negative impact on children's growth (5). It is not certain whether this is because persistent episodes are particularly devastating to nutritional status or simply because those children with persistent episodes also have especially high prevalence rates of diarrhea.

Few studies have attempted to differentiate the nutritional consequences of diarrhea by individual causative agents. In one study from Bangladesh, enterotoxigenic *Escherichia coli* diarrhea was more closely associated with reduced weight increments than other infectious causes of diarrhea, whereas shigellosis was more closely associated with impaired linear growth (5). A recent longitudinal study from west Africa found that acquisition of *Cryptosporidium* infection was not related to pre-existing nutritional status; but subsequent weight gain and linear growth were significantly reduced in infected children, especially if the infection occurred during infancy (39). No other infectious causes were specifically examined in this study. Various recent studies have focused on the nutritional impact of *Helicobacter pylori* infections, as will be discussed in more detail below.

Several investigators have described a modifying effect of diet on the relationship between diarrhea and growth. In particular, some reports indicate that diarrhea exerts less of a negative impact on the growth of breast-fed infants than on those not breast-fed (36,40). This may reflect, in part, the aforementioned protective effect of breast-feeding on diarrhea-induced anorexia and the findings that breast-fed infants have lower diarrhea incidence rates (41,42) and a shorter duration of illness (41). In addition, some investigators have found that diarrhea-induced growth impairment is reduced or eliminated in children who receive food supplements (37) and in those whose usual dietary intake is greater between episodes of illness (40). Thus, it appears that an adequate diet can provide some protection from the nutritional complications of diarrhea.

EFFECT OF HELICOBACTER PYLORI ON CHILDREN'S NUTRITION

Because of the recent profusion of publications on *H. pylori* infections and the growing appreciation of their potential importance for children's nutrition, it is worthwhile devoting special attention to this organism. *H. pylori* has been described as "probably the commonest bacterial infection of humankind" (43). During the past decade, many researchers have documented the role of this organism as a primary cause of chronic gastritis, hypochlorhydria, and peptic ulcer. Acquisition of *H. pylori* infection occurs earlier and more frequently in developing countries than in industrialized ones; in both settings, individuals of lower socioeconomic status are more likely to be infected (44–46). In industrialized countries, the prevalence of infection increases with age, from very low rates during childhood to approximately 20% in young adults. In low income countries, however, infection is often acquired by infants and young children and prevalence rates commonly reach 40% to 80% in school-aged children (44,47). Interestingly, two recent studies in South America found relations between selected dietary practices and risk of infection. In Colombia, children who consumed more milk, fruits, or vegetables were less likely to be infected (48); in Peru, the subgroup of children who avoided street foods and consumed fruits more often appeared to be protected (49).

The early age of acquisition of *H. pylori* infections in developing countries corresponds to the period of peak diarrheal incidence and growth faltering. Because the organism causes hypochlorhydria in children as well as in adults (47) and because low gastric output is associated with increased risk of bacterial colonization of the upper GI tract (50), it has been postulated that *H. pylori* may be at least partially responsible for the increased rates of diarrheal disease and secondary malnutrition observed among children in these settings (47). Some, but not all, community-based studies have found a relationship between *H. pylori* infections and children's growth or nutritional status (Table 1). However, most of the existing studies have been cross-sectional, so it is difficult to ascertain the causal direction of any association between *H. pylori* infection and nutritional status or, indeed, whether children of low income households are simply more likely to be both undernourished and more exposed to infection.

In an early study in Gambia, acquisition of *H. pylori* infection by young infants, as indicated by seroconversion, was unrelated to their pre-existing nutritional status but was associated with subsequent growth faltering during infancy (47). In a more recent study in which *H. pylori* infection status was monitored longitudinally by conducting quarterly ^{13}C-urea breath tests during infancy, children with positive breath tests on all four occasions had a significant reduction in postprandial urine acid out-

TABLE 1. *Relation between Helicobacter pylori infection and children's nutritional status*

Author	Year	Country	Reference	Age range (years)	Type of study	Results
Patel *et al.*	1994	Scotland	52	6–11	Longitudinal*	↓ Linear growth in girls infected at 11 years
Dale *et al.*	1998	Gambia	51	<1	Longitudinal	↓ W/A Z scores in infected children
Klein *et al.*	1991	Peru	46	<1–12	Cross sectional	↓ W/H and H/AZ scores in infected children
Mahalanabis *et al.*	1996	Bangladesh	54	<1–9	Cross sectional	No association
Clemens *et al.*	1996	Bangladesh	55	2–9	Cross sectional	No association
Perri *et al.*	1997	Italy	53	3–14	Cross sectional	More older (8–14 years) infected children <25% centile H/A
Goodman *et al.*	1998	Colombia	48	2–9	Cross sectional	Fewer infected children in upper (>25% centile) H/A centiles

* Height measurements at baseline and 4 years later. Anti-*H. pylori* salivary IgG measurement only at 11 years.

put (indicative of hypochlorhydria) at 6 months and significantly lower weight-for-age Z-scores at 6 and 9 months of age compared with those who had consistently negative breath tests (51). Unfortunately, the investigators did not control for potentially confounding variables in their analyses.

Patel *et al.* investigated the presence of salivary IgG antibodies to *H. pylori* in 11-year-old Scottish children whose height was measured at 6 to 7 years and again at 11 years (52). Children with positive antibody titers gained significantly less in height during the preceding interval than those without, even after controlling for socioeconomic factors. When the results were disaggregated by sex, the growth differences were statistically significant only for girls, leading the authors to hypothesize that infection may have delayed the onset of puberty.

Associations between *H. pylori* infection and reduced body size have also been identified in three cross-sectional studies, although the interpretation of these studies is complicated by the presence of possible confounding factors. A report from Italy (53) noted that the heights of a greater percentage of infected children 8 to 14 years of age (26%) were less than the 25th centile height for age compared with those of children who were free of infection (8%). However, these outcomes were not adjusted for potential confounders, and infected children were of lower socioeconomic class, which may have independently affected growth. Similarly, *H. pylori*-infected Peruvian children between 2 months and 12 years of age had lower height-for-age and weight-for-height Z-scores than those without infection (46). However, the infected children were significantly older and from families with lower incomes, so it is not possible to determine the independent effect of the infections on their nutritional status. A third study in Colombia found that fewer infected children had a height-for-age greater than the 25th centile, even after controlling for potential confounders (48). By contrast with these aforementioned results, two different sets of investigators in Bangladesh found no association between *H. pylori* infection and children's nutritional status (54,55).

In summary, several studies suggest that *Helicobacter* infections can adversely affect children's growth and nutritional status. However, limited information is available from studies using a longitudinal research design, which allows stronger scientific inferences, and no studies have yet been reported using an experimental trial design. Because of the problem of confounding factors, as discussed, it is still not possible to determine conclusively the extent to which *H. pylori* infection can affect children's growth. Moreover, little, if any information exists on the impact of these infections on children's micronutrient status, which would seem to be an important area for future research.

EFFECT OF MALNUTRITION ON SUSCEPTIBILITY TO INFECTION

As noted above, nutritional status can influence children's risk of gastrointestinal infection because of the effects of malnutrition on gastric acid production (50), immune responses (56), and intestinal mucosal regeneration following infection (57). Each of these abnormalities can increase the susceptibility to infection and the severity or du-

TABLE 2. *Studies demonstrating significant relations between anthropometric status and diarrheal incidence, duration, or severity*

Indicator of incidence of severity	Author	Year	Country	Reference	Type of study
Incidence	Tomkins	1981	Nigeria	58	Community-based
	Sepulveda *et al.*	1988	Mexico	59	Community-based
	Schorling *et al.*	1990	Brazil	60	Community-based
Duration	Tomkins	1981	Nigeria	58	Community-based
	Black *et al.*	1984	Bangladesh	64	Community-based
	Bairagi *et al.*	1987	Bangladesh	65	Community-based
Fecal excretion rate	Palmer *et al.*	1976	Bangladesh	61	Clinical
	Black *et al.*	1984	Bangladesh	62	Clinical
Case fatality rate	Bhan *et al.*	1986	India	66	Community-based
	Teka *et al.*	1996	Bangladesh	67	Clinical
	Bhutta *et al.*	1997	Pakistan	68	Clinical

ration of illness. However, the results of studies examining the relationship between nutritional status and risk or severity of infection are somewhat inconsistent, possibly because of differences in the outcome variables that were monitored, or variation in infectious causes, host micronutrient status, or other unmeasured factors. Moreover, the illness outcomes may be modified by the type of treatment provided.

Several researchers have reported increased rates of diarrhea among growth-impaired children (58–60), and others have noted increased purging rates (61,62) or more prolonged illness in malnourished individuals (58,60,63–65) (Table 2). Of greatest concern is the dramatically increased diarrhea case fatality rate that occurs in malnourished children, seen both in community-based (66) and in hospital studies (67,68).

MICRONUTRIENT STATUS AND RISK OF GASTROINTESTINAL INFECTION

In recent years, greater attention has been devoted to the possible effects of individual nutrients on risk of infection. In particular, well-designed intervention trials have been conducted to assess the impact of supplementation with zinc, vitamin A, or iron on the risk of diarrhea. The results of these trials will be considered briefly in the following section.

Because of the difficulty in assessing zinc status, the best way of determining whether a relationship exists between zinc status and risk of infection is by providing either zinc supplements or placebo to a population at high risk of zinc deficiency. Five studies using this *clinical trial* design were identified from low-income populations (Table 3). One of these studies, which was carried out in the Gambia, found no impact of zinc on the risk of diarrhea, but the morbidity information was collected by passive surveillance at a treatment center (30). The relative insensitivity of this data collection technique may have undermined the investigators' ability to detect a positive impact of supplementation. Each of the remaining studies, all of which used active domiciliary surveillance methods, found a reduced rate of diarrhea following zinc supplementation. A study in Vietnam, for example, noted a 71% reduction in diarrheal incidence among children from 4 to 36 months of age (69). Another study in northern India found a 22% reduction in diarrhea among children from 12 to 35 months of age, but no effect among those from 6 to 11 months of age (70,71). A 35% reduction in diarrheal incidence was reported from a study of children 18 to 36 months of age in Mexico (72), and a reduction of 22% was detected among children 6 to 16 months of age in Guatemala (73). The two studies that examined separately the incidence of persistent diarrhea found an even greater decrease in the occurrence of episodes lasting more than 14 days (70,73). Notably, these two studies also found that the protective effect of zinc was more pronounced in boys than in girls, although this was not true in all studies. The researchers in India reported that children with low initial plasma zinc concentration given zinc supplement had a greater reduction in morbidity than those with higher initial plasma zinc levels. Thus, most of the evidence from these trials suggests that zinc supplementation provides a powerful means of reducing diarrheal incidence among populations that have either impaired zinc status or higher zinc requirements, as may be the case among boys. To determine whether this protective effect of zinc is limited to older children requires additional research.

The effect of vitamin A supplementation on diarrhea morbidity is somewhat less consistent (Table 4). Only five of the nine studies that were identified reported a decreased incidence or duration of diarrhea (74–82). Interestingly, two studies that examined separately the effect of vitamin A on diarrheal severity found a greater impact of supplementation on more severe illness than on milder illness (76,80). Nevertheless, three of the four studies that found no benefit of vitamin A supplementation had ample study populations and were conducted in India (75,81) and Indonesia (82), countries where vitamin A deficiency had been recognized previously as a public health problem. Thus, the inconsistency of findings across studies remains unexplained.

Adequate iron status is necessary for normal immunologic function, but some evidence also suggests that excessive administration of iron can increase the risk of in-

TABLE 16.3. *Community-based trials of zinc supplementation and diarrheal morbidity*

| | | | | | | Incidence rate ratios | | |
| | | | | | | All diarrhea | Persistent diarrhea | Change in diarrheal duration (%) |
Author	Year	Country	Reference	Age (months)	n			
Bates *et al.*	1993	Gambia	30	6–27	110	(1.24)*	N/A	N/A
Ninh *et al.*	1996	Vietnam	69	4–36	146	0.29†	N/A	N/A
Sazawal *et al.*	1996	India	70	6–11	221	(1.05)	(1.24)	N/A
Sazawal *et al.*	1997	India	71	12–35	358	0.78†	0.51†	N/A
Rosado *et al.*	1997	Mexico	72	18–36	109	0.64†	N/A	(−12)
Ruel *et al.*	1997	Guatemala	73	6–16	89	0.78†	0.33†	(−2)

* Based on number of clinic visits, not active surveillance.
† Results in zinc-treated group are significantly different from control group, p <0.05; results in parentheses are not statistically significant. N/A, results not available from particular study.

TABLE 4. *Community-based trials of vitamin A supplementation and diarrheal morbidity*

						Incidence rate ratios		Change in diarrheal duration (%)
Author	Year	Country	Reference	Age (months)	n	All diarrhea	Severe diarrhea	
Bloem *et al.*	1990	Thailand	74	12–35	75	(0.76)	N/A	N/A
				36–71	56	(0.32)	N/A	N/A
Rahmathullah *et al.*	1991	India	75	6–60	15,419	(0.99)	(1.18)†	N/A
Ghana VAST	1993	Ghana	76	6–59	1,455	(0.97)‡	0.62*,§	N/A
Lie *et al.*	1993	China	77	6–36	130	0.40*	N/A	–62*
Biswas *et al.*	1994	India	78	12–71	174	(0.78)	N/A	–32*
Bhandari *et al.*	1994	India	79	12–23	374	(0.99)‡	(1.33)‡,‖	N/A
				24–60	445	(0.96)‡	(0.64)§,‡,‖	N/A
Barreto *et al.*	1994	Brazil	80	6–48	1,240	(0.97)	0.80*	N/A
Ramakrishnan *et al.*	1995	India	81	6–36	583	(1.07)	N/A	(+12)
Dibley *et al.*	1996	Indonesia	82	6–47	1,405	(1.06)	N/A	(+6)

* Results in vitamin A-treated group are significantly different from control group, p< 0.05; results shown in parentheses are not statistically significant. N/A, results are not available from a particular study.
† Incidence of persistent diarrhea.
‡ This study reported prevalence, not incidence rates.
§ Incidence of hospital admissions for diarrhea.
‖ Prevalence of diarrhea accompanied by fever.

fection (83,84). Two recent studies raise concern about the possible adverse effect of iron supplementation in populations with high rates of diarrhea. In one study, Chilean children who received iron-fortified milk containing 12 mg/l iron had a nearly 20% higher incidence of diarrhea than those who received the control milk, which contained only 1 mg/l iron (85). In the other study, Bangladeshi children from 2 to 48 months of age who received supplemental iron in addition to vitamins A, D, and C had approximately 26% more days with watery diarrhea than children who received the vitamins only, although these differences were not statistically significant (86). However, among the subgroup of infants aged less than 12 months in the latter study, the iron-treated individuals had a significant 49% increase in the rate of dysentery compared with the control subjects of the same age. One other relevant study merits brief discussion. Specifically, in the aforementioned zinc intervention trial in Mexico, the comparison group that was supplemented only with iron had a 27% greater diarrheal incidence rate than the placebo group, although this difference was not statistically significant (72).

In summary, several studies indicate that populations at high risk of zinc deficiency may have a reduced incidence of diarrheal disease if they receive supplemental zinc. It is possible that vitamin A is similarly beneficial in decreasing diarrhea, especially severe disease, in populations with vitamin A deficiency. However, the specific factors that indicate whether a population will benefit from vitamin A supplementation are still not known. By contrast with these two micronutrients, some evidence indicates that iron supplementation increases the risk of diarrhea or dysentery, although the particular populations or subgroups of children at greater risk of possibly undesirable effects of iron are still uncertain. Thus, it will be important to collect additional morbidity data from populations that are enrolled in iron supplementation programs. Studies of other nutrients and mixtures of multiple nutrients are also needed.

REFERENCES

1. Murray CJ, Lopez AD. Global and regional cause-of-death patterns in 1990. *Bull World Health Organ* 1994; 72: 447–80.
2. Bern C, Martines J, de Zoysa I, Glass RI. The magnitude of the global problem of diarrhoeal disease: a ten-year update. *Bull World Health Organ* 1992; 70: 705–14.
3. Briend A, Hasan KZ, Aziz KMA, Hoque BA. Are diarrhoea control programmes likely to reduce childhood malnutrition? Observations from rural Bangladesh. *Lancet* 1989; ii: 319–22.
4. Moy RJD, Marshall TFdeC, Choto RGAB, McNeish AS, Booth IW. Diarrhoea and growth faltering in rural Zimbabwe. *Eur J Clin Nutr* 1994; 48: 810–21.
5. Black RE, Brown KH, Becker S. Effects of diarrhea associated with specific enteropathogens on the growth of children in rural Bangladesh. *Pediatrics* 1984; 73: 799–805.
6. Hoyle B, Yunus M, Chen LC. Breast-feeding and food intake among children with acute diarrheal disease. *Am J Clin Nutr* 1980; 33: 2365–71.
7. Sarker SA, Molla AM, Karim AKMM, Rahaman MM. Calorie intake in childhood diarrhoea. *Nutr Rep Int* 1982; 26: 581–90.
8. Molla AM, Molla A, Sarker SA, Rahaman MM. Food intake during and after recovery for diarrhea in children. In: Chen LC, Scrimshaw NS, eds. *Diarrhea and malnutrition*. New York: Plenum Press, 1983: 113–23.
9. Mata LJ, Kromal RA, Urrutia JJ, Garcia B. Effect of infection on food intake and the nutritional status: perspectives as viewed from the village. *Am J Clin Nutr* 1977; 30: 1215–27.
10. Martorell R, Yarbrough C, Yarbrough S, Klein RE. The impact of ordinary illnesses on the dietary intake of malnourished children. *Am J Clin Nutr* 1980; 33: 345–50.
11. Brown KH, Black RE, Robertson AD, Becker S. Effects of season and illness on the dietary intake of weanlings during longitudinal studies in rural Bangladesh. *Am J Clin Nutr* 1985; 41: 343–55.
12. Brown KH, Stallings RY, Creed de Kanashiro H, Lopez de Romaña G, Black RE. Effects of common illnesses on infants' energy intakes from breast milk and other foods during longitudinal community-based studies in Huascar (Lima), Peru. *Am J Clin Nutr* 1990; 52: 1005–13.
13. Dickin KL, Brown KH, Fagbule D, et al. Effect of diarrhea on dietary intake by infants and young children in rural villages of Kwara State, Nigeria. *Eur J Clin Nutr* 1990; 44: 307–17.
14. Marquis GS, Lopez T, Peerson JM, Brown KH. Effect of dietary viscosity on energy intake by breast-fed and non-breast-fed children during and after acute diarrhea. *Am J Clin Nutr* 1993; 57: 218–23.
15. Brown KH, Dewey KG, Allen LH. *Complementary feeding of young children in developing countries: a review of current scientific knowledge*. Geneva: World Health Organization, 1998.
16. Brown KH, Peerson JM, Lopez de Romaña G, Creed de Kanashiro H, Black RE. Validity and epidemiology of reported poor appetite among Peruvian infants from a low income, periurban community. *Am J Clin Nutr* 1995; 61: 26–32.
17. Brown KH, Perez F. Determinants of dietary intake during childhood diarrhea and implications for appropriate nutritional therapy. *Acta Paediatr Suppl* 1992; 381: 127–32.
18. O'Loughlin EV, Scott RB, Gall DG. Pathophysiology of infectious diarrhea: changes in intestinal structure and function. *J Pediatr Gastroenterol Nutr* 1991; 12: 5–20.
19. Jonas A, Avigal S, Diver-Haber A. Disturbed fat absorption following infectious gastroenteritis in children. *J Pediatr* 1979; 95: 366–72.
20. Rosenberg IH, Solomons NW, Schneider RE. Malabsorption associated with diarrhea and intestinal infections. *Am J Clin Nutr* 1977; 30: 1248–53.
21. Brown KH, MacLean WC. Nutritional management of acute diarrhea: an appraisal of the alternatives. *Pediatrics* 1984; 73: 119–25.
22. Hammer HF, Fine KD, Santa Ana CA, Porter JL, Schiller LR, Fordtran JS. Carbohydrate malabsorption. Its measurement and contribution to diarrhea. *J Clin Invest* 1990; 86: 1936–44.
23. Sack D, Rhoads M, Molla A, Molla AM, Wahed M. Carbohydrate malabsorption in infants with rotavirus diarrhea. *Am J Clin Nutr* 1982; 36: 1112–8.
24. Castillo-Duran C, Vial P, Uauy R. Trace mineral balance during acute diarrhea in infants. *J Pediatr* 1988; 113: 452–7.

25. Paerregaard A, Hjelt K, Krasilnikoff PA. Vitamin B$_{12}$ and folic acid absorption and hematological status in children with postenteritis enteropathy. *J Pediatr Gastroenterol Nutr* 1990; 11: 351–5.
26. Isolauri E, Untunen M, Wiren S, Vuorinen P, Koivula T. Intestinal permeability changes in acute gastroenteritis: effects of clinical factors and nutritional management. *J Pediatr Gastroenterol Nutr* 1989; 8: 466–73.
27. Goto K, Chew F, Torun B, Brown KH. Prevalence and risk factors for abnormal intestinal permeability in poor Guatemalan infants. *J Pediatr Gastroenterol Nutr* 1999; 28: 282–290.
28. Lunn PG, Northrup-Clewes CA, Downes RM. Intestinal permeability, mucosal injury, and growth faltering in Gambian infants. *Lancet* 1991; 338: 907–10.
29. Roy SK, Behrens RH, Haider R, et al. Impact of zinc supplementation on intestinal permeability in Bangladeshi children with acute diarrhoea and persistent diarrhoea syndrome. *J Pediatr Gastroenterol Nutr* 1992; 15: 289–96.
30. Bates CJ, Evans PH, Dardenne M, et al. A trial of zinc supplementation in young rural Gambian children. *Br J Nutr* 1993; 69: 243–55.
31. Alam AN, Sarker SA, Wahed MA, et al. Enteric protein loss and intestinal permeability changes in children during acute shigellosis and after recovery: effect of zinc supplementation. *Gut* 1994; 35: 1707–11.
32. Martorell R, Habicht J-P, Yarbrough C, et al. Acute morbidity and physical growth in rural Guatemalan children. *Am J Dis Child* 1975; 129: 1296–301.
33. Condon-Paoloni D, Cravioto J, Johnston FE, et al. Morbidity and growth of infants and young children in a rural Mexican village. *Am J Public Health* 1977; 67: 651–6.
34. Rowland MGM, Cole TJ, Whitehead RG. A quantitative study into the role of infection in determining nutritional status in Gambian village children. *Br J Nutr* 1977; 37: 441–4.
35. Zumrawi FY, Dimond H, Waterlow JC. Effects of infection on growth in Sudanese children. *Human Nutrition, Clinical Nutrition* 1987; 41C: 453–4.
36. Rowland MGM, Goh Rowland SGJ, Cole TJ. Impact of infection on the growth of children from 0 to 2 years in an urban west African community. *Am J Clin Nutr* 1988; 47: 134–8.
37. Lutter CK, Mora JO, Habicht J-P, et al. Nutritional supplementation: effects on child stunting associated with diarrhea. *Am J Clin Nutr* 1989; 50: 1–8.
38. Morris SS, Cousens SN, Kirkwood BR, et al. Is prevalence of diarrhea a better predictor of subsequent mortality and weight gain than diarrhea incidence? *Am J Epidemiol* 1996; 144: 582–8.
39. Molbak K, Andersen M, Aaby P, et al. *Cryptosporidium* infection in infancy as a cause of malnutrition: a community study from Guinea-Bissau, West Africa. *Am J Clin Nutr* 1997; 65: 149–52.
40. Brown K, Peerson JM, Kanashiro H, et al. The relationship between diarrheal prevalence and growth of poor infants varies with their age and usual energy intake [Abstract]. *FASEB J* 1991; 5: A1079.
41. Brown KH, Black RE, Lopez de Romaña G, et al. Infant feeding practices and their relationship with diarrheal and other diseases. *Pediatrics* 1989; 83: 31–40.
42. Popkin BM, Adair L, Akin JS, et al. Breast-feeding and diarrheal morbidity. *Pediatrics* 1990; 86: 874–82.
43. Holcombe C, Omotata BA, Eldridge J, Jones DM. *Helicobacter pylori*, the most common chronic bacterial infection in Africa: random serological study. *Am J Gastroenterol* 1992; 87: 28–30.
44. Taylor DN, Blaser MJ. The epidemiology of *Helicobacter pylori* infection. *Epidemiol Rev* 1991; 13: 42–59.
45. Graham DY, Malaty HM, Evans DG, et al. Epidemiology of *Helicobacter pylori* in an asymptomatic population in the United States. *Gastroenterology* 1991; 100: 1495–1501.
46. Klein PD, Graham DY, Gaillour A, et al. Gastrointestinal Physiology Working Group. Water source as risk factor for *Helicobacter pylori* infection in Peruvian children. *Lancet* 1991; 337: 1503–6.
47. Weaver LT. Aspects of *Helicobacter pylori* infection in the developing and developed world. *Trans R Soc Trop Med Hyg* 1995; 89: 347–50.
48. Goodman KJ, Correa P, Aux HJT, et al. Nutritional factors and *Helicobacter pylori* infection in Colombian children. *J Pediatr Gastroenterol Nutr* 1997; 25: 507–15.
49. Begue RE, Gonzales JL, Correa-Gracian H, Tang SC. Dietary risk factors associated with the transmission of *Helicobacter pylori* in Lima, Peru. *Am J Trop Med Hyg* 1998; 59: 637–40.
50. Gilman RH, Partanen R, Brown KH, et al. Decreased gastric acid secretion and bacterial colonization of the stomach in severely malnourished Bangladeshi children. *Gastroenterology* 1988; 94: 1308–14.
51. Dale A, Thomas JE, Darboe MK, et al. *Helicobacter pylori* infection, gastric acid secretion, and infant growth. *J Pediatr Gastroenterol Nutr* 1998; 26: 393–7.
52. Patel P, Mendall MA, Khulusi S, et al. *Helicobacter pylori* infection in childhood: risk factors and effect on growth. *BMJ* 1994; 309: 1119–23.

53. Perri F, Pastore M, Leandro G, et al. *Helicobacter pylori* infection and growth delay in older children. *Arch Dis Child* 1997; 77: 46–9.

54. Mahalanabis D, Rahman MM, Sarker SA, et al. *Helicobacter pylori* infection in the young in Bangladesh: prevalence, socioeconomic and nutritional aspects. *Int J Epidemiol* 1996; 25: 894–8.

55. Clemens J, Albert MJ, Rao M, et al. Sociodemographic, hygienic and nutritional correlates of *Helicobacter pylori* infection of young Bangladeshi children. *Pediatr Infect Dis J* 1996; 15: 1113–8.

56. Chandra RK. Nutrition and immunity: lessons for the past and new insights into the future. *Am J Clin Nutr* 1991; 53: 1087–101.

57. Butzner JD, Butler DG, Miniats OP, Hamilton JR. Impact of chronic protein-calorie malnutrition on small intestinal repair after acute viral enteritis: a study in gnotobiotic piglets. *Pediatr Res* 1985; 19: 476–81.

58. Tomkins A. Nutritional status and severity of diarrhoea among pre-school children in rural Nigeria. *Lancet* 1981; i: 860–2.

59. Sepulveda J, Willett W, Muñoz A. Malnutrition and diarrhea: a longitudinal study among urban Mexican children. *Am J Epidemiol* 1988; 127: 365–76.

60. Schorling JB, McAuliffe JF, De Souza MA, Guerrant RL. Malnutrition is associated with increased diarrhoea incidence and duration among children in an urban Brazilian slum. *Int J Epidemiol* 1990; 19: 728–35.

61. Palmer DL, Koster FT, Alam AKMJ, Islam MR. Nutritional status: a determinant of severity of diarrhea in patients with cholera. *J Infect Dis* 1976; 134: 8–14.

62. Black RE, Merson MH, Eusof A, et al. Nutritional status, body size, and severity of diarrhoea associated with rotavirus or enterotoxigenic *Escherichia coli*. *J Trop Med Hyg* 1984; 87: 83–9.

63. James JW. Longitudinal study of the morbidity of diarrheal and respiratory infections in malnourished children. *Am J Clin Nutr* 1972; 25: 690–4.

64. Black RE, Brown KH, Becker S. Malnutrition is a determining factor in diarrheal duration, but not incidence, among young children in a longitudinal study in rural Bangladesh. *Am J Clin Nutr* 1984; 39: 87–94.

65. Bairagi R, Chowdhury MK, Kim YJ, et al. The association between malnutrition and diarrhoea in rural Bangladesh. *Int J Epidemiol* 1987; 16: 477–81.

66. Bhan MK, Arora NK, Ghai OP, et al. Major factors in diarrhoea-related mortality among rural children. *Indian J Med Res* 1986; 83: 9–12.

67. Teka T, Faruque ASG, Fuchs GJ. Risk factors for deaths in under-five-age children attending a diarrhoea treatment centre. *Acta Paediatr* 1996; 85: 1070–5.

68. Bhutta ZZ, Nizami SQ, Thobani S, Issani Z. Risk factors for mortality among hospitalized children with persistent diarrhoea in Pakistan. *J Trop Pediatr* 1997; 43: 330–6.

69. Ninh, NO, Thissen JP, Collette L, et al. Zinc supplementation increases growth and circulating insulin-like growth factor I (IGF–I) in growth-retarded Vietnamese children. *Am J Clin Nutr* 1996; 63: 514–9.

70. Sazawal S, Black RE, Bhan MK, et al. Zinc supplementation reduces the incidence of persistent diarrhea and dysentery among low socioeconomic children in India. *J Nutr* 1996; 126: 443–50.

71. Sazawal S, Black RE, Bhan MK, et al. Efficacy of zinc supplementation in reducing the incidence and prevalence of acute diarrhea a community-based, double-blind controlled trial. *Am J Clin Nutr* 1997; 66: 413–8.

72. Rosado JL, Lopez P, Munoz E, et al. Zinc supplementation reduced morbidity, but neither zinc nor iron supplementation affected growth or body composition of Mexican preschoolers. *Am J Clin Nutr* 1997; 65: 13–19.

73. Ruel MT, Rivera J, Santizo MC, et al. The impact of zinc supplementation on morbidity from diarrhea and respiratory infections among young rural Guatemalan children. *Pediatrics* 1997; 99: 808–13.

74. Bloem MW, Wedel M, Egger RJ, et al. Mild vitamin A deficiency and risk of respiratory tract diseases and diarrhea in preschool and school children in northeastern Thailand. *Am J Epidemiol* 1990; 131: 332–9.

75. Rahmathullah L, Underwood BA, Thulasiraj RD, et al. Diarrhea, respiratory infections, and growth are not affected by a weekly low-dose vitamin A supplement: a masked, controlled field trial in children in southern India. *Am J Clin Nutr* 1991; 54: 568–77.

76. Ghana VAST Study Team. Vitamin A supplementation in northern Ghana: effects on clinic attendances, hospital admissions, and child mortality. *Lancet* 1993; 342: 7–12.

77. Lie C, Ying C, En-Lin W, et al. Impact of large-dose vitamin A supplementation on childhood diarrhoea, respiratory disease and growth. *Eur J Clin Nutr* 1993; 47: 88–96.

78. Biswas R, Biswas AB, Manna B, et al. Effect of vitamin A supplementation on diarrhoea and acute respiratory infection in children. *Eur J Epidemiol* 1994; 10: 57–61.
79. Bhandari N, Bhan MK, Sazawal S. Impact of a massive dose of vitamin A to preschool children with acute diarrhoea on subsequent respiratory and diarrhoeal morbidity. *BMJ* 1994; 309: 1404–7.
80. Barreto ML, Santos LMP, Assis AMO, et al. Effect of vitamin A supplementation on diarrhoea and acute lower-respiratory-tract infections in young children in Brazil. *Lancet* 1994; 344: 228–31.
81. Ramakrishnan U, Latham MC, Abel R, Frongillo EA. Vitamin A supplementation and morbidity among preschool children in south India. *Am J Clin Nutr* 1995; 61: 1295–303.
82. Dibley MJ, Sadjimin T, Kjolhede CL, Moulton LH. Vitamin A supplementation fails to reduce incidence of acute respiratory illness and diarrhea in preshool-age Indonesian children. *J Nutr* 1996; 126: 434–42.
83. Hershko C, Peto TEA, Weatherall DJ. Iron and infection. *BMJ* 1988; 296: 660–4.
84. Keusch GT. Micronutrients and susceptibility to infection. *Ann NY Acad Sci* 1990; 587: 181–8.
85. Brunser O, Espinoza J, Araya M, et al. Chronic iron intake and diarrhoeal disease in infants. A field study in a less-developed country. *Eur J Clin Nutr* 1993; 47: 317–26.
86. Mitra AK, Akramuzzaman SM, Fuchs GJ, et al. Long-term oral supplementation with iron is not harmful for young children in a poor community of Bangladesh. *J Nutr* 1997; 127: 1451–55.

DISCUSSION

Dr. Thomas: I would like to comment on a few more issues about *Helicobacter pylori* in the Gambia. Our analyses show that acquiring *H. pylori* colonization before the age of 6 months has a negative effect on weight gain which reaches significance in the 3- to 6-month period. No matter how hard you try, you cannot correct out the association between early *H. pylori* colonization and the onset of weight and growth faltering, but we have been able to show that this is completely independent of the presence of diarrheal disease. Although I am very cautious about trying to infer causality from observational studies, even though they were reproducible in longitudinal cohort studies, one possible interpretation of these data is that they are consistent with *H. pylori* colonization being the first event that sets children on the path to undernutrition and growth faltering. Although many ways are found to leave that path, the further down you go, the harder it is to get off it. I am sure other infections do the same, but certain unique features of *H. pylori* colonization mean we stand a good chance of gaining a detailed understanding of how this particular GI pathogen might lead to undernutrition and weight and growth faltering in young children.

Dr. Brown: It was interesting to learn about these new analyses, because the original published data (1) did not discuss controlling for other potential confounders. Were birthweight, and maternal height and weight included in your model?

Dr. Thomas: Yes, they were. There were maternal factors relating to the difference in *H. pylori* colonization, but these were related to breast milk components, not to maternal height, weight, or nutritional status at all.

Dr. Wasantwisut: I have a comment about defining micronutrient status during infection. I think this is important, especially in relation to how supplementation might alter interactions between certain nutrients, for example vitamin A and zinc supplements with iron; so many factors come into play there. I was interested in seeing the difference in gender in the Guatemala study, with girls showing no effect of zinc supplementation, whereas boys did. Perhaps this reflected more severe deficiency in the boys? In relation to intestinal permeability and its effect on nutrient absorption, does this vary according to the type of organism causing diarrhea?

Dr. Brown: The issue of assessing micronutrient status in relationship to infection has been discussed by previous presenters, and I will not add to that, but I would like to say a few words about assessing zinc status. This was raised the other day, and I was not entirely in agreement with the tone of the discussion. The problems associated with assessing zinc status in the individual are well known, including the issue of using plasma zinc concentration as an indicator of status and all the factors that may influence that, including the state of fasting, the presence of infection, and so on. Having said that, however, I think that the use of an indicator such as the average plasma zinc concentration of the population, or the percentage of individuals with a low plasma zinc concentration using some cut-off, does give us insight into the status of the population. I have two pieces of evidence to support that contention. We have recently completed a meta-analysis of all the studies that we could identify looking at relationships between zinc supplementation and children's growth in different parts of the world. We looked at the relationship between the average plasma zinc concentration reported in an individual study and the likelihood of showing a response to zinc supplementation in that study. In our meta-regression analysis, the plasma zinc concentration turned out to be one of the variables that explained whether there would be a positive response to zinc in a particular study population. The other piece of evidence is related to whether plasma zinc concentration at the population level responds to supplementation, and here again we saw a very strong relationship. I think only one exception was found in all the studies of children that we looked at. That is to say, in every case but one, a significant increase in plasma zinc concentration was seen in the supplemented group but not in the control group. So, I think at the population level plasma zinc is not such a bad indicator, and it may be one more piece of evidence that we would use to establish whether a population is likely to be zinc deficient, or at least in marginal zinc status.

Regarding your question about intestinal permeability, most of the studies have been done in industrialized countries in hospitalized children, and in most of these the agent was rotavirus. I do not know whether that influences the interpretation of those studies to any great extent. In our studies in Guatemala, we did not look at the cause of the infection. We had hoped to study noninfected children, and those 10 children I was able to cite were there by accident.

Dr. Chandra: I was interested in your assessment that the recent study by Sazawal (2,3) showed a very significant effect. I have reviewed that paper recently, and I beg to differ. First, the only effect was seen in persistent diarrhea, not diarrhea in general, and persistent diarrhea never accounts for more than a small proportion of cases, even in their study. For a significant action of zinc, I would have liked to have seen an effect on all types of diarrhea. Second, the effect was seen only in boys, and only in those above 1 year of age. If you look at all the situations in which zinc did not seem to have an effect, then overall I think the study shows a marginal effect on diarrhea. Also, I do not agree with the conclusions in their abstract as published in the *Journal of Nutrition*; I think they are overstated.

Dr. Brown: One has to be very careful in the interpretation of any supplementation trial with regard to interactive models—that is, who is likely to respond? I would say the results of the Sazawal paper are exactly what you might predict in terms of which children are likely to respond to zinc supplementation, and this has also been shown in some of the vitamin A studies—that is, if not deficient initially, an individual is unlikely to respond to the supplementation unless it has some additional pharmacologic effect. Younger children in the first half of infancy are much less likely to respond to zinc supplements, presumably reflecting the fact that breast milk is probably an adequate source of zinc. The issue of a gender-specific response has not been consistent across studies, although I mentioned that the Guatemala study and the India study found an effect in boys but not girls. However, that was not true in the other trials. Regarding the issue of the response to acute versus persistent diarrhea, some consistency has been seen in the various trials, although the number of studies is quite small. Zinc supplementation appears to have a greater impact on preventing persistent diarrhea than acute diarrhea, and I believe that is exactly what you would hope for from a public health perspective. We know that persistent episodes are the ones most closely associated with secondary malnutrition and with the highest mortality. They explain an inordinately high proportion of the diarrhea-associated deaths. So, rather than interpret that pessimistically, I would interpret that optimistically in terms of what we might achieve with zinc supplementation. Overall in the pooled analysis, when we talk about a 20% reduction of diarrheal disease that may seem small to someone who is used to working with laboratory models, but in a public health setting a 20% reduction in disease is enormous. It makes us extremely excited about the potential benefits. If you compare it with what might be achieved by improved sanitation, by improved breast-feeding rates (which are only going to affect what happens in infancy), and by some of the other interventions that have been spoken of for preventing diarrheal disease, this promises to be relatively powerful in its potential effect on reducing morbidity and mortality.

Dr. Griffin: I have a comment on the anorexia that accompanies the acute phase response. To show that anorexia is responsible for weight loss, you have to show that a negative energy balance exists. Until recently, it has been very difficult to do that in people who are sick. However, using the doubly labeled water technique, it is now possible to make indirect measurements of free-living energy expenditure in someone who is ill to within $\pm$ 10%. In the acquired immunodeficiency syndrome, it has been shown that energy intake is reduced, but so too is energy expenditure considerably reduced. So, although one is in negative energy balance, this is in association with reduced energy expenditure. This, of course, confounds the view that weight loss is caused by hypermetabolism in acute or even chronic infections. So, you have to look at both sides of equation: food intake as well as energy expenditure.

My second point relates to *H. pylori*. I am not an epidemiologist, but I do believe that studies such as the ones we have been talking about are very useful in allowing us to generate hypotheses that can be tested. Some quite large epidemiologic studies have looked at *normal* C-reactive protein values–that is, the level below that of the accepted normal range of 8 mg/dl. If you stratify people into bands (8-6, 6-4, and so on), and then look at risk factors for developing certain diseases, then even within this *normal* range you find that people in the high normal range have a fivefold excess of cardiovascular disease later on. Thus, it is possible that C-reactive protein value might be useful as a chronic marker of a proinflammatory state, either caused by *H. pylori* itself or by other infections. It would be possible to use serum from the Gambia to see whether you can stratify children into these higher normal ranges consistently as a marker of inflammatory status.

Dr. Brown: Those are very nice comments and I certainly will not dispute either of them. I would just like to make one plea from the epidemiologic perspective for those of you who have expertise in the laboratory. We would love to have measures of chronic immunostimulation and chronic proinflammatory conditions, but we do not have useful markers at present. Anything that requires drawing blood frequently is not satisfactory. We need something that we can measure in urine that would be useful for assessing this condition epidemiologically.

Dr. Suskind: What are your thoughts about iron?

Dr. Brown: We have just completed a multiple micronutrient supplementation trial in Peru in children with persistent diarrhea, which included treatment of the initial presenting episode as well as 6 months of supplementation following the initial illness to see what the incidence of new disease might be, expecting that these children would be at very high risk of new infections. It was a three-cell study—placebo, zinc, or zinc plus all the other essential nutrients that we could put into a solution—the thought being that if zinc were provided and some other nutrient was limiting, the children might not be able to respond. We found a small, nonsignificant reduction in subsequent incidence of diarrheal disease in the zinc-supplemented group, but a somewhat larger and significant increase in incidence of new episodes in the group receiving multiple micronutrient supplements. The finding was consistent across all of the different symptoms of illness we examined, whether it was related to diarrheal or respiratory disease. This consistency of results leads us to believe that these findings may be real and not just because of chance, although it is hard to know for sure with the results of just one study. We do not know whether a specific component of the supplement may have explained these findings, but we wondered whether iron, which was provided at a dose of 10 mg/d, could have been responsible. We looked through the literature and found three other studies (4–6) that suggested that iron supplementation or iron fortification of milk formula resulted in increased rates of diarrheal disease, particularly in infants, although not necessarily in older children. So, all I can say is that I am concerned and I am not sure that we can draw final conclusions on the safety of supplemental iron. Does this mean that we should withhold iron? No, we know that iron is essential and that functional problems are associated with iron deficiency that we would like to prevent. At the same time, I do not think we can be so cavalier as to say that no risk is associated with iron supplements. That is an area for more research.

REFERENCES

1. Dale A, Thomas JE, Darboe MK, et al. *Helicobacter pylori* infection, gastric acid secretion and infant growth. *J Pediatr Gastroenterol Nutr* 1998: 26; 393–7.
2. Sazawal S, Black RE, Bhan MK, et al. Zinc supplementation reduces the incidence of persistent diarrhea and dysentery among low socio-economic children in India. *J Nutr* 1996: 126; 443–50.
3. Sazawal S, Black RE, Bhan MK, et al. Efficacy of zinc supplementation in reducing the incidence and prevalence of acute diarrhea—a community-based, double-blind controlled trial. *Am J Clin Nutr* 1997: 66; 413–8.
4. Brunser O, Espinoza J, Araya M, et al. Chronic iron intake and diarrhoeal disease in infants. A field study in a less-developed country. *Eur J Clin Nutr* 1993; 47: 317–26.
5. Mitra AK, Akramuzzaman SM, Fuchs GJ, et al. Long-term oral supplementation with iron is not harmful for young children in a poor community of Bangladesh. *J Nutr* 1997; 127: 1451–5.
6. Rosado JL, Lopez P, Munoz E, et al. Zinc supplementation reduced morbidity, but neither zinc nor iron supplementation affected growth or body composition of Mexican preschoolers. *Am J Clin Nutr* 1997; 65: 13–9.

Nutrition, Immunity, and Infection in Infants and Children, edited by Robert M. Suskind and Kraisid Tontisirin. Nestlé Nutrition Workshop Series, Pediatric Program, Vol. 45. Nestec Ltd., Vevey/Lippincott Williams & Wilkins, Philadelphia ©2001.

The Interaction of Acute Respiratory Infections, Measles, and Nutritional Status

Hoosen M. Coovadia and Anna Coutsoudis

Department of Paediatrics and Child Health, University of Natal, Congella, South Africa

Nutrition and infection bear the same close relationship to each other as the interdependent covariables in nature such as space and time, and mass and energy. We discuss the intricate web of relationships between nutrition, acute respiratory infections, and measles in this chapter, and conclude with suggestions for further research.

IMPACT OF ACUTE RESPIRATORY INFECTIONS ON NUTRITIONAL STATUS

Protein-Energy Malnutrition

In a longitudinal health and nutrition survey of 3,000 children (birth to 2 years of age) conducted in the Philippines, length and morbidity data were collected bimonthly over a 2-year period (1). Stunting (height for age > 2 SD below the World Health Organization [WHO] median) was found in 65% of the children, and the study showed that the likelihood of stunting was significantly increased by febrile respiratory infections. In a community-based study of 106 Kenyan children 18 to 25 months of age, being underweight (weight for age < 80% of expected) and stunted (height for age < 90% of expected) was positively associated with acute lower respiratory tract infections (2).

Vitamin A

Common acute respiratory infections have been noted to reduce vitamin A levels in various settings. Sommer *et al.* confirmed this in their prospective, community-based programs in Indonesia (3). Among rural preschool children followed-up for 18 months, those with respiratory disease were more than twice as likely to develop xerophthalmia as the children who did not have respiratory disease ($p < 0.05$). This association was not detected in those under 3 years of age; among those above age 3 years, the relative risk ranged between 3.3 and 6.2 for different age groups. Protein-energy malnutrition did not influence this risk. Among hospital cases, acute respiratory infections often occurred together with xerophthalmia; the more severe the latter, the more frequent the respiratory infections. Shenai *et al.* have reported falling levels of vitamin A among low birthweight babies in the United States who have repeated lower respiratory tract infections.

A recent study from Bangladesh examined the impact of vitamin A supplementation (15 mg each dose) given at the time of primary immunization at 6 weeks, 10 weeks, and 14 weeks after birth (4). Despite supplementation, after 3 months, 61% of 33 children remained vitamin A deficient by the relative dose-response test. Acute respiratory infection episodes were more frequent in those who remained deficient, despite vitamin A supplementation; the odds ratio for postdose vitamin A deficiency in supplemented infants was 5.4 (95% confidence interval (CI) 0.33 to 87.3; $p = 0.22$) for acute respiratory infections. The authors interpret these results to mean that frequent respiratory infections reduced vitamin A levels despite supplementation.

IMPACT OF MEASLES ON NUTRITIONAL STATUS

Protein-Energy Malnutrition

Several studies have shown that measles has a negative effect on nutritional state (5,6). Accompanying fever increases the body's need for protein and energy during a time of decreased food intake. Also seen is an increase in protein loss from the gut—it is estimated that up to 20% of protein intake is lost in the stools. A diet that was just adequate to allow growth before the illness may be inadequate to allow optimal growth during the recovery phase.

In a community study in Haiti (7) of 595 infants 6 to 12 months of age, it was shown that those infants who had serologic evidence of previous measles infection had a significantly worse nutritional status than those who had no evidence of previous measles ($p < 0.01$).

Vitamin A

The best evidence that an attack of measles profoundly affects vitamin A metabolism is the well-documented association between measles and xerophthalmia in many countries throughout the world. An acute measles episode produces a transient reduction in serum vitamin A, which recovers without supplementation once the disease is over (8–11). For example, in an Indian community-based study of 1,544 children under the age of 5 years who were prospectively followed, 318 cases of measles were seen and vitamin A concentrations measured (8). There was no supplementation with vitamin A. Serum vitamin A was lower during measles and became normal by 8 weeks after recovery. Retinol concentrations were lowest in those children with measles who also had the most severe grade of protein-energy malnutrition. The decrease in serum vitamin A during measles has been found in both developing (8–11) and industrialized countries (12). The reasons for this decline are probably multifactorial; high metabolic demand caused by widespread infection, exuberant immune responses, and vigorous catabolism are likely to be critical. Measles results both in early death and in delayed mortality. The longer term consequences of measles on the gastrointestinal tract and respiratory system can cause a gradual deterioration in vitamin A status.

IMPACT OF NUTRITIONAL STATUS ON ACUTE RESPIRATORY INFECTIONS

Protein-Energy Malnutrition

Hospital-based studies conducted in Nigeria (13) and India (14) showed that malnutrition was a strong predictor of length of hospital stay and death from acute respiratory infections. The problem with hospital studies is that measurements are made at the time of diagnosis, therefore making it difficult to ascertain whether malnutrition is an acute response to infection or a pre-existing risk factor. Community-based, prospective studies are more helpful. A study in Bangladesh of 965 children (0 to 5 years of age), followed-up once a month for 4 months, showed that, among children who developed acute respiratory infections, 63% were malnourished compared with 37% among the noninfected controls (15). A similar study in Burkina Faso showed that malnutrition was a significant risk factor for developing acute respiratory infections. Two studies in India (16,17) that followed children under 5 years of age for 1 year found that malnourished children had a significantly greater risk of acute respiratory infection.

In a 10-month prospective study of children in Kenya (6 months to 10 years of age), nutritional status and cellular immunocompetence, determined by delayed-type hypersensitivity (DTH), were related to individual attack rates of acute respiratory infection (18). When examined separately, both nutritional status and DTH responsiveness were significant predictors of individual attack rates of acute respiratory infection; however, when the effects were simultaneously tested, only DTH responsiveness was significant. These results indicate that the effect of nutritional status on the occurrence of acute respiratory infection may be mediated by cellular immune function.

Nutritional Interventions

A recent trial in Vietnam (19) used an intervention of encouraging home garden production and nutrition education in order to improve the nutritional status of children 1 to 6 years of age. Children in the intervention commune (n = 469) had a significant reduction (p < 0.0001) in the incidence of acute respiratory infections: 11.2% compared with 49.1% in the control commune (n = 251).

Vitamin A

Deficiency and Predisposition to Acute Respiratory Infections

Some early studies suggested that vitamin A deficiency may predispose to different types of respiratory infection. Several recent cross-sectional studies have also detected an association between varying degrees of vitamin A deficiency and respiratory tract infections (3,20–23). These infections include both upper and lower respiratory tract disorders. The data were derived from population-, clinic-, and hospital-based investigations in developing countries. On the other hand, some population-based projects have failed to detect an association between vitamin A deficiency and respiratory disease (24–26). A much clearer idea of this association emerges from the prospective, community-based studies conducted recently. Studies from Indonesia (27,28) and India (29,30) have shown an increased risk of respiratory disease in children with vitamin A deficiency.

Supplementation and Acute Respiratory Infections

Recent meta-analyses (31,32) have failed to detect a consistent impact of vitamin A supplementation on the incidence or mortality from acute lower respiratory tract infections. The Vitamin A and Pneumonia Working Group reviewed 12 large-scale field trials which had results available to January 1993 (32). Five of these trials had information on pneumonia incidence and prevalence. Overall, no significant impact was found of vitamin A supplementation on either the incidence or the prevalence of pneumonia (Table 1). However, a trend was seen showing a possible harmful effect of vitamin A supplementation on the incidence and prevalence of pneumonia in infants 6 to 11 month of age, and a possible beneficial effect on those 48 to 59 months of age. Most of the increased risk was contributed by data from one study. Furthermore, four of the nine studies (which had appropriate data) revealed a 5% to 10% excess of coughing in the group receiving vitamin A supplement. Only the Jumla, Nepal, study showed a significant impact of vitamin A supplements (33).

Three smaller trials, one in Thailand (23), one in China (34), and the other in Indonesia (35), showed a positive or marginal impact of vitamin A on respiratory mor-

TABLE 1. *Impact of vitamin A supplementation on pneumonia incidence*

Study	Vitamin A rate*/annum	Placebo rate*/annum	Rate ratio (CI)
Morvita *et al.* (28)	0.55	0.48	1.14 (0.99–1.32)
Bahia *et al.* (36)	0.98	1.00	0.97 (0.86–1.09)
Delhi *et al.* (37)	1.58	1.67	0.95 (0.77–1.17)
VAST Ghana Study Team (77)	0.85	0.92	0.92 (0.82–1.04)
Jumla *et al.* (33)	0.61	0.91	0.77 (0.66–0.89)
Summary	—	—	0.95 (0.89–1.01)

* Episodes of pneumonia/number of child-weeks.
CI, confidence interval.

TABLE 2. *Impact of vitamin A supplementation on pneumonia-specific mortality in children under 5 years of age*

Country (study)	Pneumonia-specific mortality	
	Rate ratio	Design effect*
Jumla *et al.* (33)	0.88	1.416 (0.38–2.05)
Madurai *et al.* (72)	0.66	1.329 (0.08–5.19)
Sarlahi (76)	1.10	1.187 (0.77–1.57)
Sudan (77)	0.43	1.000 (0.16–1.19)
Ghana (77)	1.10	2.003 (0.61–1.97)
Summary	—	0.98 (0.75–1.28)

* Where randomization was not at individual level, regression was weighted to allow for within-cluster homogeneity using design effects (31).

bidity. In China, 172 children 6 months to 3 years of age were given either a placebo or two doses (each dose 200,000 IU) of vitamin A in a 6-month period. The incidence and severity of respiratory disease were decreased in the treated group. This effect was observed only in those 12 or more months of age. The latter study has been criticized for design problems, which could have introduced bias in assessments. In the study of 269 urban Indonesian children 1 to 5 years of age, vitamin A supplementation (200,000 IU orally 6 monthly) had no effect on incidence or severity of acute respiratory infections (as defined by WHO). The duration of acute respiratory infections was slightly shorter in those in the supplemented group (35).

Five trials were conducted in which pneumonia mortality could be assessed (Table 2). The impact of vitamin A supplementation on pneumonia mortality varied, but the summary rate ratio was near unity (0.98). As pneumonia is a major cause of infant deaths, the impact of vitamin A supplementation was separately analyzed for this age group. The rate ratio for those 0 to 5 months of age was 0.88 (95% CI 0.51 to 1.51) and for those 6 to 11 months it was 1.08 (95% CI 0.57 to 2.03).

The effect of vitamin A in children aged less than 6 months remains unclear. In Indonesian infants given 50,000 IU of vitamin A at birth, the mortality was half that of the control group in the first year (38). In Tanzania (39), Fawzi showed no effect of vitamin A on pregnancy outcomes in women infected with the human immunodeficiency virus, despite a beneficial effect of multivitamin supplements on fetal mortality, low birthweight, prematurity, and fetal growth retardation. In the recent WHO/CHD randomized trial (CHD, Child Health Division), no benefit was found of vitamin A supplementation linked to immunization visits in infancy on respiratory or diarrheal morbidity, growth, or mortality (40). In our Durban studies (41), we tested the prophylactic value of vitamin A given to infants born to women infected with HIV as follows: 50,000 IU at 1 and 3 months of age, 100,000 IU at 6 and 9 months, and 200,000 IU at 12 and 15 months. Recall of morbidity was recorded monthly at each follow-up visit. Babies infected with HIV in the supplemented group had reduced diarrheal but not respiratory morbidity.

In summary, therefore, vitamin A supplementation apparently has no significant impact on pneumonia incidence, prevalence, or mortality in children between 6 months and 5 years of age. Data from these trials are insufficient to derive any firm conclusions on the impact of vitamin A on pneumonia mortality in infants of less than 6 months of age, although recent evidence strongly suggests no beneficial effect occurs. Trends showing possible detrimental effects of vitamin A supplementation (cough in all age groups; pneumonia in those 6 to 11 months of age) require further clarification.

The 1992 meta-analysis by Beaton *et al.* (31), undertaken when the results of some large trials were still incomplete, concurred with the finding that vitamin A supplementation did not reduce the incidence or duration of respiratory infections, nor had a beneficial effect on mortality from respiratory diseases.

Australian studies have suggested that preschool children with frequent respiratory infections (42), but not those with a previous respiratory syncytial virus infection (43), derived benefit from vitamin A supplementation—a 25% reduction in lower respiratory tract infections. Shenai *et al.* treated vitamin A-deficient, low birthweight infants with vitamin A and reduced the incidence of bronchopulmonary dysplasia (44). These results were not confirmed in another study of different design (45).

Various randomized, placebo-controlled studies have failed to show consistent and substantial beneficial effects of vitamin A treatment in infants and children with acute onset of lower respiratory tract infection. Some of the benefits and adverse effects are given in Table 3. These trials have been undertaken in Brazil (46), Guatemala (47), Chile (48), Peru (49), and the United States (50); they have included clinically (47) or radiologically (48) defined lower respiratory tract infections, and have assessed all-cause pneumonia (46,47) and respiratory syncytial virus specific infections (47,48). The children studied were vitamin A replete in the United States (50), Guatemala (47), and Chile (48), or marginally vitamin A deficient in Brazil (46). A bulging fontanelle, probably caused by giving vitamin A, was transient and was noted in 4% of the children treated in the Brazil study (46).

Zinc

The major associations with zinc deficiency are chronic diarrhea, growth retardation, and immunoparesis. Some studies have shown that low zinc levels are accompanied by upper respiratory tract infections. A recent study in India showed that low plasma zinc predicts the subsequent development of lower respiratory tract infection and diarrhea. Over a period of 90 days, the initial low plasma zinc predicted a 3.5 times higher mean prevalence rate of acute lower respiratory tract infection than in children with normal zinc (51).

Supplementation

The impact of zinc supplementation in children who are likely to have inadequate body zinc is primarily on (*a*) improved growth (linear growth and weight gain); (*b*) a

TABLE 3. *Vitamin A supplementation and outcome of acute respiratory infections: randomized, placebo-controlled trials*

Country (reference)	n	Age	Vitamin A dose (IU)	Disease	Outcome
Guatemala (47)	263	3 mo to 4 yr	100,000 infants 200,000 > 12 mo	ALRTI	No benefit
United States (50)	239	1 mo to 6 yr	50,000 1–5 mo 100,000 6–11 mo 200,000 > 12 mo	RSV infection	Longer hospital stay in those > 12 mo in supplemented group
Chile (48)	180	1 mo to 6 yr	50,000 1–5 mo 100,000 6–11mo 200,000 > 12 mo	RSV infection	Duration of hospital stay and tachypnea shorter in supplemented subgroup with severe hypoxemia ($p = 0.01$ and $p = 0.09$, respectively)
Brazil (46)	472	6 mo to 5 yr	200,000 infants 400,000 > 12 mo	Clinical or radiologic pneumonia	Less fever by day 3, fewer failures to first line antibiotics ($p = 0.008$ and $p = 0.054$, respectively)
Peru (49)	95	3 mo to 10 yr	150,000 infants 300,000 > 12 mo	Radiologic pneumonia	Adverse effects of vitamin A: lower O_2 saturation, higher prevalence of retractions, more consolidation, greater O_2 requirement

ALRTI, acute lower respiratory tract infection; RSV, respiratory syncytial virus.

decreased incidence, duration, and severity of diarrhea; and (*c*) restoration of immunologic integrity (52). Zinc supplements may also enhance child development and reduce malaria morbidity (52). Zinc supplementation has not been shown to reduce mortality in children. With the exception of a well-conducted, community-based, randomized double-blind controlled trial in India (53), little evidence supports the notion that zinc has beneficial effects on lower respiratory tract infection or pneumonia. It is not even clear whether zinc supplements consistently decrease the incidence of upper respiratory tract infection.

Supplementation and Respiratory Morbidity: Community-Based Studies

Results of community-based studies are summarized in Table 4. In the study in India (53), zinc-supplemented children had 0.19 lower respiratory tract infections per child per year, compared with 0.35 episodes per child per year in the control group. Pneumonia incidence was reduced (odds ratio [OR] 0.44; 95% CI 0.27 to 0.74; $p = 0.002$), as was pneumonia prevalence (OR 0.49; 95% CI 0.29 to 0.83; $p = 0.008$). In the study in Brazil (54), with the higher dose, a trend was seen toward reduced prevalence of cough and shorter duration of hospital admission. Zinc had no effect, given alone or with iron, on the incidence or duration of respiratory tract episodes among Mexican children; most of the episodes (669 of 673) were upper respiratory tract infections (55). A trend was seen toward an increased incidence and prevalence of respiratory infection (14% and 38%, respectively) in the zinc-supplemented group in Guatemala (56). A report from Vietnam (57) recorded only upper respiratory tract infections and showed a beneficial impact of zinc. The supplemented group had significantly fewer upper respiratory tract infections ($p = 0.002$); a 2.5 times reduced relative risk for these infections was found in the treated group ($p = 0.057$). Gambian children did not appear to be zinc deficient and it is unclear whether upper or lower

TABLE 4. *Randomized, double-blind, placebo-controlled trials of zinc supplementation**

Country (study)	n	Age groups (months)	Zinc dose	Level of acute respiratory infections	Follow-up	Outcome
India (53)	609	6–35	10 mg daily	LRTI	6 mo	Reduced incidence and prevalence of pneumonia
Brazil (54)	205	Low birthweight newborns	5 mg or 1 mg daily for 8 weeks	URTI/LRTI	6 mo	No significant impact
Mexico (55)	219	18–36	20 mg alone, or with 20 mg Fe daily	Mostly URTI	12 mo	No significant impact
Guatemala (56)	99	6–9	10 mg daily	URTI/LRTI	7 mo	No significant impact
Vietnam (57)	146	4–36	10 mg daily	URTI	5 mo	Reduced incidence URTI
Gambia (58)	110	6–28	70 mg twice weekly	URTI/LRTI	15 mo	No impact

* All sites were community based.
LRTI, lower respiratory tract infection; URTI, upper respiratory tract infection.

respiratory tract infections were assessed (58); in that trial, Bates *et al.* also used a bi-weekly rather than a daily dose of zinc. A trial in schoolchildren in Ohio, USA, failed to yield positive results of zinc supplementation on upper respiratory infections (59).

Supplementation and Respiratory Morbidity: Health Facility-Based Studies

Three smaller, clinic-based studies of zinc supplementation, given to moderately or severely malnourished children, do not provide any consistent evidence of a beneficial effect of zinc on lower respiratory tract infections (60–62). Two studies from Chile (60,61) showed no significant effects of zinc on lower or upper respiratory tract infections, although one reported a marginal benefit on otitis media (61). Zinc supplementation was associated with an increase in impetigo in one study (61) and a decrease in pyoderma in the other (60). Ecuadorian children experienced a short-term benefit (60 days) from zinc supplementation in reducing upper respiratory tract infection; paradoxically, cough was increased in the treated group (62). In a recent study, not yet published, from the International Centre for Diarrhea Disease Research (ICDDR), Bangladesh, a 2-week course of zinc (20 mg/d) given to 65 malnourished children with acute diarrhea had a positive impact over the next 2 months on a subgroup with stunting. In the latter, the children who received zinc supplement had fewer episodes of respiratory tract infection than controls (1.0 vs 2.4; p < 0.01), and these were of shorter duration (1.6 vs 4.2 days; p < 0.01). It is unclear whether these were upper respiratory tract or lower respiratory tract infections. Studies from the ICDDR have also made observations on respiratory disease rates in their evaluation of the effect of zinc on diarrhea. Although reductions in respiratory diseases were noted, the numbers of such cases were too few to attain significance.

In the report of a meeting on *Zinc for Child Health* held in Baltimore, Maryland, USA, on 17–19 November 1996, R. Black concluded from available zinc intervention studies that the incidence of acute lower respiratory illness or pneumonia was decreased by between 3% and 60% (average 12%). Reductions were greater in those with initial zinc deficiency and malnutrition.

Interpretation of Results of Trials

Probably many reasons exist for the failure of most of these studies to show consistent benefits of zinc supplementation on lower respiratory tract infections or pneumonias. It is possibly a true effect that zinc supplementation, as with vitamin A supplementation, may not be of benefit for respiratory diseases. On the other hand, design issues may have obscured a positive impact. Sample sizes may have been too small; the levels of zinc deficiency, stunting, and wasting too variable; associated protein-energy malnutrition and other micronutrient deficiencies may have obscured the effects of zinc replenishment; and the risks of pneumonia were probably different in the regions studied. Furthermore, the optimal dose of zinc supplementation is not clear, and there may be gender differences in response.

Iron

Controversy has existed over the role of iron in infections. On the one hand, free iron is necessary for bacterial growth; on the other hand, iron is needed by natural killer cells, neutrophils, and lymphocytes for optimal function. It is to be expected, therefore, that in iron deficiency the initial establishment of infection may be unaffected or even rendered more difficult, owing to lack of available iron for the invading microorganisms; once infection is established, however, decreased immunocompetence will make it difficult to eliminate the infection. The clinical studies investigating the role of iron in acute respiratory infections have not been very helpful and this is an area that needs continuing research.

Intervention Trials and Acute Respiratory Infections

A study was conducted in Bangladesh in 349 children 2 to 48 months of age, who were divided into a treatment group receiving a daily supplement of 15 mg iron and multivitamins for 15 months, and a placebo group given only multivitamins (63). Results showed no difference between the iron-supplemented group and the iron-free group with respect to the number of acute respiratory infection episodes and the mean duration of the episodes. It should be noted that the effect of the multivitamins may have masked any additional effect of iron. Additionally, as a word of caution on prolonged iron supplementation, it was noted, in children under 12 months of age, that those in the iron-supplemented group had a 49% increase in the number of episodes of dysentery.

In another intervention trial in Indonesia—where children received 30 mg iron/d for 2 months as opposed to 15 mg/d used in the previous trial, and control children received only vitamin C—it was shown that respiratory infections were 2.5 times more frequent in the placebo group than in the intervention group (64). It was also observed that this effect on morbidity had an indirect effect on growth, as the children in the iron-supplemented group had a greater increase in height for age.

IMPACT OF NUTRITIONAL STATUS ON MEASLES

Protein-Energy Malnutrition

Hospital studies have reported that malnourished children (weight for age < 2 SD at admission) have a higher mortality (65). However, community studies from Bangladesh, Gambia, Nigeria, Guinea-Bissau, and Benin, which had information on nutritional status before infection, have not supported this association (66–69). Only one community study has postulated higher measles mortality among malnourished children (70); in that study, 2,019 Bangladeshi children 12 to 23 months of age were followed for 2 years. Those results may be confounded because they were based on measles deaths in relation to the total population rather than in relation to the number of children contracting measles in the two nutritional groups. However, as pointed out by Aaby et al., children from large families tend to have lower weight for age and a higher risk of contracting measles because of increased exposure and, thus, a higher risk of dying from measles (68). Therefore, the association between malnutrition and higher measles case fatality rate in the hospital is likely to reflect the fact that children lose weight during the incubation period before any symptoms of measles occur.

Effect of Nutritional Interventions

During an intervention study in India (71) designed to look at the effect of a food supplement on growth (310 kcal/d plus 3 g/d protein for 1 year), a measles outbreak occurred, which provided an opportunity for an interesting observation. The control group, children who developed measles had the expected decrease in weight compared with those who did not develop measles. However, in the supplemented group the children with measles (82 of 306) had a weight gain similar to those who did not develop measles (224 of 306).

Vitamin A

Supplementation or Treatment Reduces Measles Mortality

Vitamin A deficiency renders preschool children vulnerable to severe measles and high mortality, conditions which are ameliorated or reversed by vitamin A supplements. Eight major controlled community-based trials comparing vitamin A supplements with placebo for reduction of early childhood mortality have been conducted in east Asia, south Asia, and Africa (29,33,72–77). All these trials were carried out in vitamin A-deficient populations. The cause-specific mortality is available in five of these trials (33,72,73,76,77) and a summary is provided in Table 5. The reduction in mortality from measles ranged from 18% in Ghana (77) to 76% in Nepal (33).

Three controlled trials (Table 6) have shown convincingly that treatment with vitamin A given early during the course of measles reduces mortality by about 50% (10,78,79). Most deaths were in children under 2 years of age, and the reductions in mortality across all three trials are not inconsistent when considering differences between them.

TABLE 5. *Vitamin A and measles mortality: community-based trials*

Country (reference)	Vitamin A supplement	Relative risk of measles mortality: vitamin A *vs.* control
Nepal (76)	Large dose, 4 monthly	0.24
Nepal (33)	One large dose, follow-up at 5 months	0.67
India (72)	Weekly recommended dietary allowance	0.58
Ghana (77)	Large dose, 4 monthly	0.82
Sudan (73)	Large dose, 6 monthly	*

* No measles cases reported.

TABLE 6. *Effect of vitamin A supplementation on measles mortality rate*

Country (reference)	Dose of vitamin A	Vitamin A formulation	Relative risk of mortality (control:treated)
Tanzania (78)	200,000 IU orally on admission and on next day	Oil miscible	1.9:1
Cape Town, South Africa (10)	200,000 IU orally on admission and on next day	Water miscible	4.7:1
London, UK (79)	—	1 oz cod liver oil	

The beneficial effects of prophylaxis in vitamin A-deficient populations, the measles infection-induced reduction of vitamin A levels, and the positive impact of high dose vitamin A at the onset of clinical disease all suggest that vitamin A supplementation works by improving deficient or suboptimal levels of vitamin A.

Observational studies in Zaire (9) and the United States (12) have shown that lower serum vitamin A concentrations were associated with severity of measles and higher case fatality rates. In the Zaire study, the relative risk of mortality was 2.9 (95% CI 2.3 to 6.8) in those with reduced vitamin A levels. In the Milwaukee study (12) of 114 preschool children seen during an outbreak of measles, the degree of retinol depression correlated with measles severity as measured by hospital admission rates, the presence of pneumonia, and a standard assessment of physiologic instability (the PRISM score).

Vitamin A Treatment Reduces Morbidity

Various cross-sectional studies (population, hospital, and clinic based) have detected an association between vitamin A deficiency and morbidity in measles (20,21,24,25). However, one study in Bangladesh (26) and another in the Philippines (22) did not detect such a relation.

Two studies South African studies (10,11) show clearly the reduction in complications arising from measles with vitamin A treatment. The Cape Town study (10) revealed that the group of children on vitamin A had fewer complications, a shorter hospital stay, and required less frequent intensive care than the group on placebo. The Durban study (11) provided evidence of benefit in both the short and the long term. Hospitalized children with measles who were treated with vitamin A recovered more rapidly from pneumonia, diarrhea, fever, and other complications, compared with children on placebo. This advantage of vitamin A persisted for at least 6 months.

A smaller Kenyan hospital study (80) and a village-based study in West Bengal (81) found similar benefits of therapeutic and prophylactic doses of vitamin A on severity of measles. In the Kenyan study (80), the prevalence of complications was similar between vitamin A and control groups; however, mortality was higher in the latter compared with the treated group (13% vs 7%). Most of the deaths were from respiratory diseases (*e.g.*, mortality from pneumonia was 15% in the control group and 8% in the vitamin A-treated group). This suggests that vitamin A supplementation decreased the severity of disease in these children.

The improved outcomes in children with severe measles treated with vitamin A are probably primarily mediated through immunopotentiation (82). The Durban children with measles were treated with placebo or high doses of vitamin A given on admission and on days 2, 8, and 42 thereafter (82); the serum IgG antibody response was significantly better on days 8 and 42 in the treated group. Lymphopenia, which is a good predictor of outcome in measles, was also reversed quicker in the treated children.

Meta-Analyses of Vitamin A Supplementation and Measles Mortality

Meta-analyses have confirmed the beneficial impact of supplemental vitamin A in vitamin A-deficient populations on mortality in children under 5 years of age. However, two recent meta-analyses (83,84) differed with respect to the evidence that community-based interventions with vitamin A reduce measles mortality. Glasziou and Mackerras (83) concluded that community trials show a 55% reduction in measles deaths (p = 0.017), whereas Fawzi *et al.* (84) argued that, although the results of community-based studies suggest a protective effect, the relationship between vitamin A supplementation and measles-specific mortality is not statistically significant (p = 0.30). The major difference between these meta-analyses was in the choice of trials included. Glasziou and Mackerras excluded the very large study in Sudan (which showed no significant impact of vitamin A on child mortality or measles mortality) because of bias in the method of allocation. Moreover, it can be anticipated that the effects of vitamin A supplementation on measles mortality will depend on the contribution of this disease to mortality in children under the age of 5 years. This varies from region to region. However, more detailed information on measles from Ghana continues to raise uncertainties about community-based vitamin A supplementation and measles. A recent study from the Ghana Vitamin A Supplement Trials group (VAST) (85) of measles fatalities in relation to premorbid vitamin A supplementation found no significant effect of vitamin A on measles incidence, acute measles case fatality, or delayed postmeasles mortality (median follow-up 8 months). Serum retinol concentrations were higher in the supplemented group than in the placebo group. This is a region of poor vaccine coverage, low measles vaccine efficacy, and high case fatality rates. It is also the district in which the VAST studies have previously shown a beneficial impact of vitamin A supplementation on child mortality and health services utilization.

DIRECTIONS FOR FUTURE RESEARCH

We suggest that further study is needed in the following areas.

1. The impact of vitamin A given in the late antepartum period and during infancy on maternal and child health and disease, including respiratory infections

2. Large scale, multicenter field trials in developing countries to assess the impact of zinc supplementation on respiratory and other morbidity
3. Community-based studies to evaluate the impact of other micronutrients on lower respiratory tract infections and other diseases
4. Impact of micronutrient supplementation on pneumonia and other diseases in children infected with, or exposed to HIV
5. Comparison of the impact on populations of micronutrient interventions and broader development initiatives
6. The effect of iron deficiency on immune function and whether this leads to increased severity of infection in a properly controlled large scale clinical study

REFERENCES

1. Adair LS, Guilkey DK. Specific determinants of stunting in Filipino children. *J Nutr* 1997; 127: 314–20.
2. Ballard TJ, Neumann CG. The effects of malnutrition, parental literacy and household crowding on acute lower respiratory infections in young Kenyan children. *J Trop Pediatr* 1995; 41: 8–13.
3. Sommer A, Tarwotjo I, Katz J. Increased risk of xerophthalmia following diarrhea and respiratory disease. *Am J Clin Nutr* 1987; 45: 977–80.
4. Rahman MM, Mahalanabis D, Alvarez JO, Wahed MA, Habte D, Khaled MA. Acute respiratory infections prevent improvement of vitamin A status in young infants supplemented with vitamin A. *J Nutr* 1996; 126: 628–33.
5. Bhaskaram P, Reddy V, Raj S, Bhatnagar RC. Effect of measles on the nutritional status of preschool children. *J Trop Med Hyg* 1984; 87: 21–5.
6. Smedman L, Lindeberg A, Jeppsson O, Zetterstrom R. Nutritional status and measles: a community study in Guinea-Bissau. *Ann Trop Paediatr* 1983; 3: 169–76.
7. Halsey NA, Boulos R, Mode F, et al. Response to measles vaccine in Haitian infants 6 to 12 months old. Influence of maternal antibodies, malnutrition, and concurrent illnesses. *N Engl J Med* 1985; 313: 544–9.
8. Reddy V, Bhaskaram P, Raghuramulu N, et al. Relationship between measles, malnutrition, and blindness: a prospective study in Indian children. *Am J Clin Nutr* 1986; 44: 924–30.
9. Markowitz LE, Nzilambi N, Driskell WJ, et al. Vitamin A levels and mortality among hospitalized measles patients, Kinshasa, Zaire. *J Trop Pediatr* 1989; 35: 109–12.
10. Hussey GD, Klein M. A randomized, controlled trial of vitamin A in children with severe measles. *N Engl J Med* 1990; 323: 160–4.
11. Coutsoudis A, Broughton M, Coovadia HM. Vitamin A supplementation reduces measles morbidity in young African children: a randomized, placebo-controlled, double-blind trial. *Am J Clin Nutr* 1991; 54: 890–5.
12. Butler JC, Havens PL, Sowell AL, et al. Measles severity and serum retinol (vitamin A) concentration among children in the United States. *Pediatrics* 1993; 91: 1176–81.
13. Johnson WB, Aderele WI, Gbadero DA. Host factors and acute lower respiratory infections in preschool children. *J Trop Pediatr* 1992; 38: 132–6.
14. Agrawal PB, Shendurnikar N, Shastri NJ. Host factors and pneumonia in hospitalised children. *J Indian Med Assoc* 1995; 93: 271–2.
15. Rahman MM, Rahman AM. Prevalence of acute respiratory tract infection and its risk factors in under five children. *Bangladesh Medical Research Council Bulletin* 1997; 23: 47–50.
16. Singh MP, Nayar S. Magnitude of acute respiratory infections in under five children. *J Commun Dis* 1996; 28: 273–8.
17. Pandey A, Chakraborty AK. Undernutrition, vitamin A deficiency and acute respiratory infections morbidity in under fives. *Indian J Public Health* 1996; 40: 13–16.
18. Shell-Duncan B, Wood JW. The evaluation of delayed-type hypersensitivity responsiveness and nutritional status as predictors of gastro-intestinal and acute respiratory infection: a prospective field study among traditional nomadic Kenyan children. *J Trop Pediatr* 1997; 43: 25–32.
19. English RM, Badcock JC, Giay T, Ngu T, Waters AM, Bennett SA. Effect of nutrition improvement

project on morbidity from infectious diseases in preschool children in Vietnam: comparison with control commune. *BMJ* 1997,315: 1122–5.

20. Tielsch JM, West KP, Katz J, et al. Prevalence and severity of xerophthalmia in southern Malawi. *Am J Epidemiol* 1986; 124: 561–86.

21. DeSole G, Belay Y, Zegeye B. Vitamin A deficiency in southern Ethiopia. *Am J Clin Nutr* 1987; 45: 780–4.

22. Solon FS, Popkin BM, Fernandez TL, Latham MC. Vitamin A deficiency in the Philippines: a study of xerophthalmia in Cebu. *Am J Clin Nutr* 1978; 31: 360–8.

23. Bloem MW, Wedel M, Egger RJ, et al. Mild vitamin A deficiency and risk of respiratory tract diseases and diarrhea in preschool and school children in northeastern Thailand. *Am J Epidemiol* 1990; 131: 332–9.

24. Gujral S, Abbi R, Gopaldas T. Xerophthalmia, vitamin A supplementation and morbidity in children. *J Trop Pediatr* 1993; 39: 89–92.

25. Brilliant LB, Pokhrel RP, Grasset NC, et al. Epidemiology of blindness in Nepal. *Bull World Health Organ* 1985; 63: 375–86.

26. Stanton BF, Clemens JD, Wojtyniak B, Khair T. Risk factors for developing mild nutritional blindness in urban Bangladesh. *Am J Dis Child* 1986; 140: 584–8.

27. Sommer A, Katz J, Tarwotjo I. Increased risk of respiratory disease and diarrhea in children with pre-existing mild vitamin A deficiency. *Am J Clin Nutr* 1984; 40: 1090–5.

28. Dibley MJ, Sadjimin T, Kjolhede CL, Moulton LH. Vitamin A supplementation fails to reduce incidence of acute respiratory illness and diarrhea in preschool-age Indonesian children. *J Nutr* 1996; 126: 434–42.

29. Vijayaraghavan K, Radhalah G, Prakasam BS, Sarma KVR, Reddy V. Effect of massive dose vitamin A on morbidity and mortality in Indian children. *Lancet* 1990; ii: 1342–5.

30. Milton RC, Reddy V, Naidu AN. Mild vitamin A deficiency and childhood morbidity—an Indian experience. *Am J Clin Nutr* 1987; 46: 827–9.

31. Beaton GH, Martorell R, L'Abbé KA, et al. *Effectiveness of vitamin A supplementation in the control of young child morbidity and mortality in developing countries.* Summary Report to CIDA. Toronto: University of Toronto, 1992.

32. The vitamin A and Pneumonia Working Group. Potential interventions for the prevention of childhood pneumonia in developing countries: a meta-analysis of data from field trials to assess the impact of vitamin A supplementation on pneumonia morbidity and mortality. *Bull World Health Organ* 1995; 73: 609–19.

33. Daulaire NMP, Starbuck ES, Houston RM, Church MS, Stukel TA, Pandey MR. Childhood mortality after a high dose of vitamin A in a high risk population. *BMJ* 1992; 304: 207–10.

34. Lie C, Ying C, En-Lin W, et al. Impact of large-dose vitamin A supplementation on childhood diarrhoea, respiratory disease and growth. *Eur J Clin Nutr* 1993; 47: 88–96.

35. Kartasasmita CB, Rosmayudi O, Demedts M. Plasma retinol level, vitamin A supplementation and acute respiratory infections in children 1–5 years old in a developing country. *Tubercle Lung Dis* 1995; 76: 563–9.

36. Barreto ML, Santos LMP, Assis AMO, et al. Effect of vitamin A supplementation on diarrhoea and acute lower respiratory tract infections in young children in Brazil. *Lancet* 1994; 344: 228–31.

37. Bhandari N, Bhan MK, Sazawal S. Impact of massive dose of vitamin A given to preschool children with acute diarrhoea on subsequent respiratory and diarrhoeal morbidity. *BMJ* 1994; 309: 1404–7.

38. Humphrey JH, Agoestina T, Wu L, et al. Impact of neonatal vitamin A supplementation on infant morbidity and mortality. *J Pediatr* 1996; 128: 489–96.

39. Fawzi WW, Msamanga GI, Spiegelman D, et al. Randomised trial of effects of vitamin supplements on pregnancy outcomes and T cell counts in HIV1 infected women in Tanzania. *Lancet* 1998; 351: 1477–82.

40. WHO/CHD Immunisation-Linked vitamin A Supplementation Study Group. Randomised trial to assess benefits and safety of vitamin A supplementation linked to immunisation in early infancy. *Lancet* 1998; 352: 1257–63.

41. Coutsoudis A, Bobat RA, Coovadia HM, Kuhn L, Tsai W, Stein ZA. The effects of vitamin A supplementation on the morbidity of children born to HIV-infected women. *Am J Public Health* 1995; 85: 1076–81.

42. Pinnock CB, Douglas RM, Badcock NR. Vitamin A status in children who are prone to respiratory tract infections. *Aust Paediatr J* 1986; 22: 95–9.

43. Pinnock CB, Douglas RM, Martin AJ, Badcock NR. Vitamin A status of children with a history of respiratory syncytial virus infection in infancy. *Aust Paediatr* 1988; 24: 286–9.

44. Shenai JP, Kennedy KA, Chytil F, Stahlman MT. Clinical trial of vitamin A supplementation in infants susceptible to bronchopulmonary dysplasia. *J Pediatr* 1987; 111: 269–77.

45. Pearson E, Bose C, Snidow R, et al. Trial of vitamin A supplementation in very low birth weight infants at risk for bronchopulmonary dysplasia. *J Pediatr* 1992; 121: 420–7.

46. Nacul LC, Kirkwood BR, Arthur P, Morris SS, Magalhaes M, Fink MC. Randomised, double-blind placebo controlled clinical trial of efficacy of vitamin A treatment in non-measles childhood pneumonia. *BMJ* 1997; 315: 505–10.

47. Kjolhede CL, Chew FJ, Gadomski AM, Marroquin DP. Clinical trial of vitamin A as adjuvant treatment for lower respiratory tract infections. *J Pediatr* 1995; 126: 807–12.

48. Dowell SF, Papic Z, Bresee JS, et al. Treatment of respiratory syncytial virus infection with vitamin A: a randomized, placebo-controlled trial in Santiago, Chile. *Pediatr Infect Dis J* 1996; 15: 782–6.

49. Stephenson CB, Franchi LM, Hernandez H, Campos M, Gilman RH, Alvarez JO. Adverse effects of high dose vitamin A supplements in children hospitalised with pneumonia. *Pediatrics* 1998; 101: E3.

50. Bresee JS, Fischer M, Dowell SF, et al. Vitamin A therapy for children with respiratory syncytial virus infection: a multicenter trial in the United States. *Pediatr Infect Dis J* 1996; 15: 777–82.

51. Bahl R, Bhandari N, Hambridge KM, Bhan MK. Plasma zinc as a predictor of diarrheal and respiratory morbidity in children in an urban slum setting. *Am J Clin Nutr* 1988; 68: 414–17S.

52. Black RE. Therapeutic and preventive effects of zinc on serious childhood infectious diseases in developing countries. *Am J Clin Nutr* 1988; 68: 476–9S.

53. Sazawal S, Black RE, Jalla S, Mzumdar S, Sinha A, Bhan MK. Zinc supplementation reduces the incidence of acute lower respiratory infections in infants and pre-school children: a double-blind, controlled trial. *Pediatrics* 1998; 102: 1–5.

54. Lira PIC, Ashworth A, Morris SS. Effect of zinc supplementation on the morbidity, immune function, and growth of low-birth weight, full term infants in northeast Brazil. *Am J Clin Nutr* 1998; 68: 418–24S.

55. Rosado JL, Lopez P, Munoz E, Martinez H, Allen LH. Zinc supplementation reduced morbidity, but neither zinc nor iron supplementation affected growth or body composition of Mexican pre-schoolers. *Am J Clin Nutr* 1997; 65: 13–19.

56. Ruel MT, Rivera JA, Santizo M-C, Lonnerdal B, Brown KH. Impact of zinc supplementation on morbidity from diarrhea and respiratory infections among rural Guatemalan children. *Pediatrics* 1997; 99: 808–13.

57. Ninh NX, Thissen J-P, Collette L, Gerrard G, Khoi HH, Ketelslegers JM. Zinc supplementation increases growth and circulating insulin-like growth factor (IGF-1) in growth retarded Vietnamese children. *Am J Clin Nutr* 1996; 63: 514–19.

58. Bates CJ, Evans PH, Dardenne M, et al. A trial of zinc supplementation in young rural Gambian children. *Br J Nutr* 1993; 69: 243–55.

59. Macknin ML, Piedmonte M, Calendine C, Janosky J, Wald E. Zinc gluconate lozenges for treating the common cold in children: a randomized controlled trial. *JAMA* 1998; 279: 162–7.

60. Castillo-Duran C, Heresi G, Fisberg M, Uauy R. Controlled trial of zinc supplementation during recovery from malnutrition: effects on growth and immune function. *Am J Clin Nutr* 1987; 45: 602–8.

61. Schlesinger L, Arevalo M, Arredondo S, Diaz M, Lönnerdal B, Stekel A. Effect of a zinc-fortified formula on immuno competence and growth of malnourished infants. *Am J Clin Nutr* 1992; 56: 491–8.

62. Sempertegui F, Estrella B, Correa E, et al. Effects of short term zinc supplementation on cellular immunity, respiratory symptoms, and growth of malnourished Equadorian children. *Eur J Clin Nutr* 1996; 50: 42–6.

63. Mitra AK, Akramuzzaman SM, Fuchs GJ, Rahman MM, Mahalanabis D. Long-term oral supplementation with iron is not harmful for young children in a poor community of Bangladesh. *J Nutr* 1997; 127: 1451–5.

64. Angeles IT, Schultink WJ, Matulessi P, Gross R, Sastroamidjojo S. Decreased rate of stunting among anemic Indonesian preschool children through iron supplementation. *Am J Clin Nutr* 1993; 58: 339–42.

65. Alwar AJ. The effect of protein energy malnutrition on morbidity and mortality due to measles at Kenyatta National Hospital, Nairobi (Kenya). *East Afr Med J* 1992; 69: 415–18.

66. Koster, FT. Mortality among primary and secondary cases of measles in Bangladesh. *Rev Infect Dis* 1998: 10: 471–3.

67. Heyworth B. Pathogenesis of measles. *BMJ* 1973:iii: 693.

68. Aaby P, Bukh J, Lisse IM, Smits AJ. Measles mortality, state of nutrition, and family structure: a community study from Guinea-Bissau. *J Infect Dis* 1093; 147: 693–9.

69. Sinha NP. Measles in children under six months of age: an epidemiological study. *J Trop Med Hyg* 1980; 83: 225–7.

70. Chen LC, Chowdhury AKMA, Huffman SL. Anthropometric assessment of energy-protein malnutrition and subsequent risk of mortality among pre-school aged children. *Am J Clin Nutr* 1980; 33: 1836–45.

71. Gopalan C, Swaminathan MC, Kumari VKK, Rao DH, Vijayaraghavan K. Effect of calorie supplementation on growth of undernourished children. *Am J Clin Nutr* 1973; 26: 563–6.

72. Rahmathullah L, Underwood BA, Thulasiraj RD, et al. Reduced mortality among children in southern India receiving a small weekly dose of vitamin A. *N Engl J Med* 1990; 323: 929–35.

73. Herrera MG, Nestel P, El Amin A, Fawzi WW, Mohamed KA, Weld L. Vitamin A supplementation and child survival. *Lancet* 1992; 340: 267–71.

74. Sommer A, Tarwotjo I, Djunaedi E, et al., and the Aceh Study Group. Impact of vitamin A supplementation on childhood mortality. A randomised controlled community trial. *Lancet* 1986; 1: 1169–73.

75. Muhilal, Permeisih D, Idjradinata YR, Muherdiyantiningsih, Karyadi D. Vitamin A-fortified monosodium glutamate and health, growth, and survival of children: a controlled field trial. *Am J Clin Nutr* 1988; 48: 1271–6.

76. West KP, Pokhrel RP, Katz J, et al. Efficacy of vitamin A in reducing pre-school child mortality in Nepal. *Lancet* 1991; 338: 67–71.

77. Ghana VAST Study Team. Vitamin A supplementation in northern Ghana: effects on clinic attendances, hospital admissions, and child mortality. *Lancet* 1993; 342: 7–12.

78. Barclay AJG, Foster A, Sommer A. Vitamin A supplements and mortality related to measles: a randomised clinical trial. *BMJ* 1987; 294: 294–6.

79. Ellison JB. Intensive vitamin therapy in measles. *BMJ* 1932; ii: 708–11.

80. Ogaro FO, Orinda VA, Onyango FE, Black RE. Effect of vitamin A on diarrhoeal and respiratory complications of measles. *Tropical and Geographical Medicine* 1993; 45: 283–6.

81. Sinha DP, Bang FB. The effect of massive doses of vitamin A on the signs of vitamin A deficiency in preschool children. *Am J Clin Nutr* 1976; 29: 110–15.

82. Coutsoudis A, Kiepiela P, Coovadia HM, Broughton M. Vitamin A supplementation enhances specific IgG antibody levels and total lymphocyte numbers while improving morbidity in measles. *Pediatr Infect Dis J* 1992; 11: 203–9.

83. Glasziou PP, Mackerras DEM. Vitamin A supplementation in infectious diseases: a meta-analysis. *BMJ* 1993; 306: 366–70.

84. Fawzi WW, Thomas C, Chalmers TC, Herrera MG, Mosteller F. Vitamin A supplementation and child mortality. A meta analysis. *JAMA* 1993; 269: 898–903.

85. Dollimore N, Cutts F, Binka FN, Ross DA, Morris SS, Smith PG. Measles incidence, case fatality and delayed mortality in children with or without vitamin A supplementation in rural Ghana. *Am J Epidemiol* 1997; 146: 646–54.

DISCUSSION

Dr. Fawzi: You mentioned that, in general, the vitamin A trials seem to indicate no beneficial effect on pneumonia or on its prevention. Studies even suggest that vitamin A may in some cases be harmful in pneumonia. For example, the randomized, placebo-control study in Peru showed that vitamin A supplements resulted in an increased oxygen requirement, whereas in a study from Ecuador, a significant increase was seen in respiratory infection among well-nourished children; in our study from Tanzania, a nonsignificant increased risk of mortality was found among children admitted to the hospital with pneumonia (1–4). Could you comment on the potentially harmful effects of vitamin A?

Dr. Coovadia: As you say, the evidence is that you can occasionally produce harmful effects if you give vitamin A. My understanding is that in these field trials, the incidence was extremely low ($< 2\%$), but still detectable. It is easily recognizable clinically, and it does not diminish the need for vitamin A on a public health intervention scale; the benefits outweigh the negative effects. I am, however, worried about the newborn and the infant in the first year of life, because the meta-analysis suggested that in that period mortality might increase (5). One area of further research is the impact of vitamin A in infancy. Just to emphasize how complex this subject is, Dr. Brown gave a multicomponent mixture and it had a negative impact, whereas your study showed no impact of vitamin A and yet an impact of multivitamins. I think those are very important areas of research, otherwise you will not know what to do about current recommendations for vitamin A for mothers, who are supposed to be given 200,000 IU within a few days of birth. I think we need to know a lot more about this.

Dr. Suskind: You mentioned the lower levels of vitamin A and zinc in acute respiratory infections and measles. I am wondering about the effect of infection on visceral protein synthesis, on the production of the acute phase reactants, and on zinc status. Vitamin A is transported by a visceral protein, retinol-binding protein, which has been found to be very sensitive to external influences. Perhaps the decrease in vitamin A in measles and acute respiratory infections reflects a decrease in the carrier protein. In fact, many of these patients have adequate stores of vitamin A in the liver; perhaps it is just not getting into the circulation. The same might be true for zinc. We recognize that zinc, as well as iron, is decreased in infection. The observation is an important one, but the interpretation is also important. I would like your comments on that.

Dr. Coovadia: I would like to pass this question to my co-author Dr. Anna Coutsoudis.

Dr. Coutsoudis: In our original measles trial, we did measure retinol-binding protein. A definite reduction in retinol-binding protein very closely correlated with the reduction in serum retinol. I think that would account for why we sometimes see an impact of supplementation and sometimes not. Serum retinol could be reduced purely as a marker of subclinical infection, and not necessarily because the child is deficient.

Dr. Suskind: It is worthwhile commenting on the observation that vitamin A does not necessarily have an impact on respiratory infections or diarrheal disease. I wonder if the impact of vitamin A on small bowel overgrowth has been investigated. Perhaps the impact of vitamin A on small bowel overgrowth, and other aspects of the immune system, is reflected in a decrease in mortality that is not necessarily related to a specific effect on respiratory or gastrointestinal infections.

Dr. Coovadia: One can readily imagine that vitamin A stimulates the immune system, but I know of no studies looking at small bowel overgrowth and the impact of vitamin A treatment. The field trials had minimal information on these sorts of items.

Dr. Fawzi: An animal study on rotavirus showed much more severe intestinal infection in cases of vitamin A deficiency (6).

Dr. Wasantwisut: I would like your views on the nature of supplementation. The doses of vitamin A that are given are usually massive, in contrast to zinc which is more likely to be provided on the basis of the daily required dose. Do you think this *pharmacologic* versus *physiologic* dose regimen affects the way the body responds to certain types of infection?

Dr. Coovadia: The trials vary considerably in the way they gave the vitamin A, so that was a critical variable. Some gave it at 6-month intervals, some at 4-month intervals, and I think the Indian study gave it weekly. In the meta-analysis that I referred to, this was examined and the conclusion was that giving it more frequently was probably more effective.

Dr. Meydani: I would like to emphasize the need to learn more about the mechanism of how vitamin A may protect against certain pathogens. Without that information, consistent and effective strategies cannot be developed and you end up producing more and more data that will probably just cloud the issue even more. It does seem to me that there is a lot of inconsistency.

Dr. Coovadia: That is an important question. My only difficulty is that I work in a country where I see real problems. I could spend a lifetime looking at mechanisms, but it may be better for me to gather evidence from field trials. That is the dilemma for all of us who work in the field. It is an impossible dilemma to solve. About 20 years ago, we looked at protein-energy malnutrition and thymolymphatic atrophy. Frankly, I do not think those studies have had a major impact on the welfare of children 30 years later. Children have been helped because Thailand has become a bit richer. That is the dilemma we have to find our way out of. I am sorry I am not responding to you directly, but I am trying to indicate that we need a combination of both field trials, which are imperfect, and basic research.

Dr. Meydani: I did not mean that it has to be an either or situation. I think you need to do both types of study in parallel. Ignorance of the mechanism and inconsistent results will only increase the number of people who question the need for any of this research.

Dr. Coovadia: I would certainly be very worried about continuing single nutrient studies without looking at the impact of broader interventions.

Dr. Farthing: One thing that struck me is that some of these studies look underpowered. I do not know of many major clinical intervention studies, for instance, that only have 32 subjects in them. I wonder whether with a meta-analysis with underpowered studies you end up with an underpowered meta-analysis. My other point comes out of a study that we did in adults infected with HIV with persistent diarrhea in Zambia (7). We supplemented them with vitamin A and saw no effect. This was a large study of nearly 200 individuals, so we think it was probably powerful enough to show an effect if one existed. When we looked at the vitamin A status of these individuals, as best we could, we found we had made no impact whatsoever on plasma indices, including the binding proteins, which made me wonder whether the vitamin A was actually getting where it needed to be. Vitamin A, was used, after all, as a very sensitive test of intestinal absorption in the 1940s and 1950s. My question is, are there ways in which you can assess the efficacy of your intervention not just in terms of morbidity and mortality but of whether you have actually delivered the nutrient to the body?

Dr. Coovadia: Regarding your first point about which of the studies are reliable, that was the reason why I separated all the studies into the smaller ones (hospital-based studies and clinical studies) and field trials, implying that latter were the *gold standard*. The field trials were all sufficiently powered and they have been analyzed individually and collectively, so no question exists about the sample size being insufficient to pick up the problems they were trying to detect. The reason I put up the smaller studies was precisely to show you that some may not be sufficient. Anna Coutsoudis can comment on your other question about vitamin A absorption.

Dr. Coutsoudis: I think that serum retinol is clearly not accurate enough to measure what is happening once you give vitamin A. That is why we have to use other measures. These include pool size using isotopes, and the modified relative dose response. If you want purely to measure whether the vitamin A is being absorbed, you would have to measure serum retinol within about 7 hours. It is no use coming along 3 weeks later, which most of us do; by then, if the person was actually vitamin A sufficient and infection had been cleared, probably no difference would be found in the serum retinol. However, we do know that during infection retinol is reduced.

Dr. Marini: I would like to say a word in favor of vitamin A in the lamb. The results of a multicenter study from the United States on vitamin A for the prevention of bronchopulmonary dysplasia were recently published (8), and showed that 10,000 IU of parenteral vitamin A significantly reduced the problem of bronchopulmonary dysplasia in extremely low birthweight infants.

I have a naive question for the people working in the field. Do you think that other very simple clinical tools could enhance your results? For instance, the ratio between arm circumference and head circumference, or evaluation of respiratory rate or heart rate when the baby is sleeping. You can collect these data in the field, and maybe they would give you additional information about energy wastage and so on.

Dr. Coovadia: The short answer is that it is always useful to do simple tests in the field. I spent most of my studies on measles looking for the simplest test. The lymphocyte count on admission turned out to be best. I spent a lot of time showing that it was a really good indicator and predictor (this was before the days of HIV and CD4), and that information is available in most hospitals and clinics.

Dr. Chandra: Two brief comments. First, animal data and some in humans show that large doses of vitamin A produce a period of immunosuppression, which can last for 7 to 20 days. I think it might be useful to analyze the studies in which a negative impact or higher mortality was seen after vitamin A to see if most of the problems arose shortly after giving a large dose. Second, one should remember that in all intervention studies just a visit by the child or family to a healthcare center reduces morbidity and mortality, as we learned from the Montreal Dispensary study 40 years ago and a number of other studies. So, the mere fact of contact with a health worker in these field trials may have useful benefit.

Dr. Griffin: It seems to me that if you are going to introduce something on a global scale, then it should have no adverse effects at all, but we do have some evidence of adverse effects of vitamin A—the decrease in response to hepatitis A vaccine, the transient decrease in immunity, and so on. There is another form of adverse effect as well, which I think is perhaps even more crucial. That is the concern that the introduction of an intervention such as supplementation with vitamin A could affect the childhood vaccination program. The use of vaccines may be compromised in some places where there are severe economic constraints. I was at a vaccine meeting recently where this question was addressed, and the major players in the field had no doubt that vaccination programs could be adversely affected. You then have to make a judgment of how important that would be compared with what seem to me to be the quite marginal benefits of vitamin A.

Dr. Coovadia: That is an issue for a week's discussion. I am not unaware of it, but the range of priorities is a difficult if not impossible thing for scientists to solve. But I would stress that the impact of vitamin A on mortality in certain population is so good and is achieved at such low cost that it is a really worthwhile public health intervention. I come from a country that is not giving zidovudine to pregnant women with HIV, so I know all about these priorities. For us, the use of vitamin A is not in question and in fact is going to be implemented.

Dr. Tontisirin: I believe we should apply basic research and implementation in parallel. We always need to have an understanding of mechanisms to help us avoid harmful consequences of our actions—for example, the use of large doses vitamin A may cause imbalance and create some kind of a negative effect. In terms of application, I think eventually we have to come down to community-based programs, although with nutrition, this becomes very complex.

REFERENCES

1. Fawzi WW, Msamanga GI, Spiegelman D, et al, for the Tanzania Vitamin and HIV Infection Trial Team. Randomized trial of effects of vitamin supplements on pregnancy outcomes and T-cell counts in HIV- infected women in Tanzania. *Lancet* 1998; 351: 1477–1482.
2. Stephensen C, Franchi L, Hernandez H, Campos M, Gilman R, Alvarez J. Adverse effects of high-dose vitamin A supplements in children hospitalized with pneumonia. *Pediatrics* 1998; 101:E3.
3. Sempertegui F, Estrella B, Camaniero V, et al. The beneficial effects of weekly low-dose vitamin A supplementation on acute lower respiratory infections and diarrhea in Ecuadorian children. *Pediatrics* 1999; 104: e1.

4. Fawzi WW, Mbise RL, Fataki MR, et al. Vitamin A supplementation and severity of pneumonia in children admitted to the hospital in Dar Es Salaam, Tanzania. *Am J Clin Nutr* 1998; 68: 187–92.

5. The Vitamin A and Pneumonia Working Group. Potential interventions for the prevention of childhood pneumonia in developing countries: a meta-analysis of data from field trials to assess the impact of vitamin A supplementation on pneumonia morbidity and mortality. *Bull World Health Organ* 1995; 73: 609–19.

6. Ahmed F, Jones DB, Jackson AA. The interaction of vitamin A deficiency and rotavirus infection in the mouse. *Br J Nutr* 1990; 63: 363–373.

7. Kelly P, Musonda R, Kafwembe E, et al. Micronutrient supplementation in the AIDS diarrhea-wasting syndrome in Zambia: a randomized controlled trial. *AIDS* 1999; 13: 495–500.

8. Tyson JE, Wright LL, Oh W, et al. Vitamin A supplementation for extremely low-birth-weight infants. National Institute of Child Health and Human Development Neonatal Research Network. *N Engl J Med* 1999; 340: 1962–8.

Nutrition, Immunity, and Infection in Infants and Children, edited by Robert M. Suskind and Kraisid Tontisirin. Nestlé Nutrition Workshop Series, Pediatric Program, Vol. 45. Nestec Ltd., Vevey/Lippincott Williams & Wilkins, Philadelphia ©2001.

Nutrition and Infection: Human Immunodeficiency Virus Infection, Tuberculosis, and Melioidosis

George E. Griffin and Derek Macallan

Department of Infectious Diseases, St. George's Hospital Medical School, London, UK

RODENT MODEL OF ACUTE PHASE RESPONSE: ENDOTOXIN INFUSION

Endotoxin infusion into weanling rats causes a classic acute phase response characterized by profound anorexia, acute weight loss, negative protein balance in skeletal muscle, and the appearance of acute phase proteins, produced by the liver, in the circulation (1). In this model using 55 g rats, endotoxin was infused continually through an internal jugular vein catheter. Following 18 hours of endotoxin infusion, animals lost 15% to 20% of body weight and food intake rapidly dropped to 20% of that of control animals receiving saline infusion. Indeed, no food was consumed 2 hours after starting the endotoxin infusion. To see if weight loss was a result of reduced food intake, altered metabolism, or a combination of these, intravenous nutrition was given through the indwelling internal jugular catheter and body and organ weight (Table 1), protein synthesis (Table 2), and tissue RNA content were measured (Table 3).

It was clearly shown that control animals receiving no endotoxin gained weight when given intravenous nutrition; however, administration of such intravenous nutrition to endotoxin-treated animals did not ameliorate weight loss (1). In addition, protein catabolism in skeletal muscle and in myocardium was not changed quantitatively by intravenous nutritional support. In contrast, liver weight and liver protein content increased during this endotoxin-induced, acute phase response, and the administration of parenteral nutrition exacerbated this change, doubling protein content and liver weight. Further studies of metabolic change induced by endotoxin in rats

TABLE 1. *Percentage change in body weight over the 18h treatment period**

Nutrition	Oral		Starved		TPN	
	−	+	−	+	−	+
Endotoxin	($n = 13$)	($n = 7$)	($n = 12$)	($n = 19$)	($n = 7$)	($n = 10$)
Change in wet body wt. (%)	+5.3	−6.1[a]	−19.0	−14.2	−3.9[a]	−9.4
	(1.6)	(4.8)	(3.7)	(3.7)	(1.5)	(4.6)
Change in dry body wt. (%)	+5.8	−10.5[b]	−22.5	−17.5	−8.5[b]	−12.5
	(2.4)	(5.5)	(3.4)	(3.9)	(3.2)	(2.6)

* The percentage change in wet and dry body weight over the 18-hour treatment period is shown. Values are means with SD in parentheses. Dry pretreatment body weights were calculated from weight-matched control rats ($n = 5$ for each group), killed at the start of the treatment period. Values sharing a common superscript are not statistically different at a level of $p \leq 0.02$.

TPN, total parenteral nutrition.

From Ash SA, Griffin GE *Clinical Science* 1989;76:659–66. © Biochemical Society and the Medical Research Society, with permission.

have shown a rapid fall of ribosomal RNA content in skeletal muscle (1) but the level of messenger RNA (mRNA) for myofibrillar proteins remains constant, indicating that changes in protein synthesis are largely mediated by changes in translation. However, in the myocardium, although the mRNA level for myosin is essentially unchanged, major changes occur in expression of mRNA for myosin isotypes, indicating control at transcriptional level (2). Furthermore, changes in protein metabolism in the liver have been shown to be transcriptionally controlled in that, following a single dose of endotoxin, mRNA levels for positive acute phase protein reactants α_2-

TABLE 2. *Rates of protein synthesis in vivo**

	K_s (%/day)					
Nutrition	Oral		Starved		TPN	
	−	+	−	+	−	+
Endotoxin	($n = 8$)	($n = 6$)	($n = 6$)	($n = 6$)	($n = 7$)	($n = 5$)
Heart	19.9[a]	15.5[b]	19.0[a]	15.3[b]	20.8[a]	16.2[b]
	(2.2)	(1.8)	(0.6)	(2.5)	(1.6)	(2.7)
EDL muscle	23.5	9.3[a]	12.4[b]	11.5[ab]	17.3	11.2[a]
	(2.1)	(1.2)	(1.0)	(2.5)	(1.6)	(1.3)
Soleus muscle	20.0[a]	11.8[b]	17.3	12.3[b]	22.2[a]	13.9[b]
	(1.6)	(2.4)	(1.9)	(2.9)	(3.3)	(1.9)
Liver	107.9[a]	129.4[b]	90.0	132.5[b]	109.2[a]	145.7
	(6.7)	(6.6)	(7.5)	(6.8)	(8.3)	(7.8)
Kidney	40.3[ab]	56.0[b]	35.9[a]	58.8[ab]	40.9[ab]	45.0[a]
	(3.4)	(15.7)	(4.2)	(15.2)	(7.8)	(8.1)

* Rates of protein synthesis *in vivo* in various tissues from animals in the six treatment groups, expressed as K_s (% of protein pool synthesized/day). Values are means with SD in parentheses. Values sharing a common superscript are not statistically different at a level of $p \leq 0.02$.

EDL, Extensor digitorum longus; TPN, total parenteral nutrition.

From Ash SA, Griffin GE *Clinical Science* 1989; 76: 659–66. © Biochemical Society and the Medical Research Society, with permission.

TABLE 3. *Tissue RNA content**

Nutrition	Oral		Starved		TPN	
	−	+	−	+	−	+
Endotoxin	(*n* = 8)	(*n* = 6)	(*n* = 6)	(*n* = 6)	(*n* = 7)	(*n* = 5)
Heart	16.1[a]	16.8[a]	14.9[a]	15.3[a]	16.0[a]	14.6[a]
	(3.0)	(3.4)	(1.9)	(2.7)	(2.1)	(2.5)
EDL muscle	9.1[a]	4.3[b]	5.3[b]	4.7[b]	8.3[a]	3.6[b]
	(1.8)	(1.5)	(2.7)	(1.9)	(2.7)	(1.6)
Soleus muscle	10.8[a]	6.7[b]	6.7[b]	5.5[b]	9.4[a]	7.3
	(1.3)	(0.9)	(2.9)	(1.3)	(3.5)	(1.7)
Liver	82.5[a]	78.4[a]	71.4[a]	83.9[a]	69.4[a]	73.5[a]
	(10.3)	(14.0)	(7.4)	(10.4)	(17.1)	(4.5)
Kidney	40.5[a]	39.3[a]	42.8[a]	42.3[a]	42.0[a]	41.7[a]
	(6.5)	(2.3)	(9.1)	(4.6)	(6.8)	(5.4)

RNA content (μg/mg of protein)

* RNA content of various tissues from animals in the six treatment groups is shown. Values are means with SD in parentheses. Values sharing a common superscript are not statistically different at a level of $p \leq 0.02$.
EDL, Extensor digitorum longus; TPN, total parenteral nutrition.
From Ash SA, Griffin GE. *Clinical Science* 1989; 76: 659–66. © Biochemical Society and the Medical Research Society, with permission.

macroglobulin) are increased for approximately 48 hours and that mRNA for the negative acute phase protein, albumin is decreased for some 72 hours (3).

Thus, in the acute catabolic situation caused by endotoxinemia in a rodent model, administration of intravenous nutrition does not ameliorate weight loss but fuels the acute phase response. Extrapolating these results to the acute human clinical infection situation is difficult; it is not yet clear whether giving nutritional support in the form of parenteral nutrition to the acutely septic individual has beneficial effects other than maintaining energy balance. Indeed, the time of starting parenteral nutrition and the benefit of such intervention in some clinical situations have both been questioned (4), and it is now generally accepted that parenteral nutrition is primarily of benefit in patients with pre-existing malnutrition.

HUMAN IMMUNODEFICIENCY VIRUS INFECTION

Patterns of Weight Loss

Wasting is one of the cardinal clinical features of advanced human immunodeficiency virus (HIV) infection, and the management of this condition has received much attention (5). The degree of weight loss in HIV infection is a major prognostic indicator (6). It was originally thought that the classic pattern of weight loss in HIV disease would prove to be inexorable and slowly progressive, leading to death. However, detailed prospective longitudinal studies of patterns of weight loss in HIV infection have shown that such a chronic progressive pattern is only present in approximately 20% of patients and classically in those suffering from chronic intestinal disease (7). The dominant pattern of weight change seen in HIV infection, particularly in late clinical stages, is one of intermittent acute and profound loss of weight in association with acute opportunistic infection. The magnitude of such weight loss may be great (10–15 kg) and is arrested only on successful treatment of the acute opportunistic infection. Following such periods of acute weight loss, classically occurs an anabolic phase in which, in the face of adequate nutrition, weight is restored to nearly the level before acute infection. This simple clinical observation has had great clinical significance in confounding the prevailing view that weight loss in HIV infection could not be reversed. In addition, these data showed that harnessing anabolic potential following acute opportunistic infection by optimizing nutrition is of great clinical importance.

Protein Metabolism

Protein metabolism in HIV infection has been measured using the 13-carbon (^{13}C) leucine flux technique (8). Such studies showed that in the fasting state whole body protein synthesis is accelerated, as is whole body protein degradation, compared with control subjects. Together, these changes reveal accelerated whole body protein turnover compared with controls, but with a net protein balance. However, the finding of crucial significance in these studies was that when HIV-infected subjects received a 4-hour infusion of parenteral nutrition, the net protein catabolic state was reversed to protein anabolism, and that both protein synthesis and protein degradation were changed, resulting in a net positive protein balance. Thus, in terms of whole body protein turnover, an anabolic switch still exists in HIV infection and is amenable to manipulation by nutrition. However, although useful, such whole body protein turnover studies do not indicate changes in the types of protein being metabolized, and further studies designed to look at specific proteins are clearly required.

Energy Balance

Resting energy expenditure has consistently been shown to be increased by nearly 10% in HIV-infected subjects (9), and for several years this was thought to be a dominant factor leading to weight loss seen during the clinical course of the disease. Such measurements of resting energy expenditure have classically been made using indirect calorimetry and, as such, this technique places severe logistic and technical restrictions on the patient and data interpretation. Moreover, such measurements reflect only *basal* metabolism and do not take into account the energy required for locomotion and other daily activities. A major advance in the measurement of total free-living energy expenditure in humans has been the introduction of the doubly labeled water ($^{2}H_2{}^{18}O$) technique (10). This technique involves the use of nonradioisotopically labeled water and has wide applicability in human experimentation. In this method, doubly-labeled water is given on day 0 by mouth and aliquots of urine are collected at daily intervals for 7 days. Mass spectroscopy is performed on these samples to determine the enrichment of ^{18}O, ^{2}H, in urinary water resulting from the administration of $^2H_2{}^{18}O$ and its subsequent metabolism. As some of the ^{18}O is lost in carbon dioxide ($C^{18}O_2$), the disappearance of ^{18}O is quicker than that of ^2H in water and the difference between the two disappearance curves relates to the amount of carbon dioxide produced, which is directly related to total free-living energy expenditure (11). It has been shown, using $^2H_2{}^{18}O$, that in weight-losing HIV-infected individuals, total free-living energy expenditure is reduced by some 30% to 40% (11), even in the face of the small increase in resting energy expenditure previously measured. Furthermore, in such weight-losing HIV-infected patients, when energy intake in food is prospectively measured, patients are in profound negative energy balance, resulting in weight loss. The principal mechanism of the reduced food intake is primarily anorexia; however, other simple logistic clinical problems (e.g., oral and esophageal ulceration) may be implicated and must be evaluated and corrected if possible. In addition, a simple technique using infusion of $NaH^{14}CO_3$ has been devised, which enables free-living energy expenditure to be measured in humans (12) without the need for mass spectroscopy and relatively expensive stable isotope precursors.

TUBERCULOSIS

For many years, tuberculosis (TB) has been the classic wasting disease (13); for this reason, at the turn of the century, pulmonary tuberculosis was known as *consumption*. Both undernutrition and tuberculosis result in wasting and are common in developing countries. This is now particularly pertinent in the HIV-TB pandemic in developing countries. An elegant study of protein and energy metabolism in India, in both pulmonary tuberculosis and undernutrition, clearly showed that protein and energy metabolism are perturbed in different ways when comparing conditions (14). In terms of protein metabolism, the primary finding, in the fasting state, was that protein metabolism was equivalent in normal and pulmonary tuberculosis subjects. However, when given an identical anabolic stimulus of oral food, patients suffering from tuberculosis used considerably less of their ingested amino acids for protein synthesis, as evaluated by ^{13}C leucine, than undernourished control non-TB patients. These findings strongly suggest the existence of a quantitative inhibition of normal anabolic response to food in tuberculosis. The detail of such difference clearly needs evaluation and is likely to be multifactorial. In addition to measurement of protein metabolism, resting energy expenditure was measured using ventilated hood indirect calorimetry. With this method, it was shown that resting energy expenditure was increased in pulmonary TB as it was in undernutrition when expressed per kilogram of lean body mass. This finding held true even in the presence of fever.

The primary treatment of wasting associated with tuberculosis is antimycobacterial chemotherapy. It is not unusual to see a clinical deterioration in patients on initiation of antimycobacterial therapy, and such worsening is thought to be related to a selective increase in plasma tumor necrosis factor-α (TNF-α) (15). Malnutrition very often complicates the clinical condition (16,17) and recovery in terms of nutritional state is frequently slow (17). Anabolic agents that might overcome anabolic block in TB, as demonstrated for protein metabolism, may have an important role to play in disease management and may hasten immunologic recovery and mycobacterial clearance in patients with the disease. Studies have been carried out using thalidomide, a weak anti-TNF-α agent, in patients with combined TB and HIV infection and have shown beneficial effects in terms of whole body weight gain (18). However, surprisingly no effect was shown on plasma HIV copy number in this study. Indeed, in clinical studies of patients with combined HIV-TB, no demonstrable effect was seen on plasma HIV copy number on antimycobacterial treatment, even in the face of clear clinical response in terms of weight gain and increase in hemoglobin over a 3-month period (19). These findings are of great pathophysiologic significance in combined HIV-TB infection, as in general terms intact mycobacteria and mycobacterial components elicit both proinflammatory cytokine production and HIV release from macrophages *in vitro*. It would, therefore, be predicted that reducing mycobacterial load *in vivo* might reduce plasma HIV load.

MELIOIDOSIS

Melioidosis, an infection caused by *Pseudomonas pseudomallei*, is present in Southeast Asia. In the first instance, the organism classically gains access to the body through skin or mucosal surface and causes septicemia, particularly in the immunocompromized host situation, such as in diabetes mellitus or patients receiving steroid treatment. Following an acute phase of the infection, a chronic phase occurs in which large abscesses may form in various viscera such as liver and lung. In this chronic condition, weight loss is a major feature of the disease and is not reversed until the infection has been successfully treated. In pilot experiments using ^{13}C leucine flux as a measure of protein turnover in patients with melioidosis, protein turnover has been shown to be increased by nearly 35% in both the fed and fasting state, but a quantitatively normal switch in anabolic response occurs during feeding (20). Thus, in this chronic bacterial infection, similar changes in protein metabolism are seen to those in human immunodeficiency syndrome.

CONCLUSIONS

Weight loss, as part of the acute phase response, is a common response to infection in both animals and humans. The concept of a common response to injury and inflammation has yielded much useful information since early observations. However, it is clear from the above discussion that differences are found in the pattern of metabolic response according to the type and duration of infection. Weight loss, by simple definition, is multifactorial and can result from a combination of reduced food intake, malabsorption, and inappropriate utilization of energy and protein substrates. The mechanisms driving perturbations of these three major elements are likely to differ between types of infection and will assume different proportions during acute, intermediate, and chronic phases of infection.

   Animal models of infection, to a certain extent, have given precise definition of the acute phase response (1). Such models have the advantage of tissue sampling and, therefore, enable discrete changes in organ metabolism to be compared during phases of infection and in response to therapeutic or nutritional manipulation. A dominant feature of the acute phase response in both animals (1) and humans (11) is anorexia, and it is likely that hypothalamic control of appetite resulting from the interplay of proinflammatory cytokines (*e.g.* TNF-α and IL-6), known to regulate the acute phase response, and neuropeptides (*e.g.*, cholecystokin and neuropeptide Y) will prove to be of great significance in the future. In healthy subjects, energy balance is highly regulated and despite large day-to-day variability in food intake, long-term food intake matches energy expenditure with high precision. Healthy subjects return to their usual body weight and composition after periods of overfeeding (21) and starvation (22). However, we are still ignorant of the detail in changes in body compartment composition and the relative changes in their restoration during the acute phase of infection and resolution on treatment. It is also crucial to recognize that the acute phase response to infection is preserved throughout the animal kingdom, and beneficial therapeutic manipulation of such a well-conserved pathophysiologic response requires detailed clinical studies. Both common sense and results of the types of experiments described above indicate that in treatment of wasting caused by infection, control of the infectious process and resolution of the resulting inflammation is of fundamental importance. Subsequently, manipulation of nutrition in an appropriate way is then crucial to ensure recovery.

ACKNOWLEDGMENTS

Support from the Wellcome Trust and Medical Research Council is gratefully acknowledged. Tables 1–3 are shown with kind permission of Clinical Science.

REFERENCES

1. Ash SA, Griffin GE. Effect of parenteral nutrition on protein turnover in endotoxaemic rats. *Clin Sci* 1989; 76: 659–66.
2. Macallan DC, Griffin GE. Cardiac muscle protein gene expression in the endotoxin treated rat. *Clin Sci* 1994; 87: 539–46.
3. Sharma RJ, Macallan DC, Sedgwick P, Remick DG, Griffin GE. Kinetics of endotoxin induced acute phase response in the rat. Gene regulation and its modulation by monoclonal antibody to TNF. *Am J Physiol* 1992; 262: R786–93.
4. The Veterans Affairs Total Parenteral Nutrition Cooperative study group. Perioperative total parenteral nutrition in surgical patients. *N Engl J Med* 1991; 325: 525–32.
5. Corcoran C, Grinspoon S. Treatments for wasting in patients with the acquired immunodeficiency syndrome. *N Engl J Med* 1999; 340: 1740–50.
6. Suttmann U, Ockenga J, Selberg O, Hoogestraat L, Deicher H, Muller MJ. Incidence and prognostic value of malnutrition and wasting in human immunodeficiency virus-infected outpatients. *J Acquir Immune Defic Syndr Hum Retrovirol* 1995; 8: 239–46.
7. Macallan DC, Noble C, Baldwin C, Foskett M, McManus T, Griffin GE. Prospective analysis of patterns of weight change in stage IV HIV infection. *Am J Clin Nutr* 1993; 58: 417–24.
8. Macallan DC, McNurlan MA, Milne E, Calder AG, Garlick PJ, Griffin GE. Whole body protein turnover from leucine kinetics and the response to nutrition in human immunodeficiency virus infection. *Am J Clin Nutr* 1995; 61: 818–26.
9. Grunfeld C, Pang M, Shimizu L, Shigenaga JK, Jensen P, Feingold KR. Resting energy expenditure, caloric intake, and short-term weight change in human immunodeficiency virus infection and the acquired immunodeficiency syndrome. *Am J Clin Nutr* 1992; 55: 455–60.

10. Prentice AM. Applications of the doubly labelled-water method in free-living adults. *Proc Nutr Soc* 1988; 47: 259–68.
11. Macallan DC, Noble C, Baldwin C, et al. Energy expenditure and wasting in human immunodeficiency virus infection. *N Engl J Med* 1995; 333: 83–8.
12. Paton NIJ, Elia M, Jebb SA, Jennings G, Macallan DC, Griffin GE. Total energy expenditure and physical activity measured with the bicarbonate-urea method in patients with human immunodeficiency virus infection. *Clin Sci* 1996; 91: 241–5.
13. Rubin SA. Captain of all these men of death. *Radiol Clin North Am* 1995; 33: 619–39.
14. Macallan DC, McNurlan MA, Kurpad AV, et al. Whole body protein metabolism in human pulmonary tuberculosis and under-nutrition: evidence for anabolic block in tuberculosis. *Clin Sci* 1998; 94: 321–31.
15. Bekker LG, Maartens G, Steyn L, Kaplan G. Selective increase in plasma tumor necrosis factor-alpha and concomitant clinical deterioration after initiating therapy in patients with severe tuberculosis. *J Infect Dis* 1998; 178: 580–4.
16. Kennedy N, Ramsay A, Uiso L, Guttman J, Ngowi FI, Gillespie SH. Nutritional status and weight gain in patients with pulmonary tuberculosis in Tanzania. *Trans R Soc Trop Med Hyg* 1996; 90: 162–6.
17. Onwubalili J. Malnutrition among tuberculosis patients in Harrow, England. *Eur J Clin Nutr* 1988; 42: 363–6.
18. Klausner JD, Makonkawkeyoon S, Akarasewi P, et al. The effect of thalidomide on the pathogenesis of human immunodeficiency virus type I and *M. tuberculosis* infection. *J Acquir Immune Defic Syndr Hum Retrovirol* 1996; 11: 247–57.
19. Lawn S, Shattock RJ, Acheampong JW, et al. Sustained plasma TNF-α and HIV-1 load despite resolution of other parameters of immune activation during treatment of tuberculosis in Africans. *AIDS* 1999; 13: 2231–7.
20. Paton NIJ, Angus B, Simpson A, et al. Protein metabolism in melioidosis. *Trans R Soc Trop Med Hyg* 1997; 91: 500.
21. Pasquet P, Apfelbaum M. Recovery of initial body weight and composition after long term massive overfeeding in man. *Am J Clin Nutr* 1994; 60: 861–3.
22. Heyman MB, Young VR, Fuss P, Tsay R, Joseph L, Roberts SB. Underfeeding and body weight regulation in normal-weight young men. *Am J Physiol* 1992; 263: R250–7.

DISCUSSION

Dr. Wasantwisut: I am very interested that resting energy expenditure was increased. Do you see this in other types of infection and can you comment on what may be the reason for it?

Dr. Griffin: We have only looked at this in HIV disease, and everybody who has done the same with indirect calorimetry has found this rise of 10% to 15%. I do not know the mechanism, but several possibilities exist. One thing that is very clear is that it is unlikely to be concerned with thyroid hormone status, but it is a very consistent finding in HIV.

Dr. Villamore: Was all the energy expenditure caused by physical activity in your model of reduced resting energy expenditure?

Dr. Griffin: We have not actually measured activity, although there are some very interesting ways to do that noninvasively. We assume that the reduction in free-living energy expenditure is principally through reduced activity. We know that humans and animals who are sick tend to become quiet and still as part of this adaptive response. An interesting new technique is found to assess muscle activity. When skeletal muscle contracts it makes a noise, and this can be identified using sophisticated microphonics over the forearm or the legs. Noise generated during rest at about 30 cycles per second. This is driven by the motor cortex. When you move, it increases considerably. If you do 24-hour recordings using this microphonic device, you can obtain a good measure of the amount of activity in the legs and arms. So, for the first time, it is possible to measure muscle activity easily and noninvasively.

Dr. Fjeld: You interpreted the leucine oxidation data in the TB case as meaning that the dietary intervention was ineffective in turning on an anabolic switch. Pencharz in Canada has a different way of looking at that, and I think it would be interesting to apply it in your particular case as well. That is, the excess amino acid is blown off. At the point where it is a limiting amino acid, no more peptide bonds or proteins can be built, and then any protein that is available beyond that level is blown off, as would leucine have been. I do not think you tested the hypothesis about whether a dietary intervention triggered the anabolic switch; you showed that you had too much leucine relative to the need, and that is why it was blown off, which is consistent with what we were saying this morning.

Dr. Griffin: I agree with that entirely. You may remember in my talk I mentioned all the caveats of leucine oxidation. Some people, however, do not believe leucine can be used.

Dr. Fjeld: Your data could be very interesting to interpret from the other point of view, that is, under those conditions, alterations in the amino acid substrate requirements may occur, which could be evidence exactly for that.

Dr. Griffin: Yes. We used the time in Bangalore very much as a hypothesis testing period. We were not giving intravenous nutrition under those conditions, but for obvious reasons we had to give oral nutrition that had been shown in controls to give the anabolic type of switch. In London we are looking very intensively at patients presenting to my hospital with TB and weight loss, studying body composition changes longitudinally as they put on weight, and looking at leucine oxidation at 1 month, 6 months, and 9 months. We are doing this under very controlled conditions with amino acid infusions to get a proper background, which you suggest is important.

Dr. Kennedy: You brought up a point about stimulating cells, which I would like your opinion on. As we begin to move away from phytohemagglutinin (PHA), concanavalin A, and the more classical stimulants used in immunology and start using newer agents such as leukocyte functional antigens (LFA) and anti CD3, do you think the results we are going to find will alter immunity, and how do you think that might affect nutritional immunology?

Dr. Griffin: The first point is that it is much more physiologic. I did not have time to go into details of the techniques, but you can take a primed lymphocyte, strip off its membrane, fix it with glutaraldehyde, and then add it to a macrophage infected with TB or HIV, so the lymphocyte is contributing no cytokines at all to the interaction. Under those conditions, you get exactly the same effect, and this, as we now know, is because it is primarily an intercellular adhesion molecule (ICAM)-1-LFA interaction. By plating ICAM out at different doses on the base of your Petri dish and adding macrophages you can show that you get a differential release of cytokines and so on. I do not know whether that is going to cause a different response from PHA. Quantitatively it may not, but qualitatively it might be different because if you are signaling through engagement of adhesion molecules, this is going to be through different kinase pathways. Now, the phorbol esters, I think, work through protein kinase A principally.

Dr. Kennedy: In terms of Phorbol 12–myristate 13–acetate (PMA) especially, it is unknown how it stimulates a T cell. Certainly there is calcium flux, so protein kinase (PK) is implicated, but I think it is very poorly understood at this point.

Dr. Griffin: We also tend to look at cytokines in terms of a single event. But if you look at the whole integrated cascade of the release of cytokines over a 24-hour period, for example, then in our TB model you have first a pulse of TNF, which goes away unless you have T-cell membranes, and then over about 24 hours you have a massive release of IL-8 that far exceeds the IL-8 produced by lipopolysaccharide or phorbol ester. We think that may act as a chemoattractant to bring in immune cells to form the granuloma, the host response. Then, when the granuloma is formed, you get this other surge of cytokine release as an integrated phenomenon.

Dr. Kennedy: When you look at a T cell, and to some extent probably a macrophage, they exist in the circulation in lymph nodes only in a setting of constant on-and-off excitation. Once you remove that, the T cell dies very quickly. So even in the resting state, there is a constant on-and-off stimulation of the cell. I am curious whether, in a malnourished or infected disease state where you have constant stimulation with more potent interactions than just membranes of adjacent cells, those kinds of data are going to change our view of the role of nutrition in the process.

Dr. Griffin: I believe they will. That leads me to ask, what are we looking at in plasma at any one time? We are looking at something that is trafficking, something that may be so evanescent we miss it. For example, when TNF was first looked at in meningococcal septicemia, it was only found in 15% of the patients, the reason being that people were missing the big peak. In terms of circulating cells of the immune system and their relevance, just because you have small numbers of cells in the circulation at any time does not mean you have no activity from that cell. What it might mean is a very rapid proliferation of those cells, which are leaving the circulations so fast there is a consumption. In my laboratory, Derek Macallan has worked out a very elegant technique for looking at the trafficking of immune cells in humans, whether polymorphs, lymphocytes, macrophages, or eosinophils. The idea is to label the pool of proliferating immune cells *in vivo*, using ^2H glucose, and the ^2H glucose goes into ^2H ribose which then goes into DNA. You label over about a 24-hour period with this stable isotope. Then from the peripheral blood mononuclear cells, you obtain a highly purified population of the cells you want by FACS analysis, extract the DNA, and then look at the enrichment with ^2H to enable you to work out the kinetics of those cells. Now we know, for example, that in HIV disease you have a low count of CD4 positive cells at various stages in the circulation. At one point, that is not due to rapid loss of CD4 cells, but to rapid consumption before the lysis gets going. So, using these stable isotope cell turnover techniques, we should be able to study the kinetics of these cells, in the vascular compartment at least, and by FACS analysis even work out which cells were the TB primed cells, and whether they were turning over more quickly or were just not being produced for some reason.

Dr. Fjeld: If more protein is present than the host needs, it has to be deaminated to get rid of the nitrogen. How much could that account for the increase in energy expenditure seen in patients with TB?

Dr. Griffin: That is a very good point. It is certainly possible that could account for some of the increased expenditure, although in consumption tuberculosis the muscle mass is so severely reduced that only about 50% of the oxidizing organ remains, and it might not be transaminating or oxidizing in a reasonable way at all.

Dr. Woodward: The discussion about lymphocyte trafficking triggers a comment in connection with some of McMurray's recent work at Texas A&M, in which he has a guinea pig model of infection—a pulmonary type of infection model—and a protein deficiency model. I think the simplest interpretation of his results, in which he can show depression of the ability to produce granulomas (1), is that, whereas the macrophages are capable of responding to T-cell signals if they get to the relevant place, and the T cells are capable of delivering signals if they have the chance, the two cell types cannot get together. This is because, whereas the macrophages are in the lungs, the T cells are stuck in the draining lymph nodes and cannot get to the lungs. It seems to me that rather than being so concerned about what T cells can do by way of proliferation, we might need to be concerned about how to get them to the site of infection where they are needed.

Dr. Griffin: I agree entirely. You only need to look at HIV to see that. We thought that patients who were asymptomatic and had very low viral numbers and normal CD4 cells had quiescent disease. In fact, we now know that replication in lymphoid tissue is incredibly high, with a couple of billion viral particles being produced every day. This highlights the problem of sampling blood: we are looking through a ground glass on a dark night, and it is very difficult to draw the proper conclusions.

REFERENCE

1. McMurray DN. Impact of nutritional deficiencies on resistance to experimental pulmonary tuberculosis. *Nutr Rev* 1998; 56: S147–52.

Nutrition, Immunity, and Infection in Infants and Children, edited by Robert M. Suskind and Kraisid Tontisirin. Nestlé Nutrition Workshop Series, Pediatric Program, Vol. 45. Nestec Ltd., Vevey/Lippincott Williams & Wilkins, Philadelphia ©2001.

Malnutrition and HIV Infection

Wafaie W. Fawzi and Eduardo Villamor

Departments of Nutrition and Epidemiology, Harvard School of Public Health, Boston, Massachusetts, USA

Malnutrition and the human immunodeficiency virus (HIV) infection usually overlap in adults and children. The probability of HIV infection among malnourished children is much higher than in the general population. In Africa, for example, between 12% and 25% of clinically malnourished children are infected with HIV (1–5), in contrast to about 1% in the general population (1). Micronutrient deficiency is also common in HIV infection. Deficiencies of vitamins A, B, C, and E are more prevalent among children and adults infected with HIV than in HIV-negative individuals (6–9). In these studies, HIV status as well as anthropometric or vitamin status were assessed cross sectionally. This type of study is limited by the difficulty of determining the temporal relationship between HIV infection and nutritional deficiency. HIV infection could lead to nutritional deficiency through decreased food intake, malabsorption, and increased utilization and excretion of nutrients (10). On the other hand, nutritional deficiencies may contribute to faster progression of HIV disease through an adverse impact on immune function. Longitudinal studies are better suited to examine the relations of nutritional factors and HIV infection. These are reviewed in this chapter. First, we present studies that examined how nutritional status could affect HIV-related outcomes and discuss the mechanisms associated with these relations. Next, we present data on the reverse relationship: how HIV infection affects nutritional status and the pathophysiologic mechanisms associated with it.

HOW MALNUTRITION AFFECTS HIV TRANSMISSION AND PROGRESSION

Epidemiologic Evidence

Longitudinal studies that examined the relations of nutritional status to pregnancy outcomes, mother-to-child transmission, and child morbidity and mortality will be discussed—first the prospective observational studies, then the randomized trials. Next, we will present prospective studies and trials that examined the associations between nutritional status and clinical and immunologic progression among adults. Finally, we discuss the potential mechanisms by which nutritional status can affect transmission and progression of HIV disease.

Pregnancy Outcomes and Child Health

The relations of micronutrient status, particularly vitamins, and these outcomes have been examined in several studies. We will discuss these studies first, and then examine the role of breast-feeding by HIV-positive women on the health and survival of their children.

Vitamins

Several studies suggest that low serum vitamin A levels among HIV-infected pregnant women are associated with a higher risk of morbidity and mortality among children, and with vertical transmission of HIV (Table 1). In Malawi, higher serum retinol of HIV-infected pregnant women was associated with reduced infant mortality (11); an increase of 0.45 μmol/l in serum vitamin A concentrations was associated with 50% reduction in mortality. In a study among children from the United States infected with HIV, however, no relationship was observed between serum vitamin A levels and various measures of morbidity and mortality (12). In the Malawi study, higher serum retinol of HIV-infected pregnant women was associated with a reduced risk of vertical transmission (13); an increase of 0.45 μmol/l in serum vitamin A was associated with a 44% reduction in the risk of transmission. In a study from Rwanda, mothers with normal levels of vitamin A were about half as likely to have a dead infant or an HIV-positive infant compared with vitamin A-deficient women (14). Three studies from the United States provided conflicting results: low serum vitamin A was associated with a higher risk of vertical transmission in two (15,16) studies but not in the third (17).

Various limitations need to be considered in the interpretation of these prospective studies. First, reverse causality may provide an explanation for the positive association between vitamin deficiency and health outcomes: HIV infection could lead to adverse effects on absorption and metabolism of nutrients, which could lead to biochemical deficiency. Also, serum vitamin A levels may be reduced as a result of the acute phase response to infection even in the presence of adequate liver stores of vitamin A (18). Hence, vitamin A deficiency may be a marker of, rather than a causal factor for, an advanced stage of HIV disease. Different lengths of follow-up time among vitamin deficient and sufficient groups could bias the association with disease outcomes. In an attempt to adjust for the stage of disease in some of these studies, surrogate markers of disease progression were adjusted for, including CD4 cell counts and clinical signs.

TABLE 1. Prospective cohort studies of serum vitamin A levels in relationship to pregnancy outcomes and child health

Study site (reference)	Population	Exposure: mother serum vitamin A levels	Endpoint	Measure of association		Variables adjusted
Malawi (11)	474 HIV +ve women	Increase of 0.40 µmol/l	Infant mortality	RR (95% CI)	0.47 (0.36–0.62)	Maternal age, body mass, index, CD4 cell count, birthweight, and gestational age
United States (12)	207 HIV +ve children	Increase of 1 µg/dl	Serious bacterial infections Viral infections	RR (95% CI)	0.99 (0.07–1.00) 1.00 (0.99–1.02)	Treatment (intravenous immunolglobulin) or placebo
Malawi (13)	474 HIV +ve women	Increase of 0.45 µmol/l	HIV infection in infants	RR (95% CI)	0.56 (0.37–0.85)	Maternal age, body mass index, CD4 cell count, birthweight, and gestational age
Rwanda (14)	146 HIV +ve women	≥20 vs < 20 µg/dl	Perinatal death Infant death Dead or HIV+ baby	RR (95% CI)	0.33 (0.14–0.77) 0.53 (0.27–1.00) 0.53 (0.30–0.77)	CD4 cell count, hematocrit, clinical signs
United States (15)	HIV +ve pregnant women	Mother serum levels	HIV infection in infants		Increase in serum retinol levels over time was associated with an apparent reduction in risk of transmission (see text).	
United States (16)	133 HIV +ve women	≥1.05 vs <0.70 µmol/L	HIV infection in infants	RR (95% CI)	0.22 (0.05–0.93)	(CD4 cells (%), mode of delivery, gestational age, duration of membrane rupture, race
United States (17)	90 HIV +ve women	Mother serum level	HIV infection in infants	Mean	Transmitters: 46.5 µg/dl Nontransmitters: 41.1 µg/dl	None

RR, relative risk; CI, confidence interval.

Randomized, placebo-controlled intervention studies offer the best design to assess the relations of nutrient intake to health outcomes. In a trial among HIV-infected pregnant women in Tanzania, multivitamin supplements resulted in significant reductions ($\sim 40\%$) in the risks of fetal death, low birthweight, and severe prematurity (Table 2). On the other hand, vitamin A alone had a much smaller and nonsignificant effect (19). In another study among children in Tanzania, periodic supplementation of vitamin A resulted in a large and significant reduction in mortality, overall as well as within strata of HIV-infected and uninfected children (20). In a placebo-controlled trial from South Africa among children born to HIV-positive women, vitamin A supplements resulted in approximately 50% reduction in diarrheal morbidity among HIV-infected children (21). Several trials are being carried out to examine the efficacy of varying regimens of vitamin supplements on the risk of vertical transmission of HIV in Malawi, Tanzania, South Africa, and Zimbabwe.

Breast-Feeding

Breast-feeding offers multiple benefits to both the child and the mother in developed and developing settings (22,23). Breast-fed infants are at lower risk of death; infectious disease, including diarrhea, respiratory infections, otitis media, urinary tract infections; and impaired nutritional status. Recent studies suggest that the benefits of breast-feeding on cognitive development are rather modest (24). However, in neonates born prematurely with a very low birthweight, neurocognitive development may be significantly enhanced through breast-feeding, because breast milk is rich in long chain polyunsaturated fatty acids and these compounds are highly demanded by the developing nervous system, including the retina (25). Benefits to the mother include a risk reduction in postpartum hemorrhage and maternal mortality, child spacing owing to suppression of ovarian activity, decreased risk of premenopausal breast and ovarian cancer, psychological comfort, and more rapid return to prepregnancy weight (23).

From pooled analyses of cohort studies, the risk of HIV transmission through breast-feeding has been estimated to be approximately 29% for women who acquired the virus after delivery, and 14% over and above transmission *in utero* or during delivery in prenatally infected mothers (26). A more recent study of mothers and infants in South Africa also found an excess transmission rate of 15% by subtracting the incidence among exclusively formula-fed (24%) from that among exclusively breast-fed children (39%) (27). In developed countries, both zidovudine (AZT) prophylaxis to pregnant women and newborns and formula-feeding of infants are effective strategies to reduce mother-to-child transmission of HIV through *in utero* and intrapartum routes (28). In countries with increased prevalence of HIV infection, where AZT prophylaxis is not the standard of care and the major causes of infant and child morbidity and mortality are still infectious diseases and malnutrition, the appropriateness of breast-feeding is matter of debate.

Significant uncertainty exists as to when transmission of HIV through breast milk is most likely to occur. Currently, late postnatal transmission is assumed in breast-fed

TABLE 2. *Randomized, placebo-controlled vitamin trials in relationship to pregnancy outcomes and child health*

Study site (reference)	Population	Intervention	Endpoint	RR (95 % CI)
Tanzania (19)	1,085 HIV +ve pregnant women	1085 HIV + ve pregnant women Factorial design: preformed vitamin A and β-carotene vs multivitamins other than A (multiples of RDA in both cases)		Multivitamins vs no multivitamins
			Fetal death	0.61 (0.31–0.94)
			Birthweight <2,500	0.56 (0.38–0.82)
			Birthweight <2,000	0.42 (0.18–1.01)
			Prematurity <37 weeks	0.86 (0.68–1.10)
			Prematurity <34 weeks	0.61 (0.38–0.96)
				Vitamin A vs no vitamin A
			Fetal death	0.89 (0.58–1.36)
			Birthweight <2,500	0.89 (0.61–1.29)
			Birthweight <2,000	0.89 (0.40–1.98)
			Prematurity <37 weeks	1.06 (0.83–1.35)
			Prematurity <34 weeks	1.09 (0.70–1.70)
Tanzania (20)	648 children admitted to the hospital with pneumonia, 9% were HIV +ve	200,000 (100,000 for infants) or placebo given on day 1 and 2 of hospitalization, and at 4 and 8 months after discharge	Mortality:	
			Overall	0.51 (0.29–0.90)
			HIV +ve children	0.37 (0.14–0.95)
			HIV −ve children	0.58 (0.28–1.19)
South Africa (21)	118 children born to HIV +ve mothers	50,000 IU of retinol at 1 and 3 mo, 100,000 IU at 6 and 9 mo, and 200,000 IU at 12 and 15 mo	HIV-infected children:	
			Diarrhea	0.51 (0.27–0.99)
			Total morbidity	0.69 (0.36–1.31)
			HIV-uninfected children:	
			Diarrhea	0.89 (0.37–2.10)
			Total morbidity	0.74 (0.34–1.61)

HIV, human immunodeficiency virus; CI, confidence interval; RDA, recommended dietary allowance.

children who were negative for polymerase chain reaction (PCR) or viral culture until 90 days of delivery and turned positive afterward (29). In a meta-analysis by Leroy *et al.* (30), the pooled incidence of late infection (after 2.5 months of age) was 3.2 per 100 child-years of breast-feeding. The cumulative probability of late postnatal transmission was below 1% up to 9 months and then 2.5%, 6.3%, 7.4%, and 9.6% at 12, 18, 24, and 36 months, respectively. Other prospective studies in African countries, with varying definitions of late transmission, have yielded estimates ranging from 4% after age 5 (31) or 12 months (32) through 12% after 20 months of age (33). A very high late transmission rate (32% after 15 months) was reported in a study from Nairobi (34).

The most effective measure to decrease transmission of HIV through breast-feeding is replacement feeding. However, this alternative is not always suitable for less developed countries because high-quality substitutes for breast milk are not available, and the weighted effect of replacement feeding on health outcomes of infants from HIV-positive mothers is not known. On the other hand, divergence from pre-established cultural norms of breast-feeding may expose the HIV status of a woman and contribute to the social stigmatization of the woman and her family. Strong recommendations against breast-feeding during HIV infection in developing countries could have an undesirable spillover effect among uninfected mothers. Various alternatives to complete replacement feeding have been proposed (35). Early cessation should reduce the risk of transmission, but the safest length of breast-feeding in children of HIV-positive mothers is not known. Treatment of breast milk with heat or by exposure to room temperature may be effective in inactivating HIV (36), but its feasibility in the field may be limited, given the need for sustained milk expression. Wet nursing by a tested seronegative wet nurse is likely to be effective, but there may be some risk of transmission from the child to the woman. Efficacy of the administration of antiretrovirals to the mother or the infant in reducing breast milk transmission is still unknown. The use of modified animal milk from birth as a feeding replacement requires careful and hygienic practices of preparation, the availability of safe animal milk in the household, and perhaps additional supplementation with some micronutrients.

Disease Progression Among Adults

Several longitudinal studies have examined the relations between nutritional status and disease progression among adults. We will present three groups of studies that examined the relationships of vitamins, other micronutrients, and anthropometric measurements and body composition and these outcomes.

Vitamins

In longitudinal studies, nutritional status was assessed either by using a biochemical marker of the nutrient or by measurement of dietary intake of that nutrient (Table 3).

In the San Francisco Health Study (37), a higher intake of 11 micronutrients was associated with higher CD4 counts at baseline, significantly so for six including riboflavin, thiamine, and niacin. A statistically significant protective effect of vitamin E and riboflavin against disease progression was observed, with a protective association of borderline significance with higher intakes of vitamin C, thiamine, and vitamin A. Daily multivitamin use was associated with a significant 30% reduction in the risk of developing the acquired immunodeficiency syndrome (AIDS), and a reduction of 40% in the risk of developing a CD4 cell count below 500×10^6/l during the 6 years of follow-up (37). Among homosexual and bisexual men participating in the Multicenter AIDS Cohort Study (MACS), a U-shaped relationship was noted between vitamin A intake (from diet and supplements) and risk of progression to AIDS (38), as well as risk of death (39). Levels of intake between 9,000 and 20,000 IU were associated with slower progression and lower risk of death, whereas subjects with higher levels of intake experienced no decrease in risk. Higher intakes of niacin, vitamins B_1, B_2, B_6, and vitamin C were associated with slower progression to AIDS and reduced risk of death after 8 years of follow-up. Most of the protective relationships in these dietary studies were associated with the intake of supplements rather than diet; however, there was limited statistical power to examine the association between deficiency states of these nutrients and the risk of progression because few subjects were consuming low levels. To examine the relationship between supplement use and survival independent of the effect of intake from food, the investigators included levels of supplement intake and quartiles of food intake in the same multivariate model. Supplemental use of vitamins B_1 and B_2 at levels of five or more times the recommended daily allowance (RDA) were significantly associated with an approximately 40% reduction in mortality, compared with the use at less than five times the RDA. Similarly, use of vitamin B_6 at two or more times the RDA was also associated with a significant improvement in survival, compared with intake of less than twice the RDA.

In two studies among HIV-positive intravenous drug users, low serum retinol levels were associated with a sixfold (40) and a 4.6 times (41) increase in risk of mortality compared with individuals with normal vitamin A status. In a third study carried out among HIV-positive drug users, subjects who developed biochemical vitamin B_{12} or vitamin A deficiency over an 18-month period experienced a decline in CD4 cell count, whereas higher cell counts were noted among those whose vitamin B_{12} and vitamin A levels were normalized over the same period (42). In the MACS study, men in the highest quintile of serum vitamin E levels were 34% less likely to progress to AIDS compared with those in the lowest quintile. Serum vitamin A status was not predictive of progression of HIV infection; however, the vitamin A level was in the normal range for all subjects (43). Low serum B_{12} was associated with a doubling of the risk of progression to AIDS. The median AIDS-free time was 4 years shorter in the low vitamin B_{12} group than in the higher group (44).

Given that the above studies were carried out among prevalent cohorts of seropositive persons at baseline, the duration of infection was not known and, therefore, not adjusted for in the analyses. Although baseline signs and symptoms and immuno-

TABLE 3. *Prospective cohort studies of nutritional status in relationship to progression of HIV disease among adults*

Study site (reference)	Population	Endpoint	Vitamin	Relative risk (95% CI)	Variables adjusted
United States (37)	296 HIV +ve homosexual and bisexual men	Progression to AIDS	*100% increase (doubling) in dietary intake:*		Age, smoking, energy intake, symptoms, CD4 cell count
			Carotenoids	0.93 (0.78–1.12)	
			Retinol	0.98 (0.78–1.23)	
			B_1	0.92 (0.84–1.01)	
			B_2	0.90 (0.81–1.00)	
			Folate	0.89 (0.66–1.19)	
			Niacin	0.83 (0.67–1.04)	
			C	0.90 (0.81–1.01)	
			E	0.91 (0.83–1.00)	
			Daily multivitamin use	0.69 (0.46–1.03)	
United States (38)	281 HIV +ve homosexual and bisexual men	Progression to AIDS	*Dietary intake:*		Age, symptoms, CD4 cell count, energy intake, antiretroviral use, use of prophylaxis against *Pneumocystis carinii*
			A 9,062–20,268 vs <9,062 IU/d	0.55 (0.35–0.88)	
			A >20,268 vs <9,062 IU/d	0.94 (0.56–1.57)	
			B_1 >4.9 vs <2.4 mg/d	0.60 (0.36–0.98)	
			B_2 >5.9 vs ≤5.9 mg/d	0.61 (0.38–1.00)	
			B_6 >5.7 vs ≤2.0 mg/d	0.60 (0.35–1.05)	
			C > 715 vs ≤715 mg/d	0.55 (0.34–0.91)	
			Niacin > 61.0 vs ≤ 61 mg/d	0.52 (0.31–0.86)	

Country (ref)	Subjects	Outcome	Exposure	Results	Adjustments
United States (39)	281 HIV +ve homosexual and bisexual	Mortality	*Dietary intake:* A 9,098–12,221 vs <9,098 IU/d A > 13,221–20,762 vs < 9,098 IU/d A >20,762 vs <9,098 IU/d B_1 > 5.3 vs ≤ 5.3 mg/d B_2 > 6.3 vs ≤ 6.3 mg/d B_6 >5.9 vs ≤ 5.9 mg/d Niacin > 64.0 vs ≤ 64 mg/d	0.80 (0.48–1.34) 0.72 (0.43–1.21) 1.21 (0.74–1.99) 0.60 (0.38–0.95) 0.59 (0.38–0.93) 0.45 (0.28–0.73) 0.57 (0.36–0.91)	Age, symptoms, CD4 cell count, energy intake, antiretroviral use, use of prophylaxis against *P. carinii*; for all nutrients except vitamin A, results are adjusted for β-carotene, and zinc intake
United States (40)	50 deaths; 235 controls nested in a longitudinal study of HIV +ve injection drug users	Mortality	*Serum level:* A ≥ 1.05 vs <1.05 µmol/l	0.22 (0.09–0.55)	CD4 cell count, wasting
United States (41)	126 HIV +ve drug users	Mortality	*Serum level:* A ≥ 1.05 vs <1.05 µmol/l	0.23 (0.06–0.91)	CD4 cell count, hepatitis B surface antigen
United States (42)	108 HIV +ve homosexual men	Change in CD4 cell count	*Developing deficiency in:* Serum vitamin A Serum vitamin B_{12} *Normalization of:* Serum vitamin A Serum vitamin B_{12}	−176 cells/mm^3 −112 cells/mm^3 +61 cells/mm^3 +95 cells/mm^3	AZT use, CD4 cell count
United States (43, 44)	310 HIV +ve homosexual and bisexual men	Progression to AIDS	*Serum level:* A ≥ 3.15 vs 1.82 µmol/l E > 23.5 vs <1.23 µmol/l B12 ≥ 305 vs < 105	0.73 (0.46–1.16) 0.66 (0.41–1.06) 0.55 (0.35–0.86)	Age, symptoms, CD4 cell count, antiretroviral use, serum albumin and folate, alcohol consumption

HIV, human immunodeficiency virus; AIDS, acquired immunodeficiency syndrome; AZT, zidovudine.

logic surrogates (e.g., CD4 cell counts) were taken into account, residual confounding is still a possible explanation for the findings. As mentioned, the biochemical vitamin A studies are limited by the fact that low serum vitamin A levels among individuals with infection does not necessarily mean poor vitamin A stores.

Several intervention studies have examined the hypothesis that vitamin supplementation results in slower progression of HIV infection. In a crossover study among 21 patients, those who received 180 mg of β-carotene daily for 4 weeks experienced a small increase in the total white blood cell count, change in CD4 cell count, and percent change in CD4:CD8 ratio compared with subjects on placebo; these indices decreased when the subjects on the carotene arm were switched to the placebo (45) (Table 4). However, in another study by the same investigators in which the same dose of β-carotene was used, this effect was not observed (46). In a small placebo-controlled trial among HIV-infected pregnant women in South Africa, retinol and β-carotene did not result in a change in viral load (47). Also no effect was seen of vitamin A supplementation on viral load among intravenous drug users in two studies from the United States (48,49). The lack of effect of vitamin A on immunologic endpoints was confirmed in the Tanzania study mentioned earlier. Multivitamins resulted in a significant improvement in CD4, CD8, and CD3 cell counts (19). In a study from Canada, large daily doses of vitamins C and E resulted in a significant reduction in viral load (50).

Other Micronutrients

The role of zinc and selenium in HIV disease has been examined in a few studies. In a prospective study of 95 individuals infected with HIV, low serum selenium levels were associated with higher risks of mortality and the occurrence of AIDS-defining opportunistic infections, even after adjustment for baseline CD4 count (51). In a prospective study among HIV-infected, drug-using men and women in Miami, Florida, those with low selenium plasma levels were 19.9 times at greater risk of AIDS-related mortality after adjusting for CD4 cell count less than 200 at baseline and CD4 counts during the 3.5 years of follow-up (52). When adjusting further for other indicators of nutritional status including prealbumin levels and other micronutrient levels, only selenium deficiency was significantly associated with mortality (relative risk = 10.8, p < 0.02), suggesting that selenium deficiency is an independent predictor of survival in HIV-1 infection.

Low serum zinc has been reported to be significantly correlated with a decline in CD4 cell count (53). Using a case-control design nested within the longitudinal Multicenter AIDS Cohort Study, Graham *et al.* studied zinc levels among 54 asymptomatic, HIV-positive members who subsequently progressed to AIDS, 54 men who did not progress during a mean follow-up period of 2.5 years, and 54 HIV-negative men (54). Serum zinc was significantly lower among patients who progressed compared with nonprogressors and those who were HIV negative. As zinc is an acute phase reactant, this result suggests that zinc level is a proxy for disease stage, although the possibility that it is causally related to disease progression

TABLE 4. *Randomized, placebo-controlled trials of vitamins in relationship to progression of HIV disease among adults*

Study site (reference)	Population	Intervention	Endpoint		Measure of effect	
					Intervention	*Placebo*
United States (45)	21 HIV +ve subjects: 20 men, 1 woman	180 mg β-carotene daily for 4 weeks	CD4 cell count (/mm³)	Baseline mean (range) 4 weeks mean (range)	339.5 (12–882) 352.9 (20–846)	411.5 (22–1,379) 366.6 (12–1,006)
United States (46)	72 HIV +ve subjects: 63 men, 9 women	180 mg β-carotene for 3 months All received multivitamins	CD4 cell count (/mm³)	Baseline mean (SD) 3 months mean (SD)	*Intervention* 335.4 (29.5) 296.3 (31.9)	*Placebo* 319.2 (28.5) 331.0 (33.3)
South Africa (47)	24 HIV +ve women at 28–32 weeks of pregnancy	30 mg β-carotene and 5,000 IU retinol daily for 9–13 weeks	HIV viral load (log₁₀)	Baseline mean (SD) 1 week postdelivery mean (SD)	*Intervention* 3.58 (0.98) 3.55 (0.82)	*Placebo* 4.04 (0.75) 4.35 (0.76)
Tanzania (19)	1,085 HIV +ve pregnant women	Factorial design: preformed vitamin A and β-carotene vs multivitamins other than A (multiples of RDA in both cases)	CD4 cell count (/mm³)	Baseline 6 wk postpartum 30 wk postpartum	Multivitmins 424 (207) 596 (312) 522 (278)	No multivitamins 423 (211) 520 (339) 482 (268)
				Baseline 6 wk postpartum 30 wk postpartum	Vitamin A 416 (206) 558 (376) 496 (294)	No Vitamin A 431 (212) 562 (265) 509 (252)
Canada (50)	49 HIV +ve men and women	800 IU vitamin E and 1,000 mg of vitamin C daily for 3 months	HIV viral load (log₁₀)	Week 0 Week 12 Change	Intervention 4.13 (0.27) 3.67 (0.40) −0.45 (0.39)	Placebo 4.42 (0.39) 4.92 (0.19) 0.50 (0.40)

cannot be excluded. Using a food frequency questionnaire to assess dietary zinc intake in the same study population, increased intake of zinc from food alone or from food and supplements was significantly associated with increased risks of progression to AIDS (38), and with an increased risk of mortality (39). Subjects who consumed as little as 1.3 times the recommended dietary levels of zinc had an increased progression to AIDS. Subjects in the top quartile were 2.44 times more likely to die than those in the bottom quartile of intake. In contrast, normalization of zinc was associated with higher CD4 cell counts among men who participated in another prospective cohort study (43). In the San Francisco Men's Health Study, dietary intake of zinc was positively related to CD4 cell count, but not to progression to AIDS (37).

Anthropometric Measures and Body Composition

Several longitudinal studies in children have reported associations between alterations in the nutritional status, expressed in terms of growth retardation, and accelerated progression to AIDS, shortened survival time, or both. In a study of 459 Ugandan children followed from birth up to 2 years of age, mortality during the study period was significantly higher for those who were HIV positive (54%) than for children who were HIV negative (5.6%) and seroreverters (1.6%) (55). Among those who were HIV positive, death before the second birthday was five times more likely to occur in children with a mean weight-for-age Z-score (WAZ) of less than -1.5 during the first year as compared with HIV-infected infants with WAZ ≥ -1.5. As the WAZ cut-off moved toward positive values, the risk was smaller but still significant, even comparing children below and above -0.75 WAZ (Table 5). In a longitudinal study of infants in Rwanda, WAZ and height-for-age Z-score (HAZ) at 12 months were respectively, 1.21 and 1.1 standard deviations higher among infected children who survived into the second year of life than in those who died between 12 and 24 months (56).

Among 36 HIV-seropositive hemophilic children in the United States, those with growth failure, defined as a fall of at least 15 centile units in height or weight for age during two consecutive years, were more likely to develop AIDS and subsequently die after approximately 2 years of their growth curve flattening than children who were either HIV positive without growth failure or HIV negative (57). Children with growth failure also had lower absolute CD4 lymphocyte counts after 5 years of follow-up. The small sample size and lack of control for factors such as the occurrence of opportunistic infections are limitations of the study. In a larger study of Italian children born to HIV-positive women, infected children who presented with *failure to thrive* as one of the defining nonspecific features of stage P2A had a 3.7 times greater risk of death than infected children without this condition (58). However, when secondary infections were included in a multivariate model, failure to thrive became no longer a significant predictor of death.

Malnourished HIV-infected children are at greater risk of secondary infections than HIV-positive children with better nutritional status. In a study that compared the patterns of diarrheal disease among Zairian infants, HIV-1 infected children with persistent episodes of diarrhea had significantly less weight gain in the month preceding the episode than children in whom the episode did not persist (59).

Wasting is an independent risk factor for death in HIV-infected adults as well. Early studies showed that weight loss was part of a clinical complex associated with short survival in patients with AIDS (60). The magnitude of weight loss that has been associated with shorter survival is variable. Chlebowski *et al.* found a decreased median length of survival in HIV-positive individuals who had lost more than 20% of their usual body weight (61). In a retrospective study, the risk of death was eight times greater among individuals weighing less than 90% of their usual body weight than in patients weighing more than 90% of usual body weight, after controlling for CD4 count, age, and albumin levels (62). No difference was found in the presence of secondary infections between survivors and nonsurvivors. Among HIV-infected Rwandan women, a significant association between a body mass index less than 21 kg/m^2 and mortality was noted (63). However, studies of body composition suggested that cell mass was the component actually correlated with adverse outcomes. Progressive depletion of body cell mass, independent of changes in body fat, was observed during the 3 months preceding death in a retrospective study in the United States (64); death occurred when cell mass decreased to 54% of the normal values and weight reached an average value of 66% of ideal. These findings were independent of the underlying condition of the patients, most of whom suffered from *Pneumocistis carinii* pneumonia, cytomegalovirosis, and mycobacteriosis. The results also suggested that 3 months before death, weight may not be a good indicator of the body mass composition. In another study, body cell mass less than 30% of body weight was associated with significantly decreased survival (mean survival time: 321 days vs 533 days in patients with a body cell mass of more than 30% of body weight) (65); this association was independent of the level of CD4 cells.

Potential Mechanisms

We will discuss the mechanisms by which nutritional status could affect progression of HIV disease, and then the potential mechanisms affecting the risk of transmission of the virus (Table 6).

Disease Progression

Nutritional status has been related to immune status and function, including cytokine levels, and risk of opportunistic infections, all of which are on the causal pathway to faster HIV disease progression. Use of a daily multivitamin supplement, including preformed vitamin A, B$_1$, B$_2$, B$_6$, B$_{12}$, niacin, vitamins C and D, and trace elements, reduced the risk of infection, mainly respiratory, of healthy elderly subjects who participated in a randomized, double-blind, placebo-controlled study (66). The group receiving supplement had higher numbers of natural killer cells and T-cell subsets (in-

TABLE 5. *Prospective cohort studies of anthropometric measurements and body composition in*

Study site (reference)	Population	Exposure	Endpoint
Uganda (55)	84 HIV +ve infants	Average WAZ during first year of life	Death by age 25 months
Rwanda (56)	33 HIV +ve infants	WAZ and HAZ at 12 months	Death between 12 and 24 months
United States (57)	36 HIV +ve hemophiliac boys	Growth failure: sustained decrease in ≥ 15 percentile points in height or weight for age, for two years	CD4 count at year 5 of follow-up Progression to AIDS
Italy (58)	433 HIV +ve children at stage P2A	Failure to thrive (clinical)	Death
Zaire (59)	53 HIV +ve infants	Weight gain in the month preceding diarrhea	Persistent diarrhea
United States (61)	71 AIDS adults (96% male)	% loss of usual body weight at baseline Baseline albumin	Death
United States (62)	77 HIV +ve adults (96% male)	Weight at follow-up divided by weight at baseline Baseline albumin (g/dl)	Death
Rwanda (63)	460 HIV +ve women	BMI at baseline	Death
United States (64)	32 with AIDS patients	Body cell mass divided by total body weight Body weight at or before death divided by weight at baseline	Death (moment of death or time before death)
Germany (65)	39 adults with AIDS	Body cell mass divided by total body weight at baseline Baseline albumin (g/dl)	Death

HIV, human immunodeficiency virus; AIDS, acquired immunodeficiency syndrome; WAZ weight-for-age z-score; HAZ, height-for-age z-score; BMI, body mass index.

cluding CD4), enhanced proliferation response to mitogen, increased natural cell activity and interleukin-2 production, and greater antibody response to influenza vaccine.

Vitamin A status is associated with mucosal, humoral, and cellular immune function. Impaired integrity of the epithelial linings of the respiratory and gastrointestinal systems occurs in vitamin A deficiency, leading to reduced levels of secretory IgA, decreased mucus secretion, and weakened local barriers to infection (67,68). Vitamin A supplements are associated with enhancement of cellular immune function in hu-

relationship to progression of HIV disease progression

Measure of association	Results		Variables adjusted
Odds ratio	WAZ	OR (95% CI)	None
	< −0.75 vs ≥ −0.75: 2.74 (1.12–6.67)		
	< −1.00 vs ≥ −1.00: 3.39 (1.28–8.97)		
	< −1.50 vs ≥ −1.50: 4.87 (1.27–18.7)		
Mean Z-score		WAZ HAZ	None
	Survivors	−1.84 −2.12	
	Non-survivors	−3.05 −3.22	
Mean CD4 count	Adequate growth	694 cells/mm^3	None
	Growth failure	215 cells/mm^3	
% progressing to AIDS	Adequate growth	3.7% (1/27)	
	Growth failure	55.6% (5/9)	
Odds ratio	OR (95% CI)	3.70 (2.40–5.71)	None. After adjustment for other disorders, including secondary infections, the association became nonsignificant
Mean weight gain	Not persistent	59 g/mo	None
	Persistent	348 g/mo	
Median survival time	< 10%	520 days	None
	10–20%	101 days	
	>20%	48 days	
	≥3.5	960 days	
	2.5–3.5	103 days	
	<2.5	17 days	
Odds ratio		OR (95% CI)	CD4 count, age, albumin
	<90% vs ≥90%:	8.3 (2.3–34.1)	
	< 3.5 vs ≥ 3.5 :	3.6 (1.2–10.9)	CD4 count, age, weight
Odds ratio		OR (95% CI)	Weight loss, clinical signs and symptoms of severity, secondary infections, hematocrit, leukocyte count
	≤ 21 vs > 21 :	2.3 (1.1–4.8)	
Body cell mass (%)	71% at 100 days before death		None
	54% at death		
Body weight (%)	90% at 100 days before death		
	66% at death		
Mean survival time	>30%	527	None
	<30%	335	
	>3.0	533	
	<3.0	322	None

mans, including an increase in CD4 helper cells and natural killer cells, cells expressing interleukin-2 receptors (69,70). Retinoic acid has been shown to inhibit HIV replication in infected cells (71), whereas the carotenoid halocynthaxantin had an inhibitory effect on the reverse transcriptase enzyme (72). Supplementation of retrovirally infected mice with vitamin A was associated with larger numbers of activated macrophages than in infected controls and was associated with a slower death rate for retrovirally infected mice (73).

The B vitamins are cofactors that play significant roles in many metabolic pathways. Animal and human studies have shown that vitamin B$_6$ deficiency affects both

TABLE 6. *Summary of pathophysiologic mechanisms in the interrelationship between nutritional status and HIV infection*

How malnutrition may lead to increased HIV disease progression and transmission:
  ↓ Integrity of epithelial lining:
   Respiratory system
   Gastrointestinal system
   Lower genital tract of mother
   Placenta
  ↑ Opportunistic infections
  ↑ Humoral immunity and cellular immunity
  ↑ Rate of HIV disease progression in mother
  ↑ Viral load in blood, breast milk, lower genital tract
  ↑ Prematurity and low birth weight
How HIV leads to poor nutritional status:
  Unsuccessful adaptations of energy balance
  ↓ Energy intake
  ↑ Resting energy expenditure
  ↓ Activity-related energy expenditure
  ↓ Total energy expenditure
  Reduced dietary intake
   Disturbances in chewing and swallowing
   Ulcers from esophageal HIV infection
   Dysgeusia
   Anorexia secondary to opportunistic infections.
  Nutrient malabsorption
   Enterocyte injury by opportunistic protozoans
   Infiltration of intestinal lamina propria by macrophages
   Alteration of bile salt absorption in the ileum
   Deficiency of pancreatic enzymes
   Decrease in disaccharidases specific activities
  Cytokines secretion
   ↑ Tumor necrosis factor
   ↑ Interferon-α
  Hormonal changes
   ↓ Serum testosterone, hypogonadism
   ↑ Triiodothyronine with ↓ reverse triiodothyronine
   ↓ Insulinlike growth factors/growth hormone resistance
   Disregulation in neuropeptides secretion

HIV, human immunodeficiency virus.

humoral and cellular immune function, including reduced lymphocyte differentiation and maturation, reduced delayed hypersensitivity responses, and possibly antibody production (74). Vitamin B_6 depletion in healthy elderly people significantly reduced the total number of lymphocytes, lymphocyte proliferation, and interleukin (IL)-2 production in response to T-cell mitogens. These defects were corrected following vitamin B_6 repletion (75). Vitamin B_6 deficiency in patients with rheumatoid cachexia, a wasting condition associated with increased *in vitro* production of IL-1 and tumor necrosis factor-α (TNF-α), was also associated with high levels of production of proinflammatory TNF-α (76). In clinical studies, patients with low levels of serum vitamin B_{12} had impaired neutrophil function, whereas data from *in vitro* and animal studies indicate that B_{12} supplements are associated with enhanced antibody function and mitogenic responses (74).

Vitamin C deficiency in animal models results in depressed cell-mediated immune response. T- and B-lymphocyte proliferative responses are increased following supplementation in some human studies, and enhanced vitamin C status was associated with lower rates of infections (77). In a cross-sectional study among patients with cystic fibrosis, vitamin C was directly related to indices of inflammation including IL-6 and TNF-α (78). Vitamin C also resulted in reduced reverse transcriptase activity in T lymphocytes that were chronically infected with HIV (79,80).

Vitamin E deficiency has been shown to impair T-cell–mediated function, lymphocyte proliferation, and IL-2 production in rodents, farm animals, and humans (81,82). Higher vitamin E levels are also associated with increased production of γ-interferon and IL-2 in mice with murine AIDS as well as reduced IL-6 and TNF-α (83).

Transmission

Poor nutritional status can increase the risk of vertical transmission by affecting humoral and cellular immune function that results in faster progression of mother's HIV disease. Early stages of vitamin A deficiency in rats have repeatedly been shown to result in squamous metaplasia of the simple columnar epithelium of the endocervix (84). Hence, deficiency may be associated with a higher risk of abrasions of the cervix leading to a greater risk of the baby coming in contact with infectious material during delivery. Vitamin A deficiency was found to be associated with a greater risk of viral shedding in lower genital tract secretions in two studies from Kenya (85,86), possibly leading to a higher risk of intrapartum transmission of infection. Vitamin A may also reduce the risk of vertical transmission by preventing chorioamnionitis or by enhancing placental integrity (87).

Vitamin deficiencies are also associated with greater risks for prematurity and low birthweight (19), which are associated with a higher risk of vertical transmission. Maternal vitamin A status after delivery may also be an important risk factor for postpartum transmission, given that vitamin A deficiency was associated with a higher risk of breast milk viral shedding among HIV-positive women in Kenya (88). Vitamin supplements provided to mothers during pregnancy or lactation, or both, or to babies would result in improvements of vitamin status in infants, which may be associated with enhanced development of the infant's immune system and a greater ability to prevent the establishment of HIV infection.

HOW HIV INFECTION AFFECTS NUTRITIONAL STATUS

Epidemiologic Evidence

The effect of HIV infection on the nutritional status of children is better understood along the continuum of the life cycle. We present a review of the effect of HIV infection on intrauterine and postnatal growth and body composition as indicators of the nutritional status.

Intrauterine Growth

Children born to HIV-infected mothers are at an increased risk for intrauterine growth retardation, low birthweight ($<$ 2,500 g), and prematurity (gestational age below week 37). Brocklehurst and French recently published a meta-analysis of 31 prospective studies comparing the outcome of pregnancy among HIV-infected mothers with that of noninfected mothers (89). All 17 studies, from both developed and developing settings, included reported risk estimates above unity for the analysis of low birthweight; the summary odds ratio indicates a statistically significant twofold increased risk for low birthweight associated with maternal HIV infection. Increased risk of preterm delivery was reported in 18 of 22 studies; overall, children born to infected women had an 80% excess risk of birth before term as compared with those from uninfected mothers. Confounding and several other biases were not ruled out as potentially having distorted the associations in some studies. However, the summary estimates were consistent with those reported in the best controlled studies, such as that conducted by Bulterys *et al.* in a rural area of Rwanda (90), who adjusted for sociodemographic and sexual history variables. In that study, babies from infected mothers were found to have also lower crown-to-heel length, head circumference, and chest circumference.

The difference in birth outcomes between infected and uninfected mothers may be partially attributed to the negative influences of HIV infection on the mother's health. *In utero* transmission of HIV infection is another important factor in the cause of fetal growth retardation. This is supported by the findings of the study from Rwanda mentioned above, where birthweight, head circumference, ponderal index, and weight-to-head circumference ratio were significantly lower in infants who were HIV positive than in uninfected babies of HIV-positive mothers after adjusting for a number of potential confounding covariates. No difference was found between the anthropometric variables of uninfected newborns from positive mothers and those from negative women (91). Small differences in gestational age at delivery between infected and uninfected babies did not account for the difference in birthweight.

Postnatal Anthropometric Measurements

The growth pattern of children—as measured by their expected trajectories of HAZ, WAZ, and weight-for-height (WHZ)—is often impaired during HIV infection (92,93). No differences in the growth pattern of infants born to HIV-negative women and those uninfected born to HIV-positive mothers (seroreverters) have been observed (55,56,94).

Early reports on growth alterations came from studies of prepubertal boys with hemophilia in which asymptomatic carriers of HIV were found to have a decrement of 25 centile units of HAZ compared with uninfected hemophiliacs (95). Most studies conducted subsequently among hemophiliacs have confirmed these results (57,96,97).

In the United States "Women and Infants Transmission Study" (WITS) among 282 children born to HIV-positive mothers and followed through 18 months of age, the mean values for all growth outcomes (WAZ, HAZ, WHZ, and head circumference-for-age Z-score) were lower in infected than in uninfected infants. These results were adjusted for potential confounders including the child's gender; maternal alcohol, cigarette, and drugs consumption during pregnancy; mother's education; and mean prenatal CD4 count (98). HIV infection was associated with a progressive decrease in weight and length: on average, infected infants were 0.28 kg lighter and 1.64 cm shorter at birth than exposed but uninfected infants; by 18 months, the respective figures were 0.71 kg and 2.25 cm. Body mass index of children decreased progressively from birth through 6 months and then increased until 12 months of age (98). In another prospective study from Boston among children born to infected mothers, infected children had a mean WAZ of -0.68 at 20 months of age, 0.80 Z-score units significantly lower than that of infants who remained seronegative. WHZ (-0.11 vs 0.55) and HAZ (-0.81 vs -0.50) were also lower in the group of infected children. None of the children had received retroviral therapy or supplemental feeding and all were considered *relatively healthy* on the grounds of their CD4 counts ($> 1,000$ cells/mm^3) (99).

In two studies among children from Uganda and Rwanda, HIV infection was associated with undernutrition. Berhane *et al.* (55), following Ugandan children from birth to 2 years of age, found that WAZ and HAZ curves were lower for the 84 HIV positive than for the 251 seroreverters and the 124 HIV-negative children. No differences were observed in the distribution of potential confounders such as Apgar score, gender, socioeconomic status, breast-feeding, and ethnic group among comparison groups. In a longitudinal study of children in Rwanda who were followed from birth to 4 years, WAZ and HAZ mean scores were lower among infected children than among uninfected ones; however, mean WHZ did not differ between the two groups (56).

Body Composition

Weight loss in HIV infection can occur as an unexplained phenomenon or as the result of concomitant disease. Fluctuations in total weight can represent alterations in the fat stores, hydration status, as well as changes in body cell mass. Because it is possible to lose lean cell mass without losing fat and with no alteration of total weight (100), it is important to use measurements of body composition other than simply body weight.

Very few studies have attempted to determine the changes in lean body mass in HIV-infected children. In the Boston-based study (99), arm muscle circumference at age 19 to 21 months was lower in infected children (43rd centile) compared with uninfected children (64th centile). Triceps skinfold thickness was similar between the two groups at baseline. However, an accelerated decline in fat stores (as measured by the triceps skinfold thickness) was observed after 19 to 21 months in the infected children, whereas the noninfected group experienced accelerated growth in muscle stores (according to arm muscle circumference).

Henderson et al., in a cross-sectional study of 42 asymptomatic children between 2 and 11 years of age, found that lean body mass, estimated by two methods (arm muscle area and deuterium oxide dilution), was significantly lower in HIV-infected children with growth retardation (defined using HAZ-score and WHZ-score) than in nongrowth-retarded, HIV-infected and HIV-negative children (101). Nevertheless, the decrease in lean body mass was proportional to a decrease in total body water and fat mass, suggesting that HIV-infected children did not spare fat in relation to lean body mass.

In adults, results from cross-sectional studies on body composition changes during HIV infection yielded divergent results. Some of them suggested that HIV-infected patients were in a catabolic state in which fat mass was preserved at the expense of lean body mass (100,102), whereas others reported an important depletion of fat in HIV-positive subjects compared with negative controls (103,104). The pattern of weight loss and weight gain in HIV infection has been shown to be episodic in the long term, and related to the occurrence and recovery from opportunistic infections (105). Thus, cross-sectional results may not reflect accurately the behavior of weight components during HIV infection. Paton et al. studied longitudinally the change in the weight components of 21 male patients with HIV, comparing different techniques for the analysis of body composition (skinfold thickness, dual energy x-ray absorptiometry, total body water, and bioelectrical impedance) (106). They reported that 55% to 60% of the weight loss of patients during follow-up corresponded to loss of fat-free mass, a proportion compatible with starvation rather than with a cachectic or catabolic process. Weight loss in these patients was associated with cytomegalovirus (CMV) infection, other diarrheal disease, and malignancies. These results, however, do not imply that wasting in HIV infection is always the result of starvation. The energy balance may play a fundamental role on body composition and will be discussed later. Changes in body composition during HIV infection have been reported to differ by gender. In a retrospective, cross-sectional study of 1,415 subjects, Kotler et al. found that body cell mass and fat-free mass, measured by bioelectrical impedance analysis, were significantly higher in men than in women infected with HIV in populations from Zaire as well as the United States (107). In men, one half of the difference in body weight between HIV-infected and control groups was attributable to the change in fat-free mass, whereas in women only approximately 20% to 30% of the difference was related to changes in lean body mass. The findings were in agreement with previous studies conducted among HIV-infected women that reported earlier or greater loss of body fat (108) than reported for men (104). It is suggested that HIV infection induces a state of secondary hypogonadism that results in a disproportionate loss of cell mass in men and fat mass in women, until the body converges on a common composition, reflecting the lack of action of sex hormones (107). Alternatively, higher loss of fat among women may be the consequence of a pre-existing higher content of body fat in women than in men.

Potential Mechanisms

Various mechanisms play a role in the cause of malnutrition during HIV infection, including energy balance, food intake, nutrient malabsorption, and cytokines, as well as hormonal changes.

Energy Balance

From the thermodynamic point of view, it has been proposed that wasting is the result of an imbalance between energy intake and expenditure in which an energy deficit is compensated by catabolism of body mass (109). Thus, both energy intake and expenditure should be examined in reviewing the pathophysiology of HIV-associated wasting. Most of the discussion will be based on studies conducted in adults, as research on energy balance of children infected with HIV is very limited.

Several studies have shown that resting energy expenditure (REE) in persons with HIV infection is between 3% and 34% higher than expected (103,110–116). This increment seems to be more important as the infection becomes symptomatic (115) and when secondary infections or malnutrition are present (110,111,115). An important recent finding by Mulligan *et al.* (117) is that REE is highly correlated to the HIV viral load ($r = 0.4$), indicating that the increment in REE may be part of the response to HIV replication or the result of an increased immune reaction in seropositive individuals.

However, not all the studies have produced similar results. Some have shown that HIV-infected adults seem to be in a hypometabolic state (118), whereas in others no difference in the REE was reported among infected and uninfected individuals (119). This inconsistency in results from metabolic studies may, in part, be attributable to a very important degree of between-person variability in REE among HIV-infected people (120). Even though hypermetabolism is a potential contributor to a state of negative energy balance, it has not been correlated with weight loss in HIV infection. Grunfeld *et al.*, comparing groups of HIV-infected patients, all of whom had a raised REE, showed that weight loss occurred only in AIDS patients with secondary infections who had lower energy intake (115). Macallan *et al.* reported that despite the increase in resting energy expenditure during weight loss in HIV infection, total energy expenditure was reduced, probably because as the general health status worsens, the level of physical activity tends to decrease (121). The estimate of activity energy expenditure was indeed lower in patients losing weight. In this study, energy intake again was markedly reduced during periods of weight loss.

Conclusions from the metabolic studies in adults cannot be automatically applied to children, because a proportion of the energy requirements is invested in growth. Miller *et al.* showed that infected infants who were in class P2 of HIV disease had lower arm muscle circumference and a concomitantly lower protein intake compared with children who seroreverted. The total energy intake was equivalent in the two groups (122). Henderson *et al.*, in a cross-sectional study (101), reported that HIV-positive children with growth retardation had a nonsignificant 16% higher mean value of REE than seronegative children. The lack of significance was attributed to small statistical power and increased between-person variability in the HIV-infected group. They also reported that increased resting energy expenditure was associated with reduced HAZ and WAZ scores. It was suggested that hypermetabolism may be a contributing factor to growth failure, a hypothesis that should be tested in further longitudinal designs.

Food Intake

Diminished dietary intake during HIV infection can occur through several mechanisms. The upper gastrointestinal tract is affected by HIV-related conditions in up to 70% of children (123). Infections by *Candida albicans*, CMV, and herpes simplex virus can cause ulcers and inflammation that produce pain with chewing or swallowing. Unexplained ulcers and acid-related lesions are also possible (124). Dysgeusia can be a consequence of zinc deficiency or administration of drugs. Local HIV infection of the esophagus can produce ulcers that manifest with severe odynophagia (125). Secondary anorexia could occur from secondary infections or malabsorption. Nausea, vomiting, and early satiety can be caused by pancreatic or biliary tract dysfunction or alterations in the gastric emptying rate. Depression has also been described as a factor for decreased food intake in HIV-positive patients (126), and disease of the central nervous system can affect the eating mechanics.

Nutrient Malabsorption

Inadequate absorption of nutrients, which is very common during HIV infection, contributes to further deterioration of the nutritional status, as well as to worsening the quality of life, through the generation of new secondary symptoms such as diarrhea, anorexia, and vomiting. The degree of malabsorption is usually related to the clinical stage of the disease and to the degree of immunosuppression, being more severe in advanced AIDS than in stable, uncomplicated HIV infection (127). In adults, the most common alteration related to malabsorption is enterocyte injury (128), usually as a result of intestinal infection with the *Cryptosporidium*, *Microsporidia*, and *Isospora* (129–133). The infection results in a net decrease of the functional absorptive area of the mucosa and a disproportionate acceleration in the replacement rate of enterocytes, which perform immaturely. Various morphologic changes occur in the small intestinal mucosa. The disaccharidase-specific activities in the brush border are diminished, particularly lactase-specific activity (129). In patients with AIDS and cryptosporidiosis, absorption of protein and fat is reduced in approximately 20% and 27%, respectively (128), which accounts for an energy deficit of 250 kcal/d. Infections with other agents such as *Escherichia coli* may also contribute to the malabsorptive state in AIDS by altering the absorption of bile salts in the ileum (134). In patients with AIDS and the *Mycobacterium avium* complex, absorption of chylomicrons is blocked by infected macrophages that invade the intestinal lamina propria and lymphatics. This results in loss of apoproteins as well as fat

(128). Fat malabsorption is associated with impaired absorption and, hence, deficiencies of fat-soluble vitamins, including vitamins A and E. HIV epithelial changes also result in reduced absorption of water-soluble vitamins, particularly vitamin B_{12} (135).

In children infected with HIV, persistent diarrhea is at least six times more prevalent than in HIV-negative children (136). Chronic diarrhea is accompanied by malabsorption in a significant proportion of cases, usually as a consequence of infection. Among HIV-infected children, malabsorption of carbohydrate, fat, and protein is prevalent (32%, 30%, and 17%, respectively) (137). Lactose malabsorption has been reported in 40% of HIV-infected children without a demonstrable pathogen and occurs earlier than when it affects uninfected children (138). The risk of lactose malabsorption at 36 months of age was estimated to be seven times greater for HIV-infected children than for uninfected controls (138). The prevalence of lactose intolerance seems to increase with the severity of the infection, reaching 75% in children at stage P2 (139). Disaccharide intolerance in these children is frequently associated with chronic diarrhea, even in the absence of enteric pathogens (140). Also, in the apparent absence of opportunistic infections, children with AIDS have been reported to have a deficiency of pancreatic enzymes such as elastase and chymotrypsin (141), which induces steatorrhea and worsens the problem of fat and protein absorption. Treatment of infections by *Microsporidium*, CMV, and mycobacteria that cause malabsorption results in weight gain and eventually an increase of lean body mass (133,142,143).

The microorganisms that have been associated more often with gastrointestinal dysfunction in children with AIDS include *Cryptosporidium* (144), *P. carinii*, CMV, herpes simplex virus (145), enteric viruses (137), *Giardia lamblia*, *Mycobacterium avium-intracellulare*, *Clostridium difficile*, salmonellae, shigellae, and *Campylobacter* (146). In uninfected children with an intact immune system, cryptosporidiosis induces crypt hypertrophy, atrophy of villi, and disaccharidase deficiency (147). In HIV-infected children, *Cryptosporidium* infection has been related to secretory diarrhea and subsequent dehydration and weight loss (144).

Cytokines

Cytokines are probably involved in several of the metabolic disturbances that result in altered nutritional status observed during the infection by the HIV. TNF or *cachectin* was first identified as a factor responsible for adipose tissue catabolism, hypertriglyceridemia, and weight loss among individuals with acute infections (148). Increased levels of TNF were reported in patients with AIDS and acute secondary infections (149), but subsequent studies failed to show sustained elevations of the factor along the course of the disease (150,151). Also, only marginal increases of other cytokines (e.g., IL-1, 6, and 8) have been reported among HIV-infected persons (152). In contrast, α-interferon has been found to be persistently elevated among patients with AIDS (153) and TNF receptors increase as disease progresses (154). Interleukin-1β receptor antagonist (interleukin-1Ra) has been also found at high levels among asymptomatic HIV-infected men (155) and women (152,155).

The experimental administration of TNF to human volunteers has resulted in anorexia and cachexia (156). In HIV-infected patients, increased concentrations of TNF receptors have been associated with nutritional markers. Suttmann *et al.*, in a cross-sectional analysis of data from 45 HIV-infected patients, found positive correlations between the level of sTNFR 55, a TNF receptor, and the ratio of extracellular to body cell mass (157). The rate of recent weight loss (> 5%) was also positively associated with the receptor levels. The concentration of sTNFR 55 correlated negatively with serum albumin and prealbumin levels. Arnalich *et al.* also found increased levels of TNF and TNF receptors among AIDS patients with wasting (158). However, some of the most striking metabolic alterations attributable to TNF activity (e.g., hypertriglyceridemia) do not always correlate with weight loss in patients with AIDS (159). Alpha interferon does correlate with the increased *de novo* lipogenesis and slowed triglyceride clearance observed in patients with AIDS, but it may be simply an indicator of viral activation (151).

Some of the effects of cytokines during HIV infection would include inducing anorexia; keeping protein and energy away from cell mass and shunting them into fat synthesis, thus causing wasteful energy expenditure; accelerating protein breakdown; and increasing viral replication. These mechanisms have been extensively reviewed in recently published papers (124,143,160–165). Identifying the causal pathways and precise links has yet to be done.

Various cytokine inhibitors have been found to induce weight gain and appetite, as recently reviewed by Balog *et al.* (166). Thalidomide inhibits TNF-α, increases body weight, and may also be related to an increase in muscle mass. Dietary supplementation with fish oil is associated with a reduction in tryglycerides and TNF-α production, but not with an increase in body weight (167). Pentoxifylline seems to lower the concentration of cytokines, but has not been useful in increasing weight or appetite. *N*-acetylcysteine is another inhibitor of TNF-α with a potential effect on the wasting syndrome. Clinical trials are being carried out to test the efficacy and safety of these and other agents.

Hormonal Changes

The most frequently described hormonal dysfunction in HIV infection and AIDS is a low concentration of serum testosterone (168) that may be the result of either hypogonadotropic hypogonadism or primary testicular dysfunction (143). Hypogonadism is correlated with poor prognosis in AIDS patients in terms of weight loss, reduction in lymphocyte counts, progression of the disease, and increased mortality, as reviewed by Strawford and Hellerstein (160). Loss of lean body mass and impairment in exercise capacity are correlated with androgen levels (169).

Compounds with anabolic properties have the ability to increase muscle mass. Testosterone deficiency is common in people with the HIV wasting syndrome. Some recently published randomized clinical trials suggest a positive effect of testosterone on body mass. In male patients with AIDS whose body weight was less than 90% of ideal, intramuscular testosterone injections (300 mg every 3 weeks for 6 months) produced a significant increase of fat-free mass, lean body mass, and muscle mass relative to the placebo group, without changing total body weight or fat mass (170). Reported quality of life also improved among patients treated with testosterone. In women with AIDS wasting, abdominal testosterone patches have been found to increase serum levels of the hormone and total weight after 12 weeks of administration (171).

Alterations in the thyroid function are common, often as a result of opportunistic infections or neoplasms (172). Thyroid function abnormalities, particularly hypothyroidism, have also been found in a series of HIV-infected children (173). A paradoxical elevation of triiodothyronine (T3) with low levels of reverse triiodothyronine (rT3) has been suggested as an inadequate adaptation to energy deprivation during some periods of the infection (143). Results on the levels of thyroid hormones across different studies have been conflicting (174) and the link between the thyroid function and wasting-related HIV or AIDS is still unclear. Adrenal insufficiency has been also found among patients with AIDS, which has been attributed to the acute effect of infections or drugs (143).

Resistance to growth hormone has been reported during AIDS wasting, leading to decreased levels of insulinlike growth factors (IGF) (175). However, growth hormone deficiency has not been demonstrated during HIV infection (143). Growth hormone acts by stimulating the synthesis of IGF. Besides its effect on linear growth, growth hormone promotes insulin release, protein anabolism, and mobilization of free fatty acids, and inhibits glucose uptake into the tissues. Early studies indicated the potential effect of growth hormone on the AIDS wasting syndrome. In a large, randomized, controlled trial among 178 patients with wasting, growth hormone supplementation resulted in significant weight gain, increase in lean body mass, and a reduction of 1.7 in body fat (176). Treadmill work output was also incremented among treated patients. No improvement was seen in quality of life indicators. The main adverse effects were swelling and puffiness, arthralgia, myalgia, and diarrhea, but the withdrawal rates were similar in both treatment and placebo groups. Combined treatment with both growth hormone and IGF-1 has not been shown to be advantageous in terms of gain of lean body mass over administration of growth hormone alone (177). Resistance to growth hormone in AIDS-related wasting, short-term duration of the trials, lack of knowledge of the effect on women, the possibility of adverse effects in the long term, and high costs are all factors that prevent the utilization of growth hormone as the first therapy for wasting associated with HIV infection.

Leptin, the product of the *ob* gene, secreted by adipocytes, is known to increase after the administration of TNF and IL-1 in animals, perhaps as an effect of the cytokines on adipocyte gene expression (178). TNF also prevents the normal decrease in leptin concentration that is expected during fasting (179). However, leptin has not been found to be raised in male patients with HIV infection or AIDS (180,181). Dysregulation in the secretion of neuropeptides is another potential mechanism involved in the appetite loss observed in HIV infection. Higher levels of plasma cholecystokinin and decreased concentrations of endorphin have been found in patients with HIV-associated wasting (158).

CONCLUSIONS

We have discussed published reports on the potential role of nutritional status in modulating HIV disease progression and transmission, and the mechanisms that could play a role in this. We have also reviewed the evidence that HIV infection is associated with higher risks of undernutrition, and the mechanisms that mediate this relationship. Antiretroviral drugs, including protease inhibitors and reverse transcriptase inhibitors, given to HIV-infected children have resulted in improvements in nutritional status, including weight gain (182–185). The efficacy of hormonal and cytokine therapy is being examined in a number of studies. However, these agents are expensive for use on a wide scale among infected children and adults in developing countries. The effect of relatively more cost-effective interventions, including micronutrient supplements and preventive measures against opportunistic infections, are being tested.

REFERENCES

1. Prazuck T, Tall F, Nacro B, et al. HIV infection and severe malnutrition: a clinical and epidemiological study in Burkina Faso. *AIDS* 1993; 7: 103–8.
2. De Cock KM, Odehouri K, Colebunders RL, et al. A comparison of HIV-1 and HIV-2 infections in hospitalized patients in Abidjan, Cote d'Ivoire. *AIDS* 1990; 4: 443–8.
3. Lesbordes JL, Coulaud B, Georges AJ. Malnutrition et virus de l'immunodeficience humaine (VIH) a Bangui (Centrafrique). Etude et suivi d'une cohorte de 175 enfants denutris et de 101 meres pendant 2 ans. *Med Trop* (Mars) 1990; 50: 161–5.
4. Mgone CS, Mhalu FS, Shao JD, et al. Prevalence of HIV-1 infection and symptomatology of AIDS in severely malnourished children in Dar es Salaam, Tanzania. *J Acquir Immune Defic Syndr Hum Retrovirol* 1991; 4: 910–13.
5. Mutombo T, Keusse J, Sangare A. SIDA et malnutrition en milieu pediatrique semi-rural ivoirien. *Med Trop* (Mars) 1995; 55: 357–9.
6. Beach RS, Mantero-Atienza E, Shor-Posner G, et al. Specific nutrient abnormalities in asymptotic HIV-1 infection. *AIDS* 1992; 6: 701–8.
7. Karter DL, Karter AJ, Yarrish R, et al. Vitamin A deficiency in non-vitamin-supplemented patients with AIDS: a cross-sectional study. *J Acquir Immune Defic Syndr Hum Retrovirol* 1995; 8: 199–203.
8. Baum MK, Mantero-Atienza E, Shor-Posner G, et al. Association of vitamin B_6 status with parameters of immune function in early HIV-1 infection. *J Acquir Immune Defic Syndr Hum Retrovirol* 1991; 4: 1122–32.
9. Periquet BA, Jammes NM, Lambert WE, et al. Micronutrient levels in HIV-1 infected children. *AIDS* 1995; 9: 887–93.
10. Keusch GT, Farthing MJ. Nutritional aspects of AIDS. *Annu Rev Nutr* 1990; 10: 475–501.
11. Semba RD, Miotti PG, Chipangwi JD, et al. Infant mortality and maternal vitamin A deficiency during human immunodeficiency virus infection. *Clin Infect Dis* 1995; 21: 966–72.
12. Read JS, Bethel J, Harris DR, et al. Serum vitamin A concentrations in a North American cohort of human immunodeficiency virus type 1-infected children. *Pediatr Infect Dis J* 1999; 18: 134–42.
13. Semba RD, Miotti PG, Chipangwi JD, et al. Maternal vitamin A deficiency and mother-to-child transmission of HIV-1. *Lancet* 1994; 343: 1593–7.
14. Dushimimana A, Graham NM, Humphrey JH, et al. Maternal vitamin A levels and HIV-related birth outcome in Rwanda. In: *Programs and abstracts of the Eighth International Conference on AIDS/Third STD World Conference*. Amsterdam, July 19–24, 1992: Abstract No. Poc4221.

15. Landesman S. Presentation at a forum entitled "Vitamin A relationships to mortality in HIV disease and effects on HIV infection: recent and late breaking studies." Lawton Chiles International House, National Institutes of Health, Bethesda, May 16, 1996.

16. Greenberg BL, Semba RD, Vink PE, et al. Vitamin A deficiency and maternal-infant transmission of HIV in two metropolitan areas in the United States. *AIDS* 1997; 11: 325–32.

17. Burger H, Kovacs A, Weister B, et al. Maternal serum vitamin A levels are not associated with mother-to-child transmission of HIV-1 in the United States. *J Acquir Immune Defic Syndr Hum Retrovirol* 1997; 14: 321–6.

18. Filteau SM, Morris SS, Abbott RA, et al. Influence of morbidity on serum retinol of children in a community-based study in northern Ghana. *Am J Clin Nutr* 1993; 58: 192–7.

19. Fawzi WW, Msamanga GI, Spiegelman D, et al. Randomized trial of effects of vitamin supplements on pregnancy outcomes and T cell counts in HIV-1-infected women in Tanzania. *Lancet* 1998; 351: 1477–82.

20. Fawzi WW, Mbise RL, Hertzmark E, et al. A randomized trial of vitamin A supplements in relation to mortality among HIV infected and uninfected children in Tanzania. *Pediatr Infect Dis J* 1999; 18: 127–33.

21. Coutsoudis A, Boba RA, Coovadia HM, Kuhn L, Tsai WY, Stein ZA. The effects of vitamin A supplementation on the morbidity of children born to HIV infected women. *Am J Public Health* 1995; 85: 1076–81.

22. Villalpando S, Hamosh M. Early and late effects of breast-feeding: does breast-feeding really matter? *Biol Neonate* 1998; 74: 177–91.

23. Dermer A. Breastfeeding and women's health. *J Womens Health* 1998; 7: 427–33.

24. Rogran WJ, Gladen BC. Breast-feeding and cognitive development. *Early Hum Dev* 1993; 31: 181–93.

25. Gordon N. Nutrition and cognitive function. *Brain Dev* 1997; 19: 165–70.

26. Dunn DT, Newell ML, Ades AE, Peckham CS. Risk of human immunodeficiency virus type 1 transmission through breastfeeding. *Lancet* 1992; 340: 585–8.

27. Bobat R, Moodley D, Coutsoudis A, Coovadia H. Breastfeeding by HIV-1-infected women and outcome of their infants: a cohort study from Durban, South Africa. *AIDS* 1997; 11: 1627–33.

28. Bryson YJ. Perinatal HIV-1 transmission: recent advances and therapeutic interventions. *AIDS* 1996; 10: S33–42.

29. Bryson YJ, Luzuriaga K, Sullivan JL, Wara DW. Proposed definitions for in utero versus intrapartum transmission of HIV-1. *N Engl J Med* 1992; 327: 1246–7.

30. Leroy V, Newell M-L, Dabis F, et al. International multicentre pooled analysis of late postnatal mother-to-child transmission of HIV-1 infection. *Lancet* 1998; 352: 597–600.

31. Bertolli J, St Louis ME, Simonds RJ, et al. Estimating the timing of mother-to-child transmission of human immunodeficiency virus in a breast-feeding population in Kinshasa, Zaire. *J Infect Dis* 1996; 174: 722–6.

32. Lallemant M, Le Coeur S, Samba L, et al. Mother-to-child transmission of HIV-1 in Congo, central Africa. Congolese Research Group on Mother-to-Child Transmission of HIV. *AIDS* 1994; 8: 1451–6.

33. Bulterys M, Chao A, Dushimimana A. HIV-1 seroconversion after 20 months of age in a cohort of breastfed children born to HIV-1-infected women in Rwanda. *AIDS* 1995; 9: 93–4.

34. Datta P, Embree JE, Kreiss JK, et al. Mother-to-child transmission of human immunodeficiency virus type 1: report from the Nairobi Study. *J Infect Dis* 1994; 170: 1134–40.

35. UNAIDS. *HIV and infant feeding: a guide for health managers and supervisors.* Geneva: UNAIDS, 1998.

36. Orloff SL, Wallingford JC, McDougal JS. Inactivation of human immunodeficiency virus type 1 in human milk: effects of intrinsic factors in human milk and of pasteurization. *J Hum Lact* 1993; 167: 13–17.

37. Abrams B, Duncan D, Hertz-Picciotto I. A prospective study of dietary intake and acquired immune deficiency syndrome in HIV-seropositive homosexual men. *J Acquir Immune Defic Syndr Hum Retrovirol* 1993; 6: 949–58.

38. Tang AM, Graham NMH, Kirby AJ, McCall AD, Willett WC, Saah AJ. Dietary micronutrient intake and risk progression to acquired immunodeficiency syndrome (AIDS) in human immunodeficiency virus type 1 (HIV-1)-infected homosexual men. *Am J Epidemiol* 1993; 138: 1–15.

39. Tang AM, Graham NMH, Saah AJ. Effects of micronutrient intake on survival in human immunodeficiency virus type 1 infection. *Am J Epidemiol* 1996; 143: 1244–56.

40. Semba RD, Graham NMH, Caiaffa WT, Margolick JB, Clement L, Vlahov D. Increased mortality associated with vitamin A deficiency during human immunodeficiency virus type 1 infection. *Arch Intern Med* 1993; 153: 2149–54.

41. Semba RD, Caiaffa WT, Graham NMH, Cohn S, Valahov D. Vitamin A deficiency and wasting as predictors of mortality in human immunodeficiency virus-infected injection drug users. *J Infect Dis* 1994; 171: 1196–202.

42. Baum MK, Shor-Posner G, Lu Y, et al. Micronutrients and HIV-1 disease progression. *AIDS* 1995; 9: 1051–6.

43. Tang AM, Graham NMH, Semba RD, Saah AJ. Association between serum vitamin A and E levels and HIV-1 disease progression. *AIDS* 1997; 11: 613–20.

44. Tang AM, Graham NMH, Chandra RK, Saah AJ. Low serum vitamin B-12 concentrations are associated with faster human immunodeficiency virus type 1 (HIV-1) disease progression. *J Nutr* 1997; 127: 345–51.

45. Coodley GO, Nelson HD, Loveless MO, Folk C. β-Carotene in HIV infection. *J Acquir Immune Defic Syndr Hum Retrovirol* 1993; 6: 272–6.

46. Coodley GO, Coodley MK, Lusk R, et al. β-Carotene in HIV infection: an extended evaluation. *AIDS* 1996; 10: 967–73.

47. Coutsoudis A, Moodley D, Pillay K, et al. Effect of vitamin A supplementation on viral load in HIV-1 infected pregnant women. *J Acquir Immune Defic Syndr Hum Retrovirol* 1997; 15: 86–7.

48. Semba RD, Lyles CM, Margolick JB, et al. Vitamin A supplementation and human immunodeficiency virus load in injection drug users. *J Infect Dis* 1998; 177: 611–16.

49. Humphrey JH, Quinn T, Fine D, et al. Short-term effects of large-dose vitamin A supplementation on viral load and immune response in HIV infected women. *J Acquir Immune Defic Syndr Hum Retrovirol* 1999; 20: 44–51.

50. Allard JP, Aghdassi E, Chau J, et al. Effects of vitamin E and C supplementation on oxidative stress and viral load in HIV infected subjects. *AIDS* 1998; 12: 1653–9.

51. Constans J, Pellegrin J-L, Sergeant C, et al. Serum selenium predicts outcome in HIV infection. *J Acquir Immune Defic Syndr Hum Retrovirol* 1995; 10: 392.

52. Baum MK, Shor-Posner G, Lai S, et al. High risk of HIV-related mortality is associated with selenium deficiency. *J Acquir Immune Defic Syndr Hum Retrovirol* 1997; 15: 370–4.

53. Moseson M, Seleniuch-Jacquotte A, Belsito DV, Shore RE, Marmor M, Pasternack B. The potential role of nutritional factors in the induction of immunologic abnormalities in HIV-positive homosexual men. *J Acquir Immune Defic Syndr Hum Retrovirol* 1989; 2: 235–47.

54. Graham N, Sorensen D, Odaka N, et al. Relationship of serum copper and zinc levels to HIV-1 seropositivity and progression to AIDS. *J Acquir Immune Defic Syndr Hum Retrovirol* 1991; 4: 976–80.

55. Berhane R, Bagenda D, Marum L, et al. Growth failure as a prognostic indicator of mortality in pediatric HIV infection. *Pediatrics* 1997; 100: e7.

56. Lepage P, Msellati P, Hitimana DG, et al. Growth of human immunodeficiency type 1-infected and uninfected children: a prospective cohort study in Kigali, Rwanda, 1988 to 1993. *Pediatr Infect Dis J* 1996; 15: 479–85.

57. Brettler DB, Forsberg A, Bolívar E, Brewster F, Sullivan J. Growth failure as a prognostic indicator for progression to acquired immunodeficiency syndrome in children with hemophilia. *J Pediatr* 1990; 117: 584–8.

58. Tovo PA, de Martino M, Gabiano C, Capello M, D'Elia R, Loy A. Prognostic factors and survival in children with perinatal HIV-1 infection. *Lancet* 1992; 339: 1249–53.

59. Thea DM, St Louis ME, Atido U, et al. A prospective study of diarrhea and HIV-1 infection among 429 Zairian infants. *N Engl J Med* 1993; 329: 1696–702.

60. Volberding P, Kaslow K, Bilk M. Prognostic factors in staging Kaposi's sarcoma in AIDS. *Proc Am Soc Clin Oncol* 1984; 3: 51.

61. Chlebowski RT, Grosvenor MB, Bernhard NH, Morales LS, Bulcavage L. Nutritional status, gastrointestinal dysfunction, and survival in patients with AIDS. *Am J Gastroenterol* 1989; 84: 1288–93.

62. Guenter P, Muurahainen N, Simons G, et al. Relationships among nutritional status, disease progression, and survival in HIV infection. *J Acquir Immune Defic Syndr Hum Retrovirol* 1993; 6: 1130–8.

63. Lindan CP, Allen S, Serufilira A, et al. Predictors of mortality among HIV infected women in Kigali, Rwanda. *Ann Intern Med* 1992; 116: 320–8.

64. Kotler DP, Tierney AR, Wang J, Pierson RNJ. Magnitude of body-cell-mass depletion and the timing of death from wasting in AIDS. *Am J Clin Nutr* 1989; 50: 444–7.
65. Suttmann U, Ockenga J, Selberg O, Hoogestraat L, Deicher H, Muller MJ. Incidence and prognostic value of malnutrition and wasting in human immunodeficiency virus-infected outpatients. *J Acquir Immune Defic Syndr Hum Retrovirol* 1995; 8: 239–46.
66. Chandra RK. Effect of vitamin and trace-element supplementation on immune responses and infection in elderly subjects. *Lancet* 1992; 340: 1124–7.
67. Wolbach S, Howe P. Tissue changes following deprivation of fat-soluble A vitamin. *J Exp Med* 1925; 42: 753–77.
68. Chandra RK, Vyas D. Vitamin A, immunocompetence, and infection. *Food Nutr Bull* 1989; 11(3).
69. Prabhala RH, Garewal HS, Hicks MJ, Sampliner RE, Watson RR. The effects of 13-cis-retinoic acid and beta-carotene on cellular immunity in humans. *Cancer* 1991; 67: 1556–60.
70. Watson RR, Prabhala RH, Plezia PM, Alberts DS. Effect of β-carotene on lymphocyte sub-populations in elderly humans: evidence for a dose-response relationship. *Am J Clin Nutr* 1991; 53: 90–4.
71. Nakashima H, Harada S, Yamamoto N. Effect of retinoic acid on the replication of human immunodeficiency virus in HTLV-1-positive MT-4 cells. *Med Microbiol Immunol* 1987; 176: 189–98.
72. Loya S, Kashman Y, Hizi A. The carotenoid halocynthiaxanthin: a novel inhibitor of the reverse transcriptases of human immunodeficiency viruses type 1 and type 2. *Arch Biochem Biophys* 1992; 293: 208–12.
73. Watson RR, Yahya MD, Darban HR, Prabhala RH. Enhanced survival by vitamin A supplementation during a retrovirus infection causing murine AIDS. *Life Sci* 1988; 43: xiii–xviii.
74. Benedich A, Cohen M. B vitamins: effects on specific and nonspecific immune responses. In: Chandra RK, Alan R, eds. *Nutrition and immunology*. New York: Liss, 1988: 101–23.
75. Meydani SN, Ribaya-Mercado JD, Russell RM, Sahyoun N, Morrow FD, Gershoff SN. Vitamin B-6 deficiency impairs interleukin 2 production and lymphocyte proliferation in elderly adults. *Am J Clin Nutr* 1991; 53: 1275–80.
76. Roubenoff R, Roubenoff RA, Selhub J, et al. Abnormal vitamin B_6 in rheumatoid cachexia. Association with TNF-α production and markers of inflammation. *Arthritis Rheum* 1995; 39: 105–9.
77. Benedich A. Antioxidant vitamins and immune responses. In: Chandra RK, Alan R, eds. *Nutrition and immunology*. New York: Liss, 1988: 125–47.
78. Winklohofer-Roob BM, Ellemunter H, Frühwirth M, et al. Plasma vitamin C concentrations in patients with cystic fibrosis: evidence of associations with lung inflammation. *Am J Clin Nutr* 1997; 65: 1858–66.
79. Harakeh S, Jariwall RJ, Pauling L. Suppression of human immunodeficiency virus replication by ascorbate in chronically infected cells. *Proc Natl Acad Sci USA* 1990; 87: 7245–9.
80. Harakeh S, Jariwalla RJ. Comparative study of the anti-HIV activities of ascorbate and thiol-containing reducing agents in chronically HIV infected cells. *Am J Clin Nutr* 1991; 54: 1231–5S.
81. Meydani SN, Wu D, Santos MS, Hayek MG. Antioxidants and immune response in the aged: overview of present evidence. *Am J Clin Nutr* 1995; 62 (Suppl.):1462–76S.
82. Meydani SN, Meydani M, Blumberg JB, et al. Vitamin E supplementation enhances in vivo immune response in healthy elderly: a dose-response study. *JAMA* 1997; 277: 1380–6.
83. Wang Y, Huang DS, Wood S, Watson RR. Modulation of immune function and cytokine production by various levels of vitamin E supplementation during murine AIDS. *Immunopharmacology* 1995; 29: 225–33.
84. Kuhn RH. Effect of locally applied vitamin A and estrogen on the rat vagina. *Am J Anat* 1954; 95: 309–28.
85. John GC, Nduati RW, Mbori-Ngacha D, et al. Genital shedding of human immunodeficiency virus type 1 DNA during pregnancy: association with immunosuppression, abnormal cervical or vaginal discharge, and severe vitamin A deficiency. *J Infect Dis* 1997; 175: 57–62.
86. Mostad SB, Overbaugh J, DeVange DM, et al. Hormonal contraception, vitamin A deficiency, and other risk factors for shedding of HIV-1 infected cells from the cervix and vagina. *Lancet* 1997; 350: 922–7.
87. Noback CR, Takahashi YI. Micromorphology of the placenta of rats reared on marginal vitamin-A-deficient diet. *Acta Anat* 1978; 102: 195–202.
88. Nduati RW, John GC, Richardson BA, et al. Human immunodeficiency virus type-1 infected cells in breast milk: association with immunosuppression and vitamin A deficiency. *J Infect Dis* 1995; 172: 1461–8.

89. Brocklehurst P, French R. The association between maternal HIV infection and perinatal outcome: a systematic review of the literature and meta-analysis. *Br J Obstet Gynaecol* 1998; 105: 836–48.

90. Bulterys M, Chao A, Munyemana S, et al. Maternal human immunodeficiency virus 1 infection and intrauterine growth: a prospective cohort study in Butare, Rwanda. *Pediatr Infect Dis J* 1994; 13: 94–100.

91. Weng S, Bulterys M, Chao A, et al. Perinatal human immunodeficiency virus-1 transmission and intrauterine growth: a cohort study in Butare, Rwanda. *Pediatrics* 1998; 102: e24.

92. McKinney RE, Robertson WR. Effect of human immunodeficiency virus infection on the growth of young children. *J Pediatr* 1993; 123: 579–82.

93. Saavedra JM, Henderson RA, Perman JA, Hutton N, Livingston RA, Yolken RH. Longitudinal assessment of growth in children born to mothers with human immunodeficiency virus infection. *Arch Pediatr Adolesc Med* 1995; 149: 497–502.

94. Halsey NA, Boulos R, Holt E, et al. Transmission of HIV-1 infections from mothers to infants in Haiti. *JAMA* 1990; 264: 2088–92.

95. Jason J, Gomperts E, Lawrence DN, et al. HIV and hemophilic children's growth. *J Acquir Immune Defic Syndr Hum Retrovirol* 1989; 2: 277–82.

96. Gomperts ED. HIV infection in hemophiliac children: clinical manifestations and therapy. *Am J Pediatr Hematol Oncol* 1990; 12: 497–504.

97. Kaufman FR, Gomperts ED. Growth failure in boys with hemophilia and HIV infection. *Am J Pediatr Hematol Oncol* 1989; 11: 292–4.

98. Moye JJ, Rich KC, Kalish LA, et al. Natural history of somatic growth in infants born to women infected by human immunodeficiency virus. *J Pediatr* 1996; 128: 58–69.

99. Miller TL, Evans SJ, Orav EJ, Morris V, McIntosh K, Winter HS. Growth and body composition in children infected with the human immunodeficiency virus-1. *Am J Clin Nutr* 1993; 57: 588–92.

100. Ott M, Lembcke B, Fischer H, et al. Early changes of body composition in human immunodeficiency virus-infected patients: tetrapolar body impedance analysis indicates significant malnutrition. *Am J Clin Nutr* 1993; 57: 15–19.

101. Henderson RA, Talusan K, Hutton N, Yolken RH, Caballero B. Resting energy expenditure and body composition in children with HIV infection. *J Acquir Immune Defic Syndr Hum Retrovirol* 1998; 19: 150–7.

102. Kotler DP, Wang J, Pierson RN. Body composition studies in patients with the acquired immunodeficiency syndrome. *Am J Clin Nutr* 1985; 42: 1255–65.

103. Sharpstone DR, Murray C, Ross HM, et al. Energy balance in asymptomatic HIV infection. *AIDS* 1996; 10: 1377–84.

104. Mulligan K, Tai VW, Schambelan M. Cross-sectional and longitudinal evaluation of body composition in men with HIV infection. *J Acquir Immune Defic Syndr Hum Retrovirol* 1997; 15: 43–8.

105. Macallan DC, Noble C, Baldwin C, Foskett M, McManus T, Griffin GE. Prospective analysis of patterns of weight change in stage IV human immunodeficiency virus infection. *Am J Clin Nutr* 1993; 58: 417–24.

106. Paton NIJ, Macallan DC, Jebb SA, et al. Longitudinal changes in body composition measured with a variety of methods in patients with AIDS. *J Acquir Immune Defic Syndr Hum Retrovirol* 1997; 14: 119–27.

107. Kotler DP, Thea DM, Heo M, et al. Relative influences of sex, race, environment and HIV infection on body composition in adults. *Am J Clin Nutr* 1999; 69: 432–9.

108. Grinspoon S, Corcoran C, Miller K, et al. Body composition and endocrine function in women with acquired immunodeficiency syndrome wasting. *J Clin Endocrinol Metab* 1997; 82: 1332–7.

109. Macallan DC. Wasting in HIV infection and AIDS. *J Nutr* 1999; 129: 238–42S.

110. Melchior JC, Salmon D, Rigaud D, et al. Resting energy expenditure is increased in stable, malnourished HIV infected patients. *Am J Clin Nutr* 1991; 53: 437–41.

111. Melchior JC, Raguin G, Boulier A, et al. Resting energy expenditure in human immunodeficiency virus-infected patients: comparison between patients with and without secondary infections. *Am J Clin Nutr* 1993; 57: 614–19.

112. Hommes MJ, Romijn JA, Endert E, Sauerwein HP. Resting energy expenditure and substrate oxidation in human immunodeficiency virus (HIV)-infected asymptomatic men: HIV affects host metabolism in the early asymptomatic stage. *Am J Clin Nutr* 1991; 54: 311–15.

113. Hommes MJ, Romijn JA, Godfried MH, et al. Increased resting energy expenditure in human immunodeficiency virus-infected men. *Metabolism* 1990; 39: 1186–90.

114. Suttmann U, Ockenga J, Hoogestraat L, et al. Resting energy expenditure and weight loss in human immunodeficiency virus-infected patients. *Metabolism* 1993; 42: 1173–9.

115. Grunfeld C, Pang M, Shimizu L, Shigenaga JK, Jensen P, Feingold KR. Resting energy expenditure, caloric intake, and short-term weight change in human immunodeficiency virus infection and the acquired immunodeficiency syndrome. *Am J Clin Nutr* 1992; 55: 455–60.

116. Mulligan K, Grunfeld C, Hellerstein MK, Neese RA, Schambelan M. Anabolic effects of recombinant human growth hormone in patients with wasting associated with human immunodeficiency virus infection. *J Clin Endocrinol Metab* 1993; 77: 956–62.

117. Mulligan K, Tai V, Schambelan M. Energy expenditure in human immunodeficiency virus infection. *N Engl J Med* 1997; 336: 70–1.

118. Kotler DP, Tierney AR, Brenner SK, Couture S, Wang J, Pierson RNJ. Preservation of short-term energy balance in clinically stable patients with AIDS. *Am J Clin Nutr* 1990; 51: 7–13.

119. Sharpstone D, Ross H, Hancock M, Phelan M, Crane R, Gazzard B. Indirect calorimetry, body composition and small bowel function in asymptomatic HIV-seropositive women. *Int J STD AIDS* 1997; 8: 700–3.

120. Schwenk A, Hoffer-Belitz E, Jung B, et al. Resting energy expenditure, weight loss and altered body composition in HIV infection. *Nutrition* 1996; 12: 595–601.

121. Macallan DC, Noble C, Baldwin C, et al. Energy expenditure and wasting in human immunodeficiency virus infection. *N Engl J Med* 1995; 333: 83–8.

122. Miller TL, Evans S, Morris V, Orav EJ, McIntosh K, Winter HS. Prospective study of the alterations in growth and nutritional intake in HIV infected children [Abstract]. *Gastroenterology* 1991; 100: A538.

123. Miller TL, Martin SR, Cooper ER, McIntosh K, Winter HS. Gastrointestinal inflammation and carbohydrate intolerance in HIV infected children. *Pediatr Res* 1990; 27: 650.

124. Miller TL. Malnutrition: metabolic changes in children, comparisons with adults. *J Nutr* 1996; 126: 2623–31S.

125. Kotler DP, Reka S, Orenstein JM, Fox CH. Chronic idiopathic esophageal ulceration in the acquired immunodeficiency syndrome. Characterization and treatment with corticosteroids. *J Clin Gastroenterol* 1992; 15: 284–90.

126. Lyketsos CG, Hoover DR, Guccione M, et al. Depressive symptoms over the course of HIV infection before AIDS. *Soc Psychiatry Psychiatr Epidemiol* 1996; 31: 212–19.

127. Keating J, Bjarnason I, Somasundaram S, et al. Intestinal absorptive capacity, intestinal permeability and jejunal histology in HIV and their relation to diarrhoea. *Gut* 1995; 37: 623–9.

128. Kotler DP. Human immunodeficiency virus-related wasting: malabsorption syndromes. *Semin Oncol* 1998; 25 (2 Suppl. 6): 70–5.

129. Kotler DP, Reka S, Chow K, Orenstein JM. Effects of enteric parasitoses and HIV infection upon small intestinal structure and function in patients with AIDS. *J Clin Gastroenterol* 1993; 16: 10–15.

130. Kelly P, Davies SE, Mandanda B, et al. Enteropathy in Zambians with HIV-related diarrhoea: regression modelling of potential determinants of mucosal damage. *Gut* 1997; 41: 811–16.

131. Papp JPJ, DeYoung BR, Fromkes JJ. Endoscopic appearance of cryptosporidial duodenitis. *Am J Gastroenterol* 1996; 91: 2235–6.

132. Orenstein JM, Chiang J, Steinberg W, Smith PD, Rotterdam H, Kotler DP. Intestinal microsporidiosis as a cause of diarrhea in human immunodeficiency virus-infected patients: a report of 20 cases. *Hum Pathol* 1990; 21: 475–81.

133. Leder K, Ryan N, Spelman D, Crowe SM. Microsporidial disease in HIV infected patients: a report of 42 patients and review of the literature. *Scand J Infect Dis* 1998; 30: 331–8.

134. Kotler DP, Giang TT, Thiim M, Nataro JP, Sordillo EM, Orenstein JM. Chronic bacterial entheropaty in patients with AIDS. *J Infect Dis* 1995; 171: 552–8.

135. Ehrenpreis ED, Carlson SJ, Boorstein HL, Craig RM. Malabsorption and deficiency of vitamin B_{12} in HIV infected patients with chronic diarrhea. *Dig Dis Sci* 1994; 39: 2159–62.

136. Keusch GT, Thea DM, Kamenga M, et al. Persistent diarrhea associated with AIDS. *Acta Paediatr Suppl* 1992; 381: 45–8.

137. Anonymous. Intestinal malabsorption of HIV infected children: relationship to diarrhoea, failure to thrive, enteric micro-organisms and immune impairment. The Italian Paediatric Intestinal/HIV Study Group. *AIDS* 1993; 7: 1435–40.

138. Miller TL, Orav EJ, Martin SR, Cooper ER, McIntosh K, Winter HS. Malnutrition and carbohydrate malabsorption in children with vertically transmitted human immunodeficiency virus-1 infection. *Gastroenterology* 1991; 100: 1296–302.

139. Zuin G, Fontana M, Monti S, Marchisio P, Beretta P, Principi N. Malabsorption of different lactose loads in children with human immunodeficiency virus infection. *J Pediatr Gastroenterol Nutr* 1992; 15: 408–12.

140. Yolken RH, Hart W, Oung I, Shiff C, Greenson J, Perman JA. Gastrointestinal dysfunction and disaccharide intolerance in children infected with human immunodeficiency virus. *J Pediatr* 1991; 118: 359–63.

141. Carroccio A, Fontana M, Spagnuolo MI, et al. Pancreatic dysfunction and its association with fat malabsorption in HIV infected children. *Gut* 1998; 43: 558–63.

142. Kotler DP, Tierney AR, Altilio D, Wang J, Pierson RN. Body mass repletion during ganciclovir treatment of cytomegalovirus infections in patients with acquired immunodeficiency syndrome. *Arch Intern Med* 1989; 149: 901–5.

143. Coodley GO, Loveless MO, Merrill TM. The HIV wasting syndrome: a review. *J Acquir Immune Defic Syndr Hum Retrovirol* 1994; 7: 681–94.

144. Guarino A, Castaldo A, Russo S, et al. Enteric cryptosporidiosis in pediatric HIV infection. *J Pediatr Gastroenterol Nutr* 1997; 25: 182–7.

145. Ramos-Soriano AG, Saavedra JM, Wu TC, et al. Enteric pathogens associated with gastrointestinal dysfunction in children with HIV infection. *Mol Cell Probes* 1996; 10: 67–73.

146. Lewis JD, Winter HS. Intestinal and hepatobiliary diseases in HIV infected children. *Gastroenterol Clin North Am* 1995; 24: 119–32.

147. Phillips AD, Thomas AG, Walker Smith JA. Cryptosporidium, chronic diarrhoea, and the proximal small intestinal mucosa. *Gut* 1992; 33: 1057–61.

148. Beutler B, Cerami A. Cachectin: more than a tumor necrosis factor. *N Engl J Med* 1987; 316: 379–85.

149. Lahdevirta J, Maury CPJ, Teppo AM, Repo H. Elevated levels of circulating cachectin/tumor necrosis factor in patients with acquired immunodeficiency syndrome. *Am J Med* 1988; 85: 289–91.

150. Grunfeld C, Pang M, Doerrler W, Shigenaga JK, Jensen P, Feingold KR. Lipids, lipoproteins, triglyceride clearance, and cytokines in human immunodeficiency virus infection and the acquired immunodeficiency syndrome. *J Clin Endocrinol Metab* 1992; 74: 1045–52.

151. Hellerstein MK, Grunfeld C, Wu K, et al. Increased de novo hepatic lipogenesis in human immunodeficiency virus infection. *J Clin Endocrinol Metab* 1993; 76: 559–65.

152. Thea DM, Porat R, Nagimbi K, et al. Plasma cytokines, cytokine antagonists, and disease progression in African women infected with HIV-1. *Ann Intern Med* 1996; 124: 757–62.

153. Grunfeld C, Kotler DP, Shigenaga JK, et al. Circulating interferon-alpha levels and hypertriglyceridemia in the acquired immunodeficiency syndrome. *Am J Med* 1991; 90: 154–62.

154. Godfried MH, van der Poll T, Jansen J, et al. Soluble receptors for tumor necrosis factor: a putative marker of disease progression in HIV infection. *AIDS* 1993; 7: 33–6.

155. Rimaniol AC, Zylberberg H, Zavala F, Viard JP. Inflammatory cytokines and inhibitors in HIV infection: correlation between interleukin-1 receptor antagonist and weight loss. *AIDS* 1996; 10: 1349–56.

156. Tracey KJ, Beutler B, Lowry SF, et al. Shock and tissue injury induced by recombinant human cachectin. *Science* 1986; 234: 470.

157. Suttmann U, Selberg O, Gallati H, Ockenga J, Deicher H, Muller MJ. Tumour necrosis factor receptor levels are linked to the acute-phase response and malnutrition in human-immunodeficiency-virus-infected patients. *Clin Sci* 1994; 86: 461–7.

158. Arnalich F, Martínez P, Hernanz A, et al. Altered concentrations of appetite regulators may contribute to the development and maintenance of HIV-associated wasting. *AIDS* 1997; 11: 1129–34.

159. Grunfeld C, Kotler DP, Hamadeh R, Tierney A, Wang J, Pierson RN. Hypertriglyceridemia in the acquired immunodeficiency syndrome. *Am J Med* 1989; 86: 27–31.

160. Strawford A, Hellerstein M. The etiology of wasting in the human immunodeficiency virus and acquired immunodeficiency syndrome. *Semin Oncol* 1998; 25 (Suppl. 6): 76–81.

161. Melchior JC. Metabolic aspects of HIV: associated wasting. *Biomed Pharmacother* 1997; 51: 455–60.

162. Grinspoon SK, Donovan DS, Bilezikian JP. Aetiology and pathogenesis of hormonal and metabolic disorders in HIV infection. *Baillieres Clin Endocrinol Metab* 1994; 8: 735–55.

163. Nunez EA, Christeff N. Steroid hormone, cytokine, lipid and metabolic disturbances in HIV infection. *Baillieres Clin Endocrinol Metab* 1994; 8: 803–23.

164. Grunfeld C, Feingold KR. The role of the cytokines, interferon alpha and tumor necrosis factor in the hypertriglyceridemia and wasting of AIDS. *J Nutr* 1992; 122: 749–53.

165. Grunfeld C, Feingold KR. Metabolic disturbances and wasting in the acquired immunodeficiency syndrome. *N Engl J Med* 1992; 327: 329–37.

166. Balog DL, Epstein ME, Amodio-Groton MI. HIV wasting syndrome: treatment update. *Ann Pharmacother* 1998; 32: 446–58.

167. Hellerstein MK, Wu K, McGrath M, et al. Effects of dietary n-3 fatty acid supplementation in men with weight loss associated with the acquired immune deficiency syndrome: relation to indices of cytokine production. *J Acquir Immune Defic Syndr Hum Retrovirol* 1996; 11: 258–70.

168. Christeff N, Gharakhanian S, Thobie N, Rozenbaum W, Nunez EA. Evidence for changes in adrenal and testicular steroids during HIV infection. *J Acquir Immune Defic Syndr Hum Retrovirol* 1992; 5: 841–6.

169. Grinspoon S, Corcoran C, Lee K, et al. Loss of lean body and muscle mass correlates with androgen levels in hypogonadal men with acquired immunodeficiency syndrome and wasting. *J Clin Endocrinol Metab* 1996; 81: 4051–8.

170. Grinspoon S, Corcoran C, Askari H, et al. Effects of androgen administration in men with the AIDS wasting syndrome. A randomized, double-blind, placebo-controlled trial. *Ann Intern Med* 1998; 129: 18–26.

171. Miller K, Corcoran C, Armstrong C, et al. Transdermal testosterone administration in women with acquired immunodeficiency syndrome wasting: a pilot study. *J Clin Endocrinol Metab* 1998; 83: 2717–25.

172. Lambert M. Thyroid dysfunction in HIV infection. *Baillieres Clin Endocrinol Metab* 1994; 8: 825–35.

173. Hirschfeld S, Laue L, Cutler GBJ, Pizzo PA. Thyroid abnormalities in children infected with human immunodeficiency virus. *J Pediatr* 1996; 128: 70–4.

174. Grunfeld C, Pang M, Doerrler W, et al. Indices of thyroid function and weight loss in human immunodeficiency virus infection and the acquired immunodeficiency syndrome. *Metabolism* 1993; 42: 1270–6.

175. Frost RA, Fuhrer J, Steigbigel R, Mariuz P, Lang CH, Gelato MC. Wasting in the acquired immune deficiency syndrome is associated with multiple defects in the serum insulin-like growth factor system. *Clin Endocrinol* 1996; 44: 501–14.

176. Schambelan M, Mulligan K, Grunfeld C, et al. Recombinant human growth hormone in patients with HIV-associated wasting. A randomized, placebo-controlled trial. *Ann Intern Med* 1996; 125: 873–82.

177. Waters D, Danska J, Hardy K, et al. Recombinant human growth hormone, insulin-like growth factor 1, and combination therapy in AIDS-associated wasting: a randomized, double-blind, placebo-controlled trial. *Ann Intern Med* 1996; 125: 865–72.

178. Berkowitz DE, Brown D, Lee KM, et al. Endotoxin-induced alteration in the expression of leptin and 3 adrenergic receptor in adipose tissue. *Am J Physiol* 1998; 274: E992–7.

179. Grunfeld C, Zhao C, Fuller J, et al. Endotoxin and cytokines induce expression of leptin, the ob gene product, in hamsters. *J Clin Invest* 1996; 97: 2152–7.

180. Grunfeld C, Pang M, Shigenaga JK, et al. Serum leptin levels in the acquired immunodeficiency syndrome. *J Clin Endocrinol Metab* 1996; 81: 4342–6.

181. Yarasheski KE, Zachwieja JJ, Horgan MM, Powderly WG, Santiago JV, Landt M. Serum leptin concentrations in human immunodeficiency virus-infected men with low adiposity. *Metabolism* 1997; 46: 303–5.

182. McKinney RE, Maha MA, Connor EM, et al. A multicenter trial of oral zidovudine in children with advanced human immunodeficiency virus disease. *N Engl J Med* 1991; 324: 1018–25.

183. Mueller BU, Butler KM, Stocker VL, et al. Clinical and pharmacokinetic evaluation of long-term therapy with didanosine in children with HIV infection. *Pediatrics* 1994; 94: 724–31.

184. Husson RN, Mueller BU, Farley M, et al. Zidovudine and didanosine combination therapy in children with human immunodeficiency virus infection. *Pediatrics* 1994; 93: 316–22.

185. Mueller BU, Nelson RPJ, Sleasman J, et al. A phase I/II study of the protease inhibitor ritonavir in children with human immunodeficiency virus infection. *Pediatrics* 1998; 101: 335–43.

DISCUSSION

Dr. Wasantwisut: I think it is excellent to show that in a condition such as HIV, wherein are likely to be found multiple deficiencies, a supplementation trial of a single nutrient could be very confusing. You have shown that in situations where deficiencies of more than one nutrient are probable, multivitamins are likely to be beneficial. I think it is important to stress also that when dealing with pregnancy, a couple of factors are involved: the hemodilution effect on top of infection, and whether or not deficiencies were present before pregnancy. I would like to know whether you saw any response in the lower end of your population in pregnancy. You showed that the response to placebo and vitamin A supplements was about the same, but if you stratify them do you see anything?

Dr. Fawzi: We stratified by plasma vitamin A status in 100 individuals and found no differences in effect among women with low versus normal vitamin A levels. We have just completed measuring serum retinol in all 1,000 women and we will replicate this analysis to see if we missed something with the smaller sample. We also looked at whether the efficacy of the supplements was modified by other variables such as CD4 count and body mass index, and there was no modification of effect.

Dr. Suskind: One question that we might consider as far as this meeting is concerned is as follows. With HIV, we have a chronic infection and we have heard in this workshop about the metabolic impact of infection in terms of the wastage of nitrogen and other nutrients. At the same time, I think we recognize that malnutrition itself will have an impact on the immune system. We know that the HIV virus directly attacks T lymphocytes. I wonder whether this, together with the chronic long-standing infection and nutrient wastage, has additive effects. With that wastage, a secondary impact on the immune system is seen. I wonder whether we might look at HIV as a combination of a direct viral attack on the immune system plus the long-term effect of a chronic infection leading to a secondary impact on the immune system. If this turns out to be the case, the question I would then ask is whether we could deal with the secondary loss of nutrients by nutritional supplementation, thus avoiding the nutritional component of the compromised immune system.

Dr. Fawzi: Prospective studies have found associations between protein-energy nutrition and a faster disease progression in both children and in adults (refer to chapter 19). Whether intervening with macronutrient supplements has any effect on disease progression, I am not sure. However, I do agree that a vicious circle of HIV leads to wasting and poor nutritional status, which in turn affects immune status and leads to immune suppression and faster disease progression, which, in turn, causes greater nutritional deficiency.

Dr. Griffin: In response to Dr. Suskind's point, John S. Friedland in Zambia looked at the restoration of hemoglobin as a marker of marrow function in patients who had tuberculosis (TB) and who were either HIV-positive or HIV-negative. Both groups of patients presented with pulmonary TB and had a hemoglobin on admission of approximately 5 g/dl. When they were treated for the TB, the patients who were HIV-negative eventually achieved a hemoglobin value at equilibrium of approximately 10–11 g/dl, but the HIV-positive group never managed to have above 7 g/dl. So, even with adequate nutritional repletion and a decrease in the inflammatory indices as the TB came under control, HIV was still depressing bone marrow function considerably. And, of course, a hemoglobin of 7 g/dl compared with 10 g/dl is probably going to be functionally significant in terms of the ability to do physical work.

Dr. Chandra: Do you have any information on the prevalence of hepatitis in the population you were studying? I ask this because liver is a storage organ for many nutrients, and serum levels of nutrients are affected by liver dysfunction. For instance, in one of the studies we were associated with, a high serum vitamin B_{12} was correlated with a worse outcome, and also with liver cell dysfunction as assessed by serum transaminase levels (1).

Dr. Fawzi: To be honest, I do not know, but we could find out as we have the specimens available.

Dr. Embree: I wanted to congratulate you on your study in Tanzania. I truly hope that you see some effects on transmission using the multivitamin supplements. I hope data also show improvement in child outcome, such as decreased fetal death rate and decreased prematurity among non–HIV-infected women as well, because if data exist, this would be a therapeutic intervention that could be appropriate for the entire population. You would not need to screen; you would still get the effect. That is going to be very important, particularly, in Africa. South Africa has already stated that the government cannot provide AZT in pregnancy because of the cost and other factors. The rest of Africa has not stated that so far, but it will be years, if not decades, before they will be able to institute screening in pregnancy and appropriate treatment. So, what we need in the meantime are therapeutic interventions that are useful for the entire population regardless of HIV status, so I really hope this works.

Dr. Fawzi: Thank you. I agree that it is important to see whether multimicronutrient supplements have an effect on HIV-negative women. We are planning a follow-up study among HIV-negative women in Dar es Salaam and it would be exciting to see even a small beneficial effect, as this would strengthen the case for providing these supplements to all, irrespective of HIV status.

Dr. Tontisirin: Evidence suggests that, in marginalized population groups in Thailand, supplementation with multimicronutrients does have some benefit (2). We cannot say which nutrients are the most important. In your study, you used high doses of multivitamins (e.g., 20 mg of B_1, B_2, and so on, and up to 500 mg of vitamin C). This is five or ten times higher than the RDA. What is the rationale for this?

Dr. Fawzi: The dosage was based on studies from the United States showing that multiples of the RDA were necessary to correct vitamin deficiency in HIV-positive individuals. We also wanted to use a large enough dose to ensure efficacy would be detected if it existed, while remaining in safe limits.

Dr. Tontisirin: As I mentioned previously, during the last 15 years we have had a regimen in place for multivitamin and iron supplementation to almost all pregnant women throughout the country. One tablet a day of multivitamins, composed of six to eight vitamins, in addition to iron. Our results show improved outcome in many variables, but we are not able to explain why or what nutrient or nutrients have played the major role (2).

Dr. Fawzi: I am not aware of well-designed studies that show conclusively that vitamin supplements during pregnancy are beneficial. They are given in the United States and in most developed countries, as they are in Thailand, and the rationale is probably that because they are likely to be beneficial, why not give them. This makes sense in certain settings, but where resources are limited, it is important to confirm that they are indeed beneficial before giving them on a population scale.

Dr. Coovadia: The effects of vitamin A on vertical transmission were so striking that there was even a dose-response curve. So my question is, was there any correlation with viral load? If not, is vitamin A acting as a surrogate marker for something else?

Dr. Fawzi: Studies looking at vitamin A and viral load showed no effect. For example, in a study of intravenous drug users, viral load was assessed after a does of 200,000 IU of vitamin A and no effect was seen (3). Two other studies also showed that daily doses of vitamin A during pregnancy in HIV-positive women had no effect (4,5). In the discussion of one of these papers, however, evidence was provided for the safety of vitamin A in the doses used. This is important, as concerns have been raised to whether vitamin A might even have a deleterious effect on HIV progression. Thus, the limited evidence to date suggests that vitamin A does not have an effect on viral load. It could be merely a marker of HIV infection or disease stage.

Dr. Cochran: As I recall from your slide listing all the various nutrients that can be adversely affected by HIV, among the B vitamins only one was significantly lower, going from the controls to HIV-positive to frank AIDS, and yet your supplementation levels showed a reduction in mortality with all the various B vitamins. Do you think this reflects the poor performance of serum levels as true indicators of nutrient status, or does it show that vitamin supplementation might indeed have a pharmacologic effect?

Dr. Fawzi: Other studies have shown that vitamins other than that particular one are deficient in HIV-positive individuals (6,7). But it is not clear whether there is a pharmacologic effect or whether the effect is greatest among people who are in a deficient state. Most of the studies have been observational, and it is not clear whether giving multivitamins improves the clinical outcome of HIV-positive patients. Evidence from a randomized trial shows that it does improve CD4 and CD8 cell counts and hemoglobin levels (8), but whether it improves the function of T cells or clinical outcome has yet to be determined.

REFERENCES

1. Stallings RG, Chandra RK. 2000 (*in press*).
2. Tontisirin K, Boonranasubkajorn U, Hongsumarn A, et al. Formulation and evaluation of supplementary foods for Thai pregnant women. *Am J Clin Nutr* 1986; 43:931–9.
3. Semba RD, Lyles CM, Margolick JB, et al. Vitamin A supplementation and human immunodeficiency virus load in injection drug users. *J Infect Dis* 1998; 177: 611–6.
4. Humphrey JH, Quinn T, Fine D, et al. Short-term effects of large-dose vitamin A supplementation on viral load and immune response in HIV-infected women. *J Acquir Immune Defic Syndr Hum Retrovirol* 1999; 20: 44–51.
5. Coutsoudis A, Moodley D, Pillay K, et al. Effects of vitamin A supplementation on viral load HIV-1-infected pregnant women. *J Acquir Immune Defic Syndr Hum Retrovirol* 1997; 15: 86–7.
6. Allard JP, Aghdassi E, Chau J, et al. Effects of vitamin E and C supplementation on oxidative stress and viral load in HIV-infected subjects. *AIDS* 1998; 12: 1653–9.
7. Baum MK, Shor-Posner G, Lu Y, et al. Micronutrients and HIV-1 disease progression. *AIDS* 1995; 9: 1051–6.
8. Fawzi WW, Msamanga GI, Spiegelman D, et al. Randomised trial of effects of vitamin supplements on pregnancy outcomes and T-cell counts in HIV-1-infected women in Tanzania. *Lancet* 1998; 351: 1477–82.

Nutrition, Immunity, and Infection in Infants and Children, edited by Robert M. Suskind and Kraisid Tontisirin. Nestlé Nutrition Workshop Series, Pediatric Program, Vol. 45. Nestec Ltd., Vevey/Lippincott Williams & Wilkins, Philadelphia ©2001.

The Interactions of Nutritional Status and Parasitic Diseases

D. Wakelin

School of Biological Sciences, University of Nottingham, University Park, Nottingham, UK

Parasites—protozoans and helminths—are responsible for some of the most common infections of humans and are particularly prevalent in the warmer countries of the world. With the exception of malaria, these infections are not major causes of mortality, but the sheer number of individuals infected means that these organisms make a very significant contribution to global morbidity (Table 1).

The reproductive strategies of parasites show bewildering complexities, but it is possible to identify four major routes by which the infective stages of parasites enter the human body. These are (*a*) through the activities of arthropod vectors (e.g., in malaria, trypanosomiasis, leishmaniasis, filariasis); (*b*) by active penetration (schistosomiasis, hookworm disease, strongyloidiasis); (*c*) by ingestion of cysts or eggs (amebiasis, giardiasis, toxoplasmosis, ascariasis, trichuriasis); and (*d*) by ingestion of infected food (toxoplasmosis, tapeworm infections, trichinellosis). Brief consideration shows immediately that infections by these routes are likely to be most common in those countries that have warm climates, where arthropod vectors flourish and ambient temperatures allow rapid completion of developmental cycles, and where socioeconomic factors prevent the achievement of adequate standards of hygiene and sanitation. The burden of parasitic disease, therefore, is greatest in the developing countries, although not limited to them by any means.

Epidemiologic studies show that the distribution of parasitic infections within populations living in endemic areas changes significantly with age. The prevalence of infection may remain high in all age classes, but usually the intensity of infection, or the frequency of episodes of disease, declines with age. In part, this decline reflects the altered behavior patterns seen as individuals mature, but almost certainly also involves the development of a degree of protective immunity. However, parasitic infections seem often to elicit only weak or slowly developing protective immune re-

TABLE 1. *Public health importance of major parasitic infections*

Infection	Prevalence ($\times 10^6$)	Total DALYs
Malaria	300–500	
Entamoeba	500	
Giardia	200	
Sleeping sickness	0.02–0.3	17.8
Chagas' disease	16	27.4
Schistosomias	200	45.3
Ascaris	1,000	105.2
Hookworm	500	11.4
Trichuris	900	63.1

DALY, disability-adjusted life years.
From Molyneux DH (1).

sponses, so that protection rarely becomes absolute (2). As a consequence of the socioeconomic, behavioral, and immunologic variables that determine the patterns of parasitic infection, parasitic diseases are most common and most severe in children. This is most dramatically seen in infections with the most serious form of malaria, that caused by *Plasmodium falciparum*. Infections with this parasite are acquired soon after birth, when the protective effect of maternal antibodies declines. The numbers of parasites present in the blood reach the highest values in children during the first decade of life and mortality is most severe in the first 5 years (Fig. 1a). A similar, although less dramatic, picture is seen in infections with schistosomes and with the major gastrointestinal nematodes (*Ascaris*, hookworms, *Trichuris*; Fig. 1b). Children are the most heavily infected members of the population, often carrying the bulk of the worm population, and suffering most from the debilitating consequences associated with them.

The associations between climatic and socioeconomic factors that influence the prevalence and intensity of parasitic infections, as in so many diseases, are intimately bound up with nutritional factors. Undernutrition both increases levels of susceptibility to infection and reduces the potential to express resistance mechanisms. In turn, infection can reduce levels of nutrient absorption, increase nutrient loss, and disturb homeostatic regulatory mechanisms (2). Infection is often also associated with lack of appetite. Parasites and nutrition, thus, can interact in a vicious circle, one that is exacerbated by the chronicity of many parasitic infections.

In this chapter, I focus on two groups of infection, those caused by malaria parasites and those caused by gastrointestinal parasites. The first are chosen because of their importance and because of the detailed body of published reports that now exists concerning this disease; the second are chosen again because of the reports available, but also because the interaction of these parasites with nutritional factors is somewhat different from that seen in malaria, in part because of their location in the host's body. Those interested in other groups of parasites will find useful reviews in Chandra (5), Crompton (6), Farthing and Keusch (7), Solomons (8), Solomons and Scott (9), Stephenson (10,11), and Storey (12).

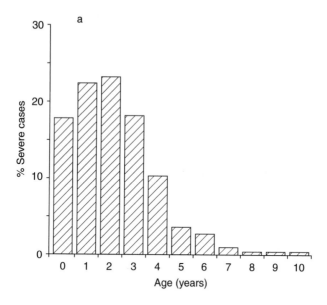

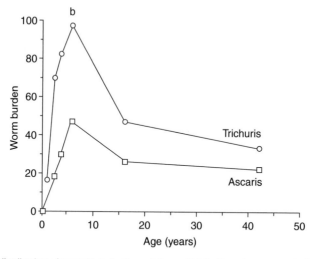

FIG. 1. Age distribution of parasitic infections. (a) age distribution of severe malaria cases. From Snow *et al.* (3); (b) age intensity profiles for *Ascaris lumbricoides* and *Trichuris trichiura* infections. From Bundy (4).

NUTRITION, SUSCEPTIBILITY, AND RESISTANCE

During evolution, parasite species have evolved to survive in the physical and physiologic environments provided by particular hosts. Some parasites are highly host specific, that is, they are adapted to survive in only one species of host (e.g., malaria and *Ascaris lumbricoides* in humans); others show low specificity and occur in many species (e.g., *Toxoplasma, Trichinella*). Survival and development in a given host species are influenced by a variety of endogenous and exogenous factors (13), of which nutrition and host immunity are two of the most important. The relationship between diet and the immune response, an area of increasing interest, is covered in some detail elsewhere in this volume. As our understanding of the ways in which the response is regulated, and as the contributions of specific cell subsets and their products (cytokines) are clarified (14), it is becoming easier to understand how dietary factors can influence specific components of the immune response and, thus, predict how particular dietary changes, rather than gross alterations, are likely to affect the outcome of particular host–parasite relations (15).

Quantitative deficiencies in diet, particularly where these involve protein-energy values or micronutrients such as zinc, can reduce the effectiveness of the immune response and, thus, promote parasite survival—that is, increase host susceptibility. However, eukaryotic parasites are almost totally dependent on the host for their own nutrient requirements, with the consequence that alterations or restrictions in the host diet can profoundly reduce parasite survival. For example, in malaria infections, nutritional deficiencies can promote resistance by denying the parasite an essential nutrient, as was shown in the early work of Hawking on para-amino benzoic acid (16). Dietary deficiencies can also enhance host resistance mechanisms indirectly (as has been shown in relation to antioxidants—see below).

The capacity of parasites to alter the host nutritional balance means that host–parasite relations are always dynamic. Chronic infections, which are characteristic of human malaria and gastrointestinal nematode infections, can lead to marked changes in host nutritional state, maintaining or increasing susceptibility to further infection. An aspect of this process which has received little attention in published reports is that changes in host nutrition induced by one species of parasite not only influence that species but influence all the other parasites to which the host is exposed. Polyparasitism, the state of infection with multiple infectious agents, is the normal condition in endemic areas and, thus, the overall interactions between nutrition and parasitism in a given host individual are likely to be very complex.

MALARIA

Malaria is the name given to infections with protozoan parasites belonging to the genus *Plasmodium*. These parasites are very host specific; those infecting humans will not develop in other host species. Infections are transmitted by the bites of anopheline mosquitoes. After a period of development in the liver, the parasites undergo repeated cycles of asexual division within the red blood cells, periodically producing sexual forms that can complete their development only if taken up again by a mosquito. The disease is caused by the development and release of the asexual stages. These must rupture infected red cells to release the next generation of invasive stages. This process not only destroys large numbers of red cells, but results in the release of toxic materials that trigger the characteristic cycles of fever and prostration. The most serious form of malaria is caused by *P. falciparum*. Developing asexual stages of this species become sequestered in the capillaries of internal organs. Those in the brain can cause cerebral malaria, a condition that is often fatal unless treated promptly. Infections are most severe, and fatalities most common, in children. The relationship between parasitemia (numbers of parasites in the blood) and the severity of malarial pathology is not always a direct one. For example, some factors, such as tumor necrosis factor (TNF) and nitric oxide, have been implicated both in protecting against infection and in causing pathology.

Protein-Energy Values

Much debate has occurred over the relationship between nutritional state and susceptibility or resistance to malaria and it is clear that this relationship is complex (17,18). Some studies in rodent models, for example (19), have shown that diets deficient in protein severely depressed the level of parasitemia in rats infected with *P. berghei*, the degree of depression being related to the level of protein supplied. Whereas infected rats fed a 17% casein diet showed 80% mortality, reduction to 8.5% prevented death altogether. Rats whose intake of the 17% casein diet was restricted to 50% of *ad libitum* fed controls similarly showed a reduction in parasitemia and mortality. In contrast, Hunt *et al.* (20) found that, although dietary restriction reduced the numbers of deaths from cerebral malaria in mice infected with *P. berghei ANKA*, it had no effects on parasitemia. These data from rodents were not supported by data from a study on malaria infection in Gambian children (21), which failed to show any relationship between protein-energy undernutrition and protection against malaria, although children experiencing clinical attacks with high parasitemias tended to have a higher weight-for-age at the start of the transmission season than children whose malaria attacks were associated with lower parasitemia.

Iron

The nature of the malaria parasite's relationship with the red cell, which is the vehicle from which the parasite derives its nutrients, means that the development of the parasite can be markedly affected, both positively and negatively, by nutritional variations in the host. Several such interactions have been described in published reports. Various interesting studies have followed the effects of dietary, particularly iron, supplementation on malaria infections in populations suffering from undernutrition and iron deficiencies. The periodic rupture of red cells, which can occur every 48 or 72 hours for prolonged periods during malarial infections, results in a significant loss of iron from the body. This infection-related iron loss contributes to the anemia often associated with infection, especially in cases where dietary intake levels are low. Early studies by Murray *et al.* (22,23) showed that levels of infection and severity of pathology could be increased by iron supplementation. These observations were corroborated later by others, for example Oppenheimer *et al.* (24) showed that intramuscular administration of iron dextran to infants increased the prevalence of malaria infections and led to lower hemoglobin and a greater reticulocytosis when infected. Intravenous infusion of iron dextran into pregnant women resulted in more perinatal malaria in women having their first child (25). These consequences of iron supplementation may reflect influences on the number of circulating reticulocytes, both *P. vivax* and *P. falciparum* preferentially developing in these or in young red cells. Similar influences of iron supplementation have been reported by other workers.

Vitamins and Antioxidants

Malaria parasites in red cells are susceptible to oxidative stress, a feature that is exploited in the design of antimalarial drugs. Dietary variation in levels of antioxidants may, therefore, significantly alter the balance between host and parasite. Antioxidant deficiencies can increase resistance to infection, presumably by increasing the activity of oxidants at the level of the infected red cell. This has been most clearly shown in experimental work using rodent and avian models, but several relevant human studies have been conducted (26). Most of the work has focused on vitamins A, C, and E, but other vitamins have also been studied. For example, Kaikai and Thurnham (27) showed that rats deficient in riboflavin had markedly lower parasitemias after infection with *P. berghei* than normal controls but suffered equivalent mortality, and Das *et al.* (28) confirmed decreased parasitemia in riboflavin-deficient humans.

Various investigators have reported decreased plasma levels of antioxidants—for example ascorbate and tocopherol (26)—in malaria patients but much discussion has arisen to the significance of these findings, as such levels are influenced by the assays used and by confounding factors such as, for vitamin E, plasma cholesterol and smoking; and, for vitamin A, the flow of plasma retinol into extravascular fluids during infection. Early experimental studies showed that vitamin E deficiency inhibited the development of *P. berghei* in mice and this has been borne out by subsequent work. Levander *et al.* reviewed (26) the interesting interactions between dietary levels of fish oils (as a source of highly unsaturated fatty acids) and vitamin E in relationship to the activity of the antimalarial qinghaosu, which imposes increased oxidative stress on the parasite. In summary, dietary fish oil, which increases the requirement for vitamin E, significantly increased resistance to infection with *P. yoelii*, even in mice fed adequate levels of vitamin E, as reflected in lowered parasitemia and enhanced survival. In mice given adequate vitamin E, feeding fish oil increased the antimalarial effects of a qinghaosu derivative and dramatically improved survival rates (0 of 10 in controls to 9 of 10 in mice given 10 mg/kg derivative when fish oil was fed, compared with 4 of 10 when lard was given as a dietary source of fat). When mice were fed a fixed level of fish oil and subjected to graded levels of vitamin E, a significant protective effect against malaria was seen in those given up to 50% of the recommended vitamin E level.

GASTROINTESTINAL INFECTIONS

Parasitic infections of the gastrointestinal tract are among the most common of all infections; the gastrointestinal nematodes alone infect a quarter of the world's population. Although some, particularly the gastrointestinal protozoans, are quite common in the developed world, gastrointestinal parasites as a whole are endemic in much of the developing world. Most are transmitted by the fecal–oral route and, thus, two factors are of prime importance in maintaining their high prevalence: climate and socioeconomic levels. Between them, these factors influence the development and survival of infective stages in the external environment, affect supplies of clean water, influence standards of sanitation and hygiene, and regulate the availability of food. The presence of parasites in the intestine is often associated with pathologic changes, enteropathy, affecting both structure and function (Table 2). These changes can be induced by the activities of the organisms themselves and by the consequences of the host's immune response. Even relatively mild pathology can impair digestion and absorption and lead to increased loss of nutrients, contributing to the vicious cycle illustrated in Figure 2.

Gastrointestinal Protozoa

Many protozoans can live in the human intestine, three in particular being of major concern—*Cryptosporidium parvum*, *Entamoeba histolytica*, and *Giardia lamblia*. *E. histolytica* can invade the mucosa, causing extensive ulceration and blood loss; *C. parvum* lives quite superficially in enterocytes; and *G. lamblia* lives attached to the luminal surface of enterocytes. Both *C. parvum* and *G. lamblia* can cause a secretory diarrhea, which can result in loss of fluid, electrolytes, and micronutrients, and both are associated with structural or functional changes in the mucosa. Flattening of villi (villous atrophy) is common in both infections and this, together with the increased turnover and immaturity of enterocytes and altered permeability, leads to impaired digestion and absorption of nutrients and increased loss of plasma protein. These are well documented in *Giardia*, where infection can be associated with impaired fat absorption and steatorrhea, and with altered disaccharidase activity that leads to lactose intolerance (29). Infections with both parasites have been associated with lower

TABLE 2. *Parasite-induced enteropathy. Intestinal changes that influence nutrition*

Villous atrophy: flattening of mucosa, reducing surface area
Altered epithelial kinetics: presence of immature enterocytes
Decreased disaccharidase activity: reduced digestion of lactose
Increased epithelial and vascular permeability: loss of protein
Altered fluid flux across mucosa: loss of fluid, electrolytes, micronutrients
Decreased transit time: reduced digestion/absorption

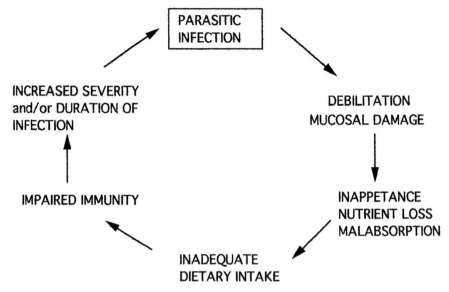

FIG. 2. Interactions between factors influencing nutrition and parasitic infections.

weight-for-height status, which is most probably a consequence of impaired nutrition (30).

Infections with gastrointestinal protozoans are normally controlled in immuno-competent individuals, but can become chronic in cases of immunodeficiency, either genetic (IgA deficiency) or infection induced. As with all parasites, gastrointestinal protozoans are likely to be common in children who are undernourished because of their decreased immune competence. A survey in Jamaica found the prevalence of *Cryptosporidium* in groups of children in the hospital to be as follows: well-nourished and nondiarrheal, 0.5%; well-nourished and diarrheal, 5.5%; malnourished and nondiarrheal, 3.5%; and malnourished and diarrheal, 23.7% (31). Sallon *et al.* (32) found that children with diarrhea who were *Cryptosporidium*-positive were significantly more malnourished than those with diarrhea but *Cryptosporidium*-negative. Severely malnourished children with infections had a significantly longer duration of diarrheal disease than a similar but uninfected group.

Gastrointestinal Nematodes

Four species of nematode can be considered under the heading of gastrointestinal nematodes—the large roundworm *Ascaris lumbricoides*, the hookworms *Ancylostoma duodenale* and *Necator americanus*, and the whipworm *Trichuris trichiura*. These *soil transmitted* nematodes are among the most common of all parasites, both in terms of the global distribution and in terms of their prevalence, which can reach 90% to 100%. Each relies on the development and survival of infective stages outside the body (eggs or larvae) and each depends on inadequate disposal of fecal material for transmission. In consequence, roundworms, hookworms, and whipworms often occur together in the same host. Although other species of gastrointestinal nematode are associated with intestinal conditions that adversely influence levels of nutrition (e.g., *Strongyloides stercoralis*, *S. fuelleborni*, and *Capillaria phillipinensis*), the prevalence of the first is lower, and the other two are much more locally distributed. Details of these species can be found in publications by Farthing *et al.* (33) and Cox *et al.* (34).

It is characteristic of gastrointestinal infections that they are aggregated in populations; that is, most individuals have small numbers of worms, whereas a few individuals harbor large numbers of parasites (Fig. 3). In most cases, the most heavily infected members of the population are the children and it is this age group that suffers most from the consequences of infection.

The gastrointestinal nematodes are large organisms and, thus, can cause physical damage to the small intestinal mucosa, in addition to the immunopathologic changes that result from infection. *Ascaris*, for example, at 30 cm in length is large enough to block the intestine of a child. Hookworms feed on blood, obtaining this by biting into the mucosa of the small intestine and secreting anticoagulants. The worms move frequently and feeding sites continue to bleed for some time after the worms leave. Loss of blood, with associated loss of protein and iron, can create serious nutritional problems in children living on marginally adequate diets. It is estimated that 25 *Ancylostoma*, the bigger hookworm, and 110 *Necator* can cause the loss of 5 ml of blood each (36), and infections are often much heavier than these values. Although iron can be recovered in the large intestine and iron stores mobilized to replace the amount

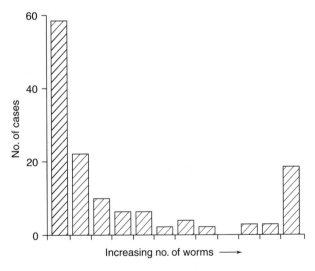

FIG. 3. Aggregated distribution of *Trichuris trichiura* infections in St. Lucia. From Bundy DAP (35).

lost, infection can lead to iron deficiency anemia unless there is an adequate iron intake. As maintenance of the red blood cell count has a high priority for the use of the body's iron, infected individuals can be under iron stress (e.g., as detected by plasma ferritin) without showing clinical anemia (37). The infection threshold at which a reduced plasma ferritin is seen is much lower than that required to reduce hemoglobin levels—300 compared with 5,000 eggs per gram of feces (38). The loss of plasma protein that accompanies the intestinal bleeding can lead to hypoalbuminemia and, thus, possibly contribute, in malnourished children, to manifestations of severe protein-energy deficiency (39). In addition to the direct loss of blood, heavy infection can cause a protein-losing enteropathy. When plasma loss is measured using radiolabeled albumin, the estimated values are approximately three times greater than the loss from feeding activities alone (40).

Heavy infections with *Trichuris* in the large intestine have also been associated with blood loss and the onset of anemia (41). Although the worm is not primarily a blood feeder, rectal bleeding occurs, in part the result of altered mucosal permeability, and the amount of blood lost in heavy infections can be significant. In a study of infected children in Jamaica, Ramdath *et al.* (42) found that those with fecal egg counts of more than 10,000/g had significantly lower hemoglobin levels than those less heavily infected, and 33% were diagnosed as anemic. Interestingly, no significant differences were found in red blood cell count or ferritin levels between the groups. The authors suggest that the absence of differences in ferritin levels may reflect the fact that ferritin is released as an acute phase protein, and the overall plasma level, therefore, may reflect a balance between parasite-induced gain and loss. Although the anemia associated with heavy *Trichuris* infections can be severe, their nutritional significance may be more directly connected with the development of inflammatory responses in the large intestine, seen at its most severe in the *Trichuris*-dysentery syndrome. The plasma loss associated with this condition has been estimated at an average of 113 ml/d compared with 17 ml/d in controls, a figure that represents about one quarter of the typical dietary intake for an infected child (40). In addition to protein loss from the inflamed large intestine, the significantly increased permeability of the mucosa results in increased absorption of test sugars (lactulose and rhamnose). Anthelmintic treatment of infected children reverses protein loss and restores normal permeability and is followed by a striking spurt in growth. This is seen even at relatively low levels of infection, but is much more dramatic in heavily infected cases (40).

Both trichuriasis and hookworm infections are associated with growth retardation and stunting, and this is the result of a combination of factors. Nutrient loss as a result of worm activity and host response is important, but loss of appetite and altered cytokine balance are also involved. Cooper *et al.* have shown that children with the *Trichuris*-dysentery syndrome have increased levels of serum TNF-α, a cytokine with pleiotropic effects on growth (43).

In contrast to hookworm and *Trichuris*, infections with *Ascaris* do not cause an appreciable degree of intestinal pathology, although villous atrophy and crypt hyperplasia have been reported. The effects of ascariasis on nutrition, therefore, are more likely to be a direct consequence of worm size and activity in the intestine. Among the observed effects are abnormal absorption of carbohydrate (especially lactose), fat, and vitamin A (39), reflected in lower plasma levels of vitamin A, C, and albumin (44).

Ascaris infection is often linked to reduced food intake, as demonstrated experimentally in pigs infected with *A. suum* (45). Chronic ascariasis causes a marked reduction in growth, especially in young children, and the risk of stunting is significantly greater in this group (46). As with hookworm and *Trichuris*, successful anthelmintic treatment leads to a spurt in growth (44). In endemic areas, treated (or uninfected) individuals showed better values for weight-for-height, weight-for-age, midarm circumference, plasma vitamins A and C, and plasma albumin, and less lactose intolerance. In a comparative study of treatments (47), vitamin A dietary supplementation was found to be more successful in restoring normal growth than anthelminthic treatment alone, particularly in children who were vitamin A deficient initially. These data suggest that the deficiencies associated with *Ascaris* infection are likely to persist unless the diet is also improved.

NUTRITIONAL FACTORS AND IMMUNITY TO GASTROINTESTINAL INFECTIONS

Several studies, primarily in experimental models using rodents, but also some in domestic animals (48), have shown that protein-energy undernutrition and micronutrient deficiencies can affect the development of immunity to gastrointestinal nematode infections. Early work using *Nippostrongylus brasiliensis* in the rat showed that iron and protein deficiencies reduced the ability of the host to mount a protective response (49), and manipulative studies implicated direct effects on lymphocytes and other bone marrow-derived cells (50,51). Maintaining rats on zinc-deficient diets has been found to reduce immunity to two other gastrointestinal nematodes in rats, *Trichinella spiralis* and *Strongyloides ratti* (52,53). In a series of studies using *Heligmosomoides polygyrus* in mice, Scott and colleagues (54–57) have shown that energy and zinc restriction limit the ability of the host to control primary and secondary infections through effects on antibody and inflammatory responses. These effects operate through altered antigen-presenting cell and T-cell function. The latter involved both Th1 and Th2 subsets and their associated cytokines, although Th2 cells—those most clearly associated with protective immunity against gastrointestinal nematodes in mice—seemed most severely affected.

Protein-deficient diets (4% protein) were found to increase levels and duration of infection with *Trichuris muris* in CBA/Ca mice (58), preventing the normal immune-mediated expulsion of worms that takes place in normally nourished (16% protein) mice of this strain during the third week of infection. Rather surprisingly, mice on the low protein diet showed greater antibody responses than protein-sufficient mice (59), perhaps reflecting the prolonged survival of antigen-releasing worms, but implying that nutritional deficiencies in this system influenced immunity through nonantibody mechanisms.

Although few comparable studies have been done in humans, zinc deficiency has been correlated with levels of infection with *T. trichiura* in Caribbean communities (60), there being a significant inverse relationship between plasma zinc concentrations and worm numbers. It was concluded that this reflected an influence of zinc deficiency on host responses rather than a direct effect on worm nutrition, and this is most likely to operate through depression of immune competence. Other studies, however, have not found improvements in levels of intestinal infections in children receiving zinc supplement (61).

PARASITIC INFECTIONS AND COGNITIVE DEVELOPMENT

Although not directly relevant to the main theme here, it is important to make the point that parasitic infections not only affect the physical development of children, but may also affect their educational development. This has been particularly well studied in the context of worm infections (62–64), and it will be clear from the data summarized above that nutritional influences on parasite burden are likely to be a significant contributory factor.

FUTURE DIRECTIONS

Controlling parasitic infections would make possible enormous progress in helping to deal with the problems of inadequate nutrition. The improvements in health, work, and educational potential gained in this way, and the eradication of the long-term nutritional drain imposed by chronic disease, would significantly alter nutritional balance at many different levels. To date, few control campaigns have had success on a global scale, although major progress has occurred in particular areas, and some parasitic diseases have been locally eradicated. No vaccine is yet available against any human parasite, although optimism remains for malaria, schistosomiasis, and filariasis. Chemotherapy remains an effective approach, but widespread drug resistance is seen in malaria, and increasing drug resistance in helminth parasites. Against the latter, selective treatment, as is currently used to target schoolaged children, has had and will continue to have remarkable success. Much remains to be learned about the intricacies of the interaction between parasites and nutrition, but it seems clear that some alteration of infection and disease status may be possible by using dietary manipulations to change, for example, levels of antioxidants and unsaturated fats. It remains clear, however, that the first consideration is to attempt to improve, or at least maintain, protein-energy levels. Without this, the insidious effects of parasitic infections will continue to reduce the physical and educational potential of a very large proportion of the world's children.

REFERENCES

1. Molyneux DH. Control of parasites, parasitic infections and parasitic diseases. In: Cox FEG, Kreier JP, Wakelin D, eds. *Topley & Wilson's microbiology and microbial infections.* Vol 5: Parasitology. London: Arnold, 1997: 85–112.

2. Cox FEG, Wakelin D. Immunology and immunopathology of parasitic infections. In: Cox FEG, Kreier JP, Wakelin D, eds. *Topley & Wilson's microbiology and microbial infections.* Vol 5: Parasitology. London: Arnold, 1997: 57–84.
3. Snow RW, Armstrong Schellenberg JRM, Peshu N, et al. Periodicity and space-time clustering of severe childhood malaria on the coast of Kenya. *Trans R Soc Trop Med Hyg* 1993; 87: 386–90.
4. Bundy DAP. Population ecology of intestinal helminth infections in human communities. *Phil Trans R Soc Lond B* 1988; 321: 405–20.
5. Chandra RK. Parasitic infection, nutrition and the immune response. *FASEB J* 1984; 43: 251–5.
6. Crompton DWT, ed. Human nutrition and parasitic infection. *Parasitology* 1993; (Suppl.):107.
7. Farthing MJG, Keusch GT. Nutrition and infection. *Am J Clin Nutr* 1986; 6: 131–54.
8. Solomons NW. Nutrition and parasitism. In: Velasquez A, Bourges H. *Genetic factors in nutrition.* Orlando: Academic Press, 1984: 225–41.
9. Solomons NW, Scott ME. Nutritional status of host populations influences parasitic infections In: Scott ME, Smith G, eds. *Parasitic and infectious diseases: epidemiology and ecology.* San Diego: Academic Press, 1994: 101–4.
10. Stephenson LS. *The impact of helminth infections on human nutrition: schistosomes and soil-transmitted helminths.* London: Taylor & Francis, 1987.
11. Stephenson LS. The impact of schistosomiasis on human nutrition. *Parasitology* 1993; 107: S107–23.
12. Storey DM. Filariasis; nutritional interactions in human and animal hosts. *Parasitology* 1993; 107: S147–58.
13. Wakelin D. Genetic and other constraints on resistance to infection with gastrointestinal nematodes. *Trans R Soc Trop Med Hyg* 1986; 80: 742–7.
14. Wakelin D. *Immunity to parasites: how parasitic infections are controlled.* Cambridge: Cambridge University Press, 1996.
15. Munoz C, Schlesinger L, Cavaillon JM. Interaction between cytokines, nutrition and infection. *Nutr Res* 1995; 15: 1815–44.
16. Hawking F. Milk diet, p-aminobenzoic acid and malaria (*P. berghei*). *BMJ* 1953; i: 1201.
17. Beisel WR. Synergism and antagonism of parasitic disease and malnutrition. *Rev Infect Dis* 1982; 4: 746–50.
18. McGregor IA. Malaria: nutritional implications. *Rev Infect Dis* 1982; 4: 798–804.
19. Edirisinghe JS, Fern EB, Targett GAT. Dietary suppression of rodent malaria. *Trans R Soc Trop Med Hyg* 1981; 75: 591–3.
20. Hunt NH, Manduci N, Thumwood CM. Amelioration of murine cerebral malaria by dietary restriction. *Parasitology* 1993; 107: 471–6.
22. Murray MJ, Murray AB, Murray MB, et al. Diet and cerebral malaria: the effect of famine and refeeding. *Am J Clin Nutr* 1978: 31: 57–61.
23. Murray MJ, Murray AB, Murray MB, et al. The adverse effect of iron repletion on the course of certain infections. *BMJ* 1978: 1113–15.
24. Oppenheimer SJ, Gibson FD, MacFarlane SB, et al. Iron supplementation increases prevalence and effects of malaria: report on clinical studies in Papua New Guinea. *Trans R Soc Trop Med Hyg* 1986; 80: 603–12.
25. Oppenheimer SJ, MacFarlane SB, Moody JB, et al. Total dose iron infusion, malaria and pregnancy in Papua New Guinea. *Trans R Soc Trop Med Hyg* 1986; 80: 818–22.
26. Levander OA, Ager AL. Malarial parasites and antioxidant nutrients. *Parasitology* 1993; 107: S95–106.
27. Kaikai P, Thurnham DI. The influence of riboflavin deficiency on *Plasmodium berghei* infection in rats. *Trans R Soc Trop Med Hyg* 1983; 77: 680–6.
28. Das BS, Das DB, Satpathy RN, et al. Riboflavin deficiency and severity of malaria. *Eur J Clin Nutr* 1988; 42: 277–83.
29. Garcia LS. Giardiasis. In: Cox FEG, Kreier JP, Wakelin D, eds. *Topley & Wilson's microbiology and microbial infections.* Vol 5: Parasitology. London: Arnold, 1997: 193–202.
30. Farthing MJG. Giardia lamblia. In: Farthing MJG, Keusch GT, eds. *Enteric infection: mechanisms, manifestations and management.* London: Chapman & Hall, 1995: 397–413.
31. MacFarlane DE, Horner-Bryce J. Cryptosporidiosis in well-nourished and malnourished children. *Acta Paediatr Scand* 1987; 76: 474–7.
32. Sallon S, Deckelbaum RJ, Schmid I, et al. Cryptosporidium, malnutrition and chronic diarrhea in children. *Am J Dis Child* 1988; 142,312–5.
33. Farthing MJG, Keusch GT, Wakelin D, eds. *Enteric infection.* 2. Intestinal helminths. London: Chapman & Hall, 1995.

34. Cox FEG, Kreier JP, Wakelin D, eds. *Topley & Wilson's microbiology and microbial infections*. Vol 5: Parasitology. London: Arnold, 1997.

35. Bundy DAP. Epidemiological aspects of *Trichuris* and trichuriasis in Caribbean communities. *Trans R Soc Trop Med Hyg* 1986; 80: 706–18.

36. Pawlowski ZS, Schad GA, Stott GJ. *Hookworm infection and anaemia*. Geneva: World Health Organisation, 1991.

37. Crompton DWT, Whitehead R. Hookworm infections and human iron metabolism. *Parasitology* 1993; 107: S137–45.

38. Pritchard DI, Quinnell RJ, Moustafa M. et al. Hookworm (*Necator americanus*) infection and storage iron depletion. *Trans R Soc Trop Med Hyg* 1991; 85: 235–8.

39. Nesheim MC. Human nutrition needs and parasitic infections. *Parasitology* 1993; 107: S7–18.

40. Cooper ES, Whyte-Alleng CAM, Finzi-Smith JS, MacDonald TT. Intestinal nematode infections in children: the physiological price paid. *Parasitology* 1992; 104: S91–103.

41. Bundy DAP, Cooper ES. *Trichuris* and trichuriasis in humans. *Adv Parasitol* 1989; 28: 107–73.

42. Ramdath DD, Simeon DT, Wong MS, et al. Iron status of schoolchildren with varying intensities of *Trichuris trichiura* infection. *Parasitology* 1995; 110: 347–51.

43. Cooper ES, Spencer J, Murch S, Venugopal S, et al. Mucosal macrophages and plasma cachectin (TNF) in *Trichuris* colitis. *Bull Soc Fr Parasitol* 1990; (Suppl. 2): 347.

44. Thein-Hlang. Ascariasis and childhood malnutrition. *Parasitology* 1993; 107: S125–36.

45. Nesheim MC. Nutritional aspects of *Ascaris suum* and *A. lumbricoides* infection. In: Crompton DWT, Nesheim MC, Pawlowski ZS, eds. *Ascaris and its public health significance*. London: Taylor & Francis, 1985: 147–60.

46. Tshikuka, JG, GrayDonald K, Scott M, et al. Relationship of childhood protein-energy malnutrition and parasite infections in an urban African setting. *Trop Med Int Health* 1997; 2: 374–82.

47. Donnen P, Brasseur D, Draimaix M, et al. Vitamin A supplementation but not deworming improves growth of malnourished preschool children in eastern Zaire. *J Nutr* 1998; 128: 1320–7.

48. Coop RL, Holmes PH. Nutrition and parasite interaction. *Int J Parasitol* 1996; 26: 951–62.

49. Bolin TD, Davis AE, Cummins AG, et al. Effect of iron and protein deficiency on the expulsion of *Nippostrongylus brasiliensis* from the small intestine of the rat. *Gut* 1977; 18: 182–6.

50. Cummins AG, Duncombe VM, Bolin TD, et al. Suppression of rejection of *Nippostrongylus brasiliensis* in iron and protein deficient rats: effect of syngeneic lymphocyte transfer. *Gut* 1978; 19: 823–6.

51. Duncombe VM, Bolin TD, Davis AE, et al. Delayed expulsion of the nematode *Nippostrongylus brasiliensis* from rats on a low protein diet: the role of a bone marrow-derived component. *Am J Clin Nutr* 1981; 34: 400–3.

52. Fenwick PK, Aggett PJ, MacDonald D, et al. Zinc deficiency and zinc repletion: effect on the response of rats to infection with *Trichinella spiralis*. *Am J Clin Nutr* 1990; 52: 166–72.

53. Fenwick PK, Aggett PJ, MacDonald D, et al. Zinc deficiency and zinc repletion: effect on the response of rats to infection with *Strongyloides ratti*. *Am J Clin Nutr* 1990; 52: 173–7.

54. Shi HN, Scott ME, Stevenson MM, et al. Zinc deficiency impairs T cell function in mice with primary infection of *Heligmosomoides polygyrus* (Nematode). *Parasite Immunol* 1994; 16: 339–50.

55. Shi HN, Koski KG, Stevenson MM, et al. Zinc deficiency and energy restriction modify immune responses in mice during primary and challenge infection with *Heligmosomoides polygyrus* (Nematoda). *Parasite Immmunol* 1997; 19: 363–73.

56. Shi HN, Scott ME, Stevenson MM, et al. Energy and zinc deficiency impair the functions of murine T cells and antigen-presenting cells during gastrointestinal nematode infection. *J Nutr* 1988; 128: 20–7.

57. Boulay M, Scott ME, Conly SL, et al. Dietary protein and zinc restrictions independently modify *Heligmosomoides polygyrus* (Nematoda) infection in mice. *Parasitology* 1998; 116: 449–62.

58. Michael E, Bundy DAP. The effect of the protein content of CBA/Ca mouse diet on the population dynamics of *Trichuris muris* (Nematoda) in primary infection. *Parasitology* 1991; 103: 403–11.

59. Michael E, Bundy DAP. Nutrition, immunity and helminth infection—effect of dietary protein on the dynamics of the primary antibody response to *Trichuris muris* (Nematoda) in CBA/Ca mice. *Parasite Immunol* 1992; 14: 169–83.

60. Bundy DAP, Golden MHN. The impact of host nutrition on gastrointestinal helminth populations. *Parasitology* 1987; 95: 623–35.

61. Grazioso CF, Isalgue M, Deramirex I, et al. The effect of zinc supplementation on parasitic reinfestation of Guatamalan schoolchildren. *Am J Clin Nutr* 1993; 57: 673–8.

62. Boivin M, Giordani B. Improvements in cognitive performance for school children in Zaire, Africa, following an iron supplement and treatment for intestinal parasites. *J Pediatr Psychol* 1993; 8: 249–64.
63. Nokes C, Bundy DAP. Does helminth infection affect mental processing and educational achievement? *Parasitol Today* 1994; 10: 14–8.
64. Simeon D, Callender J, Wong M, et al. School performance, nutritional-status and trichuriasis in Jamaican school children. *Acta Paediatr* 1994; 83: 1188–93.

DISCUSSION

Dr. Suskind: One of the points that you made at the end of your discussion was that improved growth is associated with treatment of the parasites. Is there any evidence to show why this change in growth occurs? Is it just that nutrients are no longer lost or is it connected with the relationship between infection, nutritional status, and cytokine production?

Dr. Wakelin: The evidence with experimental systems is that as soon as worms are removed, some of the depressive influences of the worms are removed as well: you immediately, or within a very short time, reverse some of the major immunopathologic changes, so then plasma protein loss certainly would be restricted and some of the consequences of enteropathy would be reduced; in mice, as you take worms away, the gut mucosa reverses the changes that the worms have induced. It has also been shown, with *Trichuris*, that one of the important cytokines associated with the mucosal inflammation is tumor necrosis factor. Presumably by removing worms, cytokine, with all its multiple effects on nutrition, is removed. So I do not think there is a simple explanation, it is probably the effect of multiple factors.

Dr. Haschke: Have similar studies been done with other antioxidants apart from vitamin E?

Dr. Wakelin: Selenium has been investigated but seems not to have that effect in the malaria system.

Dr. Mahmood: You say that children who are malnourished are more vulnerable to malaria, but in Bangladesh we observe that children in certain localized areas are affected by malaria irrespective of their nutritional status. How can you explain that?

Dr. Wakelin: I meant to be careful to say that the experimental animal data initially appeared to show very clearly that a relationship existed between malnutrition and the level of infection and the pathologic changes. The data that have come from Gambia and other parts of Africa have not shown a clear relationship between nutrition and the degree of pathology. I cannot give an explanation why a particular group in Bangladesh should have different responses to malaria from any other. There may be other factors that are relevant, such as transmission frequency, transmission intensity, and genetic characteristics.

Dr. Mahmood: We have observed that in children who come late for treatment, mortality is high irrespective of nutritional status. There are many other factors, for example a high level of parasitemia and central nervous system involvement. Malnutrition is not the only factor.

Dr. Wakelin: I hope I did not say that it was the only factor. Clearly, the time of treatment of children who have both a high level of parasitemia and the initial stages of cerebral malaria is going to influence their survival rate, without a doubt. I do not think that under those conditions nutritive status is likely to be a relevant factor at all.

Dr. Woodward: In the study from Koski's group (1,2) that we both cited, my recollection is that they applied antihelminthic drug treatment to get rid of intestinal adult stage worms between the two experimental infections. Would that not remove the skewing influence of the parasitic infection on immune function that you described?

Dr. Wakelin: I think the simple answer is no. The reason for the protocol they used is that by having a primary infection that induces a given level of immunity, and by removing that infection to allow the immunity to be expressed, an experimental system exists where host immune effects on the parasite can be very clearly measured. In that particular experimental model, if you fail to remove the parasite you will not see expression of immunity, because the parasite, as is the case in many other worms, is immunosuppressive. So, if you want to develop a model where you can compare the effects of nutritive factors on expression of immunity, you have to use a rather artificial system. Similar experiments have been done with other nematodes where that system is not used and the same effects can be demonstrated.

Dr. Keusch: From the prospective of intestinal helminths and the production of clinical symptoms, clearly a relationship exists with worm burden, if you exclude, for instance, single worm ascaris infections causing obstruction of ostia (e.g., the pancreatic duct or the hepatic duct). In addition, in looking at the distribution of worm burden in a population, the largest worm burden is carried by only a very small proportion of the population. Most individuals have relatively light loads. So, it is hard for me to understand why deworming on a population basis could have a significant impact on nutritional status in the whole of the population, when most of those individuals are carrying very light worm burdens. Also, I believe that when you do deworm the entire population and then you look for reacquisition, the individuals who had the highest worm burdens in the first place are more likely to become reinfected. Is that a reflection of potential immunosuppression from that initially heavy worm burden?

Dr. Wakelin: You are quite right that if you look at populations of individuals exposed to what one can presume is a relatively uniform level of infection, then most parasites are aggregated into a small proportion of the population. However, if you stratify the population in terms of age, then a large proportion of the aggregated worms is in the children. You are also quite correct that if you remove worms, you will get re-establishment of worms comparatively quickly if you only treat once or twice. Quite good models suggest how often and at what level you should treat to effect a permanent reduction in the population burden, as well as in individual burdens. It is true that the individuals who tend to have the most worms initially are the individuals who will have the most worms on re-infection. But I think if you look at a population stratified by age, population treatment with an effective antihelminthic will dramatically reduce the levels of infection in most children. The way to break the cycle is then to try to reduce the levels of infection in the most heavily infected people, who are the reservoirs of the infective stages.

Dr. Griffin: A question on vaccines. If I have remembered correctly, the immune response is often directed against excretory proteins such as acetylcholinesterase. Are there any meaningful immune responses that might be contrived to remove these infestations?

Dr. Wakelin: That is a very good question. If you asked me whether I could vaccinate a mouse against these parasites, I could do so very easily. If you ask me whether we can vaccinate humans, I think it is going to be very difficult. Two problems exist. One is our complete lack of understanding of the specific immunologic biology of these parasites in relationship to humans, so we do not know what the target is. Second, we have a similar lack of understanding of the mechanisms that could control these parasites in humans, although we understand how they are controlled in rodents. However, and this may justify Dr. Keusch's skepticism about animal models, I do not think it is easy to extrapolate those results to humans. But we do know there are two types of target. The first is to focus an antiparasite response on the parasite itself. This need not necessarily cause direct damage to the parasite. You can change the environment and get rid of the parasite in that way, but a problem is seen in that you may also introduce immunopathology. Secondly, some of these parasites—particularly parasites such as the hookworm—promote their own survival by releasing a multitude of factors that are immunosuppressive or anti-inflammatory. It, therefore, is a realistic possibility that you could design a protective strategy that targeted the ways in which parasites maintain themselves and, therefore, which would not be associated with the immunopathologic problems of a vaccine. The problem is that not enough money is available to fund it and not enough commercial interest to develop it.

Dr. Tontisirin: Is it true that some parasites can cause allergic manifestations? And if it is true, by what mechanism? And does it have nutritional consequences?

Dr. Wakelin: Typically, worm parasites induce an immune response that is biased toward T-helper 2 cells and type 2 cytokines. So worm parasites, be they schistosomes or intestinal nematodes, are associated with high levels of IgE, peripheral and tissue eosinophilia, and an increase in mucosal mast cells. They, therefore, create an environment for allergic responses in the intestine and also in the lungs. Whether those responses have any influence on the survival of the worm is a question that has been debated for 30 years and is not yet resolved. Certainly, I think it is true that the allergic response contributes to nutritional effects on the host by inducing inflammatory changes in the mucosa, which disturb both digestion and absorption.

Unidentified delegate: In Egypt, schistosomiasis is endemic in the rural areas and hepatitis B is found to be more prevalent among infected children. When the government implemented the antischistosomiasis program, hepatitis B incidence declined as well. It seems that immune suppression caused by the schistosomiasis encourages hepatitis B virus infection in children. These children also had a more aggressive form of hepatitis B. I am not aware of whether, following the elimination of the schistosomiasis in those children, their serum converted and they got rid of the hepatitis B virus as well. However, there seems to be value in parasite control, as the effect is more than the elimination of the parasites—it also decreases coexisting infection.

Dr. Wakelin: I think that is a very good point. The reality is that individuals are infected with many species of parasite as well as other pathogens, all of which may interact with each other or interact through the immune response. Good experimental evidence indicates that both positive and negative interactions can exist between parasites and bacteria and viruses. So, the benefit of removing parasites is not confined to the nutritional effect of simply eliminating the parasite; perhaps the resistance to a number of other infectious agents can be improved as well.

REFERENCES

1. Shi HN, Scott ME, Stevenson MM, et al. Energy restriction and zinc deficiency impair the functions of murine T cells and antigen-presenting cells during gastrointestinal nematode infection. *J Nutr* 1998; 128: 20–7.
2. Shi HN, Koski KG, Stevenson MM, et al. Zinc deficiency and energy restriction modify immune responses in mice during both primary and challenge infection with *Heligmosomoides polygyrus* (Nematoda). *Parasite Immunol* 1997; 19: 363–73.

Nutrition, Immunity, and Infection in Infants and Children, edited by Robert M. Suskind and Kraisid Tontisirin. Nestlé Nutrition Workshop Series, Pediatric Program, Vol. 45. Nestec Ltd., Vevey/Lippincott Williams & Wilkins, Philadelphia ©2001.

Concluding Discussion

The Future Perspectives and the Next 10 Years

R. M. Suskind and K. Tontisirin

The dynamic interactions between nutrition, immunity, and infection in infants and childhood have profound implications on the nutritional well-being of children, which is a major concern to all health professionals. In response to infections, the internal diversion of nutrients that occurs for the synthesis of compounds contributes significantly to the depletion of nutrient stores. A need is seen to learn more about metabolic balances, which exert marked influences on the nutritional status of children.

In terms of future needs, immunologic monitoring should be integrated into the public health management systems which, unfortunately, still have a long way to go. Evaluation of severe or acute infection helps us to know much about the host responses, which are triggered by infection and the clinical function outcomes. Although suboptimal nutrition increases susceptibility to infectious diseases, an understanding of the impact of nutrition on disease prevention requires further education. The agenda for the next 10 years must vigorously pursue practical means of acquiring evidence-based, field-level information. The potential scope and metabolic basis of the nutritional effects of chronic, subclinical infection observed in field studies needs to be explored. Health professionals must pursue the transfer of *in vitro* models and technology to practice, in addition to adopting a comprehensive, preventive approach in various field situations. This would enable counties to achieve many if not most of the child health and nutritional priorities of both the developing and the developed world.

Dr. Suskind: I think this final session could be best spent in designing what we are going to do for the next millennium. You have all had some practice now in putting together your proposals! We are very pleased that Dr. Farthing has volunteered to be our secretary and he is going to take your thoughts and put them together into a document that will be included in the Proceedings. More importantly, it will be also included in a peer-reviewed journal, to get the maximal attention to this area.

Over the course of this meeting, we have obviously discussed problems involving basic science, clinical issues, new methodologies, and interventions. With those major topics in mind, we will begin the discussion about where we are going in the next millennium. To begin the discussion I would like to call on Dr. Sorenson, who has a model he would like to share with us relating to the area of immunology. I am hoping after this meeting that Dr. Sorenson will expand his horizons to include nutrition in that important interaction that he studies in immune-deficient patients.

Dr. Sorensen: I will try to be very brief. In the Latin-American group, for primary immune deficiencies, we created a two-page form, by mutual agreement, that everybody can use. It has a demographic information component, diagnostic information, a nutrition component for immunologists, which as you see is rather short, and information about infections. It is very easy to follow and to fill in. It is an Epi-Info program that is accessible to everybody who participates in the program. Data are collected on the hard copy and then entered into the Epi-Info program. Personal data is owned individually and there is no centralized data collection, which does away with the possibility of people stealing data. However, because the data are collected in a similar way, it is easy to compare the data, by mutual agreement, between one country or one group of investigators and another. Each section of the record—demographic information, diagnostic data, infections, and so on—can be expanded at will to suit the needs of individual investigators, so this is an adaptable source of information.

The way we handle the different diagnostic components that are important in collecting data about primary immune deficiencies is by using classifications and definitions. This can be adapted easily to nutritional state, infections, the environment, or whatever you decide to use.

Lastly, because 12 countries are participating in this, we created a Web site where all this material is published (http://www.cdc.gov/epiinfo/). Anybody who has the Adobe Reader program, which is free, can download the form. It can then be adapted and shortened (in some countries the abbreviated form has been published in pediatric journals so that pediatricians can easily submit data). In that same Web site, we also publish the classifications of the different conditions we are interested in, including immune deficiencies, molecular defects, and associated diseases, as well as methods that we propose should be used by everybody studying primary immune deficiency syndromes.

To finalize the form, we shared and circulated the versions that everybody had and, after a little give and take, we came up with the issues that everybody considered essential. We then field-tested the final version of the form so that everybody could see whether it really worked and whether people could use it easily. It has now been implemented.

I think it is essential that we create ways of monitoring the changes that are occurring in our fields; having a common way of collecting essential data, allows us to compare what happens in different regions and in the same region over time.

Dr. Suskind: Thank you very much. I would like to have comments from the floor.

Dr. Fawzi: Who actually uses the form?

Dr. Sorensen: The form is made available to every investigator, that is, any physician who is interested in participating. Each one then fills it out, entering patients with primary immune deficiencies (I am just using it as an example of how things could be done). A minimum of information needs to be entered: that is, the phenotypic diagnosis and some essential laboratory results—complete blood cell count, immunoglobulin levels, and so on—so that each diagnosis is documented with the pertinent laboratory information.

Dr. Haschke: To follow-up on this proposal, how would you now implement it more generally?

Dr. Sorensen: I think implementation would need to be done by e-mail and by creating a Web site where the material can be posted and seen by everybody. I believe that implementation would probably be impossible without using electronic communication media. We have as part of our Web site an electronic journal which is very inexpensive. We did all this with very little money, because it was a volunteer job. We have no formal structure, no president or secretary or anything. The way ahead would be for people to indicate, when we leave here today, that they want to participate. I am sure that the people here, who gave such excellent talks, will be able to identify clearly what data need to be collected in relationship to nutrition in order to define the situation in a patient. I could contribute, together with several other speakers, in proposing essential data to be collected regarding immunity and allergy. We also heard what kinds of infectious diseases one should consider. The way to do it would perhaps be to announce it through this book and then start an informal group to develop the form.

Dr. Suskind: Thank you very much Dr. Sorenson. I think that is an excellent idea and it could be integrated into the entire subject matter of this meeting. Obviously, as Dr. Sorenson mentioned, the form would need to be very specific in terms of the nutritional information obtained, the standardization of both the immunologic data and any interventions, and looking at the outcome variables. I would think that something like this could be a very effective tool in developing an overall global strategy, and also in developing centers of excellence in nutrition and immunology. I am sure that many of these exist in various parts of the world, but identifying them and bringing them together by this process of standardization would be very valuable. Individuals who do not have all the technology that is associated with these centers would be able to benefit from them and be a part of an international network looking at questions to be defined in the areas of nutrition and immunology. The resources that could come from those centers of excellence in nutritional immunology could generate funding for joint studies involving different centers.

Dr. Woodward: I think something like this would be really useful and, from my perspective, for all practical purposes essential for those working with experimental animals as well. When it comes to assessing the nutritional status of our animals and relating the models that we use to categories of human disease, currently that is essentially impossible, so the first thing we would have to do would be to establish the criteria that should be applied in a standardized way to animal studies. Of course, one of the complexities of that is a database would have to be established for individual species and strains, as is the case for humans. I am not sure that is much more complex than is needed for humans anyway, as individual nations need their own standards for humans. I think the kind of format that is being suggested here could be most workable to improve the standards of animal work.

Dr. Suskind: It certainly would be a powerful tool in terms of attracting funding sources, because of the interaction that would occur between various parts of this network of nutritional immunology centers. As you point out, it would obviously include both animal models and human models in the standardization. I think one of the things that came out very clearly in this meeting is the interaction that can occur when you bring together individuals with different backgrounds to answer questions about the same problem. We all look at things in a slightly different way and I think the field could move ahead so much more effectively by the kind of interaction that might occur through a system that brought these diverse interests together.

Dr. Wasantwisut: I welcome the idea of centers of excellence in nutrition and immunology. I would like to see collaboration between centers in developed countries and developing countries, which could answer some of the important questions that we cannot tackle at present because we lack the technical expertise and equipment to do certain immunologic studies. It would be useful to identify, through e-mail networking for example, the particular interests of these centers, because it is unlikely that one center will excel in all the areas we have been covering these last three days.

My second point is to emphasize the need for standardization in the design of the field studies. We need someone to look at this and come up with recommendations about numbers of samples, the power needed, and what kind of standard protocols are required for people who want to conduct studies in the field.

Dr. Coovadia: When I first heard this proposal I was not sure about its purpose or goal and I was really skeptical. When you put it in the context of some sort of network, and if this serves as the first step, then that makes sense to me and I am in favor of it. I cannot speak for my entire continent but it is incredibly difficult to obtain this kind of information on a regular basis. I run a huge department; people such as me run departments all over Africa. To get staff to fill in an ordinary case sheet is almost impossible on a routine basis. Our notification rates for infectious diseases are dreadful. So, although it is important to try to do this, we may have to identify something equivalent to sentinel sites—you call them centers of excellence and I hope they are—and use them as markers of what is probably going on in a region.

Dr. Sorensen: Two very brief comments. First, about funding: the Latin-American group has used this system to get funding because they can now show that they will obtain better data by the collaborations that have been established. Second, a tendency exists to take an idea and develop it so much and make it so ambitious that nothing gets done. I would caution against that. If you want to start, let us start in a very modest way and get something done.

Dr. Keusch: Because we are into the phase in the meeting where sweeping generalizations are acceptable and maybe desirable, I want to pick up on something that Dr. Coovadia talked about earlier and put it in a different perspective.

Dr. Coovadia was lamenting, I think, the research perspective that lacks implementation in a public health sense. My sweeping generalization is that every intervention, in this case in nutrition, is an experimental model. If we fail to take advantage of those interventions as an experimental model, then we are doomed to repeat the errors of the past. In the context of evaluation, even if an intervention, as with vitamin A, which some think has already been proved and should just be implemented, there is ample room for continuing research in the context of: How do you deliver vitamin A? When do you deliver vitamin A? To whom do you deliver vitamin A? How often do you deliver vitamin A? At very operational levels, a need is clearly seen for ongoing research.

I would go much further than that. I think that without understanding the mechanisms by which vitamin A works, there is no way to know how that intervention could be improved. It may be that if we look at vitamin A as a transcriptional regulator and that some of the things that vitamin A does in a favorable sense may be related to transcriptional regulation of certain aspects of the immune system, then not all retinoids will act in all tissues. In addition, there may be some specificity in the nature of the retinoid metabolites that act on populations of lymphocytes or at other points in the immune system. The only way we are going to sort that out is to be actively engaged in research. It is a matter of concern that implementation agencies are concerned primarily about coverage and that as soon as you mention the word *research* they go into a panic. We should do better than that.

Dr. Gerschwin: My own perspective as an immunologist is perhaps a little different. Dr. Sorenson's form is suitable for highly defined conditions such as immunodeficiency syndromes, but based on what I have heard this week, applying it to nutritional immunology will only result in going through the law of diminishing returns all over again. I think what this group needs to do is make some standard definition of outcomes, so that everyone has some idea of what the read-outs ought to be. Then, you can compare studies properly. I think this whole conference should have the heading of "What should appropriate outcomes be?"

Dr. Chandra: Almost 15 years ago some of us who were working in this field got together and formed an international nutritional immunology group with almost no sort of funding from any central agency. The main purpose was to be able to do such simple services as providing reprints to people in developing countries where they had very poor library facilities. For quite some time we were able to sustain that, but over the years I think interest has waned and I do not know whether a central collection agency would be helpful at all. So far as research protocols are concerned, so much depends on the funding agencies, what kind of things they are looking for, what kind of questions to ask. To have some kind of a single standard form for everything would be an almost impossible goal.

Dr. Suskind: Dr. Keusch, would you like to comment as the head of the Fogarty Center at the National Institutes of Health on the potential of this approach?

Dr. Keusch: I will not speak for the US National Institutes of Health, I will just speak for myself as an individual. I think that there is value in considering the proposal of centers of excellence. In the field of nutrition, I suspect that it would require many such centers because the nutritional conditions in different countries are not identical and we would need to be able to look at a range of underlying nutritional problems and potential solutions. Because of this, it would be a costly endeavor, particularly with field studies which, as Dr. Coovadia pointed out, require a sufficient sample size to accurately assess the impact of interventions. So, I think that there is probably going to be a requirement for multiple funding sources from the developed countries that wish to invest in it, as well as from foundations, potential industry contributions, and, without a doubt, contributions from the countries themselves in which such centers might be situated. I think the idea should be pursued but it requires us to look ahead and work out how and where we can do it and what would be the research issues.

Dr. Suskind: In relation to that, do you feel that in various parts of the world, the developing as well as the developed, resources are already available which, with some modification, could apply standardized approaches to the immunologic and nutritional issues we have been talking about? I am not sure how much it would take. I think it would require the commitment of certain funding agencies to support the concept that these areas are important for future research, but fairly sophisticated laboratories are found in various parts of the world and others that could certainly be improved. One thing that is important is the implementation of programs and perhaps Dr. Tontisirin may want to talk about that.

Dr. Tontisirin: The concepts of networking in producing protocols and building up expertise through training and research are crucial. Whether we can get the funding is another matter, but we have to try. The second aspect we have to think hard about is what questions need to be answered. This meeting has provided us with a stock of knowledge and evidence to enable us to make recommendation for action to prevent and control malnutrition and infection. We can review for ourselves the key issues that need further research leading to action, and the key issues that need basic research leading to a better understanding.

Dr. Haschke: A comment on how work could be structured. Industry tries to steer clear of institutional projects. Institutions have a tendency to work together for a certain period and then new people arrive who have other interests. An efficient approach is to have *platform projects* where people meet with a certain idea on a certain platform and then go on from there. This is a project-driven approach that has been found to be very effective in covering many of the matters that have been discussed here—for example, the evaluation of nutrition and immunity, education, how studies should be designed, maybe standardization of methods, and so on. I think it would be much easier to get money from international funding agencies for such platform activities.

Dr. Fjeld: In support of what Dr. Haschke just said, I would like to mention that when we were at the Atomic Energy Agency, we had coordinated research programs built around a platform. For example, we had one on the effect of infection on amino acid metabolism and another on vitamin A. We got a group together around a common theme and we worked with developing countries and developed countries, we built partnerships, we opened up exchange, we had a network—approximately six teams of about 12 people—and sometimes we had some invited consultants who were not part of the team but who came in on an *as needed* basis. The various teams worked independently but they have all been very successful; they have contributed substantially to our knowledge as well as improved the scientific skills and technical skills of everybody involved. It was a structure that attracted a fair amount of funding and resulted in a lot of publications. I think it is a model that could be considered.

Dr. Kennedy: My experience has been very limited but for whatever it is worth I will give it to you. My work has been almost totally funded by the pharmaceutical industry. I agree with Dr. Haschke that the model he describes is probably the most utilitarian and will speed the progress of moving nutrition toward mainstream immunology the fastest. I think that a host of different ways can be used to approach this, but defining the problem, creating project teams, and somehow attracting individuals with a variety of expertise is what is going to be needed. The answers to some of these questions are going to be so complex that you are going to need to find a world class immunologist, a world class endocrinologist, and a world class nutritionist and put them altogether to solve a very specific problem. Once the project is done, you create a new project team. That, I think, is a very good idea.

Dr. Farthing: I think this has been a productive discussion. What we have not dealt with is to define what are the remaining research issues that really need to be tackled? All the speakers flagged certain areas that they regard as being important, but one thing I think would be keen for us to acknowledge is that there are some areas that no longer need to be *re-researched*. If you go to a funding agency with an enormous shopping list, they tend to use the word "unfocused" to destroy the project. I think it will be unwise for us as a group to come up with enormous shopping lists for the next 20 years. The research has to be targeted and we need to acknowledge that some areas seem to be well established now and do not need continuing enormous projects just to re-research the same area.

Dr. Suskind: I would suggest that Dr. Farthing, Dr. Tontisirin, and I put together your ideas for future priorities as a draft document. This could then be distributed electronically.

Dr. Tontisirin: We would all like to thank our Chairman for this last session.

Dr. Suskind: I think it has been a wonderful 4 days and thanks for all that you put into this and thanks to Nestlé for bringing us all together.

Subject Index

References followed by "f" indicate figures; those followed by "t" denote tables.

5-HT (serotonin), in anorexia, 310

A

Acquired immunodeficiency syndrome. *See* AIDS

Acrodermatitis enteropathica, 205

Acute phase proteins
  amino acids for, 288–289, 289f
  in inflammatory response, 47–48, 47t
  muscle proteins in, 288–290, 289f
  negative, 292–294
  protein-energy malnutrition on, 97–99

Acute phase response, 182
  animal models of, 364–365
  exercise-induced, 184–187, 185f
  protein-energy malnutrition on, 97–99
  on protein synthesis, 283
  rodent endotoxin model of, 359–361, 360t, 361t
  weight loss in, 364

Adaptive defenses, protein-energy malnutrition on, childhood, 99–108. *See also* Protein-energy malnutrition, childhood

Adenosine deaminase (ADA) deficiency, 63

Adhesion molecules, dietary fatty acids on, 144–145

Aero allergens, 267, 267f

Age, on immune function, 184–185, 185f

AIDS (acquired immunodeficiency syndrome)
  β-carotene on, 380, 381t
  global, 11
  growth hormone resistance in, 395
  insulinlike growth factors in, 395
  leptin in, 395–396
  testosterone deficiency in, 394–395
  thyroid function in, 395
  tuberculosis and, 11
  vitamin A supplements on, 377, 380
  vitamin B_{12} supplements on, 377

Allergen immunotherapy, 268–269

Allergens
  age and sensitization to, 266–267, 267f
  food
    anaphylaxis from, 269
    sensitization to, age and, 267, 267f

Allergic response
  immediate-type, 265
  modification of, 268–269

Allergic rhinitis, risk of, 269–270

Allergic sensitization, on Th1/Th2 balance, 271, 276

Allergy
  breast-feeding on, 270–271, 271t
  discussion on, 274–278
  in infections, 263
  prevention of, 271–272, 276
    in infants, 270–271, 271t
  risk of, prediction of, 269–270

α-linolenic acid, on lymphocyte proliferation, 147–148

Amino acid(s), 281–282
  for acute phase proteins, 288–289, 289f
  in infections
    metabolic effects of, 281–282
    oxidation of, 290–292
  nutritional roles of, 283
  tumor necrosis factor on, 292

Amino acid metabolism
  cytokines on, 284–286
    nutrient–endocrine interactions in, 284–285
    resetting metabolic priorities in, 285–286
    substrate competition in, 285–286
  in infection, 290–292
  tumor necrosis factor on, 292

Ancylostoma duodenale, 414–416

Anorexia
  cytokines in, 309–311, 311f
    discussion of, 314–317
    growth retardation and, 311–313, 312f
    immune activation models of, 309
    infection and inflammation models of, 310–311, 311f
    specific models of, 309–310
  infection and, 303–304
    appetite control and, in health, 304–307
      central mechanisms of, 305–306, 305f
      peripheral mechanisms of, 306–307, 306t
    in infection response, 303–307, 314–317
  in infectious disease, 49

Anorexia nervosa, 244, 245t
  cellular immune function in, 252

433

Anorexia nervosa (*contd.*)
   cytokine changes in, 253–255, 254f
   discussion on, 258–262
   disease resistance and, 246
   on immune function, 247–248
   on immunocompetent cells, 248
   on lymphocyte subsets, 249–250, 250f
Antagonism, malnutrition–infection, 45, 46t
Antibiotics
   on chicken growth, 287–288, 293, 297–298
   on immune status, 276
Antibody(ies)
   classes of, 75
   in low birthweight infants, 128
   measurement of, 60
   as opsonins, 77
   production of
      dietary fatty acids on, 151
      vitamin E supplements on, 229
Antibody dependent, cell-mediated cytotoxicity
      (ADCC), 75
Antibody-mediated immunity, Th1/Th2 balance
      in, 265–266, 266f
Antibody response, systemic
   protein-energy malnutrition on, 100
   T-cell–dependent, protein-energy
         malnutrition on, 101
   T-cell–independent
      protein-energy malnutrition on, 101
      vitamin A deficiency on, 215–216
Antigen-presenting cells (APCs), 71, 265
Antigens, protein-energy malnutrition on,
      106–107
Antioxidants. *See also* specific antioxidants,
      e.g., Malaria
   on malaria, 412–413
Appetite. *See also* Anorexia; Anorexia nervosa
   GI infections on, 320–321
Appetite control, in health, 304–307
   central mechanisms of, 305–306, 305f
   peripheral mechanisms of, 306–307, 306t
Arachidonic acid, on lymphocyte proliferation,
      148
Arcuate nucleus–paraventricular nucleus,
      neuropeptide Y pathway, 305–306,
      305f
Ascaris lumbricoides, 414–417
Ascorbate, on malaria, 412
Asthma, predicting risk of, 269–270
Atopic dermatitis, predicting risk of, 269–270
Azurophilic granules, primary, 70

B

β-carotene, on AIDS, 380, 381t
B cells (lymphocytes)
   in adaptive immune response, 175
   evaluation of, 74

   protein-energy malnutrition on, 104
   vitamin A deficiency on, 214, 214t, 215
Bacille Calmette-Guérin (BCG) vaccination, on
      allergy, 265, 277
Bacterial translocation, in protein-energy
      malnutrition, 90
Birthweight, low, 4, 15, 121–129, 132–135
   chronic disease and, 15
   discussion on, 132–135
   heterogeneity of infants with, 121–122
   hospital admission with, 122, 124
   immune system with, 127–129
      antibodies, 128
      cell-mediated immunity, 128–129
      complement, 129
      immunoglobulins, 128
      polymorphonuclear leukocytes, 129
   infection with, 122–127
      adulthood, 126
      infant and early childhood, 122–124, 123t,
         124t
      susceptibility to, 124–127
         differential, 124, 126
         mechanism of, 126–127
   morbidity with, 124, 125t
   mortality with, 122, 123t
   research on, future, 129
   vitamin E deficiency with, 228
Blood clearance activity, protein-energy
      malnutrition on, 92
Body mass index (BMI), 244
   optimum, 246t
Breast-feeding, 374
   on allergy, 270–271, 271t
   on HIV, 374, 376
   on immunity, 277
   reduced, in low birthweight infants, 127
Bulimia nervosa, 244, 245t
   cellular immune function in, 252
   discussion on, 260
   on immune function, 247
   on immunocompetent cells, 248
   on lymphocyte subsets, 250, 251f

C

C3, 76
C3a, 76
C4a, 76–77
C5a, 76
Capillaria phillipinensis, 415
β-Carotene, on AIDS, 380, 381t
CD45, 72
CD46, in measles, 189, 189f
CD antigens, 189
CD154 (CD40L), 63
CD4 cells, obesity on, 248–249
CD4+ cells, vitamin A deficiency on, 214

CD28–B7 interaction, 180
CD4:CD8 ratio, protein-energy malnutrition on, 105
cDNA analysis, in mutation detection, 64–65
CD45RA$^+$, protein-energy malnutrition on, 105
Cell-mediated immunity
  evaluation of, 60–61
  in low birthweight infants, 128–129
  malnutrition on, 29–31
  measles on, 189, 189f
  protein-energy malnutrition on, 99–102
Cellular immunity, 176–177
Chemotaxis, fatty acids in, 142–143
Chills, in infectious disease, 49
Cholecystokinin (CCK), 306
Chronic inflammatory diseases, dietary fatty
        acids on, 157–158
Common differentiated (CD) antigens, 189. *See
        also* CD
Complement
  evaluation of, 75–77
  in low birthweight infants, 129
Complement cascade, 76
Complement system
  malnutrition on, 34
  protein-energy malnutrition on, 95–97
Cow's milk, infant allergy to, 267
  prevention of, 270–271, 271t
Coxsackievirus infection, vitamin E deficiency
        on, 231
Cryptosporidium parvum, 413–414
CTLA-4, 180
Cytokine(s). *See also* specific cytokines, e.g.,
        Interleukin-1 (IL-1)
  in acute phase response, protein-energy
        malnutrition on, 97–99
  on amino acid metabolism, 284–286
    nutrient–endocrine interactions in, 284–285
    resetting metabolic priorities in, 285–286
    substrate competition in, 285–286
  in anorexia, 309–311, 311f
    discussion on, 314–317
    growth retardation and, 311–313, 312f
    immune activation models of, 309
    infection and inflammation models of,
        310–311, 311f
    specific models of, 309–310
  anorexia nervosa on, 253–255, 254f
  in chronic inflammatory disease, 157–158
  eating disorders on, 252–255, 254f
  evaluation of, 77
  exercise on, 185f, 186–187
  on feeding behavior, 310–311, 311f
  on HIV infection, 393–394
  HIV on, 153
  in immune response, 49
  in infection response, 303, 307–309, 314–317
  intracellular, evaluation of, 62–63

leptins and, 253
nutritional effects of, 283
  experimental design for, 283–284
production of
  dietary fatty acids on, 151–154
  HIV infection on, 153
protein-energy malnutrition on, 107–108
on protein synthesis and breakdown, 286–287
secretion of, detection of, 62
in vivo response to, dietary fatty acids on, 155
Cytokine-driven T-helper cell differentiation,
        177, 177f
Cytokine mRNA, 63
Cytokine receptors, dietary fatty acids on,
        145–146
Cytotoxic T cells, 73
  activity of, 74
Cytotoxicity assays, 74

D
Daycare centers, on allergy, 276–277
Defenses, host, 55–57, 56f
Delayed type hypersensitivity (DTH), 78, 177,
        177f
  dietary fatty acids on, 155–156
  Th1/Th2 balance in, 265–266, 266f
  vitamin E supplements on, 229–230
Delayed type hypersensitivity (DTH) skin
        testing, 60–61, 78
  obesity on, 251–252
  protein-energy malnutrition on, 100
  stress on, 187, 188t
  vitamin A deficiency on, 215
Dermatitis, atopic, predicting risk of, 269–270
Desaturation, 137
Diarrheal infections. *See also* Gastrointestinal
        infections
  epidemiology of, 319
  intestinal absorption in, 321–322
  on nutritional status, community-based
        studies of, 322–323
  vitamin A supplements on, 327, 328, 328t,
        332–333
    community-based mortality trials on,
        223–225, 223t
    hospital-based mortality trials on, 220–221,
        221t
Dietary intake, GI infections on, 320–321
Diets, weight loss
  on immunocompetence, 245–246
  on lymphocyte subsets, 249
  optimum, 246
Diphtheria, reemergence of, 10
DNA vaccines, 277–278
Docosahexaenoic acid (DHA), on lymphocyte
        proliferation, 148–149
DPT immunization, global, 10

E

Eating disorders
  discussion on, 258–262
  on immunity and infection, 243–256,
      259–262 (*See also* specific eating
      disorders, e.g., Obesity)
Eicosanoids, 138, 141. *See also* Fatty acids
  immune cell production of, 141–142, 142f
  metabolism of, 138f, 141
Eicosapentaenoic acid (EPA), on lymphocyte
      proliferation, 148–149
ELISA, 75
ELISPOT, 75
Endotoxin, dietary fatty acids on *in vivo*
      response to, 155
Entamoeba histolytica, 413–414
Enteropathy, parasite-induced, 413, 413t
Enzyme-linked immunosorbent assay (ELISA),
      75
Enzyme-linked immunospot (ELISPOT), 75
Epithelial mucus, protein-energy malnutrition
      on, 90
Exercise
  excess, on immune function, 184–187, 185f
  illness and, 184
Exercise immunology, 183–184

F

Fasting, neuroendocrine response to, 305–306,
      305f
Fatigue, in infectious disease, 49
Fatty acids
  endogenous synthesis of, 137–138, 138f
  polyunsaturated, 137–138
Fatty acids, dietary, 137–161, 168–172
  on acute inflammatory responses, 155
  after organ transplantation, 158
  on animal models
      of inflammatory and autoimmune disease,
        157
      of organ transplantation, 157
  on antibody production, 151
  on chemotaxis, 142–143
  in chronic inflammatory diseases, 157–158
  on cytokine production, 151–154, 155
      IL-1, 152
      IL-2, 153–154
      IL-4, 153–154
      IL-6, 152–153
      IL-10, 153–154
      tumor necrosis factor, 151–152
  on delayed type hypersensitivity, 155–156
  discussion on, 168–172
  on eicosanoid production, 141–144
  on endotoxin, response to, 155
  on γ-interferon, 153–154
  on graft *versus* host response, 156–157

  on host defense, 158–159
  on host *versus* graft response, 156–157
  on immune cell fatty acid composition, 141,
      141t
  on immune response, 139, 140f
  on inflammation and cell-mediated immunity,
      155–157
  on lymphocyte cytotoxicity, 149
  on lymphocyte proliferation, 146–149
      α-linolenic acid, 147–148
      arachidonic acid, 148
      docosahexaenoic acid, 148–149
      eicosapentaenoic acid, 148–149
      γ-linolenic acid, 147
      linoleic acid–rich oils, 147
      oleic acid, 147
      saturated, 146
  on natural killer cell activity, 149–150
  on nitric oxide, 143–144
  in pancreatic cancer, 157–158
  on phagocytosis, 143
  principal, 138, 139t
  questions on, 159–160
  on reactive oxygen species, 143–144
  on surface marker expression, 144–147
      adhesion molecules, 144–145
      cytokine receptors, 145–146
      major histocompatibility antigens, 144
Febrile response, protein-energy malnutrition
      on, 98
Feeding behavior, 304–307
  central mechanisms of, 305–306, 305f
      cytokines in, 310–311, 311f
  peripheral mechanisms of, 306–307, 306t
Female children, survival of, 12–13
Female empowerment, nutritional improvement
      from, 18
Fever, in infectious disease, 49
Folate deficiency, in expectant mothers, 11
Folic acid deficiency, global, 9
Food allergens
  anaphylaxis from, 269
  sensitization to, age and, 267, 267f
Food allergy, infant, prevention of, 270–271,
      271t
Future perspectives, 425–431

G

γ-interferon, 266, 266f
  dietary fatty acids on, 153–154
  protein-energy malnutrition on, 107–108
γ-linolenic acid, on lymphocyte proliferation,
      147
Gastric distension, 306–307
Gastrointestinal infections, 319–329, 332–335,
      413–417. *See also* Diarrheal
      infections

on appetite and dietary intake, 320–321
on cognitive development, 418
discussion on, 332–335
epidemiology of, 319, 413
Helicobacter pylori, 323–325, 324t, 332, 334
on host nutrition, 319–320, 321f
on intestinal absorption, 321–322
micronutrient status and
   iron, 327–328
   vitamin A, 327, 328, 328t, 332–333
   zinc, 326–327, 327t, 328, 332–335
nematodes, 414–417, 415f
nutrition and, 413, 414f
   immunity to, 417–418
on nutritional status, 322–323
protozoa, 413–414
susceptibility to, malnutrition on, 325–326,
   326t
Gene abnormalities, immune system, 57–58,
   58f, 58t
evaluation of, 64–65
Gene sequencing, mutation detection by, 64–65
Giardia lamblia, 413–414
Global Burden of Disease study, 16, 16t
Graft *versus* host response, dietary fatty acids
   on, 156–157
Granulocyte-macrophage colony-stimulating
   factor (GM-CSF), protein-energy
   malnutrition on, 91
Growth, cytokines on, 283
Growth hormone resistance, in AIDS, 395
Growth inhibition
   cytokines on, 311–313, 312f
   infection in, 281–285, 297–302 (*See also*
     Infection, metabolic effects of)

H

Helicobacter pylori, on children's nutrition,
   323–325, 324t, 332, 334
HIV, IgE antibodies against, 264
HIV infection. *See also* AIDS
on cytokine production, 153
differential diagnosis of, 65, 65t
malnutrition on, 371–396, 403–406
   discussion of, 403–406
   epidemiology of, 371
   transmission and progression of, 371–387
     in adults, 376–383
      anthropometric measures and body
       composition in, 382–383,
       384t–385t
      vitamins in, 376–380, 378t–379t,
       381t
      zinc and selenium in, 380, 382
     epidemiologic evidence of, 371–372
     mechanisms of, 383–387

pregnancy outcomes and child health in,
   372–376
   breast-feeding on, 374, 376
   vitamins on, 372–374, 373t, 375t
nutrition and, 361–363
   discussion on, 366–369
   energy balance, 362–363
   protein metabolism, 362
   weight loss patterns, 361–362
on nutritional status, 387–396
   epidemiological evidence of, 387–390
     body composition, 389–390
     intrauterine growth, 388
     postnatal anthropometric measurements,
      388–389
   mechanisms of, 391–396
     cytokines, 393–394
     energy balance, 391–392
     food intake, 392
     hormonal changes, 394–396
     nutrient malabsorption, 392–393
tuberculosis and, 11
vaccines against, 278
weight loss with, 304
Hookworms, 414–417
Host defenses, 55–57, 56f, 201–202, 202f, 203f
dietary fatty acids on, 158–159
in infection, 48–50
Host *versus* graft response, dietary fatty acids
   on, 156–157
Human immunodeficiency virus (HIV)
   infection. *See* AIDS; HIV infection
Humoral immune competence
malnutrition on, 33
protein-energy malnutrition on, 102–103
   childhood, 99–102
vitamin E deficiency on, 227–228
vitamin E supplements on, 229
Hyper-IgE syndrome, 268
Hypersensitivity
delayed, 78
evaluation of, 78
Hypoallergenic formula, 276

I

Immune competence
in infectious disease, 49–50
nutrition on, 188–192, 189f, 191f
protein-energy malnutrition on, 89–111,
   116–120
   adaptive defenses, 99–108
     antigen processing and presentation,
      106–107
     cytokines, 107–108
     humoral and cell-mediated responses,
      99–102
     lymphoid involution, 103–104

Immune competence (*contd.*)
    mucosal humoral immune competence,
      102–103
    T cell subset imbalances, 105–106
  discussion of, 116–120
  immunodepression, 108–109
  innate defenses, 90–99
    acute phase response, 97–99
    blood clearance activity, 92
    complement system, 95–97
    myeloid cell proliferation, 91–92
    natural killer cell, 99
    neutrophils, 91
    phagocytes
      cell numbers of, 91–92
      microbicidal and chemotactic
        capabilities of, 93–94
      respiratory burst of, 94–95
    phagocytosis, 92–93
    physical barriers, 90–91
Immune mechanisms, innate, 69–70
Immune response
  adaptive (specific), 175–181
    basic elements of, 175
    cellular immunity in, 176–177
    delayed-type hypersensitivity reaction in,
      177, 177f
    lymphocytes in, 175–176, 176t
    NK cells in, 176, 176t
    presentation in, 175
    T cells in, 176, 176t
      co-stimulatory pathways of, 180
      development of, early, 179–180
      MHC-presented antigen response of,
        178–179
      receptor signal transduction of, 178,
        178f, 179f
    Th1/Th2 differentiation in, 178
  in elderly, 274–275
Immune system, 55–68
  defects in
    differential diagnosis of, 66, 66t
    infections with, 65, 65t
    molecular, 57–58, 58f, 58t
    evaluation of, 63
  discussion on, 68
  evaluation of, in at risk hosts, 69–87
    B cells and immunoglobulins, 74–75
    complement, 75–77
    cytokines, 77
    discussion on, 83–87
    hypersensitivity, 78
    phagocytes, 70–71
    T lymphocytes, 71–74
    tier system, 78–83, 78t
      tier 1, 78t, 79
      tier 2, 78t, 79–81
      tier 3, 78t, 81–82

gene abnormalities in, 57–58, 58f, 58t
  evaluation of, 64–65
host defenses in, 55–57, 56f
immunologic phenotypes in, 57–58, 58f, 58t
  evaluation of, 59–63 (*See also*
    Immunologic phenotypes,
    evaluation of)
in low birthweight infants, 127–129
  antibodies, 128
  cell-mediated immunity, 128–129
  complement, 129
  immunoglobulins, 128
  polymorphonuclear leukocytes, 129
Immunity
  malnutrition and, 29–35
    cellular immune response, 29–31
    complement system, 34
    humoral immune response, 33
    interleukins, 31–33
    natural killer cells, 31, 73–74
    polymorphonuclear leukocyte response,
      33–34
  programming of, 126
  stress and, 173–188, 196–199 (*See also*
    Stress, immunity and)
    adaptive immune response in, 175–181
      (*See also* Immune response,
      adaptive [specific])
Immunization. *See also* Vaccines
  in sub-Saharan Africa, 10
  on Th1/Th2 balance, 271–272
Immunocompetent cells, nutritional status on,
    248
Immunodeficiency, infections with, 183, 183t
Immunodeficiency diseases. *See also* HIV
    infection
  differential diagnosis of, 66, 66t
  genotype, molecular defect, and phenotype
    of, 57–58, 58f, 58t
  infections with, 65, 65t
  from malnutrition, 65
Immunodepression
  in infection-related malnutrition
    morbidity/mortality, 89
  protein-energy malnutrition on, 108–109
Immunoglobulin (Ig)
  evaluation of, 74–75
  in low birthweight infants, 128
  protein-energy malnutrition on, 101–102
Immunoglobulin A (IgA), protein-energy
    malnutrition on, 101–103
Immunoglobulin E (IgE)
  ontogeny of, 266–268, 267f
  Th1/Th2 balance and, 265–266, 266f
  viral infections and, 264
Immunoglobulin G (IgG), vitamin A deficiency
    on, 215

Immunoglobulin M (IgM), protein-energy
    malnutrition on, 101–102
Immunologic phenotypes, 57–58, 58f, 58t
  evaluation of, 59–63
    antibodies, specific, 60
    concentrations, 59
    cytokine mRNA, 63
    cytokines
      intracellular, 62–63
      secretion of, 62
    delayed hypersensitivity skin testing,
      60–61, 78, 100
    general, 59
    lymphocyte proliferation assay, 62, 72–73
    lymphocyte subpopulations, 61–62
Immunotherapy, allergen, 268–269
India
  immunization in, 10
  maternal mortality in, 12
Infection(s). *See also* specific types, e.g.,
    Gastrointestinal infections
  allergy and, 264–265
  anorexia and, 303–304
    appetite control and, in health, 304–307
      central mechanisms of, 305–306, 305f
      peripheral mechanisms of, 306–307,
        306t
    cytokines in, 309–311, 311f
      discussion on, 314–317
      growth retardation and, 311–313, 312f
      immune activation models of, 309
      infection and inflammation models of,
        310–311, 311f
      specific models of, 309–310
  catabolic responses in, 285–286
  childhood
    malnutrition and, 34, 45–46, 46t (*See also*
      Immunity, malnutrition and;
      Malnutrition, infection and)
      nitrogen loss in, 47–48, 47t
      nutrition and, 28–29
      on nutritional status, 46–49, 47t
      prevention of, 18
  cytokines and, 303, 307–309, 314–317
  host responses to, 49
  immune activation in, 49–50
  iron in, 48–49
  metabolic effects of, 281–295, 297–302
    amino acid oxidation in, 290–292
    amino acids and functional proteins in,
      281–282
    antibiotics on chicken growth and,
      287–288
    cytokines in, 283
      experimental design on, 283–284
      nutrient–endocrine interactions and,
        284–285
      on protein synthesis and breakdown,
        286–287

      resetting metabolic priorities and,
        285–286
      substrate competition in, 285–286
    discussion on, 297–302
    modes of, 282–283
    negative acute phase proteins in, 292–294
    research on, future, 294–295
    substrate competition in, 288–290, 289f
    tumor necrosis factor in, 292
  prevention of, 271–272
  susceptibility to, malnutrition on, 325–326,
    326t
  vitamin A deficiency on, 218
  vitamin A in, 48–49
  on vitamin E status, 231
  zinc in, 48–49
Inflammatory diseases, chronic, dietary fatty
    acids on, 157–158
Inflammatory responses
  acute, dietary fatty acids on, 155
  nutrition on, 191
Innate defenses, protein-energy malnutrition on,
    90–99. *See also* Protein-energy
    malnutrition, childhood
Innate immune mechanisms, 69–70
Insulinlike growth factor-1 (IGF-1), in recovery
    from malnutrition and infection,
    299–300
Insulinlike growth factors (IGFs), in AIDS, 395
γ -Interferon, 266, 266f
  dietary fatty acids on, 153–154
  protein-energy malnutrition on, 107–108
Interleukin (IL), malnutrition on, 31–33
Interleukin-1 (IL-1)
  in anorexia, 310–311
  anorexia nervosa on, 254
  dietary fatty acids on, 152
  in infection, 308
  on metabolism and nutrition, 283
  protein-energy malnutrition on, 97–98
  in septic shock, 190
Interleukin-2 (IL-2), dietary fatty acids on,
    153–154
Interleukin-3 (IL-3), 266, 266f
Interleukin-4 (IL-4), 266, 266f
  dietary fatty acids on, 153–154
Interleukin-5 (IL-5), 266, 266f
Interleukin-6 (IL-6)
  anorexia nervosa on, 254–255
  dietary fatty acids on, 152–153
  in energy balance, 187
  growth inhibitory effects of, 284–285
  in immune response to stress, 183, 183t
  in infection, 308
  on metabolism and nutrition, 283
  protein-energy malnutrition on, 97–98
Interleukin-8 (IL-8), in infection, 308–309
Interleukin-10 (IL-10), 266, 266f
  dietary fatty acids on, 153–154

Interleukin-12 (IL-12), 268
Intestinal absorption, GI infections on, 321–322
Iodine deficiency
  on cognitive function, 17–18
  global, 7t, 8
  maternal, child mental retardation from, 17
Iron
  GI infection and, 327–328
  on host defense, 48
  on immunity, 204–205
    discussion on, 208–212
  in infection, 48
  on malaria, 411–412
  on respiratory infections, 346
Iron deficiency
  global, 7t, 8
  on immunity, 2
Iron nutritional immunity, 204

K

Keshan disease, 190
Kwashiorkor, 24–26, 25f, 26f. *See also* Protein-
        energy malnutrition, childhood
  on leukotriene synthesis, 109
  pathogenesis of, 26–28, 28f

L

Leptin, 109
  in AIDS, 395–396
  in anorexia, 311
  cytokines and, 253
  obesity on, 253
  on T-cell immune function, 191, 191f
Leucine, infection on, 291–292
Leukocytes, 71. *See also* specific types, e.g., T
        lymphocytes
Leukotriene synthesis, kwashiorkor on, 109
Linkage analysis, by restriction fragment length
        polymorphism, 64
Linoleic acid–rich oils, on lymphocyte
        proliferation, 147
α-Linolenic acid, on lymphocyte proliferation,
        147–148
γ-Linolenic acid, on lymphocyte proliferation,
        147
Lipids, dietary. *See also* Fatty acids, dietary
  on prostaglandin E_2 production, 142, 142f
Living conditions, mortality and, 13
Lymphocyte
  in adaptive immune response, 175–176, 176t
  B, evaluation of, 74–75
  T (*See* T cells)
Lymphocyte cytotoxicity, dietary fatty acids on,
        149–150
Lymphocyte proliferation
  dietary fatty acids on, 146–149

obesity on, 251
  vitamin E supplements on, 228–229
Lymphocyte proliferation assay, 62, 72–73
Lymphocyte subpopulations, evaluation of,
        61–62
Lymphoid involution, protein-energy
        malnutrition on, 103–104
Lymphoid tissues, in low birthweight infants,
        128

M

Macrophages, 70–71
  protein-energy malnutrition on, 93–94
Major histocompatibility antigens (MHAs),
        dietary fatty acids on, 144
Malaria, 410–413
  childhood mortality from, 13–14, 14f
  on cognitive development, 418
  discussion on, 421
  epidemiology of, 408, 408t
  on iron, 411–412
  protein-energy values in, 411
  vitamins and antioxidants on, 412–413
Malnutrition
  causes of, 2–4, 3f
  childhood, 23–39, 42–43 (*See also* Protein-
        energy malnutrition)
    diagnosis of, 35
    epidemiology of, 23
    GI infections and, 319–329, 332–335 (*See
        also* Gastrointestinal infections)
    treatment of, 35–38
      antibiotic therapy, 38, 38t
      dietary therapy, 36t, 37
      fluid and electrolyte, 35–37, 36t
      inpatient *vs.* outpatient, 38
  CNS, endocrine, and immune systems in,
        255, 256f
  on cognition, 17
  costs of, 16–17
  disease burden of, 16, 16t
  forms of, 2
  GI infections and, 319–320, 321f
  on immune cell response, 188–192, 189f,
        191f
  on immune response, 173, 174f
  immunity and, 29–35 (*See also* Immunity,
        malnutrition and)
  immunodeficiency from, 65, 65t
  infection and, 45–50, 46t, 51–53, 281–295,
        297–302 (*See also* Infection,
        metabolic effects of)
    discussion on, 51–53
    disease worsening from, 45–46
    host responses and immune activation in,
        49–50
    nutritional status in, 46–49, 47f
    susceptibility to, 325–326, 326t

infection and, global, 1–20
  disease reemergence and emergence in,
    10–12
  integrated approaches to, 18–20, 19f
  malnutrition–infection antagonism in, 45,
    46t
  malnutrition–infection synergism in, 1–2,
    45, 46t
  mortality from, 11–14, 12f, 13f
    neonatal, 14–15, 14f
  magnitude of, global, 4–10
    low birthweight, 4, 15
      chronic disease with, 15
    micronutrient deficiencies, 6–9, 7t
      folic acid, 9
      iodine, 7t, 8
      iron, 7t, 8
      vitamin A, 7t, 8
      zinc, 9
    obesity, 9–10
    protein-energy malnutrition, 4–6, 5t, 6f
  maternal, 14
  physical work capacity and, 17
  productivity and, 17, 17t
Marasmic kwashiorkor, 24–25, 25f. *See also*
    Protein-energy malnutrition,
    childhood
  pathogenesis of, 27–28, 28f
Marasmus, 24, 25f. *See also* Protein-energy
    malnutrition, childhood
  pathogenesis of, 27–28, 28f
Maternal mortality, 12
Maternal nutrition, low birthweight and, 15
Measles
  on cell-mediated immunity, 189, 189f
  discussion on, 354
  global, 10
  nutritional interventions on, 346–347
  on nutritional status, 338–339
    protein-energy malnutrition, 338
    vitamin A levels, 2, 338–339
  nutritional status on, 346–349
    protein-energy malnutrition, 346–347
    vitamin A supplements, 219–220, 220t,
      347–349, 347t, 348t
Meliodosis, nutrition and, 364
Memory T cells, 72
Meningitis
  bacterial, 11
  meningococcal, 11
MHC, 71–72
Micronutrient(s). *See also* specific
    micronutrients, e.g., Zinc
  on HIV, 376–382, 378t–379t, 381t
  on immunity, 202–204, 203f
    discussion on, 208–212

iron, 204–205
zinc, 205–207, 206f, 207f
Micronutrient deficiencies
  GI infection risk with, 326–329, 327t, 328t
  global, 6–9, 7t (*See also* specific
    micronutrients, e.g., Zinc)
    folic acid, 9
    iodine, 7t, 8
    iron, 7t, 8
    vitamin A, 7t, 8
    zinc, 9
  in low birthweight infants, 127
Mitogenic proliferation, vitamin A deficiency
    on, 215
Molecular and immunological evaluation, in at
    risk hosts, 69–87. *See also* Immune
    system, evaluation of
Molecular defects, immune system, 57–58, 58f,
    58t
  evaluation of, 63
Mortality
  childhood
    causes of, 13–14, 14f
    malnutrition and, 11–14, 12f, 13f
    maternal, 12
    prevention of, 18–20, 19f
    neonatal, 14–15, 14f
    from protein-energy malnutrition, 26
Mucosal humoral immune competence,
    protein-energy malnutrition on,
    102–103
Mucus, epithelial, protein-energy malnutrition
    on, 90
Myalgia, in infectious disease, 49
Myeloid cell proliferation, protein-energy
    malnutrition on, 91–92

N
Natural defenses, malnutrition mortality risk
    and, 13
Natural killer (NK) cells, 73–74
  activity of, 74
  dietary fatty acids on, 149–150
  malnutrition on, 31
  markers and distribution of, 176t
  protein-energy malnutrition on, 99
Necator americanus, 414–416
Necrotizing enterocolitis, vitamin E
    supplements on, 230
Negative acute phase proteins, 292–294
Nematodes, gastrointestinal, 414–417, 415f
Neonatal mortality, 14–15, 14f
Nepal, vitamin A deficiency in, 12
Neuroendocrine-immune interactions, 173, 174f
Neutrophils, 70–71, 214–215
  microbicidal and chemotactic capabilities of,
    93

Neutrophils, (*contd.*)
  protein-energy malnutrition on, 91, 98
  vitamin A deficiency on, 215
Nicotinamide-adenine dinucleotide phosphate
        (NADPH) oxidase, protein-energy
        malnutrition on, 94–95
Nitric oxide, fatty acids on, 143–144
Nitrogen loss, in infection, 47–48, 47t
Noel's dirty chicken hypothesis, 293, 297–298
NPY, in anorexia, 310
Nutrient deficiencies. *See* specific nutrients,
        e.g., Vitamin E
Nutrient–endocrine interactions, 284–285
Nutrition, 15–18, 17t. *See also* Malnutrition;
        specific types, e.g., Vitamin A
        deficiency
  on cell-mediated immunity, 188
  community-based programs in, 18–20, 19f
  in disease prevention, 192
  GI infections on, 319–320, 321f
  on immune cell response, 188–192, 189f,
        191f
  immunity and, 29–35 (*See also* Immunity,
        malnutrition and)
  improvement in, 18–20, 19f
  infection and, 45–50, 51–53 (*See also*
        Malnutrition, infection and)
  maternal
    on childhood cognition and activity, 15–18,
        17t
    empowerment and, 18
    low birthweight and, 15
  stress and, 188–192
Nutritional immunity, 48
Nutritional status
  infection on, 46–49, 47t, 281–295, 297–302
        (*See also* Infection, metabolic
        effects of)
  mortality risk and, 13

O
Obesity, 243–244
  on delayed type hypersensitivity, 251–252
  discussion on, 259
  global, 9–10
  on immune function, 244–246, 247–248
  on immunocompetent cells, 248
  infection in, 244–245
  leptin and cytokines in, 253
  on lymphocyte proliferation, 251
  on T-helper (CD4) cells, 248–249
Oleic acid, on lymphocyte proliferation, 147
Opsonins, antibodies as, 77
Opsonization, 76
  malnutrition on, 92
Oral tolerance, 277

Organ transplantation
  animal, dietary fatty acids on, 157
  human, dietary fatty acids after, 158
Overtraining syndrome, 184–186, 185f

P
Pancreatic cancer, dietary fatty acids on,
        157–158
Parasites, reproductive strategies of, 407
Parasitic diseases, 407–418, 421–423. *See also*
        specific diseases, e.g.,
        Gastrointestinal infections, Malaria
  cognitive development and, 418
  discussion on, 421–423
  enteropathy from, 413, 413t
  epidemiology of, 407–408, 408t, 409f
  future work on, 418
  nutrition and, 413, 414f
  susceptibility and resistance to, 410
Perspectives, future, 425–431
Phagocytes
  evaluation of, 70–71
  protein-energy malnutrition on
    cell numbers of, 91–92
    microbicidal and chemotactic capabilities
        of, 93–94
    respiratory burst of, 94–95
Phagocytosis
  fatty acids in, 143
  protein-energy malnutrition on, 92–93
Phenotypic abnormalities, of immune system,
        57–58, 58f, 58t
Physical barriers, immune system, protein-
        energy malnutrition on, 90–91
Plasmodium falciparum, 408, 408t. *See also*
        Malaria
Pneumonia. *See also* Respiratory infections
  vitamin A supplements on, 221–222
Polymorphonuclear leukocyte response,
        malnutrition on, 33–34
Polymorphonuclear leukocytes, in low
        birthweight infants, 129
Polyunsaturated fatty acids (PUFA), 137–138.
        See also Fatty acids
Popliteal lymph node assay, 156
Premature infants, vitamin E for, 230
Primary azurophilic granules, 70
Programming, 126
  fetal and postnatal, 126
Prostaglandin (PG), in immune and
        inflammatory response, 141–142,
        142f
Prostaglandin E_2 (PGE$_2$), in immune and
        inflammatory response, 141
Protein(s)
  cytokines on, 286–287
  functional, 281–282

Protein-energy malnutrition
on immune response, 173–174, 174f
on measles, 346–347
measles on, 338
on respiratory infections, 339
respiratory infections on, 337
Protein-energy malnutrition, childhood, 23–39,
42–43
classification of, 23–26
clinical criteria, 24–26, 25f, 26f
weight and height criteria, 23–24
diagnosis of, 35
discussion on, 42–43
epidemiology of, 23
experimental, study design with, 109–111
global, 4–6, 5t, 6f
on immune competence, 89–111, 116–120
(*See also* Immune competence,
protein-energy malnutrition on)
immunity and, 2, 29–35 (*See also* Immunity,
malnutrition and)
infection and, 2, 28–29
pathogenesis of, 26–28, 28f
prognosis and mortality with, 26
treatment of, 35–38
antibiotic therapy, 38, 38t
dietary therapy, 36t, 37
fluid and electrolyte, 35–37, 36t
inpatient *vs.* outpatient, 38
Protein-energy values, in malaria, 411
Protozoa, gastrointestinal, 413–414
Pseudomonas pseudomallei infection, 364

R
Reactive oxygen species, fatty acids on,
143–144
Refeeding, infection and, 246–247
Respiratory burst, phagocyte, protein-energy
malnutrition on, 94–95
Respiratory infections, acute, 337–350, 353–356
childhood mortality from, 13–14, 14f
discussion on, 353–356
nutritional interventions on, 339
on nutritional status, 337–338
protein-energy malnutrition, 337
vitamin A levels, 337–338
nutritional status on, 339–346
iron, 346
protein-energy malnutrition, 339
vitamin A deficiency, 340
vitamin A supplements, 340–342, 340t,
341t, 343t
community-based mortality trials on,
223–225, 223t
hospital-based mortality trials on,
221–223, 222t

zinc, 342
zinc supplements, 342, 344–345
research on, future, 349–350
Restriction fragment length polymorphism
(RFLP), linkage analysis by, 64
Retinoids. *See* Vitamin A
Rheumatic fever, global, 10–11
Rheumatic heart disease, global, 10–11
Roundworm, 414–417
RSV vaccine, 275

S
Saliva, in protein-energy malnutrition, 90–91
Sarcopenia, 282
Satiety regulators, 306–307
Selenium, on HIV, 380
Selenium deficiency, on immune response, 190
Sepsis, on protein synthesis and breakdown,
286–287
Serotonin (5-HT), in anorexia, 310
Skin testing, delayed hypersensitivity. *See*
Delayed type hypersensitivity
(DTH) skin testing
Southeast Asia, maternal mortality in, 12
SSCP, mutation detection by, 64
Stillbirth, 14
Stress
immunity and, 173–188, 196–199
adaptive immune response in, 175–181
(*See also* Immune response,
adaptive [specific])
discussion on, 196–199
neuroendocrine response in, 181–188
acute phase response in, 182
delayed type hypersensitivity in, 187,
188t
exercise and, 183–184
excess, 184–187, 185f
factors in, 181–182, 181f
IL-6 in, 183, 183t
models of, 182–183
overlapping mechanisms of, 184
nutrition and, 188–192
Strongyloides fuellebroni, 415
Strongyloides stercoralis, 415
Substrate competition
in childhood infection, 288–290, 289f
cytokines on, 285–286
Suppressor T lymphocytes, 73
Surface marker expression, dietary fatty acids
on, 144–147
Synergism, malnutrition–infection, 45–46, 46t

T
T-cell receptor signal transduction, 178, 178f,
179f

T-cell response, nutrition on, 188–190
T cells (lymphocytes)
    activation of, signaling components in, 178,
        179f
    in adaptive immune response, 175–176, 176t
    cytotoxic, 73
    cytotoxic activity of, 74
        dietary fatty acids on, 149
    evaluation of, 71–74
    frequencies of, 72–73
    markers and distribution of, 176t
    memory, 72
    numbers of, protein-energy malnutrition on,
        104
    subset imbalances of, protein-energy
        malnutrition on, 105–106
    suppressor, 73
    vitamin A deficiency on, 214, 214t, 215
T-helper (CD4) cells. *See also* specific types,
        e.g., Th1 cells
    obesity on, 248–249
T-helper cell differentiation, cytokine-driven,
        177, 177f
TCR, 72
Testosterone deficiency, in AIDS, 394–395
Tetanus, neonatal, 14–15
Th1 cells, 178, 265
    in elderly, 274–275
    ontogeny of, 268, 269f
    vitamin A deficiency on, 214, 215
Th2 cells, 178, 265
    in elderly, 274–275
    ontogeny of, 268, 269f
    vitamin A deficiency on, 214, 215
Th1/Th2 balance, 268, 269f, 276, 277
    IgE and, 265–266, 266f
    immunization on, 271–272
    in newborns, 268, 269f
    in pregnancy, 268
Thymulin, protein-energy malnutrition on, 104
Thyroid function, in AIDS, 395
Tier system, 78–83, 78t
    tier 1, 78t, 79
    tier 2, 78t, 79–81
    tier 3, 78t, 81–82
Tocopherol, on malaria, 412
Tolerance, oral, 277
Trace elements. *See* Micronutrient(s);
        Micronutrient deficiencies; specific
        micronutrients, e.g., Vitamin A
Transforming growth factor-b (TGF-b),
        anorexia nervosa on, 254
Trichuris trichiura, 414–417, 414f
Tuberculosis (TB)
    global, 11
    nutrition and, 363–364
        discussion on, 366–369
Tumor necrosis factor (TNF)
    adiposity on, 252–253
    on albumin, 293

on amino acid kinetics, 292
    anorexia nervosa on, 254
    dietary fatty acids on, 151–152
    in infection, 308
    on metabolism and nutrition, 283
    on protein catabolism, 287
    protein-energy malnutrition on, 97–98
Tyrosine phosphorylation, in T-cell signal
        transduction, 178, 178f

V

Vaccines. *See also* Immunization
    as allergy protection, 264–265
    DNA, 277–278
    HIV, 278
    whooping cough, 275–276
Vitamin(s)
    on HIV
        in adults, 376–382, 378t–379t, 381t
        transmission and progression of, 372–374,
            373t, 375t, 376–380, 378t–379t,
            381t
    on malaria, 412–413
Vitamin A
    on HIV, 372
        pregnancy outcomes and child health with,
            372–374, 373t, 375t
        pregnant women with, 372–374, 373t, 375t
    during infection, 48–49
    measles on, 338–339
    respiratory infections on, 337–338
Vitamin A deficiency
    comments on, 225–227
    discussion on, 239–241
    global, 7t, 8
    on immune response, 214–216, 214t
    infection and, 2, 218
    measles and, 2, 219–220, 220t
    mortality from, 11–12
    mortality trials on
        community-based, 218–225, 218t
            in children greater than 6 mos., 218, 218t
            in children less than 6 mos., 219, 219t
            diarrheal and respiratory infections,
                223–225, 223t
        hospital-based
            diarrheal infections, 220–221, 221t
            respiratory infections, 221–223, 222t
    on respiratory infections, 340
Vitamin A supplements
    on AIDS, 377, 380
    comments on, 225–227
    on GI infection risk, 327, 328, 328t, 332–333
    in HIV-infected pregnant women, 372–374,
        373t, 375t
    on immune response, 216–217
    on measles, 347–349, 347t, 348t
        mortality from, 192

on respiratory infections, 340–342, 340t,
341t, 343t
community-based mortality trials on,
223–225, 223t
hospital-based mortality trials on, 221–223,
222t
Vitamin B$_{12}$ supplements, on AIDS, 377
Vitamin E
immune response and, 227
infection and, 231–232
on malaria, 412–413
Vitamin E deficiency
comment on, 232–233
on immune function, 227–228
on infection, 231
in preterm infants, 228
Vitamin E supplementation
comment on, 233
discussion of, 239
on immune response, 228–230
infectious diseases and, 231–232

W
Weight loss, in acute phase response, 364
Wheezing, early childhood, infectious agents in,
264

Whipworm, 414–417, 415f
Whooping cough vaccine, 275–276
Women, empowerment of, nutritional
improvement from, 18
Worms, 414–417, 415f

X
X chromosome inactivation patterns, 64

Z
Zinc
GI infection and, 326–327, 327t, 328,
332–335
on HIV, 380, 382
on host defense, 48–49
on immunity, 205–207, 206f, 207f
discussion on, 208–212
during infection, 48–49
on respiratory infections, 342
supplementation of, 342, 344–345
Zinc deficiency
global, 9
on immunity and infection, 2
Zinc supplementation
childhood activity and, 18
on childhood disease, 192